Vaginal Surgery

FOURTH EDITION

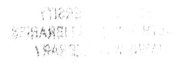

ILLUSTRATED BY

Allison Boisselle

Providence, Rhode Island

Melford D. Diedrick

Buffalo, New York

Lori Vaskalis

Portland, Oregon

FOURTH EDITION

VAGINAL SURGERY

DAVID H. NICHOLS, M.D.

Fellow, American College of Obstetricians and Gynecologists;
Fellow, American College of Surgeons; Fellow, International College
of Surgeons
Visiting Professor of Obstetrics, Gynecology, and Reproductive Biology,
Harvard University School of Medicine
Past Professor and Chairman, Department of Obstetrics and Gynecology,
Brown University, School of Medicine, Providence, Rhode Island
Lecturer, Obstetrics and Gynecology, Tufts University School of Medicine,
Boston
Chief of Pelvic Surgery, Vincent Memorial Obstetrics & Gynecological
Service, Massachusetts General Hospital, Boston, Massachusetts

CLYDE L. RANDALL, M.D. [Deceased]

Fellow, American College of Obstetricians and Gynecologists;
Fellow, American College of Surgeons; Fellow, Royal College of
Obstetricians and Gynecologists; Fellow, American Gynecological and
Obstetrical Society
Late Professor and Chairman of Gynecology and Obstetrics, State
University of New York at Buffalo
Former Chief, Gynecology and Obstetrics, SUNY Affiliated Hospitals,
Buffalo, New York
Johns Hopkins Program of International Education, Gynecology and
Obstetrics, 1975–1980

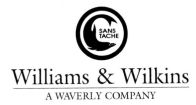

Williams & Wilkins

A WAVERLY COMPANY

BALTIMORE • PHILADELPHIA • LONDON • PARIS • BANGKOK
BUENOS AIRES • HONG KONG • MUNICH • SYDNEY • TOKYO • WROCLAW

Editor: Charles W. Mitchell
Managing Editor: Marjorie Kidd Keating
Production Coordinator: Barbara Felton
Copy Editor: Susan Zorn
Designer: Ashley Pound Design
Illustration Planner: Martha White Tenney

ISBN 0-683-06491-6

90000

9 780683 064919

Copyright © 1996
Williams & Wilkins
351 West Camden Street
Baltimore, Maryland 21201-2436 USA

Accurate indications, adverse reactions and dosage schedules for drugs are provided in this book, but it is possible that they may change. The reader is urged to review the package information data of the manufacturers of the medications mentioned.

Printed in the United States of America

First Edition 1976
Second Edition 1983
Third Edition 1989

Library of Congress Cataloging-in-Publication Data

Nichols, David H., 1925–
    Vaginal surgery / David H. Nichols, Clyde L. Randall. — 4th ed.
      p.   cm.
    Includes bibliographical references and index.
    ISBN 0-683-06491-6 (hardcover)
    1. Vagina—Surgery.   I. Randall, Clyde L.   II. Title.
    [DNLM: 1. Vagina—surgery.   WP 250 N617v 1996]
  RG104.N52   1996
  618.1′5059—dc20
  DNLM/DLC
  for Library of Congress
                              95-17805
                                 CIP

The publishers have made every effort to trace the copyright holders for borrowed material. If they have inadvertently overlooked any, they will be pleased to make the necessary arrangements at the first opportunity.

95 96 97 98 99
1 2 3 4 5 6 7 8 9 10

Reprints of chapters may be purchased from Williams & Wilkins in quantities of 100 or more. Call Isabella Wise, Special Sales Department, (800) 358-3583.

Dedicated with affection to the late Clyde L. Randall, M.D., and Edward G. Winkler, M.D., Professors and Chairmen of Obstetrics and Gynecology at the University of Buffalo, resourceful surgeons, enthusiastic teachers, and inspiration to all who would learn to master and enjoy the special responsibility and satisfaction of the vaginal approach to surgery.
Carroll E. Keating, M.D.—First and often only assistant in surgery for over a decade—whose infinite faith, patience, and encouragement helped make all these surgical things not only possible but a thoroughly enjoyable experience.

"And this is the reason why the cure of many diseases
is unknown to the physicians of Hellas,
because they are ignorant of the whole,
which ought to be studied also;
for the part can never be well
unless the whole is well."
SOCRATES IN THE CHARMIDES OF PLATO
Translated by B. Jowett, vol. i, p. 11.
From Kelly HA: *Operative Gynecology.*
New York, D. Appleton & Co, 1898

Preface

TO THE FOURTH EDITION

Coincident with the vast increase throughout the world in the number of women living longer, the need for reconstructive pelvic surgery continues to increase, despite a relative shortage of surgeons with much experience in this discipline. Restoration of quality of life is the essence of longevity and, when related to surgically correctable disorders of the urogenital system, are the responsibility of the gynecologic surgeon. This discipline is dynamic. New and different techniques are continually evolving and being rediscovered and tested. Many of the techniques that have proven to be useful are included in graphic detail in this new edition. Because coincident refinement of laparoscopic and transabdominal surgery techniques are being developed as well, the responsible surgeon will become familiar and experienced with the details and indications for each of the three routes of surgical option so that one's patient may be given an appropriate recommendation as to the best solution for her particular problem, based on a familiarity with a wide choice of procedures, not simply the only one with which the surgeon is familiar.

Many of the surgically correctable problems affect the younger patient as well as the older woman. In an era of cost containment, the length of hospitalization must be as brief as possible, the surgical complications minimal in number, and the predictable requirement for reoperation minimized by a correct choice of the initial surgical procedure, expertly performed. Implementation of this concept is not easy for most gynecologists if a broad exposure to these disciplines was not included as an integral part of one's postgraduate or residency experience, but it is remedial.

The author's lifetime and concentrated experience with the surgical definition of these problems and challenges and their solutions is explored in this new edition to considerable length, and a vast number of newer techniques reflecting the author's personal and current experience have been illustrated by the drawings of the remarkably skilled and effective medical artist Lori Vaskalis.

David H. Nichols, M.D.

Acknowledgments

Respectful and friendly appreciation is expressed to the publisher's senior editor Charles W. Mitchell for his enthusiasm and encouragement, project managers Vicki Vaughn and Margie Keating for their patient and effective persistence in keeping things moving always in a forward direction, artist Lori Vaskalis for her prompt and effective response to our needs, and to secretary Sara Goodman Mallari who patiently typed the entire manuscript.

Preface

TO THE FIRST EDITION

For untold generations women have known that vaginal relaxation may develop soon or perhaps years after childbearing. An initial sense of relaxation was known to precede a more noticeable and uncomfortable degree of prolapse. Discomforts and dysfunctions of varying degree became annoying and at times distressing, for some to a point of virtually disabling women already overburdened with the work and responsibilities of a household and family.

Without reparative vaginal surgery, the problems of those women who develop genital prolapse would have remained unchanged to this day. In many communities skillful management of vaginal delivery now usually includes prompt and adequate repair of vaginal floor and perineal damage. Although such care will minimize later need for a posterior colporrhaphy and perineorrhaphy, the most skilled management of labor and delivery is not as likely to avoid the damage which predisposes the parous woman to the later development of a cystocele, or a degree of prolapse that eventually indicates repair.

Now that the risks of elective vaginal surgery should be minimal, physicians should be mindful of the possibility that women are often annoyed or distressed by a degree of prolapse that can almost always be corrected by restorative surgery. In fact, the recognition and evaluation of indications and the performance of remedial surgery for the problems associated with genital prolapse have become a primary responsibility and major activity of the gynecologic surgeon.

We believe that successful reconstruction and relief of the discomforts of genital prolapse depend upon an accurate knowledge of the probable etiologic factors plus an appreciation of the specific principles involved in an effective repair. Success is not assured by rote repetition of a gynecologist's routine method of repair, even when the technical steps as described might be expected to result in a satisfactory repair. It is our conviction that optimal results can be assured only when the procedure selected and the technique employed is tailored to the problem recognized and the tissues available for accomplishment of the repair.

Somewhat difficult to learn, and equally difficult to teach, much of vaginal surgery seems to have been rediscovered from generation to generation. A heritage all too readily lost, the techniques of vaginal surgery must be sought for, recorded carefully, and practiced, if competence and skills are to be maintained.

Each bibliographic footnote consulted will provide valued references and is likely to enable the interested reader to develop new and improved techniques.

Simply making the vagina smaller is neither the goal, nor the purpose of vaginal reconstructive surgery. While the goal is actually a restoration to the normal of symptomatic alterations in anatomy to an anatomically correct and asymptomatic status, this implies, of course, not only restoration of anatomic relationships but also the important physiologic restoration with which the former is indelibly entwined.

This concept is not difficult to accept, but there may be differences of opinion when one seeks to establish an understanding of what the normal really is, and thus to express the definitive goals of vaginal reconstructive surgery. It was to this broad point that the concept for this book developed. The anatomic relationships, particularly of the supporting tissues of the woman's reproductive organs, so carefully detailed and examined in the anatomic texts, seem to describe an entirely different set of interorgan relationships than we have observed in the living body, and the significance of these differences will be discussed in detail in the chapters which follow.

Our investigations into the clinical significance of pelvic anatomy have disclosed some unexpected and meaningful differences in tissue interrelationships which seem responsible for the support and function of the pelvic organs in the living, as compared to the relationships previously assumed as a result of observations noted by others in the embalmed cadaver. The differences observed might well be likened to a comparison of grapes and raisins. The objectives of surgical reconstruction obviously must be designed to restore the characteristics of the living, and should, therefore, not be based upon the somewhat bizarre, somewhat unnatural and certainly nonfunctioning relationships that are apparent in the nonliving cadaver.

We believe the development of operations utilizing concepts based upon cadaver studies have led to unphysiologic and unnatural objectives of reconstruction. The modifications and new techniques suggested are attempts to emphasize physiologic reconstructions and restore the more usual and normal relationships which are characteristic of functioning gynecologic anatomy. Conclusions based upon studies of fresh gross anatomy have encouraged the evolution of certain of the technical details and the surgical procedures which we believe likely to aid in the realization of improved results. At least in our hands their use has resulted in patients realizing greater degrees of comfort than had previously been achieved by the employment of some of the older but still commonly used techniques.

There seems need to repeatedly emphasize that a protruding uterus is the result of genital prolapse and not the primary cause of the symptomatology. For this reason hysterectomy, although usually a desirable part of the surgery employed to assure a satisfactory reconstruction, is not the essential feature and does not of itself assure the success of the repair or relieve the patient of the discomforts of a prolapse. On the other hand the currently widespread use of postmenopausal estrogen replacement therapy seems certain to account for an increasing incidence of iatrogenic endometrial hyperplasia and postmenopausal dysfunctional uterine bleeding. This probability alone, we believe, provides a reasonably valid indication for coincident hysterectomy, whenever repair is indicated; and hysterectomy can be accomplished with little increased risk to the patient.

In the presentation of this material, our primary objective is to encourage others to carry on similar studies and thus help to preserve and improve a heritage of surgery for the satisfactions of succeeding generations of surgeons and their patients. We acknowledge with sincere gratitude our dependence upon the works of many others. We have drawn heavily upon such classic texts and monographs as Paramore's "The Statics of the Female Pelvic Viscera," von Peham and Amreich's "Operative Gynecology," Kennedy and Campbell's "Vaginal Hysterectomy," Malpas' "Genital Prolapse and Allied Conditions," Martius' "Gynecological Operations," Gray's "Vaginal Hysterectomy," Bandler's "Vaginal Celiotomy," Smout, Jacoby, and Lillie's "Gynecological and Obstetrical Anatomy, Descriptive and Applied," Burch and Lavely's "Hysterectomy," and Krige's "Vaginal Hysterectomy and Genital Prolapse Repair." In our own studies the influence of many teachers will be recognizable though their basic contributions to our own concepts are not being individually recognized. Gratitude is also expressed to the editors and publishers of the journals, "Obstetrics and Gynecology," "The American Journal of Obstetrics and Gynecology," "The Anatomical Record," "Postgraduate Medicine," and "Archiv für Gynaekologie" for permission to reprint portions of our studies which have appeared originally on their pages.

D.H.N.
C.L.R.
1976

CONTENTS

CHAPTER 1

Pelvic Anatomy of the Living

GENERAL CONCEPTS

Although it is agreed that distorted attachments and pathologic concentrations of pelvic connective tissues may often be restored to the normal state logically and effectively by means of pelvic surgery, there is no general agreement about what constitutes the normal state. Furthermore, there are many types of abnormalities, and they occur in various combinations at various times of life, with different etiologies and varying degrees of symptomatology and disability. Thus confusion often arises regarding concepts and definitions associated with this type of surgery.

To perform vaginal surgery successfully, the practitioner must have a detailed knowledge of the anatomy involved, must appreciate the range of individual variations that can occur, and must understand the effects of such physiologic processes as pregnancy, labor, delivery, menopause, and aging upon the tissues that require restorative surgery. Practitioners first learn about pelvic anatomy and develop their concepts of normal anatomic relationships by studying the anatomy of elderly, often debilitated, and malnourished female cadavers, and many have planned surgical reconstructions so as to recreate the anatomic relationships observed in these cadavers. These relationships are quite different from those found in the healthy, living, well-nourished, younger female, however. In addition, the standard anatomy textbook bases broad generalizations on only a small number of dissections, failing to recognize the extent of variation that occurs quite normally and frequently between individuals and at different times of life. These facts are responsible for many of the physiologic and symptomatic failures of gynecologic reconstructive surgery.

Because of the muscle paralysis that results from anesthesia and the resting or baseline under distention of the various organs, the anatomic relationships of the tissues and organs of an anesthetized patient differ from those of the patient who is wide awake. In addition, the horizontal position of the nonmoving surgical patient provides statics quite different from those of the vertical and active patient, whose pelvic organs are in varying stages of function and distention. These conditions further complicate vaginal surgery.

For example, in describing vaginal position in terms of the relationships evident in the cadaver (17, 22, 63), anatomy texts usually refer to the vagina as an almost straight and hollow tube that extends posterosuperiorly toward the sacral promontory (Fig. 1.1). This relationship is usually demonstrable on sagittal sectioning of the cadaver (Fig. 1.2). When such a concept becomes the objective of reconstructive surgery for the relief of genital prolapse, however, the result may be an unusual deviation of the vagina. In some instances, the vaginal vault has been sewn to the sacral promontory or even to the anterior abdominal wall, the latter operation causing the vaginal axis to ascend in an almost vertical or anterior direction (18, 46). Studies of the usual depth and axis of the nul-

1

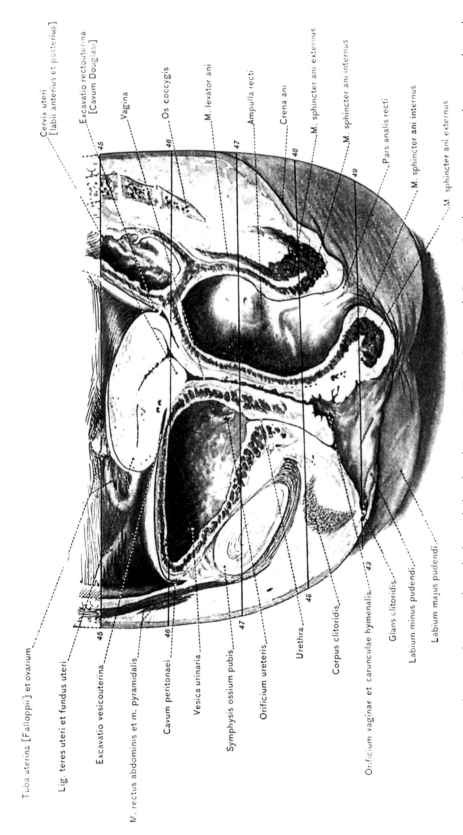

Figure 1.1. Drawing of a sagittal section through the embalmed cadaver showing the axis of the vagina to be in an almost vertical position. It is displaced anteriorly by the dilated rectum, a relationship often found in the living. (From Carter et al. Cross-sectional anatomy: computed tomography and ultrasound correlation. New York: Appleton-Century-Crofts, 1977. Used with permission.)

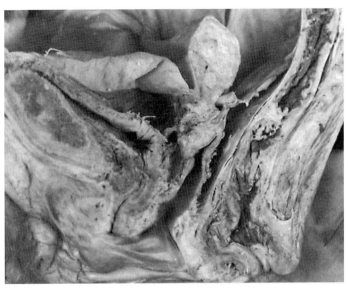

Figure 1.2. Photograph of a sagittal section of a cadaver pelvis. An almost vertical vaginal axis is shown, maintained by postmortem changes and chemical tissue fixation. (From Nichols DH, Milley PS, Randall CL. Significance of restoration of normal vaginal depth and axis. Obstet Gynecol 36:251–256, 1970. Reproduced with permission of Lippincott-Raven.)

liparous vagina in the living (Figs. 1.3 and 1.4) provide impressively different information (1, 11, 20, 38, 56, 57, 63), especially when the living patients are unanesthetized.

For years there has been heated discussion as to whether the more important factor concerned with vaginal position within the pelvis is the suspension from above (cardinal ligament complex), a view championed by Fothergill (19), or the support from below (levator ani–pelvic diaphragm), as emphasized by Paramore (47, 48) and Halban and Tandler (24). Mengert's (39) classic contribution in this area was to report an experiment whereby a tenaculum was applied to the cadaver cervix, a cord was attached to the tenaculum and run through a fixed pulley, and a 1-kg weight was attached to the opposite end of the cord. One by one, starting at the top of the fundus, the lateral supports of the uterus and vagina were cut until the uterus and vagina finally prolapsed. It was only when the paravaginal tissues had been cut that prolapse occurred. "Marked descent of the uterus mounting to actual prolapse never occurred so long as any part of the upper two-thirds of the parametrial tissues were intact." This experiment convincingly emphasized the importance of the suspensory apparatus. The conclusion was reinforced by DeLancey (12), who noted that this suspensory system of the upper vagina was continuous with the cardinal ligament of the cervix and thus served a critical role in the support of the vagina after hysterectomy.

Bonney (4) believed that both points of view were correct (that is, the vagina is suspended from above and supported from below). According to Bonney, damage to one or both systems can cause a genital prolapse, and the site or sites of primary damage determine the type of prolapse. Damage to the suspensory system can give rise to eversion of the upper vagina, often with elongation of the cervix and cul-de-sac hernia; damage to the lower supporting system is more likely to be associated with eversion of the lower vagina, including cystocele and rectocele. It is important for the gynecologic surgeon to recognize the primary site of damage and to take appropriate steps in surgical reconstruction to minimize the chance of a postoperative recurrence of the genital prolapse.

The organs of the female pelvis are readily distensible within certain maximal limits. Bladder, vagina, and rectum distend quite independently in the course of their normal functions, and each rather quickly resumes its usual or resting shape, dimension, and relationship when distention is no longer necessary. Functioning in concert, they rein-

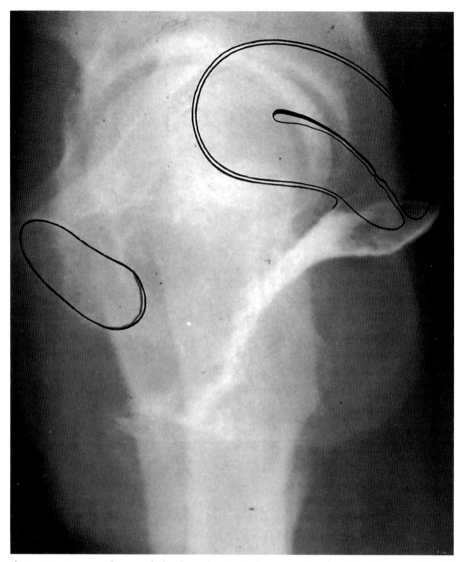

Figure 1.3. A normal vaginal depth and axis. Colpogram of a healthy 25-year-old nulli-gravida standing at rest. The vaginal walls have been painted with barium paste. The per-ineal curve of the lower vagina is shown along with the more horizontal axis of the upper vagina. The position of the symphysis is outlined to the left, and the position of the uterus outlined to the right. St. Francis Hospital, x-ray 69-3159, courtesy of Dr. Paul J. deMarovsky, Radiologist. (From Nichols DS, Milley PS, Randall CL. Significance of restoration of normal vaginal depth and axis. Obstet Gynecol 36:251–256, 1970.)

force one another; the histologic components that permit such a range of activity include combinations of varying amounts of smooth muscle, striated muscle, elastic tissue, and collagen.

Smooth Muscle

Always active, smooth muscle fibers help to maintain muscle tone. They are of lim-ited value for support, however, because the cells in these fibers lengthen readily with increased stress up to a point of maximum distention. Once they have reached their limit

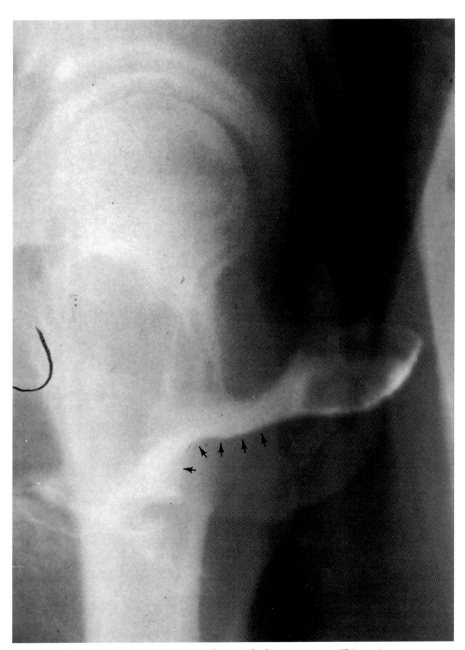

Figure 1.4. The same patient straining, as by a Valsalva maneuver. This action accentuates the horizontal axis of the upper vagina. The effect of the anterior margin of an intact levator plate is shown by the arrows. St. Francis Hospital, x-ray 69-3159, courtesy of Dr. Paul J. deMarsovsky, Radiologist. (From Nichols DH, Milley PS, Randall CL: Significance of restoration of normal vaginal depth and axis. Obstet Gynecol 36:251–256, 1970.)

of elasticity, the cells behave as those in an inactive fascial tissue do. The response of these muscle fibers to mechanical or chemical stimuli is mediated involuntarily through the autonomic nervous system and spinal reflex arcs. The syncytium of smooth muscle also evidences rhythmic contractions. The number of smooth muscle cells present within given tissues appears likely to be constant throughout the mature lifetime of the individual and does not significantly decline with age.

It appears that smooth muscle bands within the subperitoneal tissues have been consciously, although perhaps not deliberately, used in the most successful surgery for the repair of genital prolapse. In 1907 Fothergill (19) suggested that these tissues are composed primarily of smooth muscle. He was the first to suggest operating within the avascular lines of cleavage between the vagina and bladder, followed by fascial overlapping of the vesicovaginal and rectovaginal septa. An amputation of the usually elongated cervix in the repair of prolapse was later added. Apparently under the impression that he was working with layers of fascia, Fothergill was, in fact, overlapping layers that were predominantly smooth muscle fibers. He was effectively shortening and reinforcing musculofibrous groups capable of considerable support. The essential accomplishment in a successful repair operation is the restoration of the normal functioning and supportive abilities of the smooth muscle content of this "fascial layer," however, not the duplication and strengthening of a nonelastic connective tissue.

Striated Muscle

Although striated muscle lacks inherent rhythmic contractions, it responds rapidly to stress and maintains tone and equilibrium. The length of the cells tends to remain constant because the cells contract in response to strain. This maintains the equilibrium as well as the tone of supporting tissues. Smooth muscle helps to maintain tone, but, because it more readily permits elongation, smooth muscle does not effectively restore or maintain equilibrium. Thus striated and smooth muscle have complementary activities that permit and contribute to functional changes within the limitations of the pelvic supporting tissues.

Elastic Tissue

The fibers of elastic tissue are constructed in irregular networks that are especially well suited for tissues that are frequently subject to stress. These fibers respond to stress with stretching, but they resist such stretching by a natural tendency to return to their original state, much as a rubber band does. The histogenesis of these fibers is unknown, although they are apparently produced by fibroblastic cells or histocytes. They do not seem to have an innervation. The quantity of elastic tissue decreases with age, but the extent to which this is hormone-related and reversible is not known. The decrease in this tissue with aging probably accounts in part for the differences between the composition and the recurrence rate of cystoceles and other manifestations of genital prolapse in women long past menopause and those in women still in their reproductive years.

Collagen

Like elastic tissue fibers, collagen fibers are arranged in an interlacing meshwork; unlike elastic tissue fibers, they do not stretch. With age they swell, fuse, and become hyalinized. Because they are flexible, they permit movement without stretching, much like a piece of string or rope.

Bone and Cartilage

Bone and cartilage are inflexible, firm, and strong. They resist sudden strain and stress, but respond to prolonged stress and strain by gradual changes in architecture. This response appears to be both age- and hormone-related.

Wall of the Intestine

There are several layers of the large intestine, including the mucosa, the submucosa, the muscularis, and within the abdomen, the serosa. It has been shown that the submucosa is the strongest of these layers (25, 33), and some clinical significance of this fact will be discussed in Chapter 11.

ANATOMY

Relationships of Ureter to Vaginal Hysterectomy Ligatures

In order to determine why the ureter is injured less often during vaginal procedures than during abdominal procedures, even though it is more difficult to palpate or see the ureter during a vaginal procedure, Hofmeister and Wolfgram (28) used multiple consecutive roentgenographic visualizations, radiopaque ureteral catheters, and wire sutures on the uterine pedicles during vaginal hysterectomy. They demonstrated that anterior retraction through the anterior peritoneal opening lifted the ureter as much as an additional 1 cm away from the zone of danger. The actual distance demonstrated during the vaginal hysterectomy procedures varied from more than 2.1 cm at the level of the parametrial areas during the hysterectomy to 1 cm when the tube and ovary were removed by clamping the infundibulopelvic ligament. During the repair of the bladder, the needle was 0.9 cm from the ureter (28).

These studies suggest that the traction applied to the cervix during vaginal hysterectomy, in combination with adequate retraction of the anterior vesicouterine peritoneal fold, protects the ureter from trauma. Furthermore, they demonstrate that the operator's clamps are closest to the ureter at the level of the infundibulopelvic ligament during salpingo-oophorectomy and during subsequent cystocele repair.

Anatomic Systems Responsible for Pelvic Support

At least eight different anatomic systems contribute varying degrees of support to the birth canal: (a) the bony pelvis, to which the pelvic soft tissues ultimately attach; (b) the subperitoneal connective tissue retinaculum and the broad ligaments, including the smooth muscle components and round ligaments; (c) the cardinal and uterosacral ligament complex; (d) the paravaginal attachments of the vaginal sulci to the arcus tendineus; (e) the urogenital diaphragm, including the pubourethrovaginal ligaments; (f) the pelvic diaphragm, particularly the pubococcygeus component and the levator plate; (g) the fascia of Denonvilliers (rectovaginal septum); and (h) the perineum, including the perineal body. Although each of these systems is a separate anatomic unit, they are often interrelated, and additional components may exert synergistic, supportive, or even sphincterlike action. For example, contraction of the intact bulbocavernosi in concert with the pubococcygei exerts an almost sphincterlike effect on the vaginal outlet (Fig. 1.5).

It is uncommon for any of these anatomic units to be individually defective, other than by congenital anomaly. These systems can be injured or damaged separately, however, or they can be injured or damaged in various combinations. Damage may be primary, secondary, or both. Successful reconstructive surgery depends upon recognizing the specific system or systems involved. It is equally important for the physician to recognize the active etiologic agents that may require treatment.

BONY PELVIS

The bones of the pelvis are the ultimate fixed attachment of the pelvic soft tissues. As a result of either congenital anomaly (such as exstrophy of the bladder) or trauma

Figure 1.5. Effect of contraction of the levatores ani. The contraction exerts some side-to-side compression of the lower vagina. This may reinforce voluntary contraction of the intact bulbocavernosi at a somewhat lower level, steadying the perineum and constituting a sphincter-like effect.

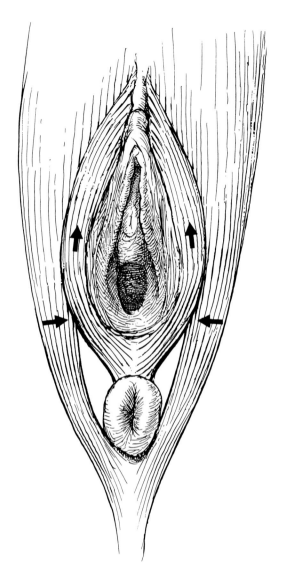

(such as fracture, avulsion, or surgery), they can be defective and thus fail to provide adequate support for the soft tissues. Any significant deficiency should be taken into consideration when a plan of repair is being formulated.

BROAD LIGAMENTS

The blood vessels and lymphatics that supply the organs of the genital system enter and exit through the broad ligaments, which sheathe those organs, unless the broad ligaments have been pathologically strengthened, for example, by severe fibrosis and scarring that has developed as a result of endometriosis, previous infection, cancer, previous surgery, or radiation therapy. Severe fibrosis may prevent the descent of the uterus. If so, prolapse of the lower birth canal and cervix may develop, often with pronounced and sometimes extreme elongation of the cervix. Some relative independence of the various levels of support may explain, in the reverse situation, why independent surgical suspension or fixation of the uterus may not arrest the development and progression of cystocele, rectocele, and descent of the cervix. The round ligaments provide only accessory support to maintain anteversion of the uterus, making it possible for the uterine axis to remain stable with a narrow angle relative to the upper vagina under normal circumstances.

CARDINAL AND UTEROSACRAL LIGAMENT COMPLEX

The ligaments in the cardinal and uterosacral ligament complex, which include a fine meshwork of muscle fibers, are part of the suspensory apparatus that serves to hold the cervix and upper vagina over the levator plate. The blood vessels and lymphatics from the hypogastric plexus enter and leave the uterus and vagina along their lateral margins, as the vessels connect with their origin from the main internal iliac (hypogastric) vessels. These vessels are surrounded by strong perivascular fibroareolar sheaths closely attached to their adventitia.

Many observers have studied the histology of these so-called ligaments. Range and Woodburne (53) found that these ligaments consist principally of blood vessels (largely veins), nerves, lymphatic channels, and areolar connective tissue; the connective tissue is more dense lateral to the cervix and vagina. Collagen bundles parallel the veins, and the connective tissue contains many smooth muscle fibers associated with the adventitia of the blood vessels. In addition, Range and Woodburne found that the loosely arranged connective tissue mesh strands become stretched or elongated longitudinally in the direction of a force applied to them (Fig. 1.6).

Von Peham and Amreich (50), Richter and Frick (58), and Luisi (34) realized that this rich network of blood vessels lateral to each side of the upper vagina and cervix is strengthened by the connective tissue and muscle sheaths that surround the valveless blood vessels. They named this the horizontal connective tissue ground bundle (50). At the cervix of an anteverted uterus, this lateral paravaginal condensation of tissues makes a rather abrupt turn anteriorly, following, as it turns, the axis of the lateral side of the cervix (Fig. 1.7); thus the cardinal ligament is in reality the same as the horizontal connective tissue ground bundle and serves to supply and to hold both cervix and upper vagina in place over the levator plate.

When Campbell (5) studied the anatomy and histology of the uterosacral ligaments, he found that they were attached to the posterolateral aspect of the cervix at the level of

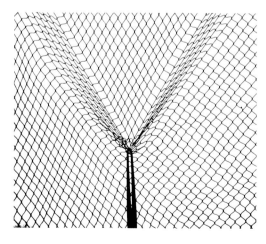

Figure 1.6. Effect of traction on the connective tissue fibers of the cardinal and uterosacral ligaments. A forceps has been applied to the center of a piece of plastic net, and traction has been applied to demonstrate the distortion of the pelvic tissues resulting from traction on the cervix. Condensation and obliteration of intra-areolar spaces account for the "ligaments" apparent at operation, which are reinforced by blood vessels, lymphatics, and nerves and their sheaths, all of which enter and exit along the lateral margin of the upper vagina. (From Nichols DH, Milley PS. Clinical anatomy of the vulva, vagina, lower pelvis, and perineum. In: Sciarra J, ed. Gynecology and obstetrics, 1977; reproduced with permission of Lippincott-Raven.)

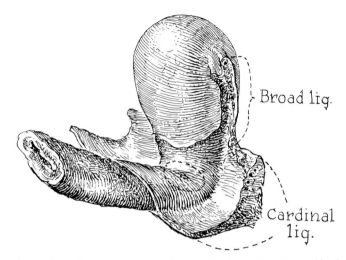

Figure 1.7. The cardinal ligament as it attaches to the lateral portions of both cervix and upper third of the vagina. The ligament follows the angulation of the intersecting axis of these two organs. (From Nichols DH, Milley PS. Clinical anatomy of the vulva, vagina, lower pelvis, and perineum. In: Sciarra J, ed. Gynecology and obstetrics, 1977; reproduced with permission of Lippincott-Raven.)

the internal os and to the lateral vaginal fornices. Although near the cervix, these ligaments are definite bands of tissue covered by peritoneum; they thin out as they course posteriorly, forming the superior boundary of the cul-de-sac of Douglas. These ligaments vary a great deal in thickness and strength, and they increase in prominence when tension or traction is applied to them. The posterior third of each uterosacral ligament is fan-shaped and consists of more delicate strands of tissue that attach to presacral fascia opposite the lower portion of the sacroiliac articulation.

Histologically, the posterior or sacral third of the uterosacral ligaments is composed almost entirely of loose strands of connective tissue with a few blood vessels, nerves, and lymphatics. The intermediate third is made up of a connective tissue network with prominent sympathetic nerve ganglia and a few scattered strands of smooth muscle and some lymphatics. The anterior or cervical third of these ligaments contains, in order of prominence: smooth muscle, fibroelastic connective tissue, blood vessels, sympathetic and parasympathetic nerves, and lymphatics. For these histologic reasons, it seems unlikely that, under physiologic conditions, the ligaments that primarily convey the pelvic parasympathetic nerve fibers from the sacral plexus to the lateral aspects of the uterus have any significant supportive function. As a general principle, nerves in the body are usually arranged in positions that limit their vulnerability to trauma. Thus it is unlikely that the primary purpose of these uterosacral ligaments is to provide for the suspensions of the uterus. They may assist in maintaining the position of the uterus and upper vagina over the levator plate, however.

The connective tissue elements of these ligaments are to a large measure enmeshed with those of the lower portion of the cardinal or transverse cervical ligaments. From a practical point of view, these elements not only are inseparable, but also constitute a surgically useful complex. The proliferation of connective tissue in this complex that is observed during surgery in patients with genital prolapse is probably a secondary pathologic hypertrophy. This hypertrophy is most likely a secondary line of defense in the body's attempt to compensate for the loss of homeostasis caused by increased intraperitoneal pressure or a result of deficient support from a weakened levator plate.

PUBOURETHROVAGINAL LIGAMENTS*
AND UROGENITAL DIAPHRAGM

After studying the connective tissue supports of the urethra, Milley and Nichols (41) confirmed the observations of Zacharin (71) that the urethra is suspended from the pubic bone (Figs. 1.8 and 1.9) for most of its length by arched, bilaterally symmetrical anterior, posterior, and intermediate pubourethrovaginal ligaments. Their studies further showed, as was suggested by Curtis and colleagues (10), that the posterior and anterior ligaments were formed by reflections of the inferior and superior fascial layers of the urogenital diaphragm (Figs. 1.10 and 1.11). The intermediate ligament represents a fusion of these fascial layers.

The posterior pubourethrovaginal ligament blends with the arcus tendineus of the levator ani. When the arcus tendineus was cut, however, the pubourethrovaginal ligament retained an attachment to the connective tissue inferior to the pelvic diaphragm. The posterior pubourethrovaginal ligament was a reflection of the superior surface of the urogenital diaphragm.

The pubourethrovaginal ligament is best demonstrated on a cadaver by sagittal section through the pelvis (Fig. 1.12) that permits its components (the anterior, intermedi-

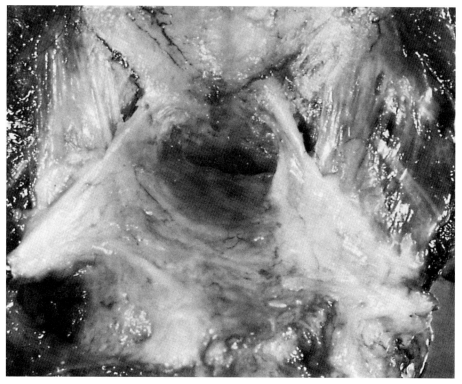

Figure 1.8. View of the cadaver pelvis from above. The symphysis pubis is at the top, and traction to the pubourethrovaginal ligament has been applied by the hemostat shown on the left, accentuating the independent origin of this ligament from the posterior surface of the pubis but showing confluence posteriorly with the fascia of the pelvic diaphragm enclosing the pubococcygeus. (From Zacharin RF. The suspensory mechanism of the female urethra. J Anat 1963;97:423–427. Reprinted with the permission of Cambridge University Press.)

*The term *ligament* is technically a misnomer, since the condensation of tissue contains a few smooth and striated muscle cells enabling the tissue to elongate and contract during the act of voiding; however, the term is accepted by common usage.

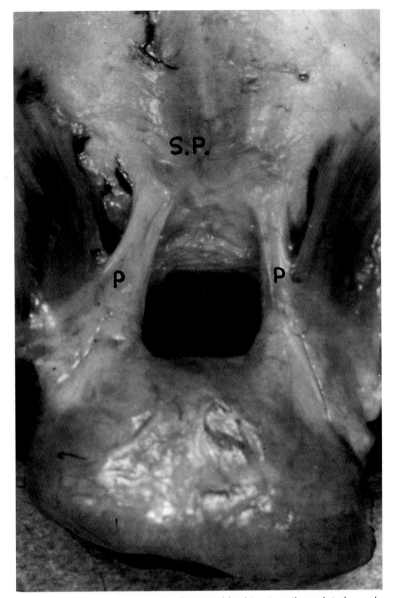

Figure 1.9. A fresh cadaver dissection is illustrated looking into the pelvis from above. The pubic symphysis (*S.P.*) is seen at the upper portion of the photograph. The bladder has been displaced posteriorly to show the posterior pubourethrovaginal ligament (*P*). The darker-colored levator ani (*L.A.*) arising from the arcus tendineus is seen lateral but distinct from the pubourethrovaginal ligaments. (From Zacharin RF, Gleadell LS. Abdominoperineal urethral suspension. Am J Obstet Gynecol 1963;86:981–994. Reproduced with permission of Mosby–Year Book, Inc.)

ate, and posterior segments) to be visualized through its entire length. The ligament is attached primarily to the lateral sides of the urethra, although some fibers are almost in apposition. Smooth muscle bundles run parallel to the long axis of the ligaments.

Histologic section has shown that the pubourethrovaginal ligaments consist of dense collagen, both smooth and striated muscle, and elastic fibers. The striated muscle may be a pubourethrovaginal continuation of some fibers of the pubococcygeus. Study by light and electron microscopy and neurohistochemistry (70) indicates that the

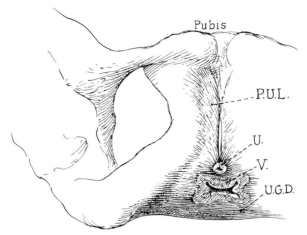

Figure 1.10. Frontal view of the urogenital diaphragm (*U.G.D.*) showing its continuity with the anterior pubourethrovaginal ligament (*P.U.L.*). The fascia of the urogenital diaphragm is reflected onto both anterior and posterior aspects of the pubis at a level more superior and medial than usually described. The sides of the diaphragm do not appear to meet anteriorly to form a transverse perineal ligament, as in the male.

tissue contains smooth muscle bundles associated with numerous nerve fibers. The enzyme content and fine structure of these nerve fibers are similar to those believed to represent cholinergic autonomic nerve tissues (acetylcholinesterase-positive). Therefore, the term *ligament* is a misnomer, since these structures contain contractile elements under neural control.

The remainder of the urogenital diaphragm is, sandwichlike, composed of superior and inferior fascial layers separated from one another by a layer of striated muscle, the deep transverse muscle of the perineum. The striated muscle that extends to the wall of the urethra in this area is minimal. In general, the sphincters of the body that are under voluntary control are formed by concentric layers of striated muscle. This is not true for the urethra, however, although some external sphincter action is provided in the midportion of the urethra by pressure from the nearby pubococcygeus muscle and in the distal urethra by pressure from the bulbocavernosi.

The urogenital diaphragm runs between the inner surfaces of the ischiopubic rami. The attachments of the urogenital diaphragm to the urethra (pubourethrovaginal ligaments) are more on the superolateral aspect of the urethra than on the vagina. The urethra and vagina pierce the urogenital diaphragm in the midline, and their attachment to it helps them to remain in place. The posterior fibers of the urogenital diaphragm are fixed to the perineal body. Because the urogenital diaphragm is almost horizontal when the woman is standing, its fixation to the perineal body contributes to the support of the urethra and vesicourethral junction, decreasing the tendency of these structures to rotate around the attachment of the pubourethrovaginal ligament to the pubis. The superficial perineal muscles, as well as the ischiocavernosus and bulbocavernosus muscles, are superficial to the urogenital diaphragm and appear to be considerably less important in urogenital support.

INTERNAL URETHRAL SPHINCTER

There is no evidence within the urethra of any significant amount of well-developed, physiologically useful, striated sphincter muscle under voluntary control. The urethral sphincter system consists primarily of smooth muscle. Curtis and colleagues described it as follows (10):

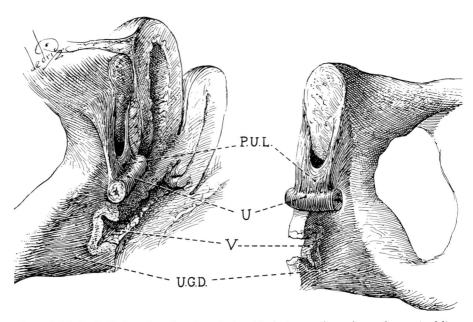

Figure 1.11. Sagittal view showing the relationship between the pubourethrovaginal ligament (*P.U.L.*) and urogenital diaphragm (*U.G.D.*) in the human female. The urethra (*U*) and
vagina (*V*) are shown in their relationship to the urogenital diaphragm. Note the bladder
sketched into the drawing at the left. (From Milley PS, Nichols DH. The relationship between pubourethral ligaments and urogenital diaphragm in the human female. Anat Rec
1971;170:281–284; reproduced with permission of John Wiley & Sons, Inc.)

The musculature of the bladder wall constitutes the internal sphincter, which is not a circular band
at the neck of the bladder but a thickening of the muscle fibers beginning at the neck of the bladder and extending throughout the urethra, reinforced by fibers from the urogenital diaphragm,
which constitute the external sphincter.

Emphasizing a bladder "base plate," Hutch analyzed the anatomy of the bladder,
trigone, and urethra and detailed theory concerning their physiology (30). He concluded:

These studies force me to conclude that the bulk of the urethra is continuous with the deep
trigone and, like the deep trigone, is derived from the Wolffian duct. It is this connective tissue that
gives the urethra its tubular shape, the tough texture of the trigone, and limits its expansibility. Fortunately, imbedded in the collagen are many rings of circularly oriented smooth muscle. It is the
tonus of this smooth muscle that keeps the lumen of the urethra constantly closed. In the female,
this collagenous tube runs from the urethral meatus to the bladder neck. Its posterior wall continues upward into the base of the bladder, where it widens to form the deep trigone. It terminates by
forming a tube-like structure at each cranial lateral border (Waldeyer's Sheath). This is an over-
simplification, because in most humans the tube fails to reach the bladder neck by about 0.5 to 0.10
cm on the anterior wall. The defect that results is filled in by detrusor loop. . . . It is this trigonal tissue that lends strength to the safety mechanism, giving form and shape and toughness to the urethra and to the bladder base. The rings of smooth muscle incorporated into the urethral portion constitute the basic primitive urethral sphincter that allows urine to accumulate in the bladder. The
superficial portion (of the trigone), on the other hand, plays no role in the dynamics of the bladder
neck, but it is primarily concerned with the competency of the urethral orifice. (pp. 78–79)

There is a difference between the distribution of the periurethral striated muscle in male and
female subjects. In both sexes, there is more striated muscle along the anterior wall than along the
posterior wall of the urethra, and in both sexes the striated muscle occupies the inferior one-half
of the anterior urethral wall. Striated muscle on the anterior wall of the urethra does not reach the
bladder neck in either male or female subjects. The junction between the smooth and striated fibers

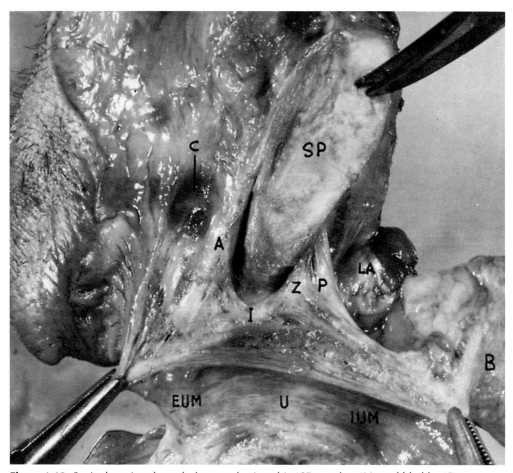

Figure 1.12. Sagittal section through the symphysis pubis (*SP*), urethra (*U*), and bladder (*B*), showing the suspensory mechanism on tension. Since traction to each end of the urethra results in some distortion, the length of the urethra is exaggerated. Continuity between the anterior ligament (*A*), intermediate ligament (*I*), and posterior ligament (*P*) is shown along with expansion of the posterior ligament (*Z*) as it runs forward to become the intermediate ligament. The levator ani (*LA*), clitoris (*C*), external urethral meatus (*EUM*), and internal urethral meatus (*IUM*) are shown. (From Zacharin RF. The suspensory mechanism of the female urethra. J Anat 1963;97:423–427. Reprinted with the permission of Cambridge University Press.)

on the anterior wall is not a sharp horizontal line, but rather an oblique line formed by the tapering, outer smooth muscle layer downward and inward, while the striated muscle moves upward and outward. Striated muscle is less prominent and less consistent along the posterior wall of the urethra. In female subjects, striated muscle is sparse along the inferior half of the posterior wall of the urethra, probably because the vagina fuses so tightly to the urethra in that area. (p. 91)

The internal sphincter is a double loop system formed by the base plate from the middle circular layer and the detrusor loop from the outer longitudinal layer. The base plate, which forms the top loop, is located in the base of the bladder, and its tonus is constantly forcing the apex of the trigone forward. The detrusor loop, which forms the bottom loop, is located in the very top of the urethra, forming most of the anterior and lateral walls of the urethra at the bladder. The loop is so positioned that the apex of the trigone fits snugly into its concave surface. Since the detrusor loop continues into the posterior surface of the bladder as the right and left lateral posterior outer longitudinal layer, its force is constantly directed backward in direct opposition to the base plate, which is pushing the apex of the trigone forward. This is the heart of the closing mechanism of the bladder neck when the bladder is at rest and passively filling with urine. (pp. 106–107)

For the internal sphincter to work properly, the base plate must be flat so that the fundus ring holds the apex of the trigone tightly into the concavity of the detrusor loop. At birth, all parts of the internal sphincter are present, but it does not function properly because the base plate is rounded. The same is true in stress incontinence. Here, the young girl is born enuretic and gains perfect control when her base plate flattens. Later in life when her anterior vaginal wall sags, the bladder descends, the bladder base becomes funneled, and she develops stress incontinence. A surgical procedure that elevates the bladder neck to a point where the base plate can flatten out restores her control. (pp. 116–117)

Any operation that opens into the urinary tract or that plicates the urinary tract in the region of the trigone, bladder neck, or urethra in an effort to narrow the caliber of these structures is harmful. In cases of stress incontinence these delicate structures are all present and will work again if they are placed in their proper position. Cutting into them or suturing them only diminishes their chance in recovery. To operate successfully for stress incontinence we must attempt to reestablish a normal relationship between the urethra, the base plate, and the symphysis (as demonstrated by a lateral cystogram) through proper positioning of the anterior vaginal wall. (p. 145)*

ARCUS TENDINEI

There are two arcus tendinei, one on each side of the pelvis. The arcus tendineus of the levator ani runs from the back of the pubis to the ischial spine. Somewhat medial to this is the arcus tendineus of the endopelvic connective tissue. The distance between

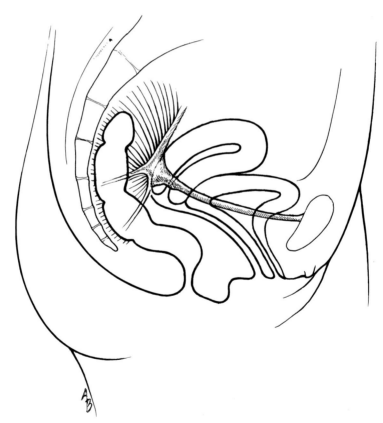

Figure 1.13. Schematic drawing showing the normal relationship between the vagina and the arcus tendinei. The arcus tendinei run between the back of the symphysis pubis to the ischial spine on each side of the pelvis.

*Hutch JA. Anatomy and physiology of the bladder, trigone and urethra. New York: Appleton-Century-Crofts, 1972; used with permission.

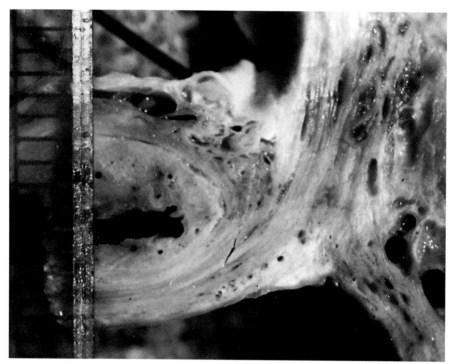

Figure 1.14. A fortuitous section through the urethra (*left*) and vagina (*below*) showing some of the distinct fibromuscular support of the urethra. Also shown is the ventral support of the anterior fornix by its attachments to the arcus tendineus and cardinal ligament (*right*).

these two arcus varies at their origin, and they may differ in their lateral extension; however, they come together at the ischial spine. The arcus tendineus of the levator ani provides a soft tissue attachment for the connective tissue bundle of fibers that is attached to the anterior vaginal sulcus (Figs. 1.13 through 1.15).

SUPPORTS OF THE URETHRA

The urethra is both suspended (by the urogenital diaphragm) and supported (by the vagina) (Fig. 1.16). Thus any hypermobility of the urethra may be surgically remedied either by suspension or by support, or by both.

PELVIC DIAPHRAGM

The levator ani, with its superior and inferior fascial covering, constitutes the pelvic diaphragm. In pronograde four-legged animals, it functions primarily as a tail wagger. When humans assumed an upright posture, they lost the tail as a functioning appendage, and the levator ani took on an entirely different purpose. The comparative anatomy of this evolution has functional significance and relevance to the physiology of pelvic statics (51, 60).

Thompson (65) wrote in his classic but not well-known treatise:

As the pubococcygeus has lost its influence as a tail wagger over the caudal vertebrae, its influence over the rectum has increased and a large number of fibers losing their connection with the coccyx pass round the rectum to form a sling; change of the commencement of which is seen in certain marsupials and carnivores.

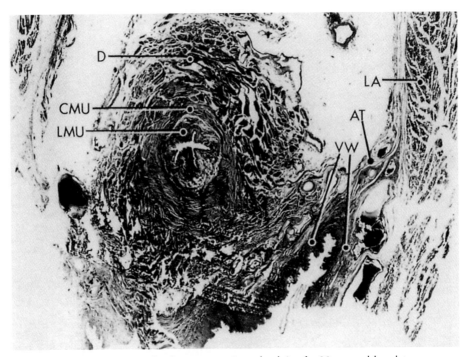

Figure 1.15. Photomicrograph of a cross section of pelvis of a 33-year-old cadaver perpendicular to the intramural urethra. Course detrusor fibers of the bladder (*D*) surround the urethra, and the outer circular smooth muscle of the urethra (*CMU*) is seen surrounding the internal longitudinal smooth muscle layer (*LMU*); note the attachment of the anterior sulcus of the vaginal wall (*VW*) to the arcus tendineus (*AT*), which overlies the levator ani (*LA*). (From DeLancey JOL. Correlative study of paraurethral anatomy. Obstet Gynecol 1986;68:91–97. Histologic sections provided by Dr. Thomas M. Oelrich. Used with permission.)

Figure 1.16. Suspension and support for the urethra. The urethra is both suspended (*central arrows* show the attachments and pull of the pubourethrovaginal ligament portions of the urogenital diaphragm) and supported (*lateral arrows* indicate the attachments of the vagina by intermediate connective tissue to the arcus tendineus).

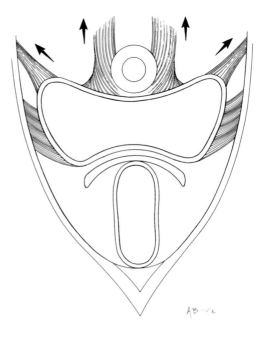

It is these detached fibers, which form a loop around the rectum, that have been called the *puborectalis* or *sphincter recti*.

Some fibers do retain their attachment to the coccyx, and they are occasionally torn during labor and delivery. When this happens, the patient may develop the unusual pain of coccydynia. As Malpas (37) pointed out, any activity that raises intra-abdominal pressure even momentarily elicits this pain in certain patients. The pain is due to the detachment of the muscle from the bone, rather than any affection of the bone itself, which explains why excision of the coccyx (coccygectomy) is generally both irrational and unrewarding. Most patients with chronic coccydynia need a perineal repair, not an excision of the coccyx. Power (51) noted the clinically significant embryology:

The recti group of thoracoabdominal muscles arise through the ventral extension of the thoracic myotomes into the body wall. As the body wall develops, extensions of the myotomes migrate ventrally into these walls and the ventral ends of these extensions fuse together to form a ventral longitudinal muscle column from which the rectus abdominis and other elements are ultimately developed. The levator ani muscle, as shown by its nerve supply, is undoubtedly derived from the fourth sacral myotome. In the view of C.P. Martin, as the cloacal membrane migrates from the umbilical cord to the extension of the linea alba, an extension of the tendency of the myo-tomes to form a longitudinal muscle column on each side of the linea also occurs. Accordingly, we might expect that in cases where the os pubis is absent or imperfectly developed, the lower end of the rectus abdominis and the ventral end of the puborectalis ought to be structurally continuous.

Power made these observations during the dissection of a stillborn fetus who had no pubis on the right side, which allowed Power to see the rectus abdominis passing without interruption into the puborectalis. Finally, Power noted that the width of the true pelvis is only about one-third that of the abdomen. Consequently, the viscera in the pelvis occupy most of the pelvic floor and separate the peritoneum from the pelvic diaphragm. The viscera are actually embedded in a mass of connective tissue that forms the layers of the endopelvic fascia. It is therefore easy to see why hernias through the pelvic floor are rare. The pelvic diaphragm is not a thin muscular layer in contact on its deep aspect with the peritoneum like the anterior abdominal wall. In fact, the vagina forms the one weak spot on the pelvic floor, and it is only in the vagina that hernias, such as cystocele, rectocele, and prolapse, occur.

The levator ani, acting reciprocally with the striated muscle of the anterior abdominal wall, is largely responsible not only for supporting both pelvic and abdominal contents, but also for maintaining the equilibrium of intra-abdominal pressure (47, 48, 66). Because of this reciprocal contraction, which has both an embryologic (51) and neurologic basis (66), any increase in intra-abdominal pressure, such as that caused by coughing and sneezing, is applied equally to all sides of the intrapelvic organs, and thus their equilibrium of position is preserved. If either the levator ani or the striated muscle of the anterior abdominal wall is pathologically weakened or temporarily inactivated (as by the splinting effect of a tight corset), the reciprocity of their action is lost, and pressure upon one side of a pelvic organ may become greater than that upon another side, permitting the organ to descend (genital prolapse). If this movement carries the organ outside the physiologically effective pelvic cavity, pressure on the content of that organ will be directed unequally. If the vesicourethral junction has been displaced outside the pelvic cavity, for example, an increase in intra-abdominal pressure, which would normally be borne equally by the intraperitoneal or intra-abdominal portion of the urethra and the bladder, will be borne by the bladder alone; as a result, the intravesical pressure would increase more than would the intraurethral pressure, and urinary incontinence would ensue (14).

Long ago, Dickinson (14) wrote:

I venture to affirm that there is no considerable muscle in the body the form and function of which are more difficult to understand than those of the levator ani, and about which such nebulous impressions prevail. The muscle sling, attached to the pubis in front, encircles like a collar the rectum and vagina. Its action in women is to drag the lower end of the vagina and rectum forward, level to the symphysis.

Sturmdorf (62) summarized its function as follows:

The levator ani diminishes the force of intra-abdominal pressure upon the pelvic contents by deflecting the direction of that pressure, augments the resistance to pressure by closing the uterovaginal angle, and obstructs the pelvic outlet against the pressure by compressing the vaginal canal. It is the tensor of the pelvic fascia, the antagonist of the diaphragm and the abdominal muscle, contracting when these opposing muscles contract and relaxing when they relax. When intact, it maintains the equilibrium of the pelvic organs; when its integrity is impaired, equilibrium is disturbed.

In their study of the periurethral and perianal parts of the levator ani, Critchley, Dixon, and Gosling used histochemical and electron microscopic techniques to make a quantitative comparison of the striated muscle fiber populations in these areas (9). They found that both regions consist predominantly of type I (slow-twitch) fibers, which maintain tone over long periods of time, with a small number of type II (fast-twitch) fibers, which contract suddenly over short periods of time. The two regions differ markedly, however, in the proportions of the two fiber types, the diameters of the constituent fibers, and the distribution of muscle spindles.

Collectively, the results of the present study have shown that the levator ani muscle cannot be considered to comprise a single morphological or functional unit since its constituent parts perform different functions according to their anatomical location. Clearly the present results are of considerable importance when interpreting electromyographic (EMG) recordings obtained from a single site in the levator ani. It is evident that the recordings obtained from one region alone do not provide an accurate indication of the functional status, either of other parts of the levator ani, or of the muscle in its entirety.

Divisions of the Levator Ani

The levator ani is composed of three general portions, each named according to its origin of insertion. The medial and anterior division is the pubococcygeus, which, from the gynecologist's clinical point of view, is the most significant component of the levator ani.

Originating on the face of the pubis, approximately 1.5 cm on each side from the center, substantial portions of the levator ani sweep downward and posteriorly along the sides of the urethra, vagina, perineal body, and rectum. These muscles appear to have clinically significant attachments to the connective tissue along the sides of the urethra, the vagina, the rectum, and the upper portions of the perineal body. Because these attachments vary considerably in strength and integrity, the support and protection that they provide to both internal and external genitalia vary as well.

There appear to be specific bundles of pubococcygeus fibers that extend medially. These bundles contribute to the posterolateral investment of the urethra (pubourethralis) and provide a slinglike posterior support to the rectum (puborectalis).

The puborectalis may be a distinct development of the most medial portion of the pubococcygeus. Bacon and Ross (2) believed the puborectalis to be a distinct muscle intimately associated anteriorly, but distinctly separated posteriorly, from the pubococcygeus; the two muscles appear to have a common origin, although the pubococcygeus arises on a higher plane. The puborectalis arises from the lowest portion of the symphysis pubis and from the deep layers of the triangular ligament. It passes downward and backward on either side of the vagina and lateral aspect of the rectum, with the two sides coming together again at the levator plate. It is continuous with the deep external anal sphincter. It fuses posteriorly in the midline, providing muscular support for the anorectal junction. Thus the puborectalis, which serves an important role in rectal continence, relates only to the lower rectum and upper anal canal along both the posterior and lateral aspects.

There is much individual variation in the nature and strength of such muscular slips, which perhaps explains the discrepancies in the literature of anatomy. Some authors deny the existence of these muscle bundles altogether, whereas others have contributed quite detailed descriptions with drawings and photographs of their relationships and distribution.

According to the careful dissections of Joachimovits (31), many women have a definite decussation of the puborectalis into clinically significant slips or prerectal bundles running from the belly of the muscles to the lateral margins of the perineal body. Superior to this area, at least in some women, muscle bundles run from the medial portion of the pubococcygeus to the posterolateral surface of the wall of the vagina and cranial toward the perineal body. These bundles have been designated the pubovaginalis muscle, but the extent of this development is quite variable. As a result, the clinical significance of the components of the pubococcygeus must vary from one woman to another. The significantly increased numbers of these muscle fibers in black women, in combination with other inherited characteristics (particularly connective tissue strengths), may help to explain the lower incidence of certain types of genital prolapse among black women.

The connective tissue attachments between the pubococcygeus and the urethra along the junction between the lower and middle third of the vagina and cranialward to the lateral portions of the central perineal body are often relatively strong. The clinical significance of these attachments appears to be primarily in the possibility that these fibers can be traumatically stretched or avulsed on either or both sides of the urethra.

Bacon and Ross (2) mentioned that the other levator components (pubococcygeus and iliococcygeus) sweep posteromedially to join each other behind the rectum and to insert into the coccyx:

At the level of the anus, the levator ends in fibromuscular extensions which join with those of the longitudinal muscle of the rectum to insert into the anal canal at the intermuscular line. Some fibromuscular extensions of the conjoined tendon also pierce the subcutaneous portion of the external sphincter to insert into the skin about the anal verge as the corrugator cutis ani.

The right and left muscle bellies of the pubococcygei fuse in the midline posterior to the rectum (Fig. 1.17) and continue to the coccyx. The fused levator ani muscles, which extend posteriorly from a point of midline fusion just behind the levator hiatus to their coccygeal insertion, form the levator plate. The rectum, vagina, and urethra pass through the levator hiatus, and both the rectum and the vagina rest on the levator plate. The normal horizontal position of this supporting levator plate accounts for the normal horizontal axis of the upper vagina. If the levator ani muscle is defective, the plate inclines downward and the hiatus sags.

Although Hadra (23) and later Halban and Tandler (24) recognized and defined the importance of the levator plate in providing pelvic support, the rectal distention and the absence of muscle tone in the cadaver made it difficult to demonstrate the function of the plate. Berglas and Rubin (3), however, were able to demonstrate this plate in the living and to relate its pathologic displacement with various degrees of genital prolapse. They did so by injecting contrast material directly into the levator muscle and plate and simultaneously placing contrast material in the vagina, uterus, and rectum. Radiograms taken of various patients while resting and while straining clearly showed the integrity and horizontal position of the normal plate, as well as the tipping of the abnormal plate with bearing down in patients with genital prolapse.

In the standing patient, the horizontal levator plate extends from the coccyx toward the midportion of the pubic symphysis, but does not reach it. The anterior margin of the

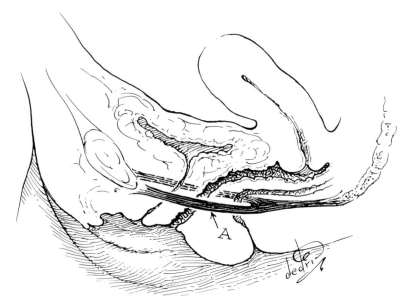

Figure 1.17. The vaginal axis of the erect or standing living female. Notice the almost horizontal upper vagina and rectum lying upon and parallel to the levator plate. The plate is formed by fusion of the pubococcygei muscles (*A*) posterior to the rectum. The anterior limit of the point of fusion is the margin of the genital hiatus, immediately posterior to the rectum. (From Nichols DS, Milley PS. Clinical anatomy of the vulva, vagina, lower pelvis, and perineum. In: Sciarra J, ed. Gynecology and obstetrics, 1977; reproduced with permission of Lippincott-Raven.)

plate is separated from the posterior margin of the pubis by the levator or genital hiatus. When the supports of the plate are damaged and it tips, not only do the organs above it "slide downhill," but also the anteroposterior diameter of the hiatus increases significantly, providing a larger portal for the egress of prolapsing organs.

Beautifully describing the function of the pubococcygeus muscle in the normal voiding mechanism, Muellner (43, 44) emphasized the importance of voluntary skeletal muscle in the mechanism of continence:

Before urination begins, the diaphragm and the muscles of the abdominal wall contract, the intra-abdominal pressure rises, and the pubococcygei relax. As the pubococcygei relax, the neck of the bladder moves downward. This downward movement activates or initiates the contraction of the detrusor. At the same time, the contraction of the longitudinal fibers of the urethra, which are continuous with those of the detrusor, shorten the urethra and thereby widen and open the internal urethral orifice. Urine is then expelled from the bladder.

At the conclusion of voiding, a contraction of the pubococcygei raises the neck of the bladder, the detrusor and urethral musculature relax, the urethra lengthens, the internal urethral orifice narrows and closes and urination stops.

Gosling (21) describes the relationship between the levator ani muscles and the urethral wall and urethral junction as follows:

The medial parts of the levator ani muscles (sphincter vaginae) are related to (but structurally separate from) the urethral wall. These periurethral fibers consist of the admixture of large-diameter fast- and slow-twitch fibers, together with muscle spindles. Therefore, unlike the rhabdosphincter, periurethral muscle possesses morphologic features that are similar to other "typical" voluntary muscles.

The levator ani plays an important part in urinary continence by providing an additional occlusive force on the urethral wall, particularly during events that are associated with an increase in intra-abdominal pressure, such as coughing and sneezing. This urethral occlusive force in the female is maximum at a level immediately distal to the maximum urethral pressure generated by the external urethral sphincter. Thus, in addition to providing support for the pelvic viscera, the periurethral parts of the levator ani also play an important active role in the urethral mechanisms that maintain continence of urine.

For micturition to occur, the pressure differential between the bladder and urethra muscle overcomes the elastic resistance of the bladder neck. Immediately before the onset of micturition, the tonus of the rhabdosphincter is reduced by central inhibition of its motor neurones located in the second, third, and fourth sacral spinal segments. Such inhibition is mediated by descending spinal pathways originating in higher centers of the central nervous system. Concomitantly, other descending pathways activate (either directly or via sacral interneurones) the preganglionic parasympathetic motor outflow to the urinary bladder. This central integration of the nervous control of the bladder and urethra is essential for normal micturition. . . . periurethral fibers are innervated by the pudendal nerves and consist of an admixture of large-diameter fast- and slow-twitch fibers.

The intermediate portion of the levator ani, the iliococcygeus, is somewhat thinner and flatter than the pubococcygeus and measures between 0.05 and 1 cm in thickness. Originating from the surface of the obturator internus fascia (from the so-called white line or tendinous arch of the levator ani, on a line running from the posterior pubis to the ischial spine), this muscle inserts along the lateral margin of the coccyx and lower sacrum.

Contrary to popular belief, the iliococcygeus is often convex in shape rather than concave (52), because fat within the ischiorectal fossa pushes on the soft belly of the muscle. This pressure, which is directed upward and medially, occurs when the woman is sitting or reclining, as these positions exert force on the ischiorectal fat from below (Fig. 1.18). A massive weight reduction that results in a loss of ischiorectal fat decreases the under support of the pelvic diaphragm, thus predisposing the levator muscle to sag, the levator plate to tip, and genital prolapse to develop subsequently.

The most posterior major division of the levator ani is the coccygeus muscle, which originates in the ischial spine and inserts along the fourth and fifth lateral margins of the

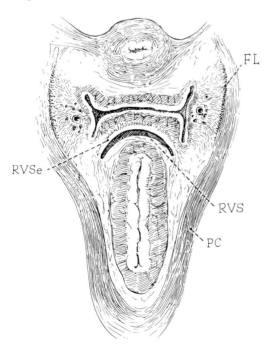

Figure 1.18. Cross section of a female pelvis through the lower midportion of the vagina. Note the convex configuration of the pubococcygeus (*PC*). The rectovaginal space (*RVS*) is indicated between the rectum and vagina, as well as the position of the rectovaginal septum (*RVSe*). The blood vessels in the connective tissue lateral to the vagina are shown. The fibers of Luschka (*FL*) attach the paravaginal connective tissue to the sheaths of the pubococcygei. These connections tend to give the vagina an H-shaped configuration. (From Nichols DH, Milley PS. Clinical anatomy of the vulva, vagina, lower pelvis, and perineum. In: Sciarra J, ed. Gynecology and obstetrics, 1977; reproduced with permission of Lippincott-Raven.)

coccyx and lower sacrum. Tandler (64) stated, "It lies intertwined with sinewy fibers on the front side of the sacrospinous ligament, and undergoes transformation into stronger more sinewy fibers at its points of insertion." The sacrospinous ligament is the "tendon" or aponeurosis of the coccygeus muscle.

The normal contraction and tonus of an intact levator ani participate in maintaining adequate pelvic venous circulation. Thus reconstitution of the levator by an appropriate colporrhaphy can be a factor in relieving perineal circulatory congestion and hemorrhoids, which will occasionally disappear several months after adequate perineal reconstruction.

Rectal Continence

When the levator ani and puborectalis muscles contract, they pull the levator hiatus toward the pubis, causing the rectum to incline at an angle that functions effectively as a valve, according to the observations of Parks (49). There is reflex reciprocity with the tone of the external anal sphincter. These muscles, which are innervated by the pudendal nerve and its accessory branches, function in synergism.

Neuromuscular pressure receptors within the striated muscle of the levator ani are responsible for mediating this tone, and they appear to communicate with the central nervous system by way of the pudendal nerve on each side of the body. The pudendal nerves generally arise from spinal cord segments S3 and S4. Either congenital or acquired pathology of the pudendal nerves can alter their efficiency and thus influence the ability and of these neuromuscular pressure receptors to maintain this responsive muscular tone. Acquired damage may result from the trauma of pelvic floor stretching during childbirth or, quite possibly, from the chronic habit of excessive straining at stool (27).

The levator ani and the external anal sphincter differ from other striated muscles of the body in that their state of tone is inversely proportional to the quantity of the rectal content. Because intestinal peristalsis continues around the clock, although at apparently various degrees of intensity, this tone is responsible for normal rectal continence.

Normal bowel function is to a large extent the product of habit. Defecation of sigmoid colon content is achieved by first voluntarily relaxing the pelvic diaphragm, unlocking the colic valve, and relaxing the external anal sphincter. A modest increase in intra-abdominal pressure, as by bearing down, forces the stool content downward. The gastrocolic reflex pattern regularly assists by promoting intestinal peristalsis. A disorder of any of these steps predisposes to or causes constipation (32). Regular and excessive bearing down may stretch the anatomic integrity of the pudendal nerve and consequently weaken the muscles that it innervates, occasionally resulting in a permanent loss of tone in the muscle of the pelvic diaphragm and external anal sphincter. The neuropathic loss of the tone of the anal sphincter permits it to relax at inopportune times, producing rectal incontinence that may be most difficult to treat surgically. The Parks group has suggested that this loss of voluntary muscle tone within the pelvic diaphragm may be associated with coincident urinary stress incontinence as well (27).

PERINEAL BODY

A pyramidal fibromuscular elastic structure, the perineal body is found in the midline between the rectum and the vagina on a line between the ischial tuberosities. Its tone, thickness, and composition vary in different individuals. It is somewhat like the hub of a wheel into which various muscles (the superficial and deep transverse muscles of the perineum, the bulbocavernosus muscle, the sphincter ani externus, and some fibers of the levator ani) are inserted like spokes. It is bounded anteriorly by the vagina and posteriorly by the rectum. Studdiford (61) found that many smooth muscles in the perineal body serve as distensible attachments to the levator ani and to the vagina. He believed that the loss of this distensibility as a result of unrepaired perineal laceration, for example, leads to rectocele and posterior vaginal eversion. Ranney (54) noted that the perineal body does not serve as a keystone, because its wide base points down, not up. If it was a keystone, it would by its very nature fall down if pressure were applied.

The large number of nerve fibers and ganglia distributed among the smooth muscle elements of the perineum indicates the functional importance of the smooth muscle. The large amount of smooth muscle within the perineal body provides it with physiologic distensibility; when this characteristic has been lost, the vaginal outlet becomes physiologically unstable.

In a thorough study of the pelvic outlet in the female perineum, Joachimovits (31) found that the size, attachments, and strength of the perineal body are subject to wide individual variations. When the perineal body appeared well developed, Joachimovits found this pyramidal tissue readily divisible into two distinct parts: (a) a distal fibrous portion practically covered by the superficial perineal muscles that penetrate the border of the urogenital diaphragm, and (b) a cranial portion that attaches to the most caudal portion of the rectovaginal septum and contains considerably more smooth and striated muscle fibers than does the distal portion. The perineal body is connected by smooth muscle bundles to the lowest portions of the anterior wall of the rectum and contains some striated prerectal muscle fibers of the levator ani and fibers of the sphincter ani.

The embryology of this structure explains the two parts of the perineal body that Joachimovits described (31). The structure develops from two vertical folds of the lateral wall of the cloaca that, early in development, grow as ventral and dorsal portions of the body. These folds fuse together in the midline to form a crescent-shaped fold of mesenchyme that is covered with epithelium (the urorectal septum) and separates the rectum permanently from the urogenital sinus. Because the lower distal portion of the perineal body arises from mesenchyme, it has only secondarily combined with the larger dorsal part. Subepithelial masses of mesoderm adjacent to the distal cloaca contribute striated muscle bundles to each side of the perineal body as derivatives of these cloacal sphincters, while the outer longitudinal muscles of the posterior vaginal wall and those of the anterior rectal wall contribute smooth muscle elements. The caudal or superficial portion of the perineal body, by its attachment to the superficial perineal muscles, becomes fixed to the ischial tuberosities; it is further fastened by its attachment to the bulbocavernosi. The external anal sphincter is anatomically weakened by its divergence into laminae about the vagina. Bacon and Ross (2) have suggested that this is the reason that the ends of the subcutaneous external sphincter tend to retract when the muscle is severed, producing anal incontinence.

Other studies have confirmed that there is considerable individual variation in the strength and composition of the perineal body and the extent to which fibers of the pubococcygeus are attached to or interspersed with fibers of the perineum. With the double embryology of the perineal body, variations in the strength of either the cranial or the caudal divisions, or both, can be genetically determined, and these differences may help determine the noticeable ethnic dissimilarity in the severity, as well as in the types, of genital prolapse.

Superficially, the pyramid of the perineal body is attached to Colles' fascia. The medial margins of the pubococcygeal muscles are in contact with the lateral surfaces of the perineal body at the border between its distal and proximal divisions. Although some prerectal fibers may insert on the lateral surface of the perineal body, the larger, more lateral bundles pass alongside the rectum and fuse into the levator plate as it extends to the coccyx.

Many smooth muscle cells extend as a ridge of variable thickness between the medial edges of the levator muscles in the midline. The attachment is greatest within the dorsal or deep division of the perineal body.

Like the perineal muscles derived from the cloacal sphincter, the prerectal bundles receive a secondary innervation. They can contract independently of the remainder of the levator complex, which helps in the process of normal defecation. The increase in their tonus (and in that of the pubovaginal bundles), accompanied by a relaxation of other levator fibers, pulls the perineal body forward and upward in a way that tends to neutralize variations in intra-abdominal pressure and helps prevent prolapse of the rectum during normal defecation. In contrast, the puborectalis bundles, those most medial portions of the pubococcygeus which come together behind the rectum in the levator plate to form an almost U-shaped sling for the rectum, contract immediately after defecation in unison with the remaining portion of the levator ani.

All of the attachments of the striated muscles to the perineal body are elastic to varying degrees. Just as the intrinsic elasticity of the connective tissues of the perineal body becomes less evident with advancing years, the elasticity of the attachments appears to vary in different phases of the woman's life cycle. The possible loss of an appreciable degree of the tissues' elasticity increases a woman's risk of obstetric damage if parturition occurs during the later years of her reproductive life. Furthermore, the relative weakness of a woman's elastic tissue may, to some degree, be correlated with the development of subcutaneous abdominal striae during her pregnancy, providing the so-called elastic index of Magdi (36). As Magdi noted, the less elastic the perineum, the larger the number of striae. Therefore, pregnant women whose tissues have lost some of their elasticity may require an earlier and larger episiotomy to prevent significant tissue damage at delivery.

Anteriorly, the attachment of the perineal body to the rectovaginal septum (see Fig. 1-27) at the site of this angle reinforces the anterior rectal wall, but disruption of this attachment between the rectovaginal septum and perineal body by tearing or attenuation contributes to the development of rectocele at this site. Generally, the perineal body is also lacerated in this case, permitting low and midvaginal rectocele; if the perineal body remains intact, however, the rectocele may occur higher within the vagina.

The length of the perineal body closely approximates the length of the urethra, since this is the level at which, under normal circumstances, the urethra, bladder, and vagina are laterally attached to the connective tissue of the pelvic diaphragm (pubococcygeus). In the case of the urethra, this support is aided considerably by the primary attachment of the pubourethrovaginal ligament, which, although primarily a portion of the urogenital diaphragm, is in a lateral relation to the fibers of the pelvic diaphragm.

SUPERFICIAL PERINEAL MUSCLES

The deep transverse perinei, arising from the inferior rami of the ischia, are enclosed within the layers of the urogenital diaphragm. The presence of the vagina interrupts the extent of the development of the urogenital diaphragm, in contrast to the male, and only a few fibers cross the midline between rectum and vagina.

The superficial transverse perinei arise from the pubic rami and attach to both the perineal body and the deep portion of the external anal sphincter, but they are not of great clinical significance.

The internal anal sphincter is the lower border of inner circular smooth muscle of the rectum and is of secondary importance in control of anal continence.

The external anal sphincter is divided into three portions.

a. The *subcutaneous* portion is continuous with fibers of the bulbocavernosus, both being derived from the cloacal sphincter and sharing common innervation and coordination of sphincter functions.

b. Unrepaired laceration will usually result in anal incontinence, because the division, the superficial portion, is weakened in its attachment to the female perineal body by the mobility of the vagina. The muscle originates from the coccyx, encircles the anus, and inserts into the perineal body.

c. The deep external anal sphincter cannot be distinctly separated posteriorly from fibers of the pubococcygeus. In fact, Courtney (8) states that the deep external sphincter is a continuation of the puborectalis formed by decussation of its fibers through the central tendinous point of the perineum. The anterior part of the anorectal ring is completed by the deep part of the external sphincter, while laterally and posteriorly it is formed by the U-shaped muscle sling of the puborectalis.

Thus he considers the levator ani, particularly on the puborectalis portion, and the deep external sphincter as anatomically and functionally one muscle, a view supported by Wendell-Smith (69).

Blood Vessels of the Female Perineum

The vascular supply of the perineal structure is derived from the branches of the internal pudendal artery, which arises from the anterior trunk of the internal iliac. The internal pudendal leaves the pelvic cavity through the greater sacrosciatic foramen. As it ascends along the pubic ramus, it pierces the posterior layer of the urogenital diaphragm, travels for a short distance within the diaphragm, and perforates the anterior layer. The terminal branches include the artery to the bulbocavernosus muscle and the dorsal artery of the clitoris. The branches within the perineum include the external or inferior hemorrhoidal arteries, and they originate as the pudendal artery rises anterior to the ischial tuberosity. The external hemorrhoidal arteries run across the ischiorectal fossa and are distributed to the anal sphincter and levator ani muscles. They are the chief sources of hemorrhage from all superficial wounds about the anus or ischiorectal fossa. These vessels have accompanying veins that empty into the pudendal veins.

The superficial perineal or vulvar artery is anterior to the external hemorrhoidal artery. It is disturbed to the vulva, with branches to the muscles, and is a source of arterial hemorrhage in wounds of the vulva.

The transverse perineal artery is smaller, supplies the cutaneous surface of the perineum, and is a source of hemorrhage from laceration of the perineal body. Another branch is the artery of the bulb, a vessel of considerable diameter but of short length. It sends branches to the bulbocavernosus muscle.

The terminal branches of the internal pudendal artery, the artery of the corpus cavernosum, and the dorsal artery of the clitoris are the vessels that supply the erectile tissue of the clitoris. When the clitoris is amputated, the two dorsal arteries may require ligation. Bleeding from the vessels of the corpora cavernosa can usually be controlled by pressure, since the trabeculae favor coagulation of blood.

The veins of the perineum are valveless and have free anastomoses with the large intrapelvic venous plexuses. Consequently, there can be alarming hemorrhage from wounds of the vulva and vagina, and massive hematomas are possible.

When the tone of the pelvic musculature is poor, venous return is impeded, and chronic congestion and varicosities, including hemorrhoids, may develop. These often improve after restoration of tone with reconstruction of the pelvic musculature.

Special properties of pelvic and perineal blood vessels include the following:

1. Although there are many large venous networks within the pelvis that are capable of considerable venous distention, these veins are almost entirely without valves.
2. Abundant smooth muscle fibers associated with adventitia of pelvic blood vessels probably account for at least part of the impressive quantity of smooth muscle found in the extraperitoneal connective tissue of the pelvis.
3. The warmth and heat of tissues undergoing erection (clitoris, bulbocavernosus muscle) demonstrate that most of the blood involved in the erectile process comes in fact from the arteriolar direction and that the venous congestion is probably a secondary phenomenon.

VAGINA

Vaginal depth and axis are maintained as a result of multiple but varying anatomic supports along the length of the vaginal walls. The lower third is supported predominantly by attachment through intermediate fibers to the pelvic diaphragm and arcus tendineus, urogenital diaphragm, and perineal body and indirectly by the same muscles and connective tissues to which the perineal body itself is attached. Support of the middle third is contributed by lateral fusion with fibers in the pelvic diaphragm. But even stronger lateral support is obtained by attachments to the inferior portions of the cardinal ligaments. The upper third of the vagina is adjacent to the rectum, which, in turn, rests on the levator plate but is not attached directly to the fibers of the pelvic diaphragm. The upper vagina and cervix are as a unit maintained in a position anterior to the levator plate by their lateral attachments to the cardinal and uterosacral ligaments.

The vagina is a fibromuscular tube, the walls of which are normally in apposition in the relaxed state; it is H-shaped in its central portion, the side walls being suspended by their attachment to the paravaginal lateral connective tissue from which they receive their blood supply and to the arcus tendineus. The vagina is lined by a stratified squamous epithelium with rugal folds, which give the epithelium accordionlike distensibility without laceration. The stratified squamous epithelium is rich in glycogen during reproductive years. A dense, thin layer of elastic fibers is found immediately beneath the epithelium. Beneath this is a well-developed fibromuscular layer. Smout et al. (60) have described a muscular meshwork of smooth muscle fibers predominantly oriented in a longitudinal direction in the innermost component but arranged circularly toward the periphery. The fibrous capsule external to this muscular coat is rich in elastic fibers and large venous plexuses.

The vagina is attached to the lateral pelvic wall by condensations of connective tissue and smooth muscle intimately adherent to the adventitia of the vaginal blood vessels. This tends to fix the position from side to side, and the muscular elements supply a certain amount of tone, permitting the vagina to adapt to changes in intravaginal and extravaginal pressure. There is a large amount of elastic tissue mingling with the fibromuscular connective tissue elements of the vaginal capsule. These permit distention and allow return to normal size. In the midline, the vagina can distend without interference from either the bladder or rectum. The relatively avascular vesicovaginal and rectovaginal spaces permit these organs to expand, contract, and slide somewhat independently of one another; thus each causes minimal interference with the function of the other. The rectovaginal septum is fused with the posterior vaginal wall as the anterior lining of the rectovaginal space. Because the vagina is a distensible organ, its depth is best measured when it is in a relaxed or resting state. The posterior vaginal wall is approximately 10 cm long. Since the cervix is incorporated in the anterior vaginal wall, the length of the anterior vaginal wall plus cervix approximates the length of the posterior wall. The connective tissue adventitia of the vagina is continuous with that of the cervix.

The vagina is normally narrowest in its lower third where it tends to be constricted laterally by the adjacent portions of the levator ani. The vagina is largest in its middle and upper thirds. The connective tissue lateral to the lower third is attached to fibers of the pubococcygeal muscle (fibers of Luschka) and to fibers fixing it to the urogenital diaphragm. Luschka (35) described the connection as follows: "In the female the fibers originating from the upper pubic ramus pass alongside the vagina and are connected with it through strong connective tissue but do not end in the vagina."

Huisman (29) believes that "the real voluntary urethral sphincter is located in the pelvic floor musculature, e.g. the pubococcygeus muscle."

Radiographic colpography has demonstrated a distinct, superiorly convex, perineal curve in the lower vagina (20, 45) (see Fig. 1.3). In the living, the upper vaginal axis lies in an almost horizontal plane when the patient is in a standing position. The upper vagina lies on the rectum, which, in turn, lies on and parallel to the levator plate. It is this almost horizontal position of the supporting levator plate that accounts for a similar axis to the upper vagina. The levator plate is formed by the fusion of the levator ani muscles posterior to the rectum, from just behind the levator hiatus to their coccygeal insertion (see Fig. 1.17). The rectum, vagina, and urethra pass through the levator hiatus, and, if the levator ani muscle is defective, the inclination of the plate will be downward and the hiatus will sag. Although the cervix and upper vagina have considerable mobility, they are more or less anchored in position over the levator plate by the cardinal ligaments. The length and flexibility of these ligaments normally permit the cervix and upper vagina to be moved in any direction over the rectum on the levator plate but not anterior to the margin of the genital hiatus.

The vagina is maintained in depth and axis by different anatomic supports at different vaginal depths. The lower third is supported predominantly by connection between fibers received from the pelvic diaphragm and the urogenital diaphragm. The most posterior portion of the lower third is further attached to the perineal body and indirectly receives contributions from the various other muscles and connective tissue thickenings to which the perineal body itself is attached (see Fig. 1.5). The middle third of the vagina receives some contribution from lateral fusion with a lesser number of fibers from the pelvic diaphragm, but even more lateral support is obtained from the lateral and most inferior portion of the cardinal ligaments that carry the main vaginal blood vessels both to and from their hypogastric origin. The upper third of the vagina receives almost no significant support from direct attachment to the fibers of the levator ani or pelvic diaphragm, but, in fact, rests on the rectum, which, in turn, rests on the fused pubococcygei of the levator plate. The upper vagina and the cervix together are maintained in position over this levator plate by their lateral attachments to the upper cardinal ligaments (50).

The vagina is "fixed" at two points, at the urogenital diaphragm and at the "cardinal ligament" at the vault, and is flexibly suspended in between with connective tissue attachments to the arcus tendineus and pelvic diaphragm.

Vessels of the Vagina

In addition to the vaginal blood supply received from branches of the internal pudendal artery, diffuse anastomoses form between these and branches of the uterine, inferior vesical, middle rectal, and vaginal arteries. The confluence of these anastomotic branches forms longitudinal azygos vaginal arteries in the midline of the anterior or posterior vaginal walls, or both, according to Smout et al. (60) and Quinby (52).

A right and left vaginal artery, or occasionally two, arise (independently in most instances) from each internal iliac artery slightly cephalad and posterior to the origin of each uterine and inferior vesical artery. Occasionally, the vaginal artery arises as a division of a short common trunk with the uterine artery. This branching, however, occurs at the lateral extremity of each cardinal ligament and has great clinical significance. Alarming arterial hemorrhage, thus, may follow laceration or surgical trauma to the vagina, especially in the vault of the vagina, even though the uterine artery has been securely ligated. Occasional postoperative arterial vaginal hemorrhage coexistent with intact ligation of the uterine artery may thus require separate isolation and ligation of the vaginal artery or, failing this, hypogastric or internal iliac ligation.

Vaginal veins communicate with rich plexuses in the paravaginal tissues, perineum, rectum, and bladder.

Normal Vaginal Depth and Axis

The vagina in the cadaver is usually depicted as an almost straight hollow tube extending vertically upward toward the sacral promontory (17, 22). As early as 1888, however, Hadra discussed the possibility that the upper vaginal axis of the living patient is more horizontal (23). In 1889, Dickinson provided objective evidence in support of this theory in his studies of impressions made in wax molds (14). Using molds of the vagina made from a rapidly solidifying dental impression paste, Morgan conducted similar studies—with similar results—in 1961 (42). Richter reported an expanded, more detailed study of this kind in 1966 (57).

Connective Tissue Planes and Spaces

Much of the beauty of soft tissue pelvic architecture derives from the abilities of the organs of the three primary systems in this area—urinary, reproductive, and rectal (gastrointestinal)—to function independently of one another. Each is capable of the limits of its normal range of function without causing permanent alteration of the anatomy or function of its neighbors; that is, the organs are capable of independent expansion and contraction.

There are connective tissue spaces (19, 50, 55, 59) between these organs that permit this relatively independent function. The connective tissue spaces to be described, it must be emphasized, are potential spaces. They are filled for the most part with loose areolar tissue, are virtually devoid of blood vessels and nerves, and are readily converted to actual spaces by blunt dissection, often with the index finger. Before dissection, they are somewhat analogous to the space inside a folded, empty paper bag. These spaces are divided by connective tissue septa that not only afford mechanical support but also provide the physical routes of blood vessels, lymphatics, and nerve tissue to and from the pelvic organs. These structures are contained within the septa along reasonably constant routes and do not trespass on the connective tissue spaces. Although their location is quite regular within the septa, they occasionally vary in their site of origin and their relative size. The anatomic ligaments form natural barriers to the spread of infection, cancer, and hematomas. The septa, on the other hand, through their blood vessels and lymphatics, form natural routes for the transmission of infection and malignancy arising from the pelvic organs. A detailed knowledge of the anatomy of these spaces and partitioning septa is essential to the understanding of their actual and potential functional importance in both health and disease. From accurate knowledge and experience, the surgeon can know not only where to find major vessels but avoid unnecessary surgical penetration of adjacent organs. This anatomic knowledge helps the gynecologic surgeon to demarcate the likely limits and routes of direct spread of malignant disease and to determine the extent of necessary extirpation. To the surgeon concerned with pelvic reconstruction, the implications are obvious because of the need to reestablish original relationships between the organs.

The connective tissue capsules or adventitia of the bladder, birth canal, and rectum are attached to the pelvis, and at certain points to one another, by condensations of connective tissue that contain the principal blood vessels and lymphatics to and from these organs. Although these septa vary in strength and thickness from person to person, their relation and position are constant.

Potential spaces exist between these septa, and the spaces are filled with fat and loose areolar tissue but are essentially free of blood vessels and lymphatics (Figs. 1.19 and 1.20). These areas become actual spaces only by dissection, but this is easily accomplished bloodlessly and bluntly once access to the space has been gained by surgical penetration through a septum.

Safe extirpation or reconstructive surgery for benign pelvic disease requires identification, penetration, and invasion of the midline anterior and posterior spaces, but the oncologic surgeon must penetrate and dissect the lateral spaces as well.

In the operative procedures to be described later, it is essential that the operator become thoroughly familiar with the pelvic connective tissue planes and spaces, especially with their relationships to one another. A relatively simple diagram of the clinically significant anatomic relationships, as illustrated in Figures 1.21 and 1.22, should be kept in mind.

The bladder, vagina, and rectum have been indicated as in the coronal section as shown (see Figs. 1.21 and 1.22). The cardinal ligament extends laterally from the central portion of the upper vagina and cervix. A vertical pillar or septum extends along each side of the three essential pelvic conduits—urinary, genital, and rectal—from the pubis to the coccyx, intersects the cardinal ligaments, and ensures both attachment and continuity with the connective tissue capsules of each of the three essential organs. Fascial

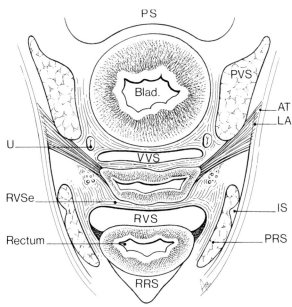

Figure 1.19. The connective tissue septa and spaces of the pelvis. The paravesical spaces (*PVS*) are shown lateral to the bladder. The ischial spine (*IS*) is in the lateral wall of the pararectal spaces (*PRS*) on each side. The prevesical space (*PS*), vesicovaginal space (*VVS*), rectovaginal space (*RVS*), and retrorectal space (*RRS*) are shown in the midline. The rectovaginal septum (*RVSe*) is also shown. Note the attachment of the vaginal sulci to the arcus tendineus (*AT*) and ventral surface of the levator ani (*LA*). The levatores ani forms the lateral wall of the pararectal spaces. The ureter (*U*) is shown. The rectal pillar separating the rectovaginal space from the pararectal space is of two layers (7), though these may be fused, as shown.

investments of striated muscle of the lateral pelvic wall form the lateral boundaries of these connective tissue spaces, now readily identifiable as the vesicovaginal, rectovaginal, and retrorectal space, the space of Retzius, and laterally, the paired paravesical and pararectal spaces. In general, these connective tissue septa and spaces are relatively constant in their relationship to one another, and the gynecologic surgeon will do well to keep such a simple diagram in mind. It will be referred to in greater detail and in a less schematic fashion later in this chapter.

VESICOVAGINAL SPACE

The vesicovaginal space lies in the midline and is bounded anteriorly by the bladder adventitia, laterally by the bladder septa or pillars, and posteriorly by the adventitia of the vagina. Superiorly, it ends at the point of fusion between the adventitia of the bladder and vagina. This point of fusion is called the supravaginal septum or vesicovaginal ligament (45). From the author's dissections he has found that this point of fusion occasionally contains multiple fasciculi, oriented in the same general direction but occurring at slightly different levels (see Fig. 1.20). Inferiorly, the vesicovaginal space is limited by the fusion of the urethral and vaginal adventitia.

SUPRAVAGINAL SEPTUM

There seems to be wide individual variation in both the strength and the extent of the supravaginal septum. At times it seems to be a nonentity, demonstrable only as the

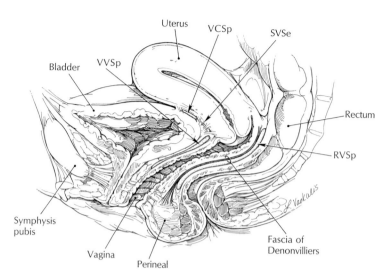

Figure 1.20. The pelvic connective tissue spaces in median sagittal view. The vesicocervical space (VCSp) is separated from the vesicovaginal space (VVSp) by fusion between the adventitia of the cervix and bladder called the *supravaginal septum* (SVSe). The rectovaginal space (RVSp) is shown between the rectum and vagina, extending from the perineal body to the bottom of the cul-de-sac of Douglas. The fascia of Denonvilliers (rectovaginal septum) is a condensation of tissue attached to the undersurface of the posterior vaginal wall along the full length of the rectovaginal space. Note its fusion to the cranial margin of the perineal body.

fascial capsule of the cervix through which the surgeon must dissect in the performance of vaginal hysterectomy in order to reach the anterior peritoneal plication. At surgical dissection, much of this tissue may be artifactual, but it represents the point of fusion between the connective tissue support of the bladder and that of the upper vagina and cervix. When a cystocele involves this area, adequate repair must involve identification and plication to ensure restoration of the fascial capsule of the cervix. It is perhaps along the long fibers of this supravaginal septum that cervical cancer may directly invade the wall of the bladder. The connective tissues of this septum may be softened considerably in pregnancy with the increase in elasticity that occurs to accommodate the necessary stretching as the uterus enlarges, as well as for the contraction of the uterus in labor with minimal alteration in bladder function. This softening accounts for the ease with which the bladder may be bluntly separated from the lower uterine segment and cervix at the time of cesarean section, contrasting sharply with the need for sharper surgical division of these organs in the nonpregnant state.

Anterior entry between the vagina and the peritoneal cavity is often through anatomic areas somewhat different, depending on whether the approach is from the vaginal or from the abdominal side. This structural difference may help explain why the surgeon who customarily operates by the abdominal route may experience unexpected difficulty in separating the bladder from the cervix when he or she approaches hysterectomy vaginally; similarly, the surgeon who is more comfortable with performing hysterectomy through the vagina may wonder why unfamiliar difficulties may arise during the course of abdominal hysterectomy.

This anatomic difference is explained in Figure 1.23. A customary route of dissection is identified by the arrows. The vaginal operator may incise directly through the point of fusion between the bladder and the vagina, providing ready access to the anterior vesicouterine perineal fold. When this is not promptly evident, it is likely that the dissection has been carried beneath the connective tissue capsule of the uterus, well

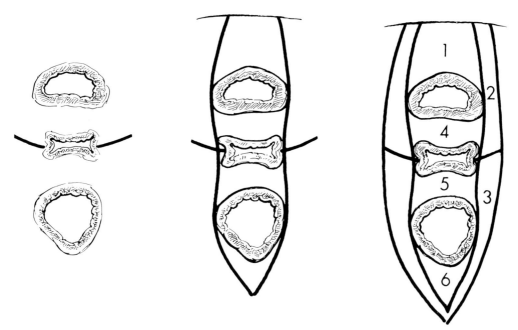

Figure 1.21. A schematic way of learning the names and relationships of the potential connective tissue spaces of the pelvis. The drawing on the *left* shows, in the center, the vagina with cardinal ligament attached. A cross section through the bladder is *above* and the rectum *below*. *Vertical lines* are drawn on either side of these three organs in the *center drawing*. They correspond to the bladder and rectal connective tissue septa and cross the cardinal ligament as shown. *Two additional lines* have been added to the drawing on the right, representing the obturator fascia and the pelvic diaphragm. The potential connective tissue spaces of the pelvis and their approximate relation to one another are labeled as follows: (*1*) the prevesical space, (*2*) the paravesical space, (*3*) the pararectal space, (*4*) the vesicovaginal space, (*5*) the rectovaginal space, and (*6*) the retrorectal space.

above the anterior peritoneal reflection. The peritoneum and the uterine connective tissue capsule will have been peeled off from the anterior surface of the uterus. The abdominal operator, on the other hand, will first enter the anterior peritoneum, continuing the dissection beneath the connective tissue capsule of the uterus beneath or through the so-called supravaginal septum to the vagina. The latter is the essence of the so-called endofascial abdominal hysterectomy (6). Recognizing these differences and becoming comfortable with both techniques will provide valuable surgical experience and enable one to find the anterior vesicouterine peritoneal fold when operating through the vagina, as well as to find the longitudinal muscle layer of the vagina more safely when operating through a transabdominal approach.

The continuity of the connective tissue capsule of the vagina and bladder is demonstrated in Figure 1.24, which shows a sagittal postmortem section through the vagina, cervix, and bladder of an aging patient with procidentia. Notice the continuity of this layer, which must be tranversed, as well as the looseness of the areolar tissues filling the potential vesicovaginal and vesicocervical spaces.

VESICOCERVICAL SPACE

The vesicocervical space is the continuation of the vesicovaginal space superiorly above the supravaginal septum. The posterior border of this space is composed of the connective tissue adventitia of the cervix and vagina. These adventitia are continuous.

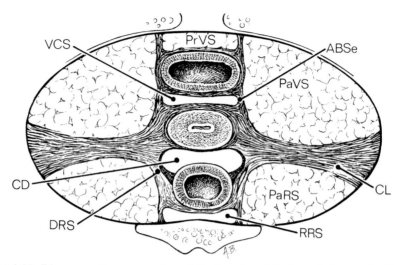

Figure 1.22. Diagrammatic cross section of the female pelvis through the cervix. The prevesical space (*PrVS*) is seen anterior to the bladder, and is separated from the paravesical spaces (*PaVS*) by the ascending bladder septa (*ABSe*). The latter also separate the paravesical spaces from vesicocervical space (*VCS*). The cul-de-sac (*CD*) is separated from the pararectal spaces (*PaRS*) by the descending rectal septa (*DRSe*), the posterior sheath of which separates the retrorectal space (*RRS*) from the pararectal spaces. Note the cardinal ligaments. (From von Peham H, Amreich J. Operative gynecology. Philadelphia: JB Lippincott, 1934. Used with permission.)

The superior border is the peritoneum lining the vesicouterine peritoneal pouch. Cutting the supravaginal septum establishes communication between the vesicovaginal space and the vesicocervical space.

ASCENDING BLADDER SEPTA

Although the ascending bladder septa are weak cephalad, they become the stronger bladder pillars (which contain efferent veins from the vesical plexus and ureter) by the addition of the lateral strong connective tissue portions of the cardinal ligament. Medially, they are loose in texture and contain fat and ureter. These septa attach to the lateral inferior extension of the bladder, connecting it to the upper surface of the cardinal ligaments, lateral to the cervix (see Figs. 1.16 and 1.19). They contain some cervical branches of the uterine artery anteriorly into the sides of the bladder base.

PREVESICAL SPACE OF RETZIUS

The prevesical space is in the form of a triangle extending from an apex at the umbilicus laterally to each lateral umbilical ligament (obliterated hypogastric artery). Anteriorly, the transversalis fascia extends from the umbilicus to the pubis; it extends inferiorly to the cardinal ligament and the supravaginal septum. It is separated from the paravesical spaces by the ascending bladder pillars or septa. The prevesical space thus includes the area between the pubis and the anterior vesical wall and is roofed by the fascia between the medial umbilical ligaments.

The ascending bladder septum above the ureter contains many blood vessels, including the inferior vesical artery and large veins of the vesical plexus. Below the ureter, however, blood vessels are scant, and the tissues between the bladder and vagina can be easily separated without hemorrhage.

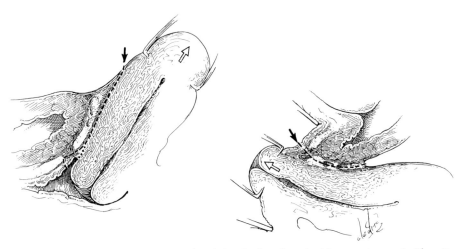

Figure 1.23. Vesicouterine incisions for abdominal and vaginal hysterectomy. **A.** The site and direction of anterior peritoneal incision often used in the so-called endofascial type of abdominal hysterectomy (*solid arrows*). This dissection, following the route of the *broken line*, is often beneath the connective tissue capsule of the uterus and must cut across the lower part of the supravaginal septum to reach the vagina, or it may enter the vagina *behind* most of the supravaginal septum, as shown by the *dotted line*. The *open arrow* shows the direction of removal of the uterus. **B.** A desirable route of incision and dissection with vaginal hysterectomy (*solid arrow*). The supravaginal septum may be incised immediately after opening the vagina, and dissection may be carried superiorly between connective tissue capsules of the uterus and bladder (the so-called vesicocervical space) until the anterior peritoneal plication is reached. If the operator dissects beneath the connective tissue capsule of the uterus, he or she will find himself or herself tunneling beneath and failing to recognize the peritoneum on the anterior surface of the uterus well above the anterior peritoneal fold. The *open arrow* shows the direction of removal of the uterus. (From Nichols DH, Milley PS. Clinical anatomy of the vulva, vagina, lower pelvis, and perineum. In: Sciarra J, ed. Gynecology and obstetrics, 1977; reproduced with permission of Lippincott-Raven.)

PARAVESICAL SPACES

The paired paravesical spaces, right and left, are natural, fat-filled, preformed spaces that lie above the cardinal ligament and its prolongation (horizontal connective tissue ground bundle); they are bounded medially by the bladder pillars and laterally by the pelvic walls, the fascia of the internal obturator muscle, and the levator ani. The roof is formed by the lateral umbilical ligament.

DESCENDING RECTAL SEPTA

The descending rectal septa or pillars run alongside the vagina from the undersurface of the cardinal ligament and its vaginal prolongation to the lateral surface of the rectum and thence to the sacrum. Each septum contains two layers, which are often fused (7). They divide the rectovaginal space from the lateral pararectal spaces.

PARARECTAL SPACES

The paired pararectal spaces are only potential and are not preformed. They lie below the cardinal ligaments and its vaginal prolongations. The medial border is formed by the rectal pillar, the lateral by the levator ani. The posterior portions extend backward above the ischial spine but under the cardinal ligament to the anterior surface of the lateral part of the sacrum. Behind the cardinal ligament the independent caudal portion of each side becomes continuous with the cranial portion of the opposite side.

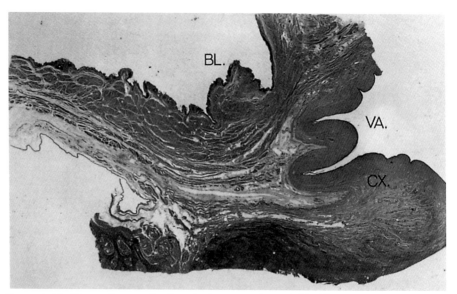

Figure 1.24. Photomicrograph of sagittal section through bladder (*top left*), vagina (*top right*), and cervix (*lower right*) of autopsy specimen of elderly patient with untreated genital prolapse. Descent of the cervix (*CX*) had drawn it and the vagina (*VA*) away from the bladder (*BL*). An attachment (supravaginal septum) of the fibromuscular connective tissue capsule of the bladder to that of the vagina is shown. (From Nichols DH, Milley PS. Clinical anatomy of the vulva, vagina, lower pelvis, and perineum. In: Sciarra J, ed. Gynecology and obstetrics, 1977; reproduced with permission of Lippincott-Raven.)

The upper rectum is surrounded by a single circular pararectal space. The boundaries of this space, formed by communication of two pararectal spaces and the retrorectal space, are formed laterally and below by the cranial surface of the levator, and above and medially by the rectum, the descending rectal septa, and the cardinal ligament. This space is made L-shaped by the horizontal part below the cardinal ligament and the cranial and ascending portion behind the cardinal ligament. The cranial portion of the space is bounded anteriorly by the cardinal ligament and posteriorly by the lateral part of the sacrum. The sheaths of the great vessels of the pelvic wall form the lateral border; the pararectal space is bordered medially by the rectal septa and ureteric sheath. The inferior or horizontal division is bounded below by the levator ani, above by the cardinal ligament, and medially by the rectal septum. The two pararectal spaces communicate with each other posterior to the rectum, where there is no limiting membrane.

RECTOVAGINAL SEPTUM

The rectovaginal septum is a distinct fibromuscular elastic tissue layer fused to the undersurface of the muscularis of the posterior vaginal wall to form the anterior border of the rectovaginal space. It was described by Tobin and Benjamin (67) as the "anterior layer of Denonvilliers' fascia" and was the subject of a special investigation by Milley and Nichols (40) in 143 specimens ranging in age from 8 fetal weeks to 100 years. It is a peritoneal fusion fascia, subject to wide individual variation in size, strength, and consistency, and is normally well formed by the 14th fetal week. In its fresh state, it is translucent and in the coronal plane parallels the sacral curvature, also curving posterolaterally to become indistinctly fused with the parietal endopelvic fascia (Fig. 1.25). The septum, representing fusion of the walls of the fetal peritoneal pouch, extends from the caudal margin of the cul-de-sac of Douglas to the proximal edge of the perineal body. It is a fixation point for the upper or proximal border of the perineal body and is of con-

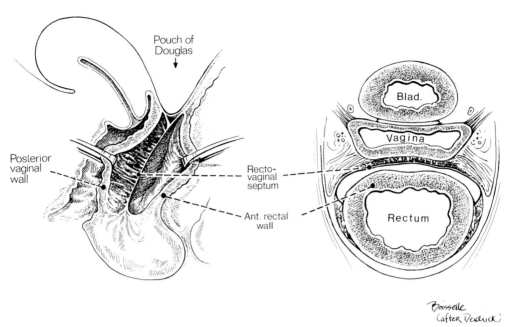

Figure 1.25. The rectovaginal septum; sections showing the partly dissected rectoseptum. The rectovaginal septum extends from the pouch of Douglas to the perineal body and forms the anterior surface of the rectovaginal space. Its adherence to the posterior vaginal wall is illustrated along with its posterolateral curve. (From Nichols DH, Milley PS. Surgical significance of the rectovaginal septum. Am J Obstet Gynecol 1970;108:217; reproduced with permission of Mosby–Year Book, Inc.)

siderable clinical significance, for if this attachment to the perineal body is avulsed, the anterior rectal wall may bulge with the straining of defecation, and the deflection of the fecal stream during normal defecation may be abolished, with resulting constipation. Midline laceration of the septum from excessive stretching during labor may cause obliteration of the rectovaginal space. Such pathologic fusion of the anterior rectal wall to the posterior vaginal wall decreases the effectiveness of defecation. Failure of this normal fusion to develop during early life may produce congenital enterocele with its inherent weaknesses. It is because of the strength contributed by the septum to the perineal body in the midline that spontaneous obstetric lacerations above the perineal body are more likely to occur in the posterolateral vaginal fornix than in the midline. Histologically, this septum consists of a fibromuscular elastic layer of dense collagen, abundant smooth muscle, and coarse elastic fibers, elements that are best demonstrated by specialized staining (Fig. 1.26). The surgical significance of reconstruction of this layer will be discussed in Chapter 11.

RECTOVAGINAL SPACE

The functional independence of the posterior vaginal wall with respect to the anterior rectal wall depends upon maintenance of the relatively avascular midline rectovaginal space, which permits the two organ walls to slide with considerable independence over one another. The anterior wall of this space is formed by the rectovaginal septum, which is attached to the posterior vaginal wall and the fat-covered rectal adventitia. The lateral walls are separated from the pararectal spaces by a descending rectal septum (rectouterine) on each side. The roof is the peritoneum and rectouterine peritoneal pouch (cul-de-sac of Douglas), and the inferior margin of this space is the perineal body.

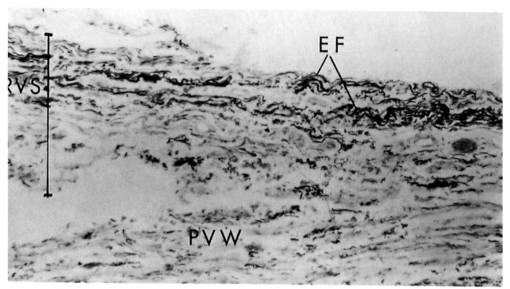

Figure 1.26. Sagittal histologic section through area of junction between the rectovaginal septum (*RVS*) and the posterior vaginal wall (*PVW*). The two have been separated at the *left* of the photograph by blunt dissection. Note the coarseness of the elastic fibers (*EF*) in the septum compared with those in the vagina. Orcein stain: × 106. (From Milley PS, Nichols DH. The human rectovaginal septum. Anat Rec 1969;163:443–447; reproduced with permission of John Wiley & Sons, Inc.)

The rectovaginal space ends where the levator ani muscles are attached to the cranial portion of the perineal body (Fig. 1.27). This coincides with the caudal attachment of the fascia of Denonvilliers to the perineal body. The relative freedom with which the vaginal wall can move independently of both bladder and rectum undoubtedly facilitates the type of segmental damage discussed in regard to the etiology of genital prolapse. This is damage concentrated principally on the lateral supports of the vagina, which permits eversion of the vault of the vagina with the development of enterocele.

RETRORECTAL SPACE

The retrorectal space lies in the midline between the sacrum and the adventitia of the rectum between the posterior portion of the rectal pillars. This space communicates with the pararectal spaces above the uterosacral ligaments. An extension of Richter and Frick's (58) third-dimensional concept of these connective tissue planes and spaces is presented in Figure 1.28.

CLEAVAGE PLANES

There are natural and potential cleavage planes (56) between organ systems in the female pelvis that, under certain stressful situations, permit segmental avulsion and pathologic sliding of one or more organ systems upon another. Although the existence of these specific segments of potential damage was well known to David B. Hart (26), their existence was demonstrated in the elegant and complex work of Halban and Tandler (24). It remained for Dickinson (13,15) to simplify and classify these characteristic segmental relationships and to draw meaningful conclusions concerning the importance of their role in the cause, type, and selective treatment of genital prolapse.

The author is in accord with Dickinson's concepts. Those which seem of practical significance may be summarized as follows:

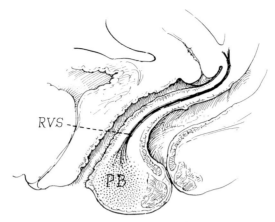

Figure 1.27. Sagittal section showing the rectovaginal septum (*RVS*) as it blends with the superior border of the perineal body (*PB*).

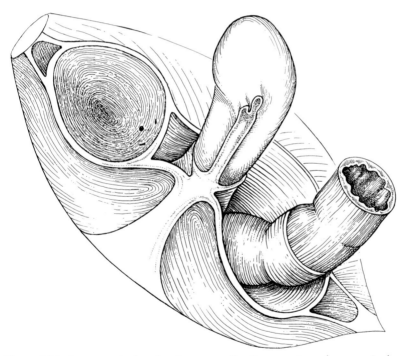

Figure 1.28. Stereograph showing the connective tissue septa and paravaginal spaces in relation to the bladder, uterus, and rectum. The spaces permit these three organs to function independently of one another (58).

1. There is a retropubic plane between the pubis and the urethra that is of clinical significance when the pubourethrovaginal ligament of the urogenital diaphragm becomes avulsed or stretched. This displacement permits the proximal urethra to rotate from its usual location, with consequent "wheelings" and rotational descent of the bladder neck (Fig. 1.29).

2. Another potential plane of cleavage exists between the posterior vaginal wall and the anterior wall of the rectum, that is, in the rectovaginal space. The organ systems anterior to this space are to a large extent interconnected, especially in the upper

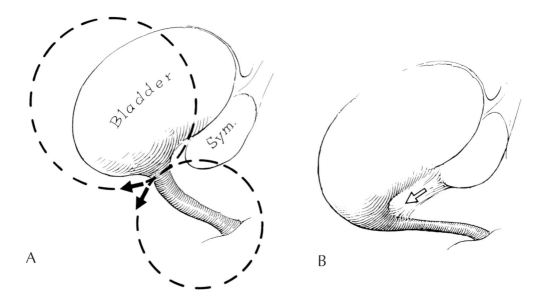

Figure 1.29. "Wheeling" or rotational descent of the vesicourethral junction. **A.** Rotational descent. **B.** This descent may result at rest from pathologic elongation of the pubourethral ligaments, with obliteration of the posterior vesicourethral angle forming one contributing factor for urinary stress incontinence.

two-thirds of the musculoelastic investments. There may be eversion of the upper vagina and cervix as a result of an overstretching of the cardinal and uterosacral ligaments. These structures together may first pull upon the anterior leaf of the cul-de-sac, causing a traction enterocele. As they slide over the anterior rectal wall, a sliding hernia is produced; if the hernia is progressive, it will pull upon the anterior wall, aiding in the development of high rectocele. This development is further favored by the following mechanisms: high rectocele often coexists with enterocele because the peritoneal fusion fascia of Denonvilliers (rectovaginal septum) is missing above the lower point of the enterocele. This results in a loss of support to the anterior rectal wall and the posterior vaginal wall. Whenever a high rectocele is present, enterocele should be suspected. Its presence or absence should be determined with certainty; if found, repair should be accomplished as a separate step during high posterior colporrhaphy.

References

1. Aronson MP, Lee RA, Berquist TH. Anatomy of anal sphincters and related structures in continent women studied with magnetic resonance imaging. Obstet Gynecol 1990;76:846–851.
2. Bacon HE, Ross ST. Atlas of operative technic: anus, rectum and colon. St. Louis: CV Mosby, 1954.
3. Berglas B, Rubin IC. Study of the supportive structures of the uterus by levator myography. Surg Gynecol Obstet 1953;97:677–692.
4. Bonney V. The sustentacular apparatus of the female genital canal, the displacements from the yielding of its several components and their appropriate treatment. J Obstet Gynaecol Br Emp 1914;45:328.
5. Campbell RM. The anatomy and history of the sacrouterine ligaments. Am J Obstet Gynecol 1950; 59:1–12.
6. Contamin R, Leger P. Anatomic principles of major gynecologic surgery: abdominal hysterectomy. Int J Gynaecol Obstet 1970;8:522–525.
7. Contamin R, Bernard F, Ferrieux J. L'Hysterectomie vaginale intrafasciale avec reconstitution de la paroi vaginale posterieure. Gynecologie Pratique 1972;23:17–30.
8. Courtney H. Anatomy of the pelvic diaphragm and anal rectal musculature as related to sphincter preservation in anal rectal surgery. Am J Surg 1950;79:155.

9. Critchley HOD, Dixon JS, Gosling JA. Comparative study of the periurethral and perianal parts of the human levator ani muscle. Urol Int 1980;35:226–232.

10. Curtis AH, Anson BJ, McVay CB. The anatomy of the pelvic and urogenital diaphragms in relation to urethrocele and cystocele. Surg Gynecol Obstet 1939;68:161–166.

11. DeLancey JOL. Correlative study of paraurethral anatomy. Obstet Gynecol 1986;68:91–97.

12. DeLancey JOL. Anatomic aspects of vaginal eversion after hysterectomy. Am J Obstet Gynecol 1992;166:1717–1728.

13. Dickinson RL. Genital prolapse: its operative correction based on a new study of cleavage lines and sliding segments. Am J Obstet Dis Wom 1910;17:17–35.

14. Dickinson RL. Studies of the levator ani muscle. Am J Obstet Dis Wom 1889;22:897–917.

15. Dickinson RL. The vagina as a hernial canal. Am J Obstet Dis Wom 1889;22:692–697.

16. Enhorning G. Simultaneous recording of intravesical and intraurethral pressure. Acta Chir Scand 1961;276:4–12.

17. Eycleshymer AC, Schoemaker DM. A cross section in anatomy. New York: Appleton-Century-Crofts, 1983:5.

18. Ferguson WH. New functional repair of post hysterectomy vaginal vault prolapse with Marlex mesh. Am Surg 1964;30:227.

19. Fothergill WE. On the pathology and the operative treatment of displacements of the pelvic viscera. J Obstet Gynaecol Br Emp 1907;13:410–419.

20. Funt MI, Thompson JD, Birch H. Normal vaginal axis. South Med J 1978;71:1534–1536.

21. Gosling JA. The structure of the female lower urinary tract and pelvic floor. Urol Clin North Am 1985;12:207–214.

22. Grant JCB. An atlas of anatomy. 2nd ed. Baltimore: Williams & Wilkins, 1943:123.

23. Hadra BE. Lesions of the vagina and pelvic floor. Philadelphia: Records, McMullin, 1888.

24. Halban J, Tandler J. Anatomie und Ätiologie der Genitalprolapse beim Weibe. Vienna and Leipzig: Wilhelm Braumuller, 1907.

25. Halsted WS. Circular suture of the intestine: an experimental study. Am J Med Sci 1887;94:436–461.

26. Hart DB. The structural anatomy of the female pelvic floor. Edinburgh: Maclachlan & Stewart, 1880.

27. Henry MM, Swash M. Coloproctology and the pelvic floor. London: Butterworths, 1985.

28. Hofmeister FJ, Wolfgram RC. Methods of demonstrating measurement relationships between vaginal hysterectomy ligatures and the ureters. Am J Obstet Gynecol 1962;83:938–948.

29. Huisman AB. Aspects on the anatomy of the female urethra with special reference to urinary continence. In: Ulmsten U, ed. Contributions to gynecology and obstetrics. Basel: Karger, 1983;10:1–31.

30. Hutch JA. Anatomy and physiology of the bladder, trigone and urethra. New York: Appleton-Century-Crofts, 1972.

31. Joachimovits R. Das Beckenausgangsgebiet und Perineum des Weibes. Vienna: Wilhelm Maudrich, 1969.

32. Lennard-Jones JE. Constipation. In: Henry MM, Swash M, eds. Coloproctology and the pelvic floor. London: Butterworths, 1985.

33. Lord MG, Valies P, Broughton AC. A morphologic study of the submucosa of the large intestine. Surg Gynecol Obstet 1977;145:55–60.

34. Luisi M. Anatomica Clinica Ginecologica. Milano: E Ambrosiana, 1978:64.

35. Luschka HV. Die Anatomie des Menschen. Tubingen: H Lauppsche Buchhandlung, 1869:143–149.

36. Magdi L. Obstetric injuries of the perineum. J Obstet Gynaecol Br Commonw 1942;49:687–700.

37. Malpas P. Genital prolapse and allied diseases. New York: Grune & Stratton, 1956.

38. McCarthy S, Vaqueno E. Gynecologic anatomy with magnetic resonance imaging. Am J Obstet Gynecol 1986;155:255–259.

39. Mengert WF. Mechanics of uterine support and position. Am J Obstet Gynecol 1936;31:775.

40. Milley PS, Nichols DH. A correlative investigation of the human rectovaginal septum. Anat Rec 1969;163:443.

41. Milley PS, Nichols DH. The relationship between the pubourethral ligaments and the urogenital diaphragm in the human female. Anat Rec 1971;170:281–283.

42. Morgan KF Jr. Casts of the vagina as a means of evaluation of structural changes and treatment. Calif Med 1961;94:30–32.

43. Muellner SR. The anatomies of the female urethra. Obstet Gynecol 1959;14:429.

44. Muellner SR. The etiology of stress incontinence. Surg Gynecol Obstet 1949;88:237–242.

45. Nichols DH, Milley PS, Randall CL. Significance of restoration of normal vaginal depth and axis. Obstet Gynecol 1970;36:251–256.

46. O'Leary JA. Ventrofixation in the management of vaginal vault prolapse. Surg Gynecol Obstet 1965;120:1296.

47. Paramore RH. Some further considerations on the supports of the female pelvic viscera, in which the intra-abdominal pressure is still further defined. J Obstet Gynaecol Br Emp 1908;14:173–189.

48. Paramore RH. The supports-in-chief of the female pelvic viscera. J Obstet Gynaecol Br Emp 1908;13:391–409.

49. Parks AG. Anorectal incontinence. Proc Roy Soc Med 1975;68:21.

50. Peham H von, Amreich J. Operative gynecology. Philadelphia: JB Lippincott, 1934.
51. Power RMH. Embryological development of the levator ani muscle. Am J Obstet Gynecol 1948;55: 367–381.
52. Quinby WC. The anatomy and blood vessels of the pelvic. In: Meigs JV, ed. Surgical treatment of cancer of the cervix. New York: Grune & Stratton, 1954:32.
53. Range RL, Woodburne RT. The gross and microscopic anatomy of the transverse cervical ligament. Am J Obstet Gynecol 1964;90:460–467.
54. Ranney AL. The topographical relations of the female pelvic organs. New York: Wood, 1883:107–110.
55. Ricci JV, Thom CH, Kron WL. Cleavage planes in reconstructive vaginal plastic surgery. Am J Surg 1948;76:354–363.
56. Richter K. Lebendige Anatomie der Vagina. Geburtshilfe Frauenheilkd 1966;26:1213.
57. Richter K. Die Physiologische Topographie der Weiblichen Genitale in Moderner Sicht. Zentralbl Gynakol 1967;89:1258.
58. Richter K, Frick H. Die Anatomie der Fascia Pelvis Visceralis aus Didaktischer Sicht. Geburtshilfe Frauenheilkd 1985;45:282–287.
59. Sims, JM. Clinical notes on uterine surgery. London: Robert Hardwick, 1866, pp 305–306.
60. Smout CFV, Jacoby F, Lillie EW. Gynecological and obstetrical anatomy. Baltimore: Williams & Wilkins, 1969.
61. Studdiford WC. The involuntary muscle fibers of the pelvic floor. Am J Obstet 1909;60:23.
62. Sturmdorf A. Gynoplastic technology. Philadelphia: FA Davis, 1919:109–114.
63. Sultan AH, Nicholls RJ, Kamm MA, et al. Anal endosonography and correlation with in vitro and in vivo anatomy. Br J Surg 1993;80:508–511.
64. Tandler J. Lehrbuch der systematischen Anatomie. Leipzig: Vogel, 1926;1:370–371.
65. Thompson P. The myology of the pelvic floor. London: McCorquodale, 1899.
66. Tilney F, Pike FH. Muscular coordination experimental studies in its relation to the cerebellum. Arch Neurol Psychiatry 1925;13:289–334.
67. Tobin CE, Benjamin JA. Anatomical and surgical restudy of Denonvilliers' fascia. Surg Gynecol Obstet 1945;80:373–388.
68. Uhlenhuth E: Problems in the anatomy of the pelvis. Philadelphia: JB Lippincott, 1953:161.
69. Wendell-Smith CP. The homologues of the puborectalis muscle. J Anat Aust N Z 1964;98:489.
70. Wilson PD, Dixon JS, Brown ADG, et al. Posterior pubourethral ligaments in normal and genuine stress incontinent women. J Urol 1982;130:802–805.
71. Zacharin R. The suspensory mechanism of the female urethra. J Anat 1963;97:423–427.

CHAPTER 2

Reduction of Maternal Injuries Associated with Childbirth

Although improvements in treatment during the 20th century have certainly improved the general health of all United States citizens, measures designed to prevent problems have been the most effective means of improving the gynecologic health of United States women during this period. Prophylactic measures now spare all but a very few women in the United States from the life-threatening or disabling consequences of obstructed labor or obstetric hemorrhage and from the development of eclampsia or puerperal sepsis. Similarly, the measures employed to ensure the earlier diagnosis of sexually transmitted disease and of carcinoma of the cervix, rather than more effective new treatments, have been largely responsible for improving the gynecologic health of United States women during this century.

Although the effectiveness of preventive measures has been generally recognized, obstetric practices seem to have largely neglected opportunities to minimize anatomic injuries in the maternal reproductive tract and to reduce disabilities that can frequently be attributed to the conduct of childbirth (17, 18). It seems that there has been a rather general acceptance of the probability of injury and the need for subsequent repair of maternal tissues as unavoidable consequences of human parturition (1, 4).

The surgical repair of varying types and degrees of maternal injury has been described thoroughly, but relatively little has been spoken or written about techniques and procedures recommended to reduce the frequency and extent of maternal injuries (3). For example, the well-documented study of Curtis and Anson (5), published in 1942, did not indicate any major factors in the management of parturition that might account for the injuries to maternal soft tissues that the authors described.

In the literature of the United States, however, there have been a few noteworthy exceptions. Writing a review from a clinician's perspective, Gustafson entitled his 1940 report "The Prevention and Treatment of Cystocele in the Reproductive Age" (11). He related several variations in the management of labor and delivery to maternal injuries that had been recognized postpartum.

The first truly significant, objectively documented study that correlated the management of labor and delivery with subsequent evidence of maternal soft tissue injuries was reported by Gainey (9) in 1943. No equally significant study appeared in the United States literature until 1955, when Gainey reported the results of his comparison of specific, documented injuries in two series of 1000 patients each (10). In both series, Gainey personally delivered each patient and assessed the postpartum evidence of injury. There was, however, an essential difference in the management of labor in the two series. He performed an episiotomy in the first group only when there was a maternal or fetal indication for it—either to avoid "impending" perineal laceration or to hasten delivery because of "fetal distress." In every instance in the second series, he performed an episiotomy at the outlet station of the presenting part, after which he accomplished all deliveries by low or outlet forceps (except in 27 instances that required forceps rotation and 40 "breech assists" with forceps to the after-coming head). Gainey found that performing the episiotomy and controlling the delivery of the fetal head by "outlet" or "prophylactic" forceps provided significant protection for the vagina, urogenital diaphragm, and perineum (Table 2.1).

In spite of the studies made and reported by DeLee in 1920 (7) and by Gainey in 1943 and 1955 (9, 10), the literature contains few indications of efforts to prove or disprove the effects of the factors that those observers had recognized and reported. Their studies still await either confirmation or denial through objective observation at least as well documented as the data that DeLee and Gainey presented. This failure to consider the relationship between obstetric events and maternal injury and to study the possible effectiveness of prophylactic measures does not seem compatible with usual professional points of view.

Every obstetrician in training should study Gainey's two reports carefully, not because they indicate the virtues of so-called routine episiotomy and prophylactic application of forceps, but because they illustrate the obstetrician's ability to predict, assess, and record the damage that labor and delivery may do to soft tissues. Clearly, the concerned obstetrician can develop the ability to correlate maternal injuries during parturition with the events that have preceded them. However, a review of the obstetric literature and of the annual reports of the teaching services suggests that most of the residency training programs in the United States have not been teaching or encouraging the Gainey type of objective and systematic postdelivery appraisal of maternal injuries.

Table 2.1.

Comparison of Pelvic Soft Tissue Damage between Primiparous Obstetric Patients without Laceration and Those with Episiotomy

	Series 1 Para I without Laceration (209 cases) (%)	Series 2 Para I with Laceration (590 cases) (%)
Detached urethra	6	5.6
Relaxation	9	1.9
Left pubococcygeus	10	1.9
Right pubococcygeus	19	6.4
Left iliococcygeus	3	0
Right iliococcygeus	2	1.2
Total levator atrophy	27	11.2
Detached urethra	6	5.6
Relaxation	28	10.3
Anovaginal damage	29	1.2
Cystocele	15	6.1
Obliteration of fornix	17	3.6
Rectocele	7	<1
Detached retrovaginal septum	8	<1
Anal sphincter damage	0	<1

Adapted from Gainey HL: Postpartum observation of pelvic tissue damage: Further studies. *Am J Obstet Gynecol* 70:800, 1955.

It is an undeniable fact that the "teachers" of obstetric practice at the undergraduate, graduate, and continuing education levels have, for the most part, failed to emphasize ways to manage labor and delivery in order to avoid or minimize maternal tissue damage. For generations, dedicated teachers of obstetrics have emphasized and personally practiced conservative obstetrics. A virtually universal willingness to perpetuate the conviction that "nature does it best" has ensured that each medical student and resident in training observes a sufficient number of spontaneous deliveries to appreciate the satisfactions of the "natural" delivery of a normal child, as well as to recognize and remember the factors that permit such a delivery (2, 14).

In their efforts to improve the management of labor and delivery, obstetricians and gynecologists may well find Gainey's approach a reliable means of recording injuries. Although DeLee and Gainey both directed their attention, or at least seem to have directed their reports, to the obstetrician's management of the actual delivery and the consequences of that management for mother and child, the use of their methods in conjunction with today's sophisticated data collection systems may well make it possible to determine the relation of the conduct of both the first and second stages of labor with the subsequent degrees and sites of maternal injury.

Obstetricians and gynecologists may have raised too few questions in regard to the management of the first stage of labor. Operative interference by means of such procedures as Voorhees bags to tamponade intrapartum bleeding, Dührssen incisions to expedite completion of the first stage, or vaginal hysterotomy to effect delivery before completion of the first stage are, fortunately, no longer considered useful techniques to be learned by the obstetrician in training. On the other hand, the quality of myometrial action during the first stage of labor, in terms of the effectiveness of uterine contractions, is now receiving a great deal of attention.

Although immediately evident injuries to maternal soft parts during labor and delivery, such as laceration, avulsion, or inversion, may account for an alarming amount of bleeding and require the obstetrician's immediate attention, some types of obstetric injury, ranging from a minor degree of relaxation to a disabling degree of procidentia, are slow to develop. It is this latter type of maternal injury, which may not occur until months or years after the birth of a child, with which the gynecologic surgeon usually gains an extensive experience.

FACTORS THAT ACCOUNT FOR UTERINE PROLAPSE

A few years after a single uncomplicated pregnancy and labor that results in the delivery of an average-sized infant, one woman may develop a virtually complete prolapse of the uterus, with perhaps equally evident eversion and prolapse of the vagina. Another woman of the same age, in no better general health, many develop no demonstrable prolapse of the uterus and may have surprisingly well supported vaginal walls and well preserved perineum after delivery of one or several large infants. Why do the forces of "normal labor" produce extensive injuries in one woman and no demonstrable injuries in another woman when the bony pelvis and soft tissue in both women seem adequate, comparable, and normal? The fact that a woman who has never been pregnant and has no history of unusual trauma or weight bearing occasionally develops uterine and vaginal prolapse indicates the presence of a neurogenic or congenital factor. Such a "predisposition" has, of course, been noted in association with multiple sclerosis and spina bifida occulta. In the majority of instances, however, the trauma of labor and delivery appears to be the only probable cause.

The most obvious possible explanation for the subsequent uterine prolapse in women who have presumably been exposed to the same forces of labor and delivery as have women who do not later suffer such a prolapse is that all labors do not actually involve the same stresses and strains on the tissues that support the uterus, cervix, and vagina. The factors that account for the resistance offered may be as important as the factors that account for the strength and effectiveness of uterine contractions. A better understanding of both types of factors may lead to the resolution of resistance and an increasingly reliable means of controlling or regulating the strength of contractions.

The means of decreasing resistance through the encouragement of relaxation and the means of augmenting the forces of labor through the accurately regulated infusion of an oxytocic are now universally available. Both are controllable and may be helpful to mother and child when administered appropriately. Psychologic preparation for labor, as well as sedation, analgesia, or regional blocking, not only may relieve the pains of childbirth but may also improve the progress of labor. Fatigue, impaired morale, and tissue depletion secondary to prolonged pressure and strain decrease tissue response and elasticity, however, and the oversolicitous administration of sedatives may prolong labor harmfully. Furthermore, the well-meaning but ill-advised coaching of the woman in labor by "supporting" personnel, whether an apprehensive but fatigued friend or the less personally concerned labor room attendant, may increase the risk of maternal injury.

Fortunately, the majority of patients in labor do not seem to feel a desire to bear down with their uterine contractions until the presenting fetal part begins to distend the pelvic floor. When the woman in active labor bears down as forcefully as she can before her cervix is fully dilated and before the presenting part can readily descend in the vagina in response to the pressures being applied, the tissues that support both the fundus and the cervix in normal anatomic relationships with the bony pelvis and adjacent viscera must either succeed in resisting the woman's efforts to "deliver her uterus with the baby in it," or will stretch and detach considerably more than if there had been no such premature bearing-down effort. By the same mechanism, when the fetus is disproportionately large; has a poorly flexed, unfavorably presenting vertex; or is in the breech position (so that the passageway must be molded or adapted before descent can occur), voluntary bearing-down efforts can increase the stress and stretch on the tissues that normally support the uterus and vagina within the maternal pelvis. Without intelligent management, the forces of labor under these circumstances can result in injuries that will predispose the patient to the later development of uterine prolapse (18).

INJURIES TO THE VAGINA

Although it is obvious that overdistention of the vaginal walls during the birth of a large fetus may leave the vaginal walls stretched beyond the ability of tone-regaining involutionary processes to restore them to their original caliber and may lead to the development of a cystocele or rectocele, the mechanism of injury that results in the detachment of the vaginal wall from its supporting tissue is not so generally understood. The vagina can be damaged obstetrically by a single event or a combination of two events. Overstretching by the presenting part of the fetus that damages the elasticity and integrity of the vaginal wall itself is one event. The other is stretching or avulsion of the lateral connective tissue segments that attach the vagina to the pelvic side walls (Fig. 2.1).

Injuries to the Vaginal Wall

Laceration of the vaginal wall can be expected when the forces that distend the vagina are unevenly applied, as when a poorly flexed vertex or a compound presentation results in maximal distention of only one segment within the circumference of the vagina. The occurrence of so-called superior sulcus tears is perhaps the best example of a laceration of the vaginal wall due to maximal need for or maximal resistance to distention in a segment of the vaginal circumference.

Simple overdistention of the vaginal circumference may thin the vaginal wall to the point that it is unable to resist any natural bulging tendency of the bladder or rectum to sacculate into the vaginal lumen; as a result, a cystocele or rectocele may develop. At

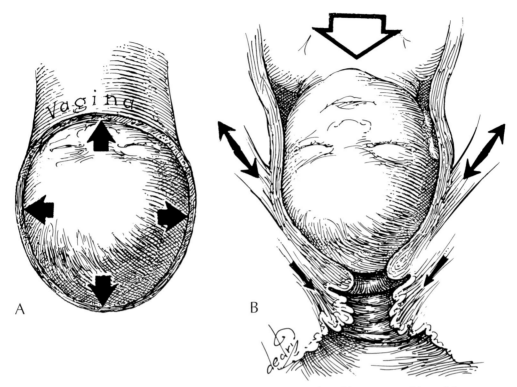

Figure 2.1. Types of cystocele. **A.** A distention cystocele produced by overstretching of the walls of the vagina itself during childbirth is most often related to long labor or the development of some pressure necrosis, or occasionally to a short, precipitous labor in which distention was so rapid that the vagina was not given time for elastic adaptation and distention. Defective connective tissue and elastic tissue in a wall of the vagina may also be a factor. Progression is usually slow until accentuated by the nutritional changes after menopause, when estrogen withdrawal seems associated with more rapid progression. This type of cystocele can be recognized by the lack of rugal folds. **B.** A translocation or displacement cystocele is associated with the vaginal descent that occurs as a result of an overstretching or attenuation of the lateral connective tissue support to the vagina. The lateral attachments of vagina and cervix are being stretched as they are pushed in front of the baby's head. In this traction type of cystocele, the rugal folds of the anterior and posterior walls of the vagina are about the same size as those on the lateral vaginal walls.

the opposite end of the spectrum of myometrial behavior, when labor seems arrested in the second stage or when disproportion impedes the progress of labor after full dilation of the cervix, the relatively prolonged pressure of a large fetal vertex in the vagina may cause ischemia and lead to eventual focal necrosis within the musculoconnective tissue layer of the vaginal wall. The weakening of the vaginal wall by such events during parturition may also allow the subsequent development of a cystocele or rectocele.

If laceration or overdistention represented the extent of the vaginal injuries that occur so frequently in childbirth, repair of the damage would be no problem, and the results of vaginal repairs would be uniformly good. The more significant types of vaginal injury, however, result from the detachment of the vaginal wall from the supporting tissues that maintain the vagina in its normal relation to the bony pelvis and to the adjacent rectum, uterus, and bladder.

In order to understand and anticipate the vaginal injuries commonly associated with parturition, it is necessary to realize that, normally, the presenting fetal part does not first emerge from the cervix and begin to descend into and through the vagina only when the cervix is fully dilated. Rather, the fully engaged presenting part, almost completely covered by the thinned, beginning-to-dilate cervix, has in all probability occupied the upper third to half of the vagina for 2 or more weeks. As a result, the distention of the upper vagina to accommodate the engaging vertex or breech has occurred very gradually, so gradually, in fact, that the patient may be unaware of the descent until she notices a new heaviness, low backache, and, at times, rectal pressure; at the same time, her breathing becomes somewhat easier, for "lightening" has occurred. Although such gradual positioning or settling of the presenting part, particularly its descent into the upper vagina, does not always occur in the multigravida who is approaching term, it usually occurs in the primigravida days or weeks before painful contractions (labor) begin. With the onset of effective labor, therefore, the contractions do not push the presenting part out of the cervix, but rather tend to draw the cervix up and over the presenting part while the station of the vertex or breech changes relatively little during the process.

Injuries to the vaginal walls are more likely to occur in the multigravida who experiences a hard, but short, labor than in the primigravida who begins a labor of 8 or more hours' duration with the presenting part well engaged. Even though evidence that parturition had damaged the vaginal walls and supporting tissues of the primipara may be expected, examination several weeks postpartum often reveals that the contour of the upper vaginal walls is well preserved and the vaginal fornices and sulci are well supported. The vaginal caliber and fornices may not be equally well preserved, however, if the primipara went into labor before the presenting part was well engaged. Should such a patient's cervix be approaching full dilation with the presenting part still not engaged, her obstetrician may suspect disproportion, abnormality, or malpresentation and may elect to perform delivery by cesarean section. Although there may have been no disproportion or abnormality that would have jeopardized the fetus, cesarean section under such circumstances would probably preserve the integrity of the mother's pelvic supporting tissues and spare her the subsequent development of a prolapse that would eventually require an extensive gynecologic repair.

Injuries to the Vaginal Supporting Tissues

Vaginal damage may occur when an unengaged presenting part begins to descend rapidly into the vagina as the second stage of labor begins. The forces of labor may shred congenitally weak or inadequate fascial attachments until so little support remains that the vagina eventually appears detached, redundant, and "prolapsing." In other instances, however, the fascial support of the upper vagina is so strong that it actually resists dilation of the vagina by the presenting part. Under these circumstances, the force of uterine contractions may tend to push an undilating, contracting, ringlike segment of the vagina ahead of the presenting part (Fig. 2.2). If this situation persists, the forces of labor are exerted not so much on the vagina as on the supporting fascia that is trying to hold that segment of the vagina in its normal position within the maternal pelvis. Whether because of their congenital weakness or their excessive stretching, these tissues are no longer able to maintain the concavity of the superior vaginal fornices after postpartum involution is complete. Such superfluous or redundant vaginal wall tissues eventually give way to clinically evident vaginal eversion, often with associated uterine prolapse.

As a rule, the apparent obliteration of the vaginal fornices and the bulging of the vaginal walls down along the cervix at the time of the postpartum examination are signs of the descent and lack of upper vaginal support, and the upper vagina is likely to have been detached coincident with the disruption (or at least a noninvoluting degree of lengthening) of uterine and cervical support. Under such circumstances, prolapse to procidentia can be expected sooner or later, although, fortunately, few women experience such an extreme degree of supporting tissue injury.

Even though there is no sign of prolapse and the upper vagina may appear well supported with well-preserved fornices, the patient may develop a marked cystocele, recto-

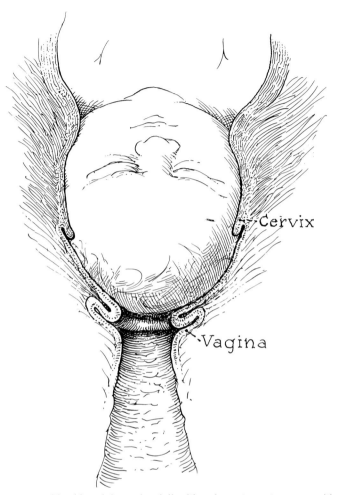

Figure 2.2. Descent of fetal head through a fully dilated cervix against an undilated vagina. As the presenting part descends through the vagina, in addition to the marked thinning out of the vaginal wall due to the very considerable increase in the diameter of the vagina, more potentially significant changes may be occurring in the connective tissue strands that normally maintain the position, relationships, and contour of the upper vagina. Effective uterine contractions serve to draw the lower uterine segment and cervix up over the presenting part. Such cervical dilation may occur without earlier or simultaneous descent of the presenting part into the upper vagina. When this occurs, an abrupt or precipitous descent of the presenting part into an undilated vagina may result in a segment of undilated vaginal wall being pushed into an intusseceptionlike doubling of the thickness of the vaginal wall. A segment of vaginal wall so thickened results in still greater resistance to further descent of the presenting part.

cele, or both. As a matter of fact, it is not unusual to find this type of injury at the time of postpartum examination in the para 1 whose labor began after the vertex had been deeply engaged for 2 weeks and whose completely effaced cervix was dilated 2 cm at the onset of labor. Under such circumstances, the upper vagina has been dilated slowly, and the descent of the presenting fetal part does not subject the vaginal supporting tissues to the stresses that develop when a presenting vertex begins to descend rapidly through an undilated upper vagina. Although it is true that cystocele, rectocele, and prolapse are often observed in the same patient and there may be no history or earlier record to suggest that one type of relaxation occurred before the other, it is equally true that a rather marked cystocele, rectocele, or both may develop without significant descensus or prolapse of the uterus.

As explained earlier, the voluntary bearing down that is traditionally encouraged throughout the second stage of labor can appreciably increase the risk of the vaginal injury that is most to be avoided: the overstretching and disruption of the connective tissues that normally maintain the concavity of the upper vaginal fornices and the support of the upper vaginal walls in their normal relationship to the bony pelvis, bladder, and rectum. Admittedly, the patient's bearing-down effort generally seems beneficial to progress in the second stage of labor and is certainly of psychologic importance to both the parturient and those attending her. However, no one can predict, and very few can determine during labor, whether such voluntary efforts actually facilitate the descent of the presenting part through dilating, relatively nonresisting vaginal walls.

If it could be determined with certainty that the vaginal walls were, in fact, offering little resistance to dilation, it would be appropriate to encourage voluntary bearing-down efforts as soon as the cervix is fully dilated and descent begins. Under such circumstances, the contractions of the uterus would cause the presenting part to descend readily through the upper vaginal segment, especially if the upper vagina had previously been gradually dilated during engagement (preceding the onset of labor). Too often, however, even when the first stage of labor has been completed and the second stage is beginning, the vagina is not adequately distended and may, in effect, actually be resisting dilation and therefore the descent of the vertex or breech. A noticeable lack of progress during the earlier part of the second stage is likely to be due to such vaginal resistance.

Ideally, the force behind the descending fetus is sufficient to cause the resisting segment of the vagina to dilate and yield. If the vagina continues to resist dilation and the descent of the presenting fetal part, a ringlike segment of vaginal wall may form around all or part of the circumference of the vertex or breech. With each contraction and bearing-down effort, this resisting ring of vagina remains ahead of the presenting vertex or breech. Adding appreciably (through voluntary bearing down) to the forces that are pushing the presenting vertex or breech against the ring of the vagina that is resisting descent is likely to increase ischemia, reduce tissue elasticity, and augment the occurrence of such a ring. Under such circumstances, the presenting part can descend only by pushing the undilated segment or ring of the vaginal wall ahead of it.

In all probability, once a resisting ringlike segment of vagina has been pushed ahead of the presenting part, the damage to vaginal supporting tissue has been done. As the fascial attachments give way, the rim or roll of resisting, undilated vaginal wall irons out rapidly, and the presenting part descends to the perineal stage. Only weeks later, when postpartum examination reveals the loss of the vaginal rugae and of the concavity of the superior vaginal fornices, is the damage evident. The persistence of redundant vaginal wall and the development of eversion (with or without uterine prolapse) confirm that the vaginal wall support has not necessarily reattached spontaneously during involutionary tightening of the pelvic fascial planes.

If those attending the parturient could determine the moment when the disruption of the planes of connective tissue that support the vaginal walls begins, it seems theoretically possible that an episiotomylike incision of the rolled-up, nondilating segment of vaginal wall would relieve the obstruction and allow the presenting part to descend without tearing or loosening the lateral attachment of the tissues supporting that portion of the vagina. For several reasons, however, this appears to be a procedure of no practical value. Whether the parturient is a primigravida or a multipara, if she nears the second stage of labor before the presenting part is engaged, the segment of vagina likely to be torn from its attachments is the pericervical upper third, where fascial attachments are strongest; an obstructing rim of undilating vagina would be difficult to visualize and incise in this area. Of even greater significance is the probability that, by the time a nondilating ridge of vagina became evident, the forces of labor would already have begun shredding or loosening the connective tissue supporting that segment of the vagina. Finally, disruption of the fascial support of the vagina is the injury that the obstetrician is most anxious to avoid, since the permanent detachment of the fascial support of the vagina in the posterior and lateral pericervical fornices is likely to result in a prolapsing vagina.

When it appears that the presenting part is not descending into the vagina as full dilation of the cervix is near, the parturient should be cautioned not to bear down until told to do so. Careful appraisal of the situation is essential. Regional blocking anesthesia is not likely to alter the pattern of myometrial contractions significantly. If uterine contractions at this stage are hard, long, and frequent, there is a risk that fetal oxygenation will become inadequate. If the perineal outlet is tight, a partially asphyxiated fetus cannot tolerate prolonged compression of the head on the perineum. Precipitous second-stage descent of the fetus and prompt delivery will give attendants an opportunity to resuscitate the infant, but the cost will probably be considerable maternal "childbirth damage." If the problems have been anticipated and delivery can be accomplished by cesarean section before vaginal supporting tissues are damaged, the infant will also benefit. There are very few situations in which a cesarean section is indicated (before an impending vaginal delivery can occur), but, when the presenting part is unengaged at full dilation and the uterine contractions are frequent and long, the risks to the fetus and to the mother's pelvic supporting tissues warrant such "interference" to prevent an eventual prolapse.

INJURIES TO THE PERINEUM

The vulnerability of perineal tissue to permanent damage from stretching or tearing during parturition (15) appears to correlate directly with the number and width of the striae gravidarum of the patient's abdominal skin at term. When these striae are broad and coarse, laceration of the perineum is likely, and early episiotomy is indicated; when there are no or few striae, there may be little risk of perineal laceration and no need for "routine" episiotomy (13).

PROPHYLACTIC MEASURES

Those attending the woman in labor must recognize and minimize the factors that are likely to cause excessive stresses and possible damage to uterine and vaginal supporting tissues. They should assure the parturient that her contractions will do the work, and they should often encourage relaxation rather than voluntary bearing-down efforts. In the interests of preserving the integrity of uterine and vaginal supporting tissues, it is particularly important to urge the parturient not to bear down and not to work with her pains at least until the cervix is fully dilated and, almost equally important, until the presenting fetal part has traversed the upper vagina, descent is evident, and the presenting part is beginning to distend the perineum.

Management of Labor

It is possible to reduce the degree of vaginal wall injury, protect the integrity of the venous sinuses, and maintain adequate circulation in the fetal cranium by managing labor in a way that avoids a tumultuous, precipitous labor that is likely to damage the musculofibrous layers responsible for the circumference of the vagina and that ensures that any arrest of progress in the second stage is not neglected. Management will have a more evident effect on the site and degree of maternal injury, however, if it focuses on efforts to minimize damage to the uterine and vaginal supporting tissues, for significant damage in this area can account for the eventual development of uterine prolapse or vaginal eversion.

The shape of the bony pelvis significantly affects the probability and the type of maternal soft tissue injury (Fig. 2.3). Obstetricians have traditionally and consistently regarded the classic gynecoid bony pelvis as desirable for childbearing. Postpartum patients who show extensive anterior vaginal wall damage, particularly a cystocele and urethrocele (sometimes associated with a small rectocele) frequently have the wide infrapubic arch that is characteristic of the gynecoid pelvis, however. In contrast, the structures of the anterior vaginal wall usually suffer relatively little damage in patients with the narrow infrapubic arch of an android type of pelvis, because the fetal head was obliged to distend the pelvic floor and perineum to a greater degree than a vertex of the same size would have required to emerge through a gynecoid type of bony outlet. Consequently, "urethrocele" (or vesico-urethral hypermobility) are less frequent, but lacerations of the pelvic floor and perineum are more common in a patient who has an android type of bony pelvis.

The dimensions and type of the patient's bony pelvis determine whether the problem of disproportion is likely to arise in the management of labor and delivery. Faced with a potential disproportion, some obstetricians favor the induction of labor before the fetal head becomes as large as it may become at full term. The majority, however, prefer to await the onset of labor, appraise the situation, and then decide whether vaginal delivery or cesarean section is indicated.

There are few actions that the obstetrician can take during the perineal stage of labor to alter the stress of vaginal dilation on the anterior wall relative to the stress on the pos-

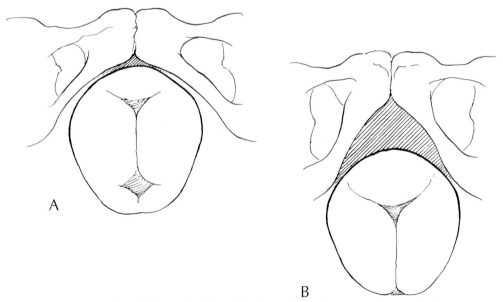

Figure 2.3. Effect of the angle of the subpubic arch on the site and degree of obstetric damage in the lower vaginal walls and perineum. **A.** A widely arched gynecoid pelvis facilitates delivery of the baby's head, but a wide bony arch, as shown here, provides little or no protection to the anterior vaginal wall and infrapubic tissues supporting the trigone and urethra. **B.** The relatively uncommon narrow angled arch of an android pelvis holds the descending and extending head away from the soft tissues supported above the anterior vaginal wall. A narrow bony arch forces the presenting part to require and cause greater distention posteriorly. As a result, when the bony pelvis is android, the posterior vaginal wall, perineum, and rectum will be at greater risk, whereas relatively little damage should occur anteriorly.

terior wall. The most frequently indicated "interference" is the rotation of a persistently posterior vertex to an occiput anterior presentation. This rotation permits the normal mechanism of flexion and extension as the vertex emerges beneath the pubic arch to proceed with much less distention of the posterior wall than would occur during delivery of the head as an occiput posterior. There is no way to alter the presentation so as to protect the anterior vaginal wall and the tissues supporting the trigone and urethra, however. Although the performance of an adequate episiotomy decreases the extent of injuries to the supporting tissues in the anterior vaginal wall, it is effective only if it is done before the perineum has held the extending vertex against the infrapubic structures long enough to cause anterior wall damage.

Episiotomy

In 1878, Broomall (3) documented that episiotomy was an effective method of preventing perineal ruptures during labor. A posterolateral episiotomy directed toward the ischial tuberosity was recommended.

Gainey's careful studies clearly demonstrate the effectiveness of episiotomy as a means of decreasing the extent of maternal soft tissue injuries that can be associated with specific events during vaginal delivery. It is important to remember that the very considerable pressure that develops around the entire circumference of the vaginal wall as the presenting part dilates the vagina increases when the musculature of the perineum reinforces the posterior vaginal wall. Although the android type of bony pelvis, which has a relatively narrow infrapubic arch, reduces the distention of the anterior vaginal wall beneath the trigone and urethra by holding the descending fetal vertex away from it, the gynecoid type of bony pelvis, which has a wide infrapubic arch, does not protect the fascial support in this area from the distention that occurs when the presenting part is forced anteriorly against the bony pelvis as the extending vertex comes against the musculature of the perineum.

Most obstetricians consider episiotomy a means of protecting the lower posterior vaginal wall and perineum from a laceration that cannot be repaired as satisfactorily as can an elected incision. It is particularly valuable in minimizing damage to the support of the lower urethra and the musculature that encircles the introitus. An adequate episiotomy immediately decreases the resistance of the perineal musculature to lower vaginal dilation. Therefore, in a parturient who has an android type of pelvis, an episiotomy is indicated to protect the pelvic floor and perineum from the laceration that is likely because of the greater distention necessary posteriorly before the vertex can emerge from beneath the infrapubic arch. Although there is less distention posteriorly as the vertex comes under the wider infrapubic arch of a parturient who has a gynecoid pelvis, an adequate episiotomy spares the tissues that support the trigone and urethra from the damage likely to occur anteriorly if an episiotomy is not performed.

It is not clear whether episiotomy itself reduces the incidence of uterine prolapse and eventual procidentia. It would be difficult to assemble convincing data on this point, because the factors that determine how the first and second stages of labor are managed also determine whether an episiotomy is performed. Therefore, the obstetrician who attends the woman in labor is likely to recognize, minimize, or avoid altogether the factors that increase the probability of eventual prolapse well before the stage of labor when an episiotomy is indicated. Although it may appear that routine episiotomy reduces the frequency of prolapse, a direct relationship should not be assumed.

The objective of an episiotomy, no matter what the site or the type, is the same. When repaired in an anatomically correct manner, the result of either a mediolateral or a midline episiotomy seems satisfactory to those who prefer one over the other. Difficulties sometimes arise in association with both types of episiotomy, however. After a mediolateral episiotomy (i.e., an episiotomy that begins at the 4 or 8 o'clock position), for example, it may be difficult to realign the severed tissues properly. A generous midline episiotomy (i.e., an episiotomy that begins at the 6 o'clock position) extended from the vaginal wall to the margin of the posterior fornix, if performed before the presenting vertex distends the lower vagina, pelvic floor, and perineal musculature, may protect the vaginal and urethral supporting tissues, but it may leave the anterior rectal wall vulnerable to laceration when the vertex and the fetal face descend to the outlet. The anterior wall of the anal canal and the external anal sphincter may even remain intact while such a split in a segment of anterior wall occurs (12, 16, 19).

Midline episiotomy has been documented to be associated with an increased risk of third- and fourth-degree perineal lacerations in operative vaginal deliveries (12). The midline episiotomy has at least two advantages that make it worth the admittedly greater risk of third-degree laceration through the anal sphincter or even a fourth-degree laceration into the anal canal (12, 19). First, the anatomic realignments are simpler; the "two sides always match." Second, perineal scarring after repeated midline episiotomies is much less than that after repeated mediolateral episiotomies, and the thin midline raphe that tends to develop following repeated incisions and repairs at the same midline site only rarely leads to dyspareunia. Finally, when it appears that the midline episiotomy is likely to extend into the anal canal, an adequate incision performed cleanly through the anal sphincter and the anal wall (6, 8) ensures that, in the subsequent repair, there will be no need to perform the difficult task of realigning tissues that are separated and irregularly edged by a laceration (which could have been avoided by adequate extension of the midline episiotomy into the anal canal). It has been shown that postpartum incontinence of flatus is six times more common among women who have experienced a third- or fourth-degree perineal laceration which was repaired than by those without anal sphincter rupture (4). A midline episiotomy, anatomically closed with fine polyglycolic acid or chromic catgut and usually "running sutures," causes very little discomfort and needs very little attention during the puerperium.

ADVANTAGES OF ROUTINE EPISIOTOMY

Vaginal delivery causes partial denervation of the pelvic floor (with consequent reenervation) in most women having their first baby. This is influenced by the length of the second stage of labor and the weight of the baby (1, 20). Denervation is apparently not affected by forceps delivery and perineal tears, but shortening of a long, active second stage of labor by an episiotomy may minimize the risk of denervation damage to the pelvic floor. A comprehensive repair, skillfully accomplished, becomes an objective worthy of the gynecologist's time and the patient's period of disability. Since not even the patient knows with certainty how many pregnancies she will experience in her lifetime, it is difficult to deny the reasonableness and the desirability of providing the best care of each immediate problem with each confinement. In the minds of many the question remains: Does the best care involve or require "routine" episiotomy?

The advantages of virtually routine episiotomy greatly outweigh the frequently heard objections to making every delivery an operative procedure. Although it can be shown that episiotomy is not always necessary, it is not possible to predict which patients will suffer a significant degree of soft tissue injury if all patients are permitted— and this usually means encouraged—to deliver spontaneously without episiotomy (14). To minimize soft tissue damage, episiotomy can be performed during the end of the second stage of labor before crowning of the fetal head, particularly in older parturients in whom tissue elasticity is limited (13, 14). An Argentine study concluded that routine episiotomy should be abandoned, and the operation used selectively in less than 30 percent of parturients (2). It is possible to state with confidence, however, that not every parturient will achieve spontaneous delivery without evident, regrettable, and largely preventable soft tissue injury at the outlet. A sizable proportion (in Gainey's studies, no fewer than one in four primigravida [9, 10]) suffer significant soft tissue damage of the type that can often be avoided by the routine administration of regional anesthesia for relaxation of the musculature of the pelvic floor and perineum, and adequate prophylactic episiotomy, anatomically repaired, and the completion of delivery by outlet forceps or a breech assist. Furthermore, the injuries that result from the infrequent extensions of routine episiotomies into the sphincter or rectum are more readily repaired than are the lacerations that most certainly occur during deliveries in which episiotomy is not performed. There is little current enthusiasm for prophylactic complete perineotomy (6, 8), because the increased postpartum perineal discomfort is unacceptable.

ADMINISTRATION OF REGIONAL ANESTHESIA

It is difficult to evaluate the effects of adequate regional anesthesia without consideration of episiotomy, for the two are almost invariably employed together. The use of regional anesthesia significantly reduces soft tissue outlet trauma; it does not simply alleviate the pain that the parturient would otherwise experience during the incision and repair of an episiotomy. To realize the maximal benefit, regional anesthesia should be administered before the descent of the presenting fetal part has subjected the pelvic floor to maximal distention, well before damage to the perineum and to the soft tissues of the vaginal outlet can occur.

Regional anesthesia and episiotomy are more effective and protective in combination than is either alone. The disadvantage of administering regional anesthesia is that it often interferes with the effectiveness of uterine contractions. The primary reason for the decreased expulsive effort associated with regional anesthesia, however, may be the fact that the patient is more comfortable and no longer contributes the maximal type of voluntary bearing-down effort that the unanesthetized patient would make in her determined effort to complete her delivery.

Use of Outlet Forceps

Many obstetricians are convinced that the use of outlet forceps and the delivery of either a presenting vertex or an after-coming head between pains provide better control and minimize maternal soft tissue injury. It is difficult to determine how frequently this is true, however, because the administration of anesthesia often decreases the parturient's expulsive effort and thus prolongs the second stage of labor undesirably if outlet forceps are not used. Whenever the pros and cons of episiotomy and the prophylactic use of outlet forceps are being discussed, it is essential to remember that regional anesthesia is not used primarily to permit the use of episiotomy and forceps, but rather to decrease maternal soft tissue injuries; similarly, that objective alone warrants the use of outlet forceps. Although the effects of the anesthesia necessitate the use of outlet forceps, there are other appreciable advantages to be gained by the prophylactic use of forceps. It is, therefore, the combination of regional anesthesia, episiotomy, and outlet forceps that is of established and significant value in minimizing the extent of maternal injuries due to childbirth.

AVOIDANCE OF IATROGENIC INJURY

Those obstetricians who adopt a protocol for vaginal delivery that involves the degree of operative interference inherent in the administration of regional anesthesia, the performance of episiotomy, and the prophylactic use of outlet forceps must remain aware of the ever-present risk of iatrogenic injury, which may require prompt, objective appraisal and the best of reparative skills (2, 3). Obstetricians must balance the advantages against the risks of prophylactic measures before they assume that their interventions will be as helpful as their intentions. Moreover, episiotomy is but one measure available to obstetricians in their efforts to minimize the maternal soft tissue injuries that may result from vaginal delivery. Other equally effective measures should be more widely recognized.

The possible effects of the management of the third stage of labor on the site or degree of maternal injury have been subjected to relatively little study. During the centuries when labor attendants simply did not consider manually exploring the uterine cavity and manually removing the placenta after childbirth, their efforts to aid in the expulsion of the placenta consisted almost exclusively of applying pressure or "massaging" the uterine fundus through the thickness of the abdominal wall. Although the forces that they applied to the fundus were probably seldom of a magnitude comparable to that of a myometrial contraction plus a voluntary bearing-down effort, the virtually frantic efforts of an occasional attendant to "credé out the placenta" could have resulted in added trauma (disruption) of the uterine and cervical supporting tissues. In more modern times, if the placenta does not separate promptly, the attendant usually terminates the third stage of labor (within a few minutes after the delivery of the infant) by manual intrauterine removal of the placenta. At that time, the lower uterine segment and cervix are not likely to offer any significant resistance to the procedure. Today, therefore, there are very few, if any, circumstances that justify applying sufficient pressure to the uterine fundus to increase the traumatic stretching of the ligamentous support of the fundus and cervix.

Some authorities refer to the several hours immediately after delivery of the placenta as the fourth stage of labor. During this potentially critical period, alert attendants should observe the patient repeatedly to ensure that the myometrium remains contracted and blood loss is not excessive. There is also a possibility during this period that overly vigorous massage of the fundus in ill-advised attempts to keep the uterus contracted will injure the now relatively loosely arranged connective tissues of the cardinal and uterosacral ligaments and disrupt the thin-walled, poorly supported, and engorged venous channels in the parametrium.

During World War II, when the physical activities of many women, especially those working in industry and transportation, were altered and increased, early ambulation following childbirth became a virtually universal practice. Older obstetricians in particular were skeptical, and many opposed early ambulation after delivery. They believed that the puerperal uterus, only 12 to 48 hours postpartum, would be heavy enough to place additional stress on the uterine supports, which had already been strained during the delivery; that parametrial involution would be at least delayed; and that any subsequent tendency to descensus would be aggravated. Five decades later, however, there is no documentation to suggest that early ambulation will increase the frequency or the degree of uterine or vaginal wall prolapse or that it is anything but beneficial to the parturient.

Throughout the past three decades, some of those who advocate natural childbirth have suggested that obstetricians feel threatened by women's awakened awareness that they can give birth safely without professional guidance and help. Generally improved maternal health and adequate nutrition during pregnancy are indeed certain to result in the births of healthier babies. Furthermore, an informed and confident parturient often delivers normally and satisfactorily without professional aid of any kind. It would be remarkable, however, if the problems and the risks of childbirth that created the obstetric profession generations ago did not reappear should most women decide to give birth without professional assistance and at home. As the need for professional help again becomes evident, the obstetrician's skills should be directed not only toward ensuring a safe delivery of the child, but also toward minimizing the incidence of those maternal injuries that not infrequently occur in an unmanaged and unaided spontaneous delivery.

The art of obstetrics is in the experienced obstetrician's ability to appraise the parturient's needs and to ensure that labor is as efficient and nontraumatic as possible. Good clinical judgment is essential in the administration of analgesics or sedation to help the patient's morale and in the use of measures to improve the effectiveness of her uterine contractions, since such interventions can either help or hinder the progress of labor. Clearly, the type and degree of maternal tissue damage are related not so much to the patient's parity as to the presentation and the position of the presenting fetal part near completion of the first stage of labor. Of virtually equal importance are the character, duration, and frequency of uterine contractions.

The conduct of labor can, to a significant degree, determine the site and the extent of any maternal soft tissue injury. This is true whether the labor and delivery are accomplished by a confident, intelligent parturient who believes in the advantages of natural childbirth or by a cooperative parturient who seeks the support and assistance of understanding attendants and an obstetrician's management of either dystocia or precipitous labor. In either instance, immediate recognition of the forces in labor that may damage maternal soft tissues and lead to later prolapse of the uterus or detachment of vaginal wall supports, together with the initiation of measures to decrease these forces, can reduce the incidence of maternal soft tissue damage to a minimum. This should be a major objective in the conduct of every labor and delivery. When the obstetrician is motivated and effective, or the woman delivering unaided is fortunate, there will be less frequent need for the gynecologic surgeon's careful assessment and skillful repair of the vagina.

References

1. Allen RE, Hosker GL, Smith ARB, Warrell DW. Pelvic floor damage and childbirth: a neurophysiological study. Br J Obstet Gynaecol 1990;97:770–779.
2. Argentine Episiotomy Trial Collaborative Group. Routine vs. selective episiotomy: a randomized controlled trial. Lancet 1993;342:1517–1518.
3. Broomall AE. The operation of episiotomy as a prevention of perineal ruptures during labor. Am J Dis Wom Child 1878:517–527.
4. Crawford LA, Quint EH, Pearl ML, DeLancey JOL. Incontinence following rupture of the anal sphincter during delivery. Obstet Gynecol 1993;82:527–531.
5. Curtis AH, Anson BJ. Perineal birth injuries: pathogenesis and surgical correction. Q Bull Northwest Univ Med Sch 1942;16:275–284.
6. Cunningham CB, Pilkington JW. Complete perineotomy, Obstet Gynecol 1960;16:172.
7. DeLee JB. The prophylactic forceps operation. Am J Obstet Gynecol 1928;1:43–44.
8. Fleming AR. Complete perineotomy. Obstet Gynecol 1960;16:172.
9. Gainey HL. Postpartum observation of pelvic tissue damage. Am J Obstet Gynecol 1943;45:457–466.
10. Gainey HL. Postpartum observation of pelvic tissue damage: further studies. Am J Obstet Gynecol 1955;70:800–807.
11. Gustafson GW. The prevention and treatment of cystocele in the reproductive age. Urol Cutaneous Rev 1940;144:160–161.
12. Helwig JT, Thorp JM Jr, Bowes WA Jr. Does midline episiotomy increase the risk of third- and fourth-degree lacerations in operative vaginal deliveries? Obstet Gynecol 1993;82:276–279.
13. Magdi I. Obstetric injuries of the perineum. J Obstet Gynaecol Br Emp 1942;49:687–700.
14. Nichols DH (ed). Gynecologic and obstetric surgery, St. Louis: Mosby-Year Book, 1993:1048–1049.
15. Power RMH. The pelvic floor in parturition. Surg Gynecol Obstet 1946;83:296–311.
16. Rageth JC, Buerklen A, Hirsch HA. Long-term sequelae of episiotomies. Z Geburtshilfe Perinatol 1989;193:233.
17. Randall CL. Foreword: prolonged and difficult labor. Clin Obstet Gynecol 1959;2:271–360.
18. Randall CL. Childbirth without fear of interference. Clin Obstet Gynecol 1959;2:360.
19. Shiono P et al. Midline episiotomies: more harm than good? Obstet Gynecol 1990;75:765.
20. Snooks SJ, Swash M, Henry MM, Setchell M. Risk factors in childbirth causing damage to the pelvic floor innervation. Int J Colorect Dis 1986;1:20–24.

CHAPTER 3

Instruments and Sutures

Effective and successful surgery is more dependent upon the surgeon's judgment and technical competence than upon the design or the quality of the instruments used. No set of instruments will consistently be associated with a satisfactory surgical result without the skills of the surgeon. The carpenter is more important than his or her tools, but fine tools may help improve the carpenter's work. There are significant choices available in the surgeon's armamentarium, and the right choices will enable the operator to accomplish with greater ease and efficiency the best of which he or she is capable.

The operating room should be of an adequate and comfortable size, in a quiet location, and with elbowroom and moving space around the table for the surgeon and assistants, the anesthesiologist and his or her equipment, and the nursing staff and instrument tables (Fig. 3.1). Continuous suction equipment is desirable, including one weighted speculum equipped with a suction tip. A separate, hand-held suction device with tube

Figure 3.1. Arrangement of personnel within the operating room. The surgeon is in the central position at the foot of the operating table with the second assistant to the right and the first assistant to the left. There is a spotlight over a right-handed surgeon's shoulder illuminating the perineum, and the instrument table is to his or her back and somewhat to the right. The instrument nurse is behind the instrument table, facing the back of the surgeon. This enables him or her to share in a full view of the operative field and to follow visually the progress of the surgical procedure. The positions of the spotlight, the nurse, and the instrument table are reversed if the surgeon is left-handed.

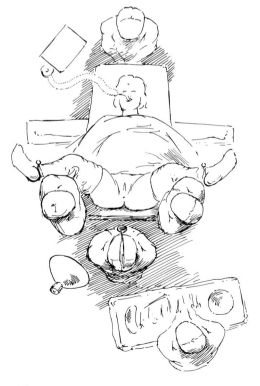

should be provided. The trap for each suction device provides a quick and accurate estimate of surgical blood loss.

Adequate modern anesthesia equipment provides for continuous monitoring of the patient's pulmonary and cardiac status. Adequate amounts of appropriate suture material and sterile supplies, including any packing that might be called for, should be at hand, where they can be provided on short notice without the necessity of sending out a hurried call for additional supplies. Efficiency in surgery is developed not through rushing but through effectively using each minute of operative time and through avoiding the necessity of waiting for special instruments or sutures that are needed but were not requested ahead of time. Blood loss during surgery is the product of milliliters per minute times the number of minutes. Fearing AIDS and hepatitis, most patients are frightened by blood transfusion. When operative blood loss is minimized, so is the need for transfusion.

The greatest care must be taken when handling suture needles to avoid glove perforation from the sharp tips of the needle. Surgical glove perforation places the surgeons at risk for blood-borne infectious diseases. In one study (10), the overall perforation rate was measured at 13.3 percent, and 62 percent of these perforations were unrecognized during the surgical procedure. Most perforations occurred in the gloved fingers of the nondominant hand, suggesting that perforation was due to direct grasping of the needle. More frequent use of tissue forceps to grasp the needle should reduce this incidence. Among 2166 operations in another study (4), there was an incidence of 5.5 percent inadvertent injuries, of which 95 percent were a result of needle sticks. Most occurred at the time of wound closing, and 72.3 percent occurred on the left hand. Visible blood has been reported found on the hands of 38 percent of gynecologic surgeons wearing single gloves, but on only 2 percent of double-gloved surgeons (1). Double-gloving does significantly increase protection against needle puncture during surgery, and thus offers some measure of protection against exposure to unexpected AIDS or hepatitis infection. A cut resistant glove liner is available (2).

When double gloves are worn, it is more comfortable for the surgeon if one of the pairs is a half size larger than that regularly worn. The larger glove is put on first, and then the glove of one's usual size.

SUTURE MATERIAL

Basic requirements concerning the suture materials to be used in the closing of surgical wounds are indicated in the following quotation (3):

The purpose of a surgical suture is to maintain approximation of tissues until the healing process has progressed to the point where artificial support is no longer necessary for the wound to resist normal stresses. Beyond this point, the sutures serve no useful purpose, and may, in fact, be the source of irritation or serve as a nidus for persistent infection. Thus, the ideal suture should persist and maintain tensile strength until the tissue has healed sufficiently, and then disappear.

RELATIONSHIP OF SUTURES TO WOUND HEALING

The strength of a closed surgical wound is the sum of the scar plus the suture material. Immediately after the wound has been closed and for the next 3 or 4 days, the suture material provides all the strength of the wound. This strength has been estimated at about 40 percent of the original strength of the tissues before surgery. As healing develops and scar tissue is formed, the strength increases. In the absence of infection, it has been estimated that the wound is about one-third healed on the 6th postoperative day and two-thirds healed by the 10th. The remaining one-third may require several months. Variances from these generalizations may be caused by many factors, including the tension applied to the margins of the wound, the biochemistry and physical condition of the particular patient and of the suture material, and the presence of infection. The suture material has become superfluous once wound healing has finished and a strong scar is produced. In the presence of infection, sutures may be absorbed with unusual speed and fail to supply adequate support during the initial and critical healing. When non-absorbable suture has been used in the presence of infection, a sinus may form postoperatively. The suture behaves as an infected foreign body. The sinus will close only after the sutures or foreign body is extruded or surgically removed.

Tissue reaction to suture material does not determine wound strength, although it is proportional to the bulk of the suture material present in the wound. Knot pull strength (Fig. 3.2) is important. Time should not have to be taken in replacing sutures that break while being tied, but there is little additional advantage and there are distinct disadvantages to the routine use of the larger sizes of suture material. Larger sizes of absorbable suture permit greater tissue injury because their greater strength permits knots to be tied too tightly without breaking. Because the larger sizes incite more intensive phagocytic activity, those of catgut may not maintain their tensile strength any longer than the smaller sizes. Thus the use of larger sizes of suture may actually result in a weaker scar than that associated with the use of smaller suture sizes. In most situations, 0 size or 2-0 will suffice, and occasionally 3-0 or 4-0 is preferable, particularly in the repair of a fistula. Although a traditional past choice of suture material has been chromic catgut, the delayed absorption of the new synthetic sutures, polyglycolic acid (Dexon) and polyglactin (Vicryl), has proven to be a clearly superior advantage when using similar sizes of suture material.

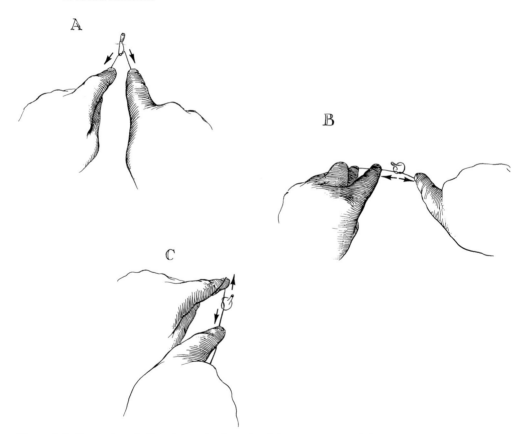

Figure 3.2. Knot tying. **A.** Traction to both ends of the suture toward the operator and against the point to be ligated is incorrect and dangerous, since there is considerable risk of pulling the thread and knot off the point or vessel being tied. **B.** Instead, traction should be applied to each thread in an equal and opposite direction around the point of ligation. **C.** Deep within a body cavity, the tips of the index fingers safely provide the fulcrum, lessening the chance of slippage or avulsion.

The newer synthetic sutures are strong, permitting the use of smaller sizes; quality control manufacturing ensures lack of batch-to-batch variability. The suture holds its strength in the tissue in which it is placed longer than does catgut, permitting wound healing to have a better start by the time the sutures are absorbed, and there is less tissue reaction in the scar produced during healing, resulting in a stronger scar. The sutures appear to remain stable, even in the presence of infection. Some knot-tying practice is necessary in learning to use these newer sutures effectively. Monofilament sutures require an extra throw to the first cast for effective knot security, and three or four additional standard casts. There is a marked reduction in the formation of postoperative vaginal granulation tissue when synthetic sutures are used. We now almost exclusively use these new synthetics for vaginal surgery. Braided polyglycolic acid-type sutures maintain much of their tensile strength for up to a month postoperatively, and the even newer long-acting absorbables, monofilament polydioxanone (PDS) or polyglyconate (Maxon), which we use with increasing frequency, seem to retain their strength for up to 3 months.

Polybutester (Novafil) is a unique copolymer monofilament nonabsorbable synthetic suture material that has the unique qualities of high breaking strength, similar to that of similar-sized nylon, combined with stretchability proportional to the force applied, and prompt elastic recovery. It is twice as flexible as nylon or polypropylene of similar size, yet secure knots can be formed with three or four throws. These qualities, particularly that of elastic stretching once it is in place, make it ideal for wound closure, especially when a single buried layer technique is chosen. As postoperative edema and swelling develop in the tissues in which the suture is placed, the suture stretches temporarily up to 10 to 15 percent of its length, to lessen the chance that it will tear or strangulate the tissues in which it has been placed. As postoperative edema and swelling subside, the stretched suture contracts, taking up any slack that was produced, and holding the tissues in approximation during their long healing phase. This should lessen the chance of postoperative wound dehiscence. Dehiscence unrelated to suture breakage occurs not at the suture site itself, but lateral to the suture line (6, 7, 8).

It is important to pull up on the slack in the suture before tying the knot. This will ensure prompt apposition of tissue, bringing contiguous structures together without the risk of a suture bridge. The knots must be tied square, beginning with the first cast, or there is a risk of fraying that contributes to suture breakage, which is always inopportune. While one is tying a square knot, the first cast may loosen up; but by putting tension on one end of the suture, the second cast will slide down and remain in place.

When a surgeon's knot is tied, a double throw with the first cast will remain in place; but after the second cast is made, the knot will slide down no further. A third cast, for safety and knot security, is usual practice.

As already stated, a wound that does not become infected is approximately one-third healed by the 6th postoperative day, two-thirds by the 10th. The remaining one-third of healing may require several months. Many factors, including the degree of tension applied to the margins of the wound, the biochemistry and physical condition of the particular patient, and the type of suture material used, may produce variances from these generalizations (9).

SUTURING TECHNIQUE

Good primary healing occurs best when the edges of the wound are approximated without tension. If tension is inevitable, either relaxing incisions can be made (see Chapter 20) or a simple myocutaneous graft can be developed to bridge the defect in the vaginal skin.

The various methods of suture placement in bringing two edges together are noted in Figure 3.3, which shows the path taken by the suture during placement and the effect of tying the suture.

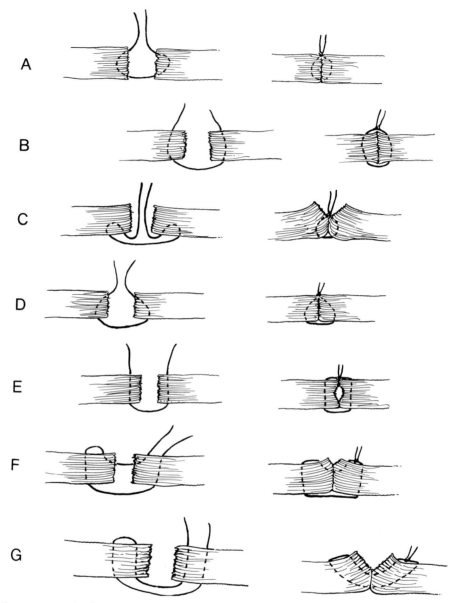

Figure 3.3. Methods of suture placement of a tissue layer after placement (*left*) and the effect of approximation after the knot has been tied (*right*). **A.** A subcuticular stitch placed with a round needle. **B.** The effects of a through-and-through suture placed with a round needle. **C.** A buried mattress stitch placed with a round needle. This stitch tends to evert the superficial portion of the wound, and yet takes up some slack in the deeper portion of the approximated layers. **D.** A subepithelial stitch. When tied, this stitch leaves a portion of the suture exposed on the undersurface of the wound. **E.** A through-and-through stitch with a straight needle. When this has been tied, a potential gap is left in the center of the layer of the tissues being approximated. **F.** A vertical mattress stitch placed with a straight needle. After the knot has been tied, the suture material is exposed beneath the tissue layer. **G.** A vertical mattress stitch after two through-and-through passes of the straight needle on each side of the layer being approximated. When this knot has been tied, the tissue will have been plicated, but there may be some gaping of the superficial portion of the wound.

In Figure 3.3, *A* to *E*, a curved needle of the proper size is used, and in *F* and *G*, a straight one is used. The choice is determined by the tension to which the layer will be subjected, as well as by its importance in providing essential wound support. Some suture bits clearly take up greater tissue slack than others and help influence vaginal size when used during colporrhaphy. Collagenase may be liberated by the epithelial trauma of through-and-through suture placement, and will penetrate the full thickness of the wound and may interfere with healing. This trauma-producing elaboration is probably less when subepithelial sutures are used, which is another reason for the recommended subcuticular closure of the vaginal wall and of the perineal skin. Daily doses of 500 mg of ascorbic acid may reduce collagenase production. Failure to approximate tissues creates a suture bridge (Fig. 3.4) and greatly weakens the scar and its effectiveness.

Various methods of closing a hollow viscus such as bladder or bowel are illustrated in Figure 3.5, showing how sutures can be placed either into the wall or through the wall, and knots tied inside or outside the lumen. A second intramural layer of suture serves to reduce the tension on the first layer. The mucosal layer may be included or excluded as desired. A separate mucosal layer may be used, primarily when mucosal hemostasis is required.

Two methods of subcuticular suture placement are noted in Figure 3.6; a choice may be made according to whether or not the full thickness of the subepithelial tissue is to be used to provide maximal strength, or whether the goal is close approximation of the most superficial layer for a cosmetic effect.

Thick skin edges from flap transplantation may be approximated by Allegoewer-type mattress sutures, as shown in Figure 3.7, whereas thinner skin is better brought together by the Donati type of mattress suture, provided that the vulvar skin can be mobilized on at least one side of the defect to be closed (Fig. 3.8). These stitches are not hemostatic, and should be tied only tightly enough to bridge the gap (5).

A pulley stitch may be used to bring two tissues, one fixed and one movable, together within a cavity or confined space (Fig. 3.9). The free end of the pulley stitch suture must be through the nonmovable tissue, and traction upon this end will bring the movable tissue (through which the suture has been passed and tied) to the fixed tissue. When the tissues are brought into direct contact with one another, a firm, strong scar will develop, which might not develop in the presence of only a suture bridge.

A

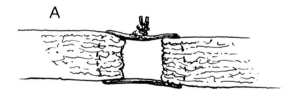

B

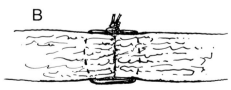

Figure 3.4. A. Failure to approximate tissue layers directly during reconstruction. This gives rise to a suture bridge, often productive of a weak scar, particularly when there is any tension upon the layers being approximated. **B.** The desirable result of layer approximation. This provides the opportunity for strong scar development between the edges of the closely approximated tissues.

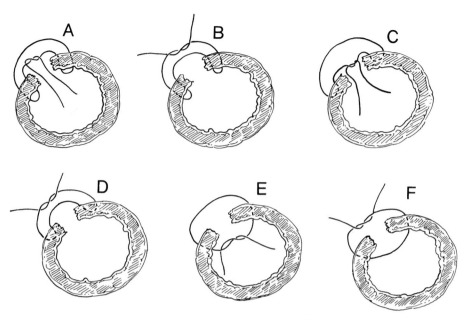

Figure 3.5. Methods of applying sutures to the wall of a hollow viscus. **A.** Mattress suture extending through all layers with an intraluminal knot. **B.** Mattress suture with an extraluminal knot. **C.** Sutures placed in a submucosal fashion with the knot buried. **D.** Sutures placed in a submucosal fashion, with an external knot. **E.** Simple through-and-through stitch with intraluminal knot. **F.** Simple through-and-through stich with extraluminal knot. Knots involving the wall of the rectum should be intraluminal, and those involving the wall of the genitourinary system should be extraluminal.

Various methods of suture-ligating a pedicle are shown in Figure 3.10. One's choice depends upon various factors, which include the contents of the pedicle, the risk of slippage, the tension to which it will be subject, and its surgical accessibility.

Technical facility in surgery is enhanced when the surgeon learns to use both hands equally well. This is especially helpful in suture placement, application and removal of hemostatic forceps, and knot tying. This is an acquired skill, and with frequent practice one can become technically ambidextrous.

LIGHTING

There should be adequate lighting. When this is directed over the right-handed surgeon's left shoulder, illumination should be shadow-free. Most operating room lighting has been designed to illuminate the operative field during a laparotomy and is often not adaptable and will not provide adequate illumination into the horizontal axis of a relatively deep pelvic cavity, such as the vagina. When adequate overhead lighting adaptable for vaginal surgery is not available, movable spotlights are necessary, but these often have an inherent and annoying tendency to move or slide out of focus as a result of the movements of operating room personnel. A surgeon may find it useful to wear a fiberoptic or tungsten headlight, which will provide a shadowless spot of from 2 to 4 inches of very bright light in the center of the operative field (Fig. 3.11). Because the wearer is in control of the position of the light from the headlight at all times, it can be quite helpful.

OPERATING TABLE

The operating table to be used for vaginal surgery should be equipped with adjustable stirrups that can be extended at least a foot or more according to the length of the patient's

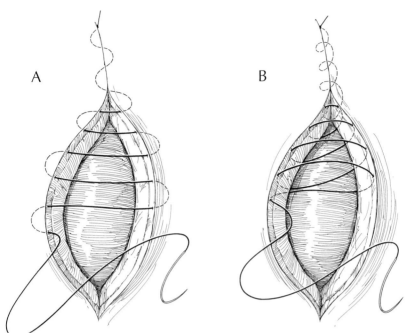

Figure 3.6. Two methods of subcuticular closure. **A.** The full thickness of the subepithelial layer is used by a spiral type of suture placement. This is particularly useful within the walls of the vagina, where the maximal strength of this fibromuscular layer will provide essential support to a healing colporrhaphy. **B.** A snakelike or zigzag suture placement is used immediately beneath the epithelial layer, which produces a superior cosmetic result that is not as strong. This is useful when subepithelial tissue layer strength is not a specific requirement and is particularly helpful in closing perineal skin or epithelial incisions elsewhere in the body. To avoid overlaps or wrinkling of the skin edges, care should be taken to make each point of entry beneath the epithelial layer accurately opposite the point of emergence of the last suture on the opposite side of the incision.

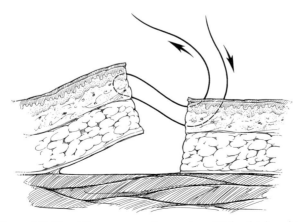

Figure 3.7. The Allegoewer mattress suture (5) for thicker skin.

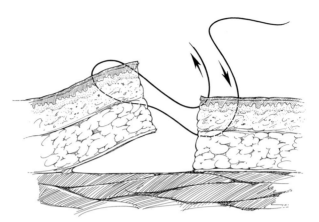

Figure 3.8. The Donati mattress suture (5) for thinner skin.

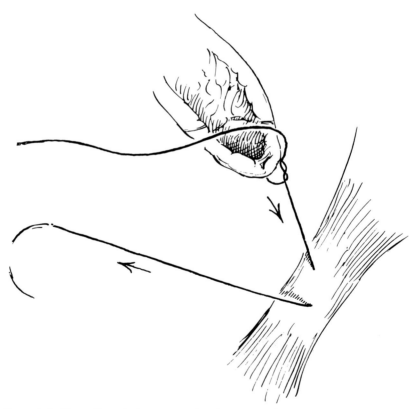

Figure 3.9. The pulley stitch. A suture has been passed through and tied to a tissue previously mobilized, which is to be brought and fixed to the surface of an immovable structure. Traction on the free end of the suture after it has been passed through the immovable tissue will bring the mobilized tissue against the surface of the immovable tissue, where the suture is to be tied. (From Nichols DH. Repair of enterocele and prolapse of the vaginal vault. In: Barber H, ed. Goldsmith's practice of surgery. Reproduced with permission of Cine-Med, Woodbury, CT, 1981.)

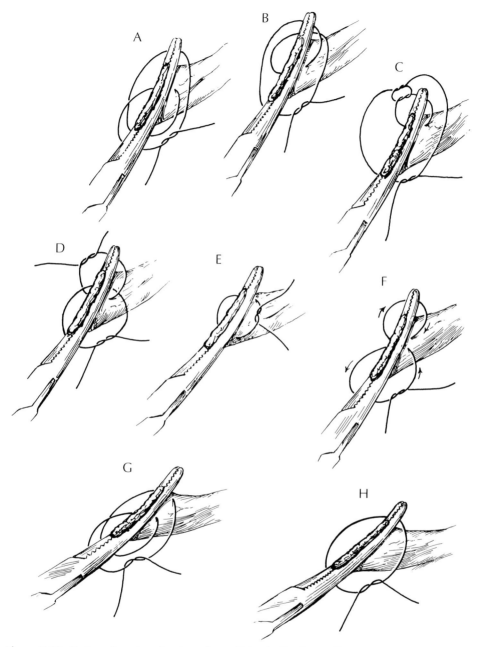

Figure 3.10. Options in suture ligation of a pedicle. **A.** Single needle penetration of the pedicle but with the base doubly ligated. **B.** Single needle penetration of the pedicle with the toe doubly ligated. **C.** After a small loop over the toe of the hemostat has been tied, a second loop goes around the entire pedicle. **D.** Interlocking loops provide security but require a double penetration of the pedicle by the needle. **E.** A double penetration that leaves a small portion unligated. **F.** This arrangement provides security but also requires a double penetration. **G.** The suture is fixed at two points. **H.** A single free tie, which is most likely to slip under certain circumstances. The suture ligation shown in **B** is recommended for the infundibulopelvic ligament, reinforced by a free tie. The suture ligation shown in **G** represents the Heaney stitch, which is especially useful for the cardinal or uterosacral ligament. It is unlikely to slip but does require a double penetration of the pedicle. (From Nichols DH. A technique for vaginal oophorectomy. Surg Gynecol Obstet 1978;147:765. Used with permission.)

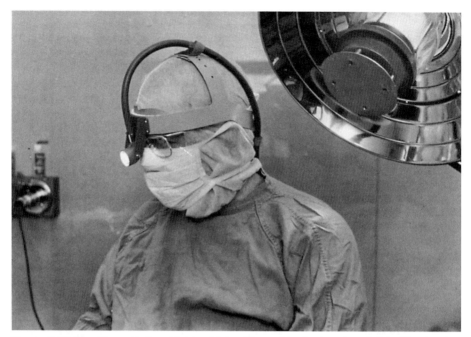

Figure 3.11. The fiberoptic headlight, which will provide shadow-free, bright illumination to the depths of a body cavity, even in a horizontal plane.

legs. These should be placed in such a fashion that when the patient's ankles are suspended from the stirrups, acute angulation of the leg will be avoided to ensure unobstructed venous return (see Fig. 8.3). Excess external rotation of the hip should be carefully avoided to lessen the chances for pathologically stretching the sciatic, peroneal, or femoral nerves.

The patient should be so positioned on the operating table that an imaginary line drawn between the two stirrups will intersect each acetabulum or hip socket. The operating table should also be equipped to ensure rapid adjustment into varying degrees of Trendelenburg and reverse Trendelenburg positions, as individual and occasionally emergency circumstances may require. The table height should be sufficiently adjustable to permit the operator either to stand during the operative procedure or to be seated if that is his or her preference.

If a lithotomy sheet is used, it should have ample casings for the feet, so that it can be placed in position readily even though the patient's legs are placed somewhat vertically in the extended leg holders or stirrups.

Elastic stockings for the patient are advisable and should be in place before the start of the anesthesia. Whether their use will significantly reduce postoperative pulmonary embolism may be debatable, but they do provide venous compression. When the patient's legs are taken out of the stirrups and are lowered into the horizontal recumbent position at the conclusion of the operative procedure, the resultant rapid pooling of blood into the large venous beds of the legs has been reduced. Lowering the legs without compression as they come down out of the stirrups may result in a precipitous and significant drop in blood pressure as a result of what, in effect, has been a sudden increase in the size of the venous pool into which a fixed volume of blood is circulating. Intermittent compression boots are recommended for the patient with a history of previous phlebitis of the lower extremity or pelvis.

SPECIAL INSTRUMENTS

Vaginal surgeons usually develop preferences for a few special instruments that are well designed for vaginal work. Although it is desirable that the surgeon have two assistants for vaginal operations, this is not always possible. When one must occasionally work with a single assistant, the large Rigby retractor (Fig. 3.12*h*) is of considerable help, freeing the assistant's hands for knot cutting, sponging, and holding the movable retractors. A weighted speculum usually will be found quite helpful for the frequent situation in which virtually all of the surgical dissection must be accomplished within the vagina. A modification of the standard weighted speculum, which provides for built-in continuous suction (Fig. 3.12*a*), has been our preference for many years. The suction tubing may be built into the retractor blade, further increasing operative exposure (Fig. 3.13). The wall-mounted trap of the suction apparatus helps one keep track of estimated blood loss during surgery.

The instruments attributed to N. Sproat Heaney were especially designed for use within the vagina. The Heaney needle holder is particularly valuable because it provides for a considerable range of angles at which the needle can be grasped (Fig. 3.14*c*). This variability facilitates placement of curved needles and sutures at almost any conceivable angle with relative ease when placing sutures deep within the pelvis (Fig. 3.15). The Heaney hemostats have a desirable "pelvic curve," which ensures placement and a grip on tissues that provides security with minimal risk of slippage. In the hysterectomy in which there might not be much prolapse at the start of the operation, the Heaney-Ballantine hysterectomy forceps (Fig. 3.14*b*) are valuable. They have both an upward curve and a lateral curve adapted to both the right and left sides of the patient, as is stamped on the forceps. The Heaney-Ballantine hysterectomy forceps (Fig. 3.14*a*) are useful, as are the Masterson forceps and the Maingot. The Merz hysterectomy forceps (Fig. 3.16) has the standard Heaney curve and uses the principle of the Glassman noncrushing jaws, causing minimum trauma to the tissue to which it has been applied. It, or the Masterson clamp (not shown), is useful for clamping the mesovarium during oophorectomy because it neither slips nor tears tissue even when traction is necessary.

During a vaginectomy or a Schauta radical vaginal hysterectomy, the long mouse-toothed forceps of Krobach (Fig. 3.14*d*) provides an effective means of retracting or tem-

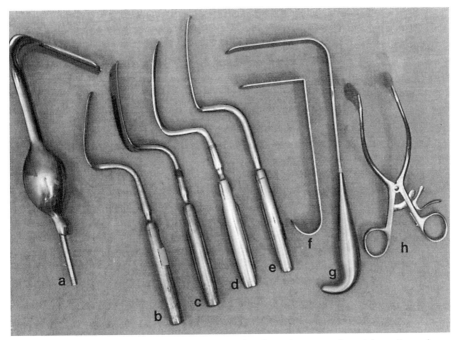

Figure 3.12. Various retractors: a Remine weighted suction speculum (*a*); various shapes and sizes of Briesky-Navratil vaginal retractors (*b–e*); a small Heaney retractor (*f*); a long-handled Heaney retractor (*g*); and a large-sized Rigby self-retaining retractor (*h*).

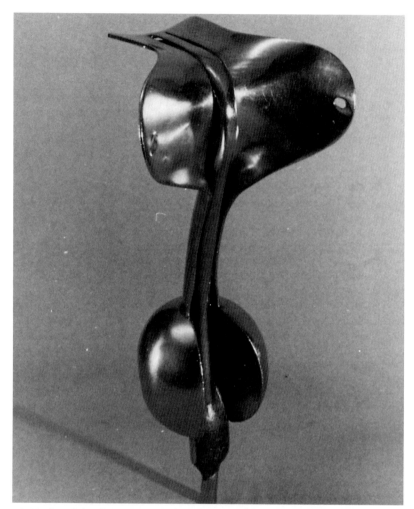

Figure 3.13. A weighted suction speculum for the posterior wall of the vagina. The suction tubing has been buried in the posterior blade of the retractor, improving the exposure in the operative field. It is available from BEI Medical Systems/Zinnanti Surgical Instruments, Chatsworth, California, 91311; and the custom order department of Codman-Shurtleff, New Bedford, Massachusetts.

porarily occluding the vagina. When the operator is familiar with their use, one or two of these can be of considerable help for traction and retraction during a usual type of perineorrhaphy and posterior colporrhaphy and for transvaginal sacrospinous colpopexy.

Bonney forceps (Fig. 3.17b) are highly recommended, since they combine a rat tooth for holding the tissues with occlusive serrated edges for grasping the needle deeply placed in tissues. Long Singley forceps (Fig. 3.17c) are particularly desirable for handling peritoneum and intra-abdominal organs with minimal trauma. So-called Russian forceps (Fig. 3.17a) are comfortable to use on the vaginal surface of the bladder during anterior colporrhaphy because they distribute the compression given the tissue within their grasp equally over a wide area.

Heaney retractors (see Fig. 3.12f) are easier to hold than the narrow Deaver retractors. The short-handled Heaney retractor is lightweight, the handle is unobtrusive, and it can be very helpful during colporrhaphy. The long-handled Heaney retractor (see Fig. 3.12g) is particularly helpful during vaginal hysterectomy as a means of holding the

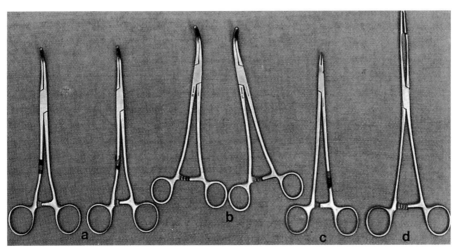

Figure 3.14. Clamps and needle holders: A pair of Heaney-Ballentine forceps are shown in (*a*); a pair of Heaney-Glenner hysterectomy forceps, with right and left curves (*b*); a Heaney needle holder (*c*); and Krobach mouse-toothed clamps (*d*).

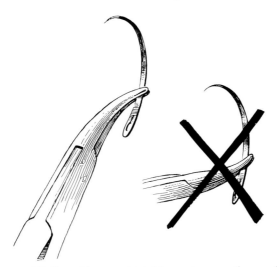

Figure 3.15. The correct (*left*) and incorrect (*right*) way to grasp the needle with a Heaney needle holder.

bladder safely out of the way after the anterior vesicouterine peritoneal fold has been identified and opened.

Briesky-Navratil retractors (see Fig. 3.12, *b–e*) come in an almost limitless assortment of sizes. They are widely used in vaginal surgery on the European continent, but are not very well known in America. An assortment in the varying widths and depths available will provide useful retraction in an infinite variety of clinical circumstances.

The handle of the retractor, being parallel to the blade, may be grasped easily and securely, much like a dagger. Thus it can be held comfortably with less tendency toward slippage or wandering and without obstructing the surgical team's view of the operative field. Even greater exposure may be provided in the depths of the wound by the flat blade retractor with the handle angled as shown in Figure 3.18, which should be held as shown in Figure 3.19.

Figure 3.16. The Merz hysterectomy forceps, showing the Glassman-type jaws and the Heaney curve.

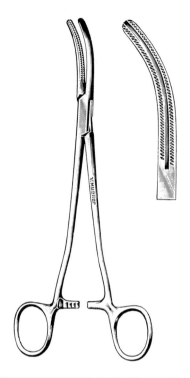

Figure 3.17. Tissue forceps: Russian forceps (*a*); Bonney forceps (*b*); and Singley forceps (*c*).

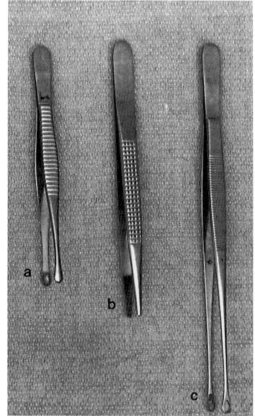

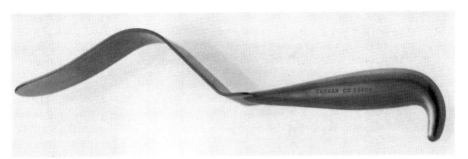

Figure 3.18. Flat-bladed vaginal retractor. Available in various sizes from BEI Medical Systems/ Zinnanti Surgical Instruments, Chatsworth, California, 91311; the special order department, Codman-Shurtleff Inc, CD 1106 or 09804, New Bedford, Massachusetts; or Mr. William Merz, Baxter V. Mueller, Chicago, Illinois.

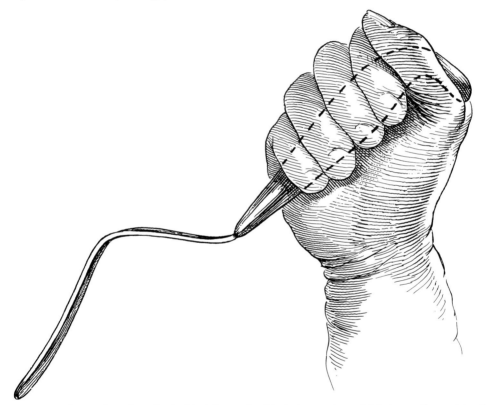

Figure 3.19. The preferred method of holding a flat-bladed retractor, which keeps the assistant's hand out of the operator's field of view.

The 28-cm Deschamps ligature carrier for the right hand is particularly useful during a sacrospinous fixation procedure, but it is also useful during oophorectomy, because the blunt point tends to push adjacent blood vessels to one side, thus avoiding the lacerations that would be more likely to occur with a sharp-pointed needle. Some various modifications of the Deschamps and other useful ligature carriers of special usefulness during sacrospinous colpopexy are shown in Chapter 16. A long hook to grasp the suture after it has penetrated the tissue is a desirable accessory. The Shutt suture punch is also illustrated in Chapter 16.

These instruments are available from various American and European makers and distributors, and may be obtained, for instance, on order from Zinnanti Surgical Instruments in Chatsworth, California; from Mr. William Metz of American V. Mueller of Chicago, Illinois; or from the custom instrument department of Codman-Shurtleff in New Bedford, Massachusetts.

References

1. Cohn GM, Seifer DB. Blood exposure in single versus double gloving during pelvic surgery. Am J Obstet Gynecol 1990;162:715.
2. Diaz-Buxo JA. Cut resistant glove liner for medical use. Surg Gynecol Obstet 1991;172:312.
3. Hermann JB. Changes in tensile strength and knot security of surgical procedures in vivo. Arch Surg 1973;106:707–710.
4. Hussain SA, Latif ABA, Choudhary AA. Risks to surgeons: a survey of accidental injuries during operations. Br J Surg 1988;75:324.
5. Knapstein PG. Principles of reconstructive surgery. In: Knapstein PG, Friedberg V, Sevin B-U, eds. Reconstructive surgery in gynecology. New York: Thieme, 1990:8–9.
6. Nichols DH, ed. Gynecologic and obstetric surgery. St. Louis: Mosby-Year Book, 1993.
7. Rodeheaver GT, Nesbit WS, Edlich RF. Novafil: a dynamic suture for wound closure. Ann Surg 1986;204:193.
8. Rodeheaver GT, et al. Unique performance characteristics of Novafil. Surg Gynecol Obstet 1987;164:230.
9. Sanz L, Smith S. Mechanisms of wound healing, suture material, and wound closure. In: Sanz LE, ed. Gynecologic surgery. Oradell, NJ: Medical Economics Books, 1988.
10. Serrano CW, Wright JW, Newton ER. Surgical glove perforation in obstetrics. Obstet Gynecol 1991;77:525.

CHAPTER 4

Minor and Ambulatory Surgery

Some minor gynecologic surgery is regularly performed in an office setting, whereas that requiring more surgical dissection may be performed in an operating room of an ambulatory care center or hospital.

The simplest maneuvers, such as endometrial biopsy, may often be performed without anesthesia, but effective anesthesia should be provided, often by local infiltration, if the discomfort is likely to be severe or more than momentary.

BIOPSY OF THE VULVA

Biopsy of a suspicious lesion of the vulva should be accomplished under local anesthesia. A sample of the full thickness of the vulvar skin can be obtained using the Keyes skin biopsy drill (Fig. 4.1). Alternatively, a sharp biopsy punch can be used to obtain one or more specimens. The base of the donor site should be coagulated to minimize bleeding. When large lesions of the vulvar skin have been excised, the remaining skin defects may be obliterated by the harvest and rotation of flaps from the neighboring skin as noted by Julian and associates (27). Knapstein describes useful techniques for closing skin gaps of different shapes (30). The closure of a large rectangular defect is shown in Figure 4.2; oval and round defects can be covered as shown in Figure 4.3. A flap can also be used in covering a triangular defect (Fig. 4.4) (30).

CHRONIC VULVAR PRURITUS

Subcutaneous injection of triamcinolone acetonide (Kenalog) provides relief of symptoms of incapacitating, chronic vulvar pruritus. After malignancy had been excluded by biopsy of any suspicious areas, local applications of betamethasone valerate cream or lotion are prescribed for a period of 2 weeks. If these topical steroids alleviate the symptoms for a period of 30 to 60 minutes during this trial, then the subcutaneous injection is recommended. A 25-gauge needle injects a small quantity of local anesthetic into the midportion of the labia majora of each side lateral to the clitoris. Then, using a long needle, 15 to 20 mg of triamcinolone acetonide is slowly injected as the needle is directed posteriorly toward the anal orifice (Fig. 4.5). The area is massaged thoroughly so that the agent is diffused throughout the labia. The patient should be instructed to take a cool sitz bath the following evening for 15 to 20 minutes and to expect that it will take 24 to 48 hours after the injection for the agent to be effective. Most patients will be improved, and the procedure may be repeated if necessary (29).

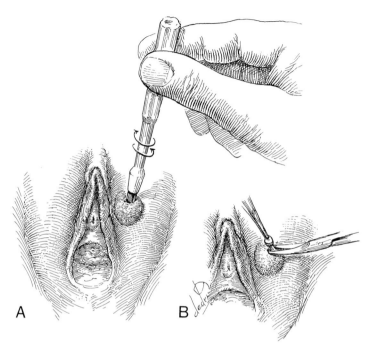

Figure 4.1. Biopsy of vulvar skin using a Keyes punch. The site has been infiltrated with a local anesthetic and the cutting end of the punch applied to the site selected for biopsy. Pressure is applied lightly and the punch rotated back and forth (see *arrows*) to drill a hole through the full thickness of the skin. The specimen disk is elevated with fine pointed forceps and cut away from the subcutaneous tissue. The wound is cauterized for hemostasis. (From Nichols DH, Sweeney PJ, eds. Ambulatory gynecology. 2nd ed. Philadelphia: Lippincott-Raven, 1995. Used with permission.)

VULVAR AND VAGINAL INTRAEPITHELIAL NEOPLASIA

Excisional rather than ablative electrosurgical techniques provide tissue for complete histopathologic evaluation of specimens obtained from the vulva, vagina, or cervix. This reduces the possibility of doing an inadequate preoperative sampling of the lesion and then inappropriately treating a microinvasive or frankly invasive lesion by destroying it without having tissue for diagnosis (6).

Vulvar intraepithelial neoplasia in the patient under 40 years of age appears to be a less aggressive lesion than in a patient over 40, and may be treated by laser thin section (as opposed to vaporization), which when peeled away provides an abundant sample of tissue for histologic study. Baggish has provided an excellent description of the technical details of these procedures (2, 3). Close lifetime follow-up is, of course, essential. Vaginal intraepithelial neoplasia responds well to CO_2 laser therapy, and more than one treatment is usually required. After malignant change has been excluded by representative biopsy(s), CO_2 laser vaporization may be used to vaporize grossly visible vulvar condyloma acuminata.

EXCISION OF THE VAGINAL APEX

A precancerous lesion of the posthysterectomy vaginal apex may be treated by full-thickness excisional biopsy (Fig. 4.6). It may represent vaginal intraepithelial neoplasia in a patient with previous surgical intraepithelial neoplasia treated previously by hysterectomy, but the tissue must be studied in the laboratory to exclude unexpected invasion of the subepithelial tissues.

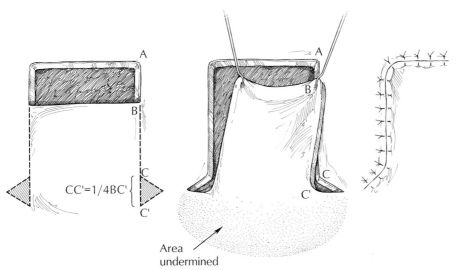

Figure 4.2. Closure of a large rectangular defect. When skin flaps are used, the width of the base should generally be twice that of the length to preserve the blood supply of the flap. To cover the rectangular defect *AB*, the tissue embraced by *BCC'* must be mobilized. Two triangles measuring one-fourth the distance of the flap *BC* must be excised, as shown in the drawing to the *left*. To preserve blood supply, the skin underlying the flap must be mobilized as shown in the *center* drawing, and the defect closed with interrupted stitches as shown in the drawing to the *right* by bringing *point B* to *point A* and *point C'* to *point C*, and the flaps united by interrupted mattress stitches, as shown (30).

SURGERY OF BARTHOLIN GLAND

A Bartholin cyst is a cyst of the duct and not of the gland, which is usually compressed around the deep periphery of the cyst and not necessarily visible to the naked eye. After surgical excision of a cyst, often a formidable procedure associated with an unexpectedly high blood loss due to the vascularity of the tissues in this area, the future secretions of the remaining and buried but functional glandular tissue can reaccumulate and, without an opening to the external skin, may recreate a new and often symptomatic cyst requiring reexcision.

Acute initial Bartholin abscess can be treated by aspiration through a no. 19 needle and syringe. The aspirate should be sent for bacteriologic identification, culture, and sensitivity. The patient, meanwhile, should be started on 400 mg of metronidazole twice daily and 250 mg of penicillin four times daily, both for 7 days. If it is later determined that the offending organism is of gonorrhea, the patient should be given 1 g of probenecid and 3.5 g of ampicillin. When tissue edema subsides, the patency and function of the duct will return in about 80 percent of cases (10).

A Bartholin duct cyst may be successfully ablated with a CO_2 laser under local anesthesia as an office procedure (12, 24, 32). Incision and drainage of a Bartholin abscess can be performed in the vestibular area close to the hymen through an area of fluctuation. The incision should be between 1 and 2 cm in length, and a drain or wick inserted for 24 hours. Because the skin heals and seals itself rapidly, reoccurrence is not uncommon, particularly if the duct has been damaged by the infection.

An alternative method of great simplicity is offered by the placement and inflation of a Word catheter through a stab wound into the cyst cavity (Fig. 4.7), where it will remain for 3 to 4 weeks until the tract of the wound has become epithelialized, forming a new duct (36). The bulb should always be inflated with saline rather than air, since the latter may permit premature deflation. During this 3- to 4-week period, the protruding

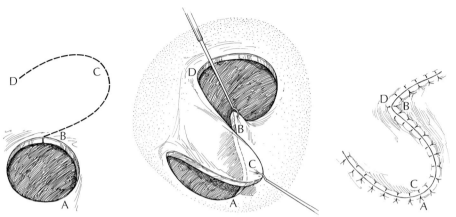

Figure 4.3. Closure of oval and round defects. Oval and round defects can be covered by an oval transposition graft of the same size, as identified in the drawing to the *left*. The extent by which the donor and recipient site are undermined and mobilized is identified by the *dotted area* in the *center* drawing. When hemostasis has been achieved, *point C* is sewn to *point A*, and *point B* sewn to *point D* as shown. The defect between these stitches is closed with interrupted mattress sutures, as shown (30).

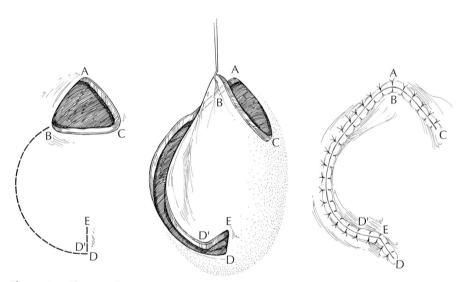

Figure 4.4. Closure of a triangular defect. A transposition flap covering a triangular defect *ABC* is shown. The dashed line indicates the preliminary outline of the incisions. When the flap has been thoroughly undermined as shown in the *center* drawing, *point B* is brought to *point A*, and the remainder of the incision closed with interrupted mattress sutures as shown in the drawing to the *right*. Notice the now linear relationship of points *D'*, *E*, and *D* (30).

proximal end of the small catheter can be tucked out of the way into the vagina. At the end of 3 to 4 weeks, the bulb on the catheter is deflated and the catheter removed. This procedure is particularly useful in the presence of infection. A small Foley catheter can be used instead of the Word. The bulb is inflated and the entire catheter tightly ligated about 3 inches from where it enters the skin. It may be transected just distal to the point of ligation, which has occluded both the central and side lumens, and the free end should be tucked into the vagina.

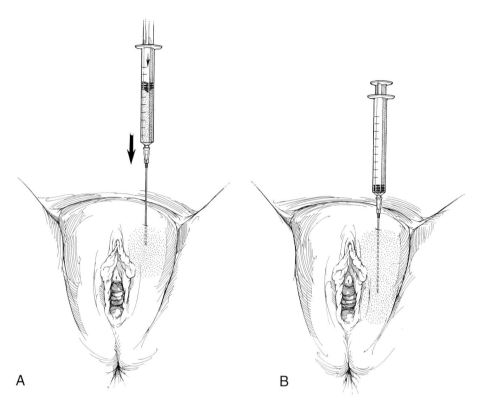

Figure 4.5. Subcutaneous injection of triamcinolone acetonide (Kenalog) to relieve disabling vulvar pruritus. **A.** Following the production of the small wheal of local anesthetic, a long needle attached to the syringe with the Kenalog is injected into the subcutaneous tissue. **B.** The contents of the syringe are expressed *in advance* of the needle as a slow injection is made through the full length of the labia majora. A similar injection is made on the opposite side, and the tissues massaged to ensure widespread dispersion of the agent (29).

A Bartholin cyst may also be marsupialized when large and uninfected. A window may be cut from the vestibular skin that includes the cyst wall. The edge of the residual cyst lining may be sewn to the vestibular skin by a series of interrupted through-and-through stitches. When healing has been completed, a permanent fistula will have been created between the cyst cavity and the skin, essentially becoming a new "duct." The size of the ostium will gradually contract over a period of months and in time will become scarcely visible, though still functional.

A solid lesion within Bartholin gland should be sampled by needle biopsy or surgical excision (1) to exclude the presence or absence of malignancy, which can be either adenocarcinoma if the tumor is of the gland, or transitional or squamous cell carcinoma if it is a malignancy of the duct. Bartholin carcinoma is serious and is generally treated by radical vulvectomy and bilateral groin dissection.

TREATMENT OF AN OBSTRUCTED HEMIVAGINA

A hemivagina associated with a didelphic uterus or a bicornuate or septate vagina may be completely or partially obstructed. When completely obstructed, there will be dysmenorrhea from the accumulated monthly blood and a mass will be palpated in the lateral wall of the vagina (50). Congenital urinary abnormalities may coexist. Diagnosis is confirmed by aspiration of old blood from the mass, and treatment is by prompt marsupialization, creating a large vaginal window connecting the cavities of the two vaginas.

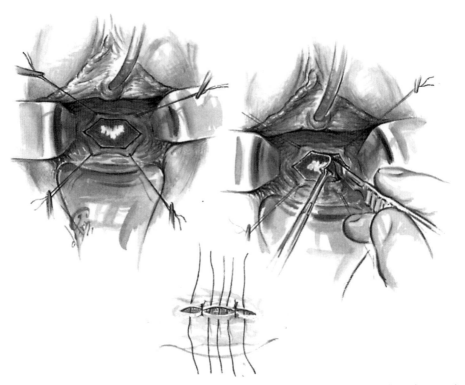

Figure 4.6. Excision of the vaginal apex. The lesion is carefully demarcated, such as with Schiller stain, and four guide sutures are inserted as shown. The subepithelial tissue may be infiltrated by 0.5% lidocaine in 1:200,000 epinephrine solution for hemostasis, and the tissue to be excised indicated by incision through the full thickness of the vaginal wall as shown. This is excised by sharp dissection and the vaginal edges brought together by a series of interrupted polyglycolic acid sutures placed as shown. If there is concern about preserving vaginal depth, a closure may be made in a vertical rather than horizontal direction.

LESIONS OF THE PROXIMAL URETHRA

Prolapse of the urethra is not uncommon, particularly in postmenopausal women but occasionally in newborns. If asymptomatic, it need not be treated. It rarely causes bleeding, but if it is a source of annoyance to the patient, it may be treated by excision of the circular area, and the wall of the urethra can be sewn to the skin of the circumferential tissue by a series of interrupted sutures. When a lesion of the distal urethra is associated with bleeding, differentiation must be made between the benign and relatively harmless urethral caruncle and the much more ominous invasive carcinoma of the urethra. The carcinoma tends to be harder when palpated and somewhat more friable, but the distinction is made by histologic examination of biopsy material. The treatment of caruncle is by simple excision, but the treatment of carcinoma varies between interstitial radiation and radical surgery, depending upon the circumstances.

SURGERY OF THE HYMEN

Incision and hymenectomy is the treatment of choice and will be curative for an imperforate hymen. A small but rigid hymen producing obstruction to the vagina may be treated by hymenotomy at the 4 and 8 o'clock positions and kept open during the healing phase by digital stretching performed by the patient. A rigid, inelastic perineum may be overcome by midline perineotomy, sufficient to admit three finger breadths into the

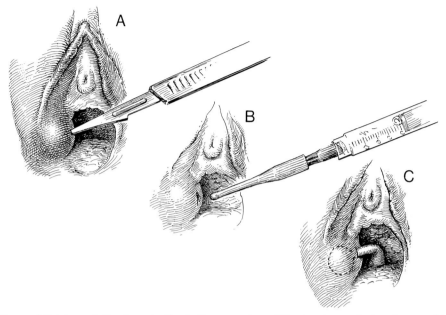

Figure 4.7. Marsupialization of a Bartholin cyst using a Word catheter. **A.** A stab wound is made through the full thickness of the right Bartholin cyst at the site chosen for the new duct. **B.** A Word catheter is attached to a syringe containing 2 ml of sterile saline and the tip of the catheter is quickly introduced into the cyst cavity. **C.** The catheter bulb is inflated with saline, the syringe removed, and the free end of the catheter tucked back into the vagina. The catheter should remain in place for several weeks, until the new duct has become epithelialized. Then the bulb is deflated and the catheter removed. (From Nichols DH, Sweeney PJ, eds. Ambulatory gynecology. 2nd ed. Philadelphia: Lippincott-Raven, 1995. Used with permission.)

vagina. The edges of the incision should be sewn to the perineal skin transversely, at right angles to the original incision.

When recurrent postcoital cystitis occurs, examination should be made for the presence of a congenital anomaly of thick lateral bands connecting the urethral meatus to the hymenal margin. External urethrolysis at this site is curative (Fig. 4.8).

PERINEOTOMY

Painful stenosis of the introitus may be relieved by a midline perineotomy (Fig. 4.9). Introital stenosis, usually postmenopausal and too inelastic to permit relief by perineotomy, will respond effectively to Z-plasty (Fig. 4.10).

VULVAR VESTIBULAR SYNDROME (FOCAL VULVITIS, VESTIBULAR ADENITIS)

There is no evidence that infection causes vulvar vestibulitis, and although the specific etiology remains unknown, hormonal factors such as early oral contraceptive use may be involved (5). Although some have suggested that the condition may be related in some patients to infection with human papillomavirus (HPV) (19, 48). This infection, which is acetowhite, demonstrates multiple papillae that may cover the entire mucosal surface of the labia minora, and is sometimes asymptomatic, may represent a different disease. Unlike vulvar vestibular syndrome, this disease may respond to laser vaporization. There appears to be some ill-defined, suggested relationship between human

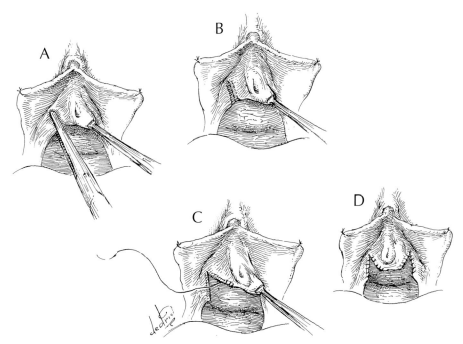

Figure 4.8. External urethrolysis. **A.** The site of the hymenal attachment to the urethra is being crushed in a forceps, first on one side and then on the other. **B.** An incision is made through the crushed tissue (*broken line*). **C.** The cut edge of the incision is overcast by a running locked suture. **D.** The end result. (After C. Wood, the Mason Clinic, Seattle, WA.)

papillomavirus in vulvar vestibulitis patients and their treatment with interferon (48). Essential vulvodynia describes a condition of constant, unremitting vulvar burning in the absence of any significant findings on physical examination. The patients are usually postmenopausal. Low doses of tricyclic antidepressants have proven helpful in treatment (35).

This condition may be suspected from an abrupt onset of severe dyspareunia, usually in a young Caucasian patient with no visible outlet obstruction or palpable endopelvic pathology. The patient may have one or more areas of exquisite tenderness that have been identified in the vestibule, most commonly in the posterior portion between the hymen and the vulvar skin (51). Gently touching these areas with the end of a cotton-tipped applicator will produce instant discomfort, and the sites can be sharply demarcated. The condition has been identified from time to time for over 100 years (44), and the most recent interest has been initiated since 1981 (16, 17, 38, 52–54). The vestibule is of endodermal origin from the urogenital sinus, making it embryologically quite distinctive from the other tissues of this area. Four percent aqueous lidocaine on a cotton ball applied to this area for 10 minutes, three times daily, and again some 15 minutes before coitus will often provide sufficient temporary anesthesia for coitus. Lidocaine ointment may be applied to the area during the day to obtain temporary relief. Because the taking of oral contraceptives may exacerbate the condition, for reasons unknown, they should be stopped for at least 6 months. Remission will occur in about one-half of the cases during this time.

If the syndrome is persistent after 6 months of observation and treatment as described above, including perhaps alternative or noncoital means of sexual gratification, a surgical approach of vestibulectomy and perineoplasty may be expected to provide relief in most cases. Diagnosis is reconfirmed preoperatively by examination of the vestibule with a magnifying glass or low-power colposcope, and often a cluster of raised pinkish or yellowish papules will be present in the area of pain. This specific site of pain

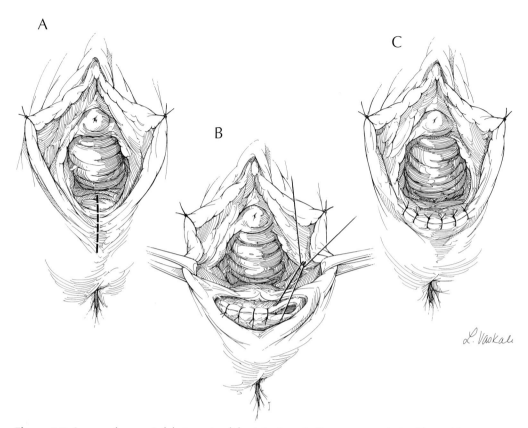

Figure 4.9. Surgery for a painful stenosis of the introitus. **A.** Surgery may start with a midline incision through the skin of the lower vagina and perineum (*dashed line*). **B.** The skin is freed from the underlying scar tissue by sharp dissection, and the deeper tissues of the perineum are united transversely by a series of through-and-through interrupted sutures. **C.** The skin of the fourchette is reapproximated by a series of interrupted sutures.

may be carefully mapped out with a marking pen immediately preoperatively and before anesthesia so that the affected area may be totally excised (Fig. 4.11). General or regional anesthesia should be employed, and the full epithelial thickness, including the adjacent hymen of this sensitive area within the vestibule, should be excised. The full thickness of the posterior vaginal wall should be mobilized for 2 or 3 cm so that it can be brought down to cover this raw area at the conclusion of the operation, where, after hemostasis has been obtained, the vaginal wall is attached to the skin of the perineum by two layers of interrupted sutures (53). Because postoperative oozing and pain at this site are common, the patient should be kept in the hospital for a day postoperatively. Ice packs are applied to the perineum for comfort and to help hemostasis in the initial postoperative period. Laxative stool softeners are given, and if prompt, spontaneous voiding does not occur, the patient is catheterized and given a 10-mg capsule of phenoxybenzamine (Dibenzyline) and an alpha blocker to temporarily relax the urethral musculature. Sitz baths may be given starting on the third postoperative day. Postoperatively, the perineal skin will be permanently altered by the transposed posterior vaginal wall.

CULDOCENTESIS

This procedure, usually performed at a site in the midline of the upper posterior vaginal wall between the uterosacral ligaments, is useful in identifying the nature and character of fluid distending the cul-de-sac of Douglas (Fig. 4.12). When abscess

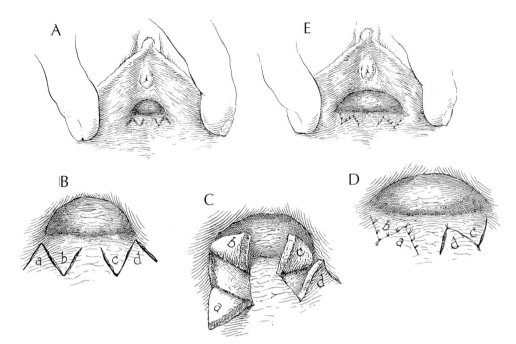

Figure 4.10. Z-plasty. **A.** View of preoperative introital stenosis showing the lines of incision. **B.** The full-thickness flaps are undermined. **C.** The flaps are rotated. **D.** The flaps are sewn in place. **E.** View of the completed operation showing the introital enlargement.

is suspected, the culdocentesis should take place in an operating room and the procedure performed at the site of fluctuation as determined by the bimanual abdominal-rectal-vaginal palpation. If the patient is awake, the needle may be poised for penetration of the vagina and the patient asked to give a hard cough (which will increase her intra-abdominal pressure); at that moment, the needle is quickly thrust into the cul-de-sac as shown. The nature of the fluid distending the cul-de-sac of Douglas is identified, and, if purulent, the needle is left in place, the entry into the cavity enlarged by surgical colpotomy, and drainage promptly instituted. The abscess contents are sent for prompt bacteriological identification, culture, and sensitivity. Other aspirates are treated appropriately.

POSTERIOR COLPOTOMY

Provided the uterus is movable and the cervix can be drawn to the introitus, a posterior colpotomy, as shown in Figure 4.13, will provide ready, transvaginal, surgical access to the tubes and ovaries following preliminary anesthesia.

EXCISION OF ENDOMETRIAL OR ENDOCERVICAL POLYP

A polyp protruding through the external cervix should be excised in its entirety and sent for prompt laboratory study. The base of a small polyp can be grasped within the jaws of a small hemostat and twisted off. Larger polyps are better removed by excision of their entire stalk. Because the site of origin and attachment to the endocervix or endometrium is usually invisible, the polyp can be fed through the loop of a tonsil snare (Fig. 4.14). The loop is advanced within the endocervical or endometrial cavity until its progress stops, at which point the snare is slowly tightened so that the pedicle of the polyp is crushed and transected. The polyp is sent for laboratory examination. The patient should be reexamined after a month to determine whether other polyps might be present that should also be removed and studied.

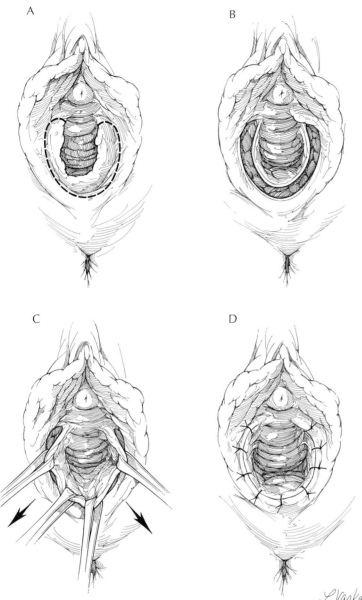

Figure 4.11. Vestibulectomy. **A.** The painful area of vestibular skin is carefully demarcated preoperatively and an incision made lateral to this line of demarcation (*dashed line*). **B.** The full thickness of the skin, including the adjacent hymen, is removed, and any bleeding vessels clamped and ligated or electrocoagulated. **C.** The posterior vaginal wall is mobilized and pulled down (*arrows*) to cover the raw area. **D.** The full thickness of the vagina is sewn to the skin of the vulva by two layers of interrupted synthetic absorbable sutures. Raw areas anterior or lateral to the urethra may be left open to granulate and avoid stricture.

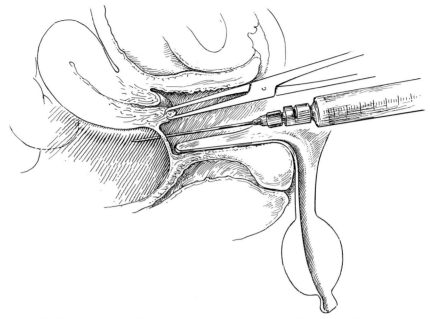

Figure 4.12. Culdocentesis. The cervix has been steadied with a tenaculum, and a sharp, pointed no. 18 needle attached to a syringe inserted directly into the bulging cul-de-sac. The fluid is then aspirated and examined. (From Nichols DH, Sweeney PJ, eds. Ambulatory gynecology. 2nd ed. Philadelphia: JB Lippincott, 1995. Used with permission.)

TREATMENT OF A WOLFFIAN DUCT CYST

Large Wolffian duct cysts are occasionally found along the side walls or beneath the lateral surface of the vaginal apex. They are anatomically separate from the urethra and bladder and are filled with clear mucus (41). If they are enlarging or are a source of dyspareunia, they should be treated. Marsupialization is preferable to excision because excision is occasionally accompanied by unexpectedly profuse bleeding and risks ureteral ligation when hemostatic deep sutures are placed at the base of the cyst cavity to control bleeding.

OFFICE ENDOMETRIAL BIOPSY FOR AMBULATORY PATIENTS

Fortunately, the technique of endometrial biopsy, done as an office procedure on a fully ambulatory patient, will often identify a malignancy in the endocervix or in the uterine cavity. It is best, however, to consider that such an endometrial biopsy is dependable only when it is histologically positive. One may plan therapy of endocervical or endometrial malignancy when the pathology report of an endometrial biopsy identifies malignancy. As a first step of such planned therapy, the operator should not neglect a careful appraisal of the clinical stage of the malignancy based on the findings (*a*) on examination under anesthesia and (*b*) during a fractional curettage of the cervix and cavity of the uterus. It is equally important when biopsies taken in the office or clinic are negative and there is any clinical suspicion of malignancy that operating room fractional curettage be performed that involves a thorough exploration of first the endocervical canal and then the uterine cavity. In the uterus, both the polyp forceps and a curette, usually larger than that employed in the cervix, ensure detection of a pedunculated polyp, as well as an infiltrating malignancy.

For endometrial biopsies, many gynecologists are now using flexible plastic "Pipelle-type" curettes instead of rigid, hollow, steel curettes of varying sizes (Fig. 4.15). In young women conventional diagnostic dilatation and curettage can be replaced by endometrial biopsy (43), and the Pipelle DeCornier and the Curelle cause the least pain (33). The overall cost savings, should this be implemented, are enormous (11). Because the outer diameter is only 3.1 mm, in outer diameter, its insertion without preliminary dilatation or anesthesia is virtually painless. The Pipelle is an inexpensive and disposable unit. After its tip is inserted into the cavity of the uterus, suction is applied by traction on a built-in plunger, and the tip is moved back and forth several times within the cavity as the hollow tube is rotated so that the four quadrants of the endometrial cavity are sampled quickly. The curette is removed from the uterus and the tip is cut off. One expresses the contents of the hollow tube into a specimen jar by pushing the plunger to its original position.

HYSTEROSCOPY

Hysteroscopy permits direct visualization and resection of endometrial pathology or anomaly, but the potential for tumor dissemination has prevented its widespread use in the diagnosis and staging of uterine cancer. Operative hysteroscopy is an excellent method of lysing interuterine adhesions or resecting a uterine septum that has been thought to interfere significantly with past pregnancies. Hysteroscopic septum resection has virtually replaced transabdominal metroplasty for this indication. Removal of endometrial polyps can be accomplished, as well as resection of certain symptom-producing submucous leiomyomas up to 5 cm in diameter. March has described the techniques, and notes that acute pelvic infection is the only absolute contraindication (34). Great caution must be taken to avoid uterine perforation during hysteroscopy, since subsequent uterine rupture during pregnancy following perforation has been reported (56).

ENDOMETRIAL ABLATION

The principal indication for endometrial ablation is for the treatment of intractable hypermenorrhea. There is, however, a 5 to 10 percent failure rate that the patient must be willing to accept. Hysteroscopy combined with ultrasound is safer that an IUD hook for removing an embedded or "lost" intrauterine device. Endometrial ablation is an alternative to hysterectomy when other modalities have failed, are contraindicated, or are undesirable. Most ablations are done in an ambulatory setting, and postoperative discomfort is minimal, though the patient can expect some bloody discharge for up to 10 days (34).

Endometrial ablation for the treatment of hypermenorrhea and polymenorrhea, after a cause of this symptom from malignancy has been ruled out, may be accomplished by using the rollerball electrode followed by the resectoscope or the laser. The risk of burying or leaving behind a small nidus of endometrium is ever present, and little is yet known of the magnitude of the eventual risks involved. Postablation endometrial malignancy has been reported (39), stressing the need for long-term careful follow-up in patients treated by this medium (18). The risk of complication is greater among patients under the age of 40 years and in those with multiple leiomyomata.

Uterine perforation has been associated with endometrial ablation. Damage to bowel, bladder, and large blood vessels may occur, demonstrating the necessity for adequate training before undertaking any type of operative hysteroscopy (26).

CERVICOPLASTY

This plastic repair of the cervix may be considered for a patient with a healed but unrepaired previous cervical laceration that has exposed the endocervical canal to the vaginal bacterial flora. This causes chronic glandular inflammation with mucopurulent leukorrhea and loss of cervical integrity. The condition requires freshening of the edges, excision of scar tissue, and reapproximation in layers.

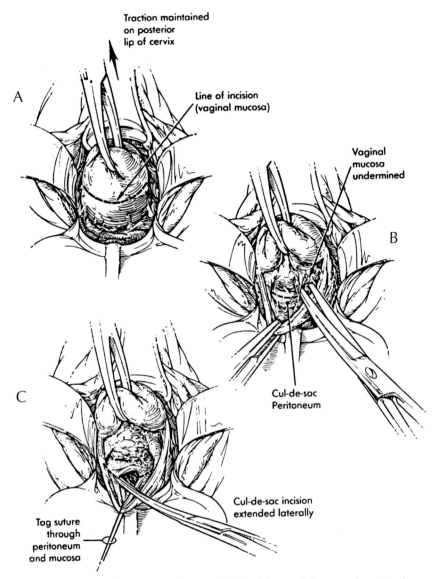

Figure 4.13. Posterior colpotomy. **A.** The posterior lip of the cervix is grasped by a Jacobs tenaculum, traction is applied, and the cul-de-sac is palpated. An incision will be made along the path of the *dashed line*. **B.** The vaginal wall is pushed back and the Jacobs clamp repositioned so that the posterior jaw is beneath the cut edge. The vaginal wall is pushed back further to expose the peritoneum of the cul-de-sac, which may be opened along the pathway of the *dashed line*. **C.** A guide suture holds the posterior margin of the peritoneal opening, which may be enlarged by a transverse incision (*dashed line*). The uterosacral ligaments are not usually cut.

TREATMENT OF CERVICAL INTRAEPITHELIAL NEOPLASIA

When a patient with cervical intraepithelial neoplasia wishes to preserve her uterus and its reproductive function, treatment other than hysterectomy can be (*a*) cryosurgery, (*b*) laser surgery, (*c*) electrocoagulation, (*d*) loop excision, or (*e*) conization. All these techniques require the following:

1. The abnormal epithelium is visualized completely.
2. Endocervical curettage is negative.

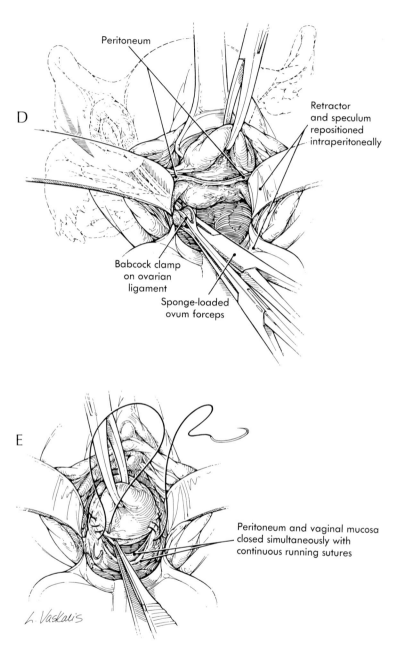

Peritoneum

D

Retractor
and speculum
repositioned
intraperitoneally

Babcock clamp
on ovarian
ligament

Sponge-loaded
ovum forceps

E

Peritoneum and vaginal mucosa
closed simultaneously with
continuous running sutures

L. Vaskalis

Figure 4.13. D. The ovary or tube may be grasped by the ring forceps or Babcock clamp.
E. Following the completion of the intraperitoneal surgery, the incision is closed by a single layer of running through-and-through sutures that include both margins of the vaginal wall and peritoneum. If desired, a drain may be placed at the 6 o'clock position. (From Nichols DH. Gynecologic and obstetric surgery. St. Louis: Mosby–Year Book, 1993. Used with permission.)

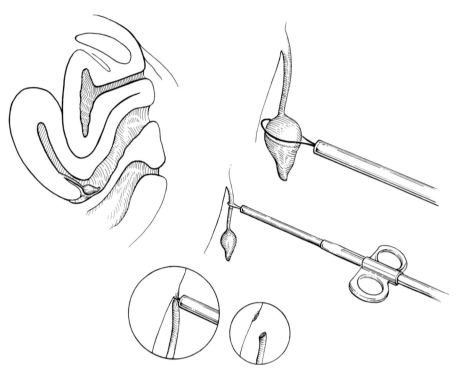

Figure 4.14. Removal of an endocervical or endometrial polyp. The polyp protruding through the cervix is seen in sagittal section through the pelvis. It is threaded through the eye of the wire of a tonsil snare, which is advanced along the stalk as far as it will go. The snare is tightened slowly (*insert*) to first crush and then transect the stalk, and the polyp is removed for laboratory examination.

3. There is agreement between the findings of cytology and colposcopy.
4. The patient is willing to participate in long-term and adequate follow-up activity.

CRYOSURGERY AND LASER THERAPY

Coincident with careful cytologic interpretation of the screening Papanicolaou (Pap) smear, experienced colposcopy added to the usual armamentarium of gynecologists has made it possible to locate with specificity the site of epithelial abnormalities of the cervix, vagina, and vulva, and to take biopsies of these suspicious areas under colposcopic guidance for histologic study to rule out invasive cancer. Obviously invasive malignancy should be confirmed by the examination of tissue obtained by punch biopsy. When a premalignant condition has been identified and the entire lesion visualized colposcopically, a spectrum of definitive treatment can be offered to the patient. When the endocervical extent of a lesion cannot be estimated with certainty and the endocervical curettage is inconclusive, conization will provide adequate material for study. Although laser conization is popular with some gynecologists, our experience has found the so-called cold-knife conization to be entirely effective.

Premalignant lesions can be treated by cryosurgery (15, 37, 45, 47) or laser vaporization (4, 9, 28, 40, 43, 45–47, 55) as alternatives to surgical excision.

When a colposcopically directed biopsy is reported as showing microinvasion of a malignancy, or possible microinvasion, conization becomes necessary for a study of the entire lesion (8). When microinvasion is discovered during pregnancy and the squamocolumnar junction everts, a shallow "coin biopsy" type of conization avoids the poten-

A

B

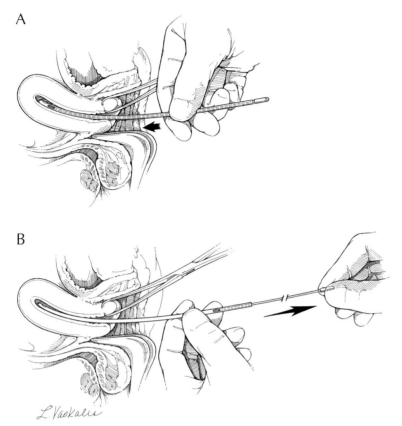

L. Vaokalii

Figure 4.15. Endometrial biopsy using the Pipelle or Curelle. **A.** The plastic curette with sheath fully advanced is inserted through the cervix into the full depth of the endometrial cavity. A tenaculum may be used to steady the cervix if necessary. **B.** While the sheath is held, the piston is then quickly and fully withdrawn from it until the piston is stopped and "locked" in position. The sheath is rotated as it is moved back and forth several times to sample the endometrium; it is then withdrawn and the tip cut off and discarded. The contents of the hollow tube are expressed into a specimen jar by pushing the plunger to its original position.

tially dangerous excision of the endocervix (13, 14). Eversion of the squamocolumnar junction and excessive blood loss is reduced by six hemostatic pursestring sutures placed close to the vaginal reflection (2).

Large-loop excision of the transformation zone (LLETZ) has been shown to be an effective alternate to cone biopsy. Most patients can be managed as outpatients under local anesthesia (6, 22).

Carbon dioxide laser vaporization for treating cervical intraepithelial neoplasia (7) has been displaced by large-loop electrical excision, which supplies a specimen for histologic evaluation. Laser is faster in skilled hands and provides an excellent specimen for histologic study, but a loop electrical excision cone (LEEC) requires less technical skill. It may be performed under local anesthesia, and hemostasis is achieved by preliminary intracervical injection of a "liquid tourniquet." Complications of the laser vaporization to the cervix are uncommon. For extensive lesions of cervical intraepithelial neoplasia (i.e., involving three or four cervical quadrants and extending into the vaginal fornices), a "combination cone" may be useful. This combines vaporization of the exocervical lesion with a narrow cylindrical endocervical cone (2).

CONIZATION OF THE CERVIX

In recent years, gynecologists have discontinued the routine preoperative shaving of vulvar and suprapubic hair before a conization or dilatation and curettage (D&C) (or most other vaginal surgery). It is sometimes helpful to clip long hair to keep it out of the way (49).

Although diagnostic conization has been largely replaced by colposcopically directed biopsy, it is of value in the investigation of patients with a malignant noninvasive lesion or an abnormal Pap smear in whom the squamocolumnar junction is too high to be visualized and sampled for a biopsy. Although the procedure is primarily diagnostic, it may be therapeutic under certain circumstances, such as when an entire noninvasive lesion of the cervix may be visualized and included within the surgical specimen. (Because intraepithelial neoplasia is commonly multicentric, this does not preclude the future development of other areas of dysplasia or carcinoma in situ.)

Technique

A simple technique that provides acceptable hemostasis consists of infiltration of the cervical stroma with not more than 50 ml of 0.5% lidocaine (Xylocaine) in 1:200,000 epinephrine (Adrenalin) solution. This produces marked spasm of cervical blood vessels, confirmed by a visible blanching of the cervix. With a no. 11 pointed scalpel for the incision, a cone of tissue of the proper size is removed, up to but not including the internal cervical os.

It is absolutely essential that the axis of the cone parallel the axis of the vagina and cervix; perforation of the uterus at the apex of the cone can damage the neighboring organs and tissues. The 12 o'clock position on the operative specimen may be marked for orientation by a suture. Bleeding or oozing points should be coagulated with the electrosurgical unit. An alternative procedure for preliminary hemostasis requires the insertion of deep hemostatic sutures of absorbable material placed in the 3 and 9 o'clock positions. After the cone of cervix is obtained, bleeding points are coagulated, and the cervix is packed for 24 to 48 hours with 1/4-inch iodoform gauze. If significant oozing is immediate, which is rare, a second and more hemostatic "hot" electroconization may follow. The difficulty with this as a routine procedure is that if the initial cone has not removed the entire lesion, there is no more fresh adjacent tissue to study by immediate biopsy. Because of tissue destruction, postoperative cervical scarring will be great. When a D&C and conization are to be performed on the same patient at the same time, the D&C is done immediately after the conization, never before.

Complications

Hemorrhage may be seen either at surgery or within the first postoperative weeks after conization. Visible bleeding points should be electrocoagulated, and if there is a general ooze, the area should be suture-ligated. Mild bleeding may be stopped by application of the tip of a silver nitrate stick, or a cotton applicator soaked in Monsel solution. If this is not successful, packing the affected area with microfibrillar collagen (Avitene) is generally effective. (Avitene exerts its hemostatic effect by attracting functioning blood platelets, which adhere to the microfibrils, triggering the formation of thrombi in the adjacent tissue. Although more expensive, it is more effective than Gelfoam or Surgicel.) A "pulsating" ooze should be treated by a carefully placed suture. If bleeding recurs, bilateral transvaginal ligation of the uterine artery may be required. Rarely, hysterectomy or internal iliac ligation may be indicated to control excessive recurrent postoperative bleeding, particularly if the conization has transected a major branch of the uterine artery that has subsequently retracted into the substance of the cervix or lower uterine segment.

Premature labor and delivery appears to be a significant risk in the patient who has experienced prior conization (31). Cervical stenosis is the principal long-range complication after unintended resection or trauma to the internal cervical os. Because cervical conization heals by scar formation, contraction will cause the diameter of the canal to become smaller, inducing a stenosis or stricture in some patients. The gynecologist who does a conization of the cervix must assume a responsibility to make certain that the patient's cervical canal does not become stenotic a few weeks or several months after the operation. The patient must be advised to return for postoperative examinations at regular intervals for at least 6 months. At each visit during this time, the gynecologist should test the patency of the cervical canal by carefully passing a small dilator or sound through the canal and internal os. To let stenosis develop and progress to occlusion will lead to amenorrhea, hematometria, possibly endometriosis, and certainly to a rightfully dissatisfied patient. The cervix tending to stenosis cannot always be dilated sufficiently without anesthesia to alter the progressive tightening of scar tissue. If the os cannot be dilated in the office without intolerable discomfort, the use of a *Laminaria* tent for 24 hours has been recommended (21). The operator must be careful not to let the tent slip into the uterine cavity, however, for it will become swollen, stuck, and difficult to remove without reinsertion of a second tent to dilate the cervix. If a stenosis does develop, dilating the canal under anesthesia and suturing an old-fashioned stem pessary in the canal to be worn for several months (or until it falls out) may be preferable to occasional, but usually futile, sounding or dilatation in the office or clinic. A stenosis may require long-term treatment by periodic endocervical dilatation until the surface of the cervix has been reepithelialized and scar formation and healing have stabilized.

There is little place for "hot" conization in the treatment of chronic cervicitis. The procedure is not cost-effective and carries additional risks, including scar tissue with formation retraction and its troublesome sequelae. When endocervicitis causes a chronic leukorrhea that has become sufficiently troublesome to the patient to require treatment, strip cauterization or electrocoagulation of the affected area of the cervix may be the procedure of choice. Because infection often involves the depths of the endocervical glands, superficial cauterization of the cervix by local applications of a caustic or of silver nitrate is not very useful.

Conization and Curettage: Preferred Sequence

Results will usually be better if the conization is done *after* the cervix and uterus have been "sounded" but *before* the curette is used in the canal or uterine cavity. The indications for conization and fractional curettage do not often coexist, but the procedures are not mutually exclusive. An external mucocutaneous junction around the margin of an "erosion" can, of course, be removed with a large biopsy loop without coagulating the endocervix. Even when a usual conization includes excision of 1 or 2 cm of the endocervix, the small, sharp curette can still be used to determine if malignancy is suggested by the presence of friable tissue in a softened area in the lower uterine segment adjacent to the inner os. When such curettage of the endocervix does not suggest carcinoma, it will probably be necessary to dilate the internal os to admit a larger curette and polyp forceps to the uterine cavity. If careful conization precedes curettage, a satisfactory fractional curettage can still be accomplished (25).

DILATATION AND CURETTAGE (D&C)

The most frequently performed surgical procedure in gynecology is cervical dilatation and uterine curettage. Referred to universally as a D&C, this operation is often the first surgical procedure to be undertaken by the doctor preparing to be a specialist in obstetrics and/or gynecology. It is generally recognized that the technique of D&C is not difficult or tricky to learn. Few surgical procedures are as straightforward or more suitable for unvaried routine performance (20).

Conventional D&C of the uterus is indicated under the following circumstances (42):

1. To evaluate abnormal uterine bleeding in patients in whom the cervical os is so tight that an endometrial biopsy cannot be performed.
2. To evaluate and diagnose the cause of postmenopausal uterine bleeding when a diagnosis has not been made clear by endometrial biopsy. Knowledge of the presence of an endometrial polyp or malignant tumor is essential to the patient's treatment.
3. Immediately preceding hysterectomy in a patient with abnormal uterine bleeding, because positive or suspicious endometrial findings may influence the operative decision.
4. To empty the uterus of its contents when unwanted products of conception remain, as after an incomplete abortion.
5. For the patient with intractable menorrhagia and an enlarged uterus, to distinguish between adenomyosis interna and uterine leiomyomas, particularly submucous leiomyomas, clarifying a recommendation for treatment.
6. As part of the work-up of an infertility patient with leiomyomas when a hysterogram has not clarified the location and types of leiomyomas present (e.g., submucous).
7. In the evaluation of a patient with an abnormal Pap smear, when there is no gross or colposcopically visible lesion of the cervix.
8. To treat known or suspected intrauterine synechiae (Asherman syndrome). Adhesions may be freed and an intrauterine device inserted to keep the walls of the uterine cavity apart during the healing process.

Although D&C of the uterus may be performed with the patient under analgesia only, or under local anesthesia using paracervical block, it is generally performed with the patient under brief general or regional anesthesia to provide the opportunity for careful examination of the internal genitalia at a time when all painful stimuli have been removed. D&C is ideally suited to an ambulatory setting.

There is both dogma and confusion in operating room procedure manuals concerning the degree of surgical "prep" needed for a D&C. What has been recommended seems to have been determined principally by the site at which the procedure will take place. In all instances, cleansing or bacteriostatic douches, pubic shaving, and enemas are not only unnecessary and serve no useful purpose but also add to the patient's discomfort.

Ambulatory Surgical Center

For D&C in an ambulatory setting, the vagina and cervix are painted with a solution of povidone-iodine (Betadine). Instruments are sterile, draping is minimal, and the surgeon, whose hands have been washed but not necessarily scrubbed, wears sterile gloves.

Hospital Operating Rooms

D&C in the hospital operating room is generally done under maximum aseptic techniques. This is important because, in certain patients, the gravid uterus is readily prone to infection and is easily perforated. The atrophic or cancerous uterus also may be easily perforated. The patient is prepared with nonabrasive perineal and vaginal wash and then the operative area is painted with povidone-iodine (Betadine). The patient is fully draped and instruments are sterile. The surgeon is fully gowned, masked, capped, and gloved (23).

Technique

Suction curettage may be used to complete an abortion. When curettage is to be performed in a recently pregnant uterus, intramuscular or intravenous injection of an oxytocic should produce a helpful, firm contraction of the myometrium, increasing its resistance to perforation. When outpatient curettage of the nonpregnant uterus is performed with a suction apparatus, the procedure can be preceded by administration of some analgesia or a paracervical block. The majority of cases of diagnostic uterine curettage should be accomplished in a fractional manner using the sharp curette.

A careful examination with the patient under anesthesia should be first performed. This always provides unexpected and vital information concerning diagnosis and future clinical management. It may also provide valuable information about the choice of the route and technical details of a possible future hysterectomy; one should note the size, shape, and mobility of the uterus, the location and size of the cul-de-sac, and the strength and elasticity of the uterosacral ligaments, the cardinal ligaments, and the urogenital diaphragm.

After the axis and size of the uterus have been determined, the anterior cervical lip should be grasped by a tenaculum for traction and the endocervical canal carefully scraped with a small, sharp curette (such as the Duncan), up to but not beyond the internal cervical os. One may start curettage at the 12 o'clock position and proceed in a careful clockwise or counterclockwise direction around the circumference of the cavity. The curettings are saved on a piece of Telfa or gauze to be processed separately from the specimen obtained later from the endometrial cavity. The malleable sound should then be bent to accommodate the anteflexion, anteversion, retroflexion, or retroversion of the uterus. The sound is best grasped at its round shaft rather than held firmly by the flat part of the end, because the latter practice would impede the tendency of the sound to follow the path of least resistance, the axis of the uterus. The minimal force exerted on both sound and curette during the process of their introduction should be similar to that required to hold a pencil or a pen; forceful insertion is to be avoided to decrease the risk of perforation.

After a blunt-tipped, malleable Simpson uterine sound has been gently inserted into the axis of the uterine cavity, careful note is made of the depth of the cavity from the external cervical os to the top of the fundus. Not only is this important in establishing the size of the endometrial cavity, but it also tells the operator precisely the depth beyond which the curette should not be passed during the curettage. The cervical canal and internal cervical os are then expanded by the passage of the graduated dilators to a size large enough to permit the introduction of the largest size of curette and/or polyp forceps that will be used during the procedure. Gradual dilatation with the patient under anesthesia markedly reduces the risk of rupture or permanent damage to the musculature of the cervix. A sharp curette is gently grasped and introduced into the endometrial cavity to the top of the fundus. The handle is then firmly grasped, and, by firm traction against the resisting uterus, the curette is made to scrape the endometrial cavity down to but not through the presumed basal layer. In an orderly clockwise or counterclockwise direction, the endometrium is scraped from all segments and quadrants. Scraping is stopped when the passage of the sharp edge of the curette across the surface of the endometrium produces the delicate sensation of a "grating" resistance, characteristic of the basal layer.

Curettage and Asherman Syndrome

As soon as the entire circumference of the endocervix has been curetted, the cervix should then be dilated sufficiently to admit the polyp forceps easily. A larger curette and the polyp forceps should then be used to remove the tissue lining the uterine cavity carefully but thoroughly and systematically. However, the operator must always be mindful of the possibility that an over-thorough curettage can remove literally all of the endometrium over areas sufficient to result in amenorrhea. This most unfortunate result of a curettage, known as Asherman syndrome, is most likely to follow a particularly thorough effort to clean out an aborting uterus. Usually the deeper invaginations of endometrial tissue into the myometrium are not removed during even a thorough curettage of the nonpregnant uterus. This is important to remember, because it is these undisturbed portions of endometrium that serve as the foci from which the endometrium will proliferate rapidly after a curettage. It is not the technique of curetting as much as the status of the myometrium that largely determines the risk of removing too much endometrium. The myometrium of the pregnant or aborting uterus is relatively soft and relaxed, and in that state offers little resistance. Under such circumstances the curette tends to spread myometrial fibers more readily and superficially, but, significantly, it scrapes out endometrial tissue at a greater depth than if the myometrial tone was the tonic or firmly contracted state of the nonpregnant uterus. Therefore, when curettage of an aborting uterus is indicated, measures should be taken to decrease the risk of removing too much endometrium. Firm contraction of the myometrium can be ensured by an intravenous or intramuscular injection of an oxytocic (Ergotrate, Methergine, Pitocin, Syntocinon, etc.) 2 or 3 minutes before curettage of the uterine cavity.

When the endometrium has been adequately curetted in this orderly fashion, and the presence of any submucous irregularities, diverticula, or septa in the cavity of the uterus has been noted, the curettings are separately saved on a piece of Telfa or gauze. The specimen is carefully examined and palpated. Benign tissue is soft and spongy and, when squeezed, is somewhat elastic and resists shattering. In contrast, the tissue of malignancy tends to be hard and rather fragile. When gently squeezed, it will fragment and shatter. The cavity of the uterus should then be explored with polyp or kidney stone forceps, because an endometrial polyp of almost any size may be missed by the curette, particularly if the polyp has a narrow base. After the polyp forceps have been introduced, the jaws are opened and then closed in various quadrants in the cavity of the uterus, and after each closing a tug is made to see if any resistance is encountered. If one finds a narrow-based polyp of a size sufficient to negotiate the dilated cervical canal, it can safely be removed by twisting of the forceps.

After all instruments are removed, the uterus and cervix are carefully inspected. If significant fresh bleeding from the endometrial cavity is noted, the uterine cavity should be carefully sounded to ensure that neither perforation of the uterus nor laceration of the endocervix has occurred. Should either of these circumstances be noted, appropriate observation and treatment should be instituted. Excessive bleeding from tenaculum marks on the cervix can be cauterized or a gentle and temporary packing can be placed against the face of the cervix.

The operative report should be dictated immediately while all the details of each procedure are fresh in the surgeon's mind. A plan should be made for the removal of any packing that may have been placed. One should convey to the patient or her family the operative findings and discharge instructions, and arrange for postoperative office evaluation.

Complications

Although a minor surgical procedure, a D&C must be accomplished with delicacy and precision if it is to be effective. Done carelessly, forcefully, or thoughtlessly, the procedure can cause serious damage to the patient.

Perforation of the wall of the uterus by either a sound or a curette is generally a result of failure to identify the proper axis of the cavity of the uterus, which may often be in anteflexion or retroflexion (Fig. 4.16). The perforating instrument is forced through the wall of the uterus, often on the presumption that it is negotiating a somewhat stenotic internal os. Some possible sites of uterine perforation and the lateral proximity of nearby arteries are shown in Figure 4.17. When the myometrium is compromised by softness due to pregnancy or invasion by malignant tumor, perforation becomes quite easy. It is recognized by the passage of the tip of the sound or curette deeper than the cavity of the uterus. The instrument may be introduced all the way to its handle without any resistance.

When perforation occurs with the sound, the instrument should be promptly withdrawn. Little of consequence will usually follow. The position of the uterus should be carefully determined by bimanual examination and the sound bent an appropriate amount to negotiate the uterine cavity safely. If the sound has been reinserted in the axis of the uterine cavity, the insertion will generally stop when the top of the instrument has reached the fundus of the uterus and the procedure continued to completion. The instruments must be inserted gently, with no more force than would be required to hold a pencil or pen for the purpose of writing. If, following perforation, the proper axis of the uterus cannot be determined, it is best to discontinue the procedure and schedule it for some future date, at which time the myometrium will have had an opportunity to heal.

The patient should be told postoperatively of the event and should be watched for tachycardia, hypotension, abdominal tenderness, fever, and other signs of intraperitoneal bleeding or uterine or pelvic infection. Any of these signs will be known within 24 hours.

If the tip of the sharp curette has been made to perforate the uterus, and this has not been recognized by the surgeon, great damage may be done to the visceral contents of the pelvis by curettage. If the curette brings forth evidence of perforation by recovery of intestinal epithelium, bowel wall, or bowel contents, immediate laparotomy is essential to repair whatever damage has been produced. If the operator has a strong suspicion that intestinal damage has been produced but the character of the curettings fails to confirm this suspicion, the observations of a preliminary diagnostic laparoscopy may be of value. If it is suspected that no damage to the bowel has been done, the patient may be observed only.

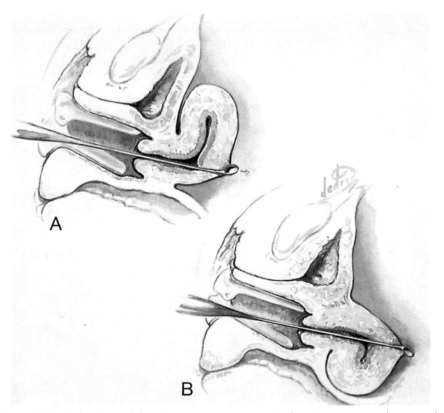

Figure 4.16. Perforation of the uterus at curettage. **A.** Failure to recognize the axis of a markedly anteflexed uterus may result in the curette perforating the posterior wall of the uterus. **B.** Similarly, perforation of the anterior wall of the uterus may occur when retroflexion is present. (From Nichols DH, Sweeney PJ, eds. Ambulatory gynecology. 2nd ed. Philadelphia: Lippincott-Raven, 1995. Used with permission.)

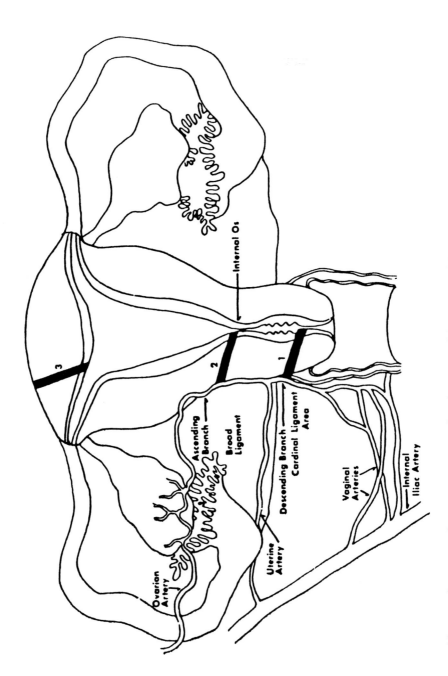

Figure 4.17. Possible sites of uterine perforation. Low cervical perforation with laceration of descending branches of uterine artery (1). Perforation at junction of cervix and lower uterine segment with laceration of ascending branch of uterine artery (2). Fundal perforation (3). (From Berek JS, Stubblefield PG. Anatomical and clinical correlations of uterine perforations. Am J Obstet Gynecol 1979;135:181. Used with permission.)

If it is evident initially that a severe endocervical stenosis is present in a patient who is about to have a D&C, and it is possible to insert only a small and very narrow sound or probe and not possible to dilate the endocervical canal significantly, a small *Laminaria* tent may be inserted along the path of the sound and the patient rescheduled for the D&C 24 hours later. At that time, the tent may be removed; the cervix will be sufficiently dilated to permit insertion of a small curette.

Examination of Curettings

The experienced clinician often recognizes the evidence of endocrine dysfunction by the gross appearance of the endometrial fragments obtained by a sampling technique. However, the therapy to be instituted should be based upon the histologic appraisal. It is also true that the gynecologist often recognizes evidence of malignancy in uterine curettings, but therapy should not be initiated before histologic confirmation. Fragments of normal endometrium, proliferative and premenstrual or secretory, can usually be smoothed out on a sponge and will appear as a fragment of relatively thin or thick membrane. Fragments of tissue from an area infiltrated or replaced by malignancy, however, appear as little chunks of tissue that have more of a third dimension and when placed on a sponge will probably fragment, rather than smooth out like a membrane.

References

1. Axe S, Parmeley T, Woodruff JD, et al. Adenomas in minor vestibular glands. Obstet Gynecol 1986;68:16.
2. Baggish MS. Extraperitoneal laser surgery. In: Nichols DH, ed. Gynecologic and obstetric surgery. St. Louis: Mosby–Year Book, 1993:273–285.
3. Baggish MS. Management of cervical intraepithelial neoplasia by CO_2 laser. Obstet Gynecol 1982; 60:378.
4. Baggish MS, Dorsey JH. CO_2 laser for the treatment of vulvar carcinoma-in-situ. Obstet Gynecol 1981;57:371.
5. Bazin S, Bouchard C, Brisson J, et al. Vulvar vestibulitis syndrome: an exploratory case-control study. Obstet Gynecol 1994;83:47–50.
6. Bloss JD. The use of electrosurgical techniques in the management of premalignant diseases of the vulva, vagina and cervix: an excisional rather than an ablative approach. Am J Obstet Gynecol 1993;169:1081–1085.
7. Burke L. The use of carbon dioxide laser in the therapy of cervical intra-epithelial neoplasia. Am J Obstet Gynecol 1982;144:337.
8. Burkhardt E, Girardi F. Conization of the uterine cervix. In: Nichols DH, ed. Gynecologic and obstetric surgery. St. Louis, Mosby–Year Book, 1993:264–272.
9. Capen CV, Masterson BJ, Magrine JF, et al. Laser therapy of vaginal intra-epithelial neoplasia. Am J Obstet Gynecol 1982;142:973.
10. Cheerham DR. Bartholin's cyst: marsupialization or aspiration? Am J Obstet Gynecol 1985; 152:569–570.
11. Coulter A, Klassan A, MacKenzie IZ, McPherson K. Diagnostic dilatation and curettage: is it used appropriately? BMJ 1993;306:236–239.
12. Davis GD. Management of Bartholin duct cysts with the carbon dioxide laser. Obstet Gynecol 1985;63:279–280.
13. DiSaia PJ. Microinvasive cancer of the cervix in pregnancy. In: Nichols DH, ed. Clinical problems, injuries and complications of gynecologic surgery. 2nd ed. Baltimore: Williams & Wilkins, 1988:239–340.
14. DiSaia PJ, Creasman WT. Clinical gynecologic oncology. 2nd ed. St. Louis: CV Mosby, 1984:483–484.
15. Draeby-Kristiansen JD, Garsaae M, Bruun M, Hansen K. Ten years after cryosurgery treatment of cervical intraepithelial neoplasia. Am J Obstet Gynecol 1991;165:43–45.
16. Friedrich EG. The vulvar vestibule. J Reprod Med 1983;28:773.
17. Friedrick EG. Vulvar vestibulitis syndrome. J Reprod Med 1987;32:110–114.
18. Garcia C-R, Pfeifer SM. Myomectomy. In: Nichols DH, ed. Gynecologic and obstetric surgery. St. Louis: Mosby–Year Book, 1993:620.
19. Goetsch MF. Vulvar vestibulitis: prevalence and historic features in a general gynecologic practice population. Am J Obstet Gynecol 1991;164:1609–1616.
20. Grimes DA. Diagnostic dilatation and curettage: a reappraisal. Am J Obstet Gynecol 1982;142:1–6.
21. Hale RW, Pion RJ. Laminaria: an under utilized clinical adjunct. Clin Obstet Gynecol 1972;15:829–850.

22. Hallam NF, West J, Harper C, Edwards A, Hope S, Merriman H, Pandherk S, Pinches P, Slade R, Marsh G, Charnock M, Gray W. Large loop excision of the transformation zone (LLETZ) as an alternative to both local ablative and cone biopsy treatment: a series of 1000 patients. J Gynecol Surg 1993;9:77–82.

23. Haskins A. Questions and answers. JAMA 1979;241:623.

24. Heah J. Method of treatment for cysts and abscesses of Bartholin's gland. Br J Obstet Gynecol 1988;195:321–322.

25. Helmkamp GF, Denslow BL, Bonfiglio TA, Beecham JB. Cervical conization: when is uterine dilatation and curettage also indicated? Am J Obstet Gynecol 1983;146:893–894.

26. Itzkowic D. Uterine perforation associated with endometrial ablation. Aust N Z J Obstet Gynecol 1992;32:359–361.

27. Julian CG, Callison J, Woodruff JD. Plastic management of extensive vulvar defects. Obstet Gynecol 1971;38:193–198.

28. Kaufman RH, Friedrich EG. The carbon dioxide laser in the treatment of vulvar disease. Clin Obstet Gynecol 1985;28:220.

29. Kelly RA, Foster DC, Woodruff JD. Subcutaneous injection of triamcinolone acetonide in the treatment of chronic vulvar pruritus. Am J Obstet Gynecol 1993;169:568–570.

30. Knapstein PG. Principles of reconstructive surgery. In: Knapstein PG, Friedberg V, Sevin B-U, eds. Reconstructive surgery in gynecology. New York: Thieme Medical Publishers, 199:1–9.

31. Kristensen J, Langhoff-Roos J, Kristensen FB. Increased risk of preterm birth in women with cervical conization. Obstet Gynecol 1993;81:1005–1008.

32. Lashgari M, Keene M. Excision of Bartholin duct cysts using the CO2 laser. Obstet Gynecol 1986;67:735–736.

33. Lewis BV. Diagnostic dilatation and curettage in young women. BMJ 1993;306:225–226.

34. March CM. Hysteroscopy. In: Nichols DH, ed. Gynecologic and obstetric surgery. St. Louis: Mosby–Year Book, 1993:750–767.

35. McKay M, Frankman O, Horowitz BJ. Vulvar vestibulitis and vestibular papillomatosis: report of the ISSVD Committee on Vulvodynia. J Reprod Med 1991;36:413–415.

36. Nichols DH, McGoldrick KL. Minor and ambulatory surgery. In: Nichols DH, Sweeney PJ, eds. Ambulatory gynecology. 2nd ed. Philadelphia: JB Lippincott, 1995.

37. Ostergard DR. Cryosurgical treatment of cervical intra-epithelial neoplasia. Obstet Gynecol 1980;56:231.

38. Peckham BM, Maki DG, Patterson JJ, Hafez G-R. Focal vulvitis: a characteristic syndrome and cause of dyspareunia. Am J Obstet Gynecol 1986;154:855–864.

39. Ramey JW, Koonings PP, Given FT, Acosta AA. The process of carcinogenesis for endometrial adenocarcinomas could be short: development of a malignancy after endometrial ablation. Am J Obstet Gynecol 1994;170:1370–1371.

40. Raphael SI, Burke L. Laser and cryosurgery. In: Nichols DH, Evrard JR, eds. Ambulatory Gynecology. Philadelphia: Harper & Row, 1985:328–349.

41. Rock JA, Azziz R. Wolffian duct cyst at the vaginal vault. In: Nichols DH, ed. Clinical problems, injuries and complications of gynecologic surgery. 2nd ed. Baltimore: Williams & Wilkins, 1988:144–146.

42. Smith JJ, Schulman H. Current dilatation and curettage practice: a need for revision. Obstet Gynecol 1985;65:516–518.

43. Stafl A, Wilkinson EJ, Mattingly RF. Laser treatment of cervical and vaginal neoplasia. Am J Obstet Gynecol 1977;128:128.

44. Thomas TG. Hyperaesthesia of the vulva. In: The Diseases of Women. Philadelphia: Henry C. Lea, 1880:145–146.

45. Townsend DE. Cryosurgery for CIN. Obstet Gynecol Surv 1979;34:828.

46. Townsend DE, Levine RU, Crum DP, et al. Treatment of vaginal carcinoma-in-situ with the CO_2 laser. Am J Obstet Gynecol 1982;143:565.

47. Townsend DE, Richart RM. Cryotherapy and the carbon dioxide laser management of cervical intraepithelial neoplasia: a control comparison. Obstet Gynecol 1983;61:75.

48. Umpierre SA, Kaufman, Adam E, et al. Human papillomavirus DNA in tissue biopsy specimens of vulvar vestibulitis patients treated with interferon. Obstet Gynecol 1991;78:693–695.

49. Walton LA, Baker VV. Mechanical and chemical preparation of the abdomen and vagina. In: Buchsbaum HJ, Walton LA, eds. Strategies in gynecologic surgery. New York: Springer-Verlag, 1986:46–47.

50. Wiser WL: Mass in the lateral wall of the vagina. In: Nichols DH, DeLancey JOL, eds. Clinical problems, injuries and complications of gynecologic surgery. 3rd ed. Baltimore: Williams & Wilkins, 1995.

51. Woodruff JD. Vestibular adenitis. In: Quilligan EJ, Zuspan FP, eds. Current therapy in obstetrics and gynecology. Philadelphia: WB Saunders, 1990:145–148.

52. Woodruff JD, Friedrich EG. The vestibule. Clin Obstet Gynecol 1985;28:134–141.

53. Woodruff JD, Genadry R, Poliakoff S. Treatment of dyspareunia and vaginal outlet distortions by perineoplasty. Obstet Gynecol 1981;57:750–754.

54. Woodruff JD, Parmley THG. Infection of the minor vestibular gland. Obstet Gynecol 1983;62:609.

55. Wright CV, Cavies E, Riopelle MA. Laser surgery for cervical intra-epithelial neoplasia: Principles and results. Am J Obstet Gynecol 1983;145:181.

56. Yaron Y, Shenhar M, Jaffa AJ, Lessing JB, Peyser MR. Uterine rupture at 33 weeks gestation subsequent to hysteroscopic uterine perforation. Am J Obstet Gynecol 1994;170:786–787.

Types of Prolapse

Genital prolapse may result when normal pelvic supports are subjected to chronic increases in intra-abdominal pressure or when congenitally defective genital support responds to even normal intra-abdominal pressure. The single most common etiologic factor of genital prolapse is parturition, and the increased intra-abdominal pressure and the softening of the pelvic connective tissues and smooth muscle as a result of hormonal influences during pregnancy may be contributing factors. The trauma of labor and the increased weight of the uterus during the period of involution may also be contributing factors. Types as well as degrees of genital prolapse may be evident singly or in combination as a result of damage to any one or more of the following seven separate supportive systems:

1. The bony pelvis to which the soft tissues ultimately attach
2. The subperitoneal retinaculum and smooth muscle component of the broad ligaments
3. The cardinal-uterosacral ligament complex
4. The pelvic diaphragm, as well as the levator ani and its fibromuscular attachments to the pelvic organs
5. The urogenital diaphragm
6. The perineal body
7. The walls of the vagina, with essential loss of tone and evident weakness as a result of both pathologic stretching and the attenuating changes of aging

In each patient with a genital prolapse, the surgeon must determine the mechanism that is responsible for the prolapse in order to plan the reconstruction and overall medical management that will remedy the specific defect. For example, the restoration of normal intra-abdominal pressure alone may relieve the genital prolapse and urinary stress incontinence associated with ascites or large ovarian tumors if the degree of pelvic strain has not yet become irreversible. Although the usual anatomic or morphologic classifications of degrees of genital prolapse do not take into account the significant differences in the various causes of prolapse, it is essential for the surgeon to recognize these etiologic differences; they affect the likelihood that the displacement will progress, the rate at which it will progress, and the chances of surgical cure or recurrence. Therefore, the surgeon must take the etiology into consideration if postoperative results are to be optimal.

Either excessive intra-abdominal pressures or inherent weaknesses in the supporting tissues may lead to varying degrees of genital prolapse; in the extreme degree, the vagina may be turned virtually inside out. These forces may work alone or in combination and at quite different times in life. It is essential to recognize both the primary condition and the components involved in the secondary damage when evaluating the patient's problem. The most important single step in surgical treatment is to recognize and correct, or at times overcorrect, the primary damage or weakness. Unless the correction of the primary condition is adequate, the prolapse is likely to recur in spite of an initially successful surgical repair of the more obvious damage.

CLASSIFICATION OF VAGINAL RELAXATION

As Ricci (21) has pointed out, a classification of the degrees of prolapse has not always been clear to all authorities, the terms *prolapsus uteri*, *descensus*, and *procidentia* often being used synonymously. Sabatier (23) in 1757 called the slightest degree, or first stage, a relaxation of the uterus; a greater degree, prolapse; and protrusion through the vulva, procidentia. Cooper (4) in 1813 adhered to the classification of "first-, second- and third-degree prolapse." Today we essentially follow the system described in 1980 by Beecham (2) to describe the degree of prolapse of the contributing elements, there being no instruments of any kind within the vagina. Including our modifications, it is as follows:

Cystocele

1. First degree: The anterior vaginal wall is visible at the introitus from the urethral meatus to the anterior fornix.
2. Second degree: The inferior bladder wall and its attached vaginal wall extend outside the introitus.
3. Third degree: This cystocele is part of a third-degree uterine prolapse or total prolapse of a posthysterectomy vaginal apex. The entire bladder is outside the introitus.
4. Fourth degree: The full length of the urethra and the entire bladder are outside the introitus.

Rectocele

1. First degree: When the perineum is depressed, a saccular protrusion of the vaginorectal wall is visible.
2. Second degree: The sacculation is visible at the introitus without depressing the perineum.
3. Third degree: The sacculation protrudes or extends outside the introitus.

Uterine Prolapse

1. First degree: The cervix is visible when the perineum is depressed.
2. Second degree: The cervix extends over the perineal body, i.e., through the introitus.
3. Third degree: The cervix and corpus uteri totally extend outside the introitus, but there is no significant hypermobility of the urethra.
4. Fourth degree: Same as third degree, but with hypermobility of the urethra. There is more than a 90-degree change in the urethral axis.

Enterocele

This saccular defect of the posterior cul-de-sac and vaginal wall may be part of a high rectocele. The peritoneal sac, which dissects down the rectovaginal septum, contains bowel, in contradistinction to the condition of the deep cul-de-sac, which does not contain bowel.

1. First degree: The sac is visible in the vagina when the perineum is depressed.
2. Second degree: The sac extends just through the introitus.
3. Third degree: The sac extends out of the introitus and generally contains small and/or large bowel.

Prolapse of the Vaginal Apex

Following total or incomplete hysterectomy the apical vaginal scar or remaining cervix can prolapse. This can occur alone or in combination with a cystocele, enterocele, rectocele, or all three.

1. First degree: The vaginal apex is visible when the perineum is depressed.
2. Second degree: The apex extends just through the introitus.
3. Third degree: The upper two-thirds of the vagina is outside the introitus. The sac will contain bladder, urethra, ureters, and small and/or large bowel. The evagination is cranial to the urogenital diaphragm, and hypermobility of the urethra is not significant.
4. Fourth degree: The entire vagina is outside the introitus and includes the tissues caudal to the urogenital diaphragm. Hypermobility of the urethra is present with more than a 90-degree change in the urethral axis.

The patient is examined first while at rest in the lithotomy position, then while straining as by a Valsalva maneuver, and then when standing, first at rest and then while straining. The maximal displacement of each element of the prolapse is noted.

VAGINAL PROLAPSE

Bonney pointed out in 1914 that the relationship of the vagina to the peritoneal cavity is the same as the inturned finger of a rubber glove which may be turned out by closing the mouth of the glove and compressing air locked within it (3). (In the instance of the rubber glove, he pointed out, the pressure is purely gaseous and depends upon the amount of force supplied by the hand compressing it. Intra-abdominal pressure is more complicated, however, depending partly on the intestinal gas pressure, which acts equally in all directions; partly on the contraction of muscles surrounding the abdominal cavity; and partly on the weight of the movable viscera, which are dependent upon gravity and therefore move downward.) Why does the rubber glove evert so readily, whereas the vagina does not (Fig. 5.1)?

The fascial strands that maintain the position of the vagina in the pelvis become stretched and elongated longitudinally in the direction of any force applied to them. Progressive normal labor usually thins and stretches the strands of fascial support, but does not disrupt them. Obviously, the precipitous force is more likely to disrupt the attachments and continuity of fascial fibers than is more moderate and repeated stress. Precipitous descent of the fetal presenting part into the vagina that is resisting rapid dilation is also likely to disrupt connective tissue support, with or without laceration of the vaginal wall.

Basically, vaginal vault prolapse falls into one of two groups: prolapse of the upper vagina or eversion of the lower vagina. These may occur separately or together, and they are produced by quite different etiologic factors. Prolapse of the upper half of the vagina results primarily from a weakening of the upper vaginal supports (Fig. 5.2B), usually because of the forces and damages of labor and delivery, but sometimes because of chronically increased intra-abdominal pressure that allows the upper vagina gradually to evert within itself. Such a prolapse, with its consequent vaginal telescoping, shortens the length of the vagina and increases the width of the anterior vaginal wall. There is usually an enterocele and generally some degree of cystocele; an accompanying rectocele is uncommon, however, since the pelvic and urogenital diaphragms often remain intact.

The cardinal and uterosacral ligaments function as the "stays" and provide the principal suspension of the upper vagina and cervix, holding them over the levator plate. The pelvic diaphragm and its levator plate may be intact, but if the "stays" have become permanently stretched or elongated, the cervix will have a degree of mobility sufficient for it to slide or fall through the levator hiatus and over the edge of the levator plate, with consequent prolapse of the upper vagina. When, in addition, the patient is observed while straining or bearing down, it will be noted that, although the upper vagina prolapses, the lower vagina is not involved, and neither moves nor tends to evert so long as there is demonstrable integrity of the pelvic and urogenital diaphragms. Because the damage is

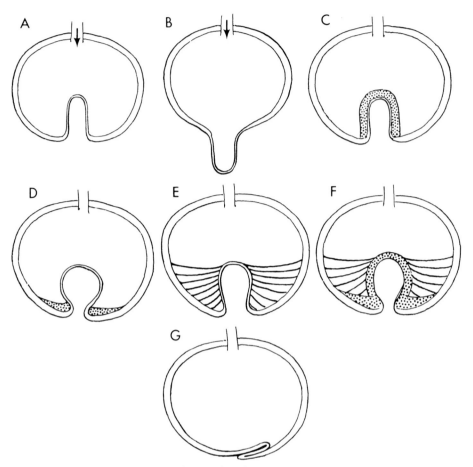

Figure 5.1. Bonney's description of vaginal prolapse.
   As an approach to the problem, let us first take the case of an artificial cul-de-sac in-
   truding into an artificial, closed gas-containing cavity (**A**) and consider what steps could
   be taken to prevent the cul-de-sac from turning inside out when the pressure in the
   closed cavity is raised (**B**).
1. Because the ease with which a cul-de-sac can be turned inside out depends largely on
   the resistance of its wall and the relation between the thickness of the wall and caliber
   of the lumen, turning inside out could be prevented either by making the wall of the cul-
   de-sac rigid or by thickening it so much in relation to the caliber of its lumen that turning inside out would be impossible, as in the case of a piece of pressure tubing (**C**).
2. If the outlet of the cul-de-sac were sufficiently narrowed, complete turning inside out
   would be rendered impossible for, although the cul-de-sac might collapse down as far
   as the constriction, it could not pass through it. This is really a special case of the general principle enunciated under 1 (**D**).
3. If the cul-de-sac, instead of being straight, were sharply bent, the effect of raising the pressure in the closed cavity would be to increase the bend and make turning inside out more
   difficult or impossible (**G**).
4. The out-turning effect could be combated by attaching the wall of the cul-de-sac to the
   wall of the closed cavity, either directly or by some intermediary structure, as for example a series of threads (**E**) or by a combination of the devices mentioned (**F**). When we
   come to consider that which obtains in the case of the vagina and uterus we find that
   nature has anticipated us in all of these devices. (After Bonney V: The sustentacular
   apparatus of the female genital canal, the displacements that result from the yielding of
   its several components, and their appropriate treatment. *J Obstet Gynaecol Br Emp*
   45:328, 1914.)

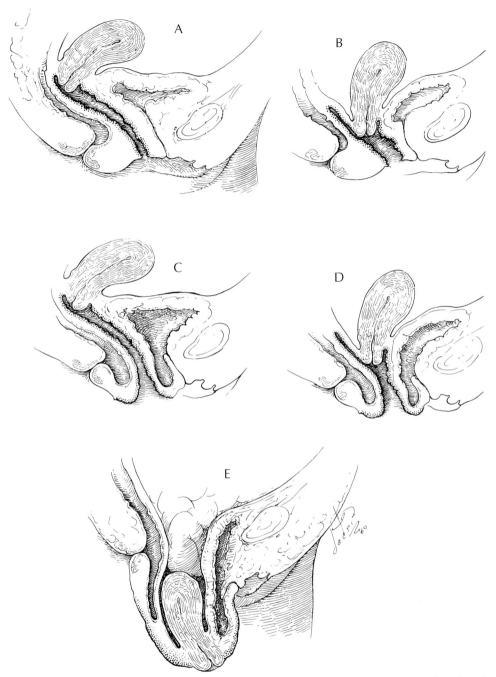

Figure 5.2. Degrees of prolapse. **A.** Sagittal section after Bonney (3) of a normally positioned vagina. **B.** Prolapse of the upper vagina may result from weakening of the upper vaginal supports, the cardinal and uterosacral ligament complex. **C.** Eversion of the lower vagina results from damage to the pelvic and urogenital diaphragms. **D.** Simultaneous vault prolapse and eversion may occur. **E.** Procidentia may evolve as the result of unrestrained progression of any of the above types of prolapse. (Reproduced with permission of Postgraduate Medicine from Nichols DH. Types of genital prolapse. Postgrad Med 1969;46(5):183–187.)

anterior to the rectum, rectocele is not necessarily associated even though the cul-de-sac is being pulled downward, producing a traction type of enterocele.

Eversion of the lower vagina (Fig. 5.2C), characterized by cystocele and rectocele, results from loss of support because of damage to the soft tissues attaching the vagina to the pelvic and urogenital diaphragms and, although usually the result of obstetric trauma, may occur as part of a general postmenopausal atrophic weakening of the pelvic supporting tissues or of coincident neuropathy. A third possibility is that of the two conditions being simultaneous, in which case the vagina will be prolapsing above and rolling out or everting below (Fig. 5.2D). Which of these two mechanisms is the dominant or initial one can usually be determined by manual replacement of the prolapsed organs and, without touching the patient, asking her to bear down and then observe which segment of vagina seems to prolapse first. If a cystocele and rectocele appear first, followed by the cervix and vaginal vault, the primary site of damage is probably the lower supporting tissues and lower vaginal eversion is dominant. If, on the other hand, the cervix and vaginal vault appear first, followed by the cystocele and rectocele, the primary site of damage in that circumstance is probably the upper vaginal suspensory tissues. Unrestrained progression of either eversion of upper or lower vagina or both may continue so that the result may be a vagina turned completely inside out (Fig. 5.2E). When the cervix and uterus extend completely outside the bony pelvis, the condition is termed procidentia (Fig. 5.3). As organs drop, traction is applied to previously uninvolved supporting tissue attached to neighboring organs, and extensive secondary damage will result.

The rate of progression has a great deal to do with the symptomatology and the opportunity to recognize the etiology. When prolapse is rapidly progressive, acute discomfort or concern is likely to bring the patient promptly to the physician for evaluation, whereas degrees of descensus that are static, chronic, or slowly progressive are more likely to be first noted without the strong complaint of the patient at the time of a routine pelvic examination. In the latter situation, pertinent symptoms may have developed so slowly that the patient has accepted them matter-of-factly without recognizing their relevance.

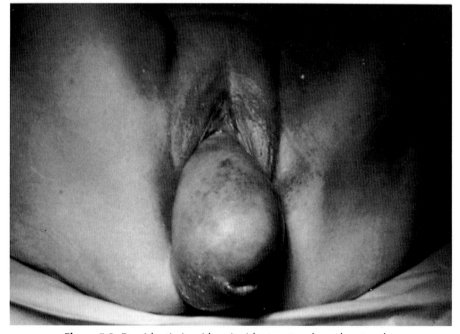

Figure 5.3. Procidentia is with coincident cystocele and rectocele.

Malpas (17) has described a nonprogressive postobstetric genital prolapse characterized by mild degrees of relaxation, in which the lateral supporting tissues of the vagina and uterus, although stretched and torn, apparently become refused to the lateral walls of the pelvis but at a lower level. This refusion is sufficiently stable in most instances to relieve the patient of troublesome symptoms, provided the urogenital diaphragm remains relatively well preserved. If the pelvic diaphragm is not damaged, the lesion may remain nonprogressive and not require operative repair. Absence of progression between periodic examinations tends to identify this type of genital prolapse.

Slowly progressive uterovaginal prolapse is usually due to damage to the lateral supports of the cervix and upper vagina, whereas rapidly progressing prolapse is due in all probability to primarily atrophic failure of all of the supporting tissues, including the pelvic floor. Relatively asymptomatic progression of a noted degree of prolapse is far more ominous than is a static condition, because the progression suggests a transient phase inevitably advancing toward more complete prolapse. Detection of prolapse progression from one annual visit to another is more likely when such periodic examinations have involved the same examiner and is less apparent when there has been a different examiner on each visit. The extent of each component of a prolapse will be more convincingly demonstrated by examination of the relaxed and then straining patient in the standing position, which adds the effects of gravity (preferably at least 6 months postpartum, when involution should be complete).

Involution does not reattach fascia to the sites of original attachment, and if such damage has occurred, it may be evident postpartum. Whenever an examiner first notes the loss of the normal concavity of the vaginal fornices, there is reason to expect that vaginal eversion will eventually develop.

Magdi (16) coined the term *elastic index* of a patient, suggesting that when the striae gravidarum are broad and coarse, there is less integrity of elastic tissue and the tendency toward prolapse is greater; conversely, when the striae are fine and narrow, both stretch and involution are adequate and neither laceration nor loss of tone is as likely to occur.

RACIAL DIFFERENCES IN GENITAL PROLAPSE

There may be individual and racial differences in connective tissue strengths, as noted by the relative infrequency with which black women sustain lacerations from spontaneous delivery and their relative immunity from uterine prolapse. After studying the Bantu, for example, Geldenhuys believed it was not so much environment that influenced the occurrence of prolapse but rather inherent racial constitutional factors, such as the size and form of the pelvis, the quality of the connective tissue and pelvic supports, and the tendency to fibrosis (5, 6).

Heyns (10) maintains that excess intra-abdominal pressure is a primary cause of genital prolapse in women and has observed the absence of prolapse in Bantu women as a fundamental racial difference. The Bantu woman, by not wearing corsets and by eating but one meal per day, has developed accommodation to a wide range of day-to-day changes in intra-abdominal pressure, even during pregnancy.

The racial incidence of genital prolapse and its significance were reported by F.G. Goldenhuys (5, 6) of the Department of Obstetrics and Gynecology, University of Pretoria, South Africa, who observed that during a 5-year period, from January 1945 through December 1949, 6302 European gynecologic inpatients were admitted to the Pretoria General Hospital. Of these patients, 410 underwent operations for genital prolapse, an incidence of 6.5 percent. During the same period, 3478 Bantu gynecologic patients were admitted, of whom only 21 were operated on for prolapse, an incidence of 0.6 percent. Direct communication with other institutions in South Africa indicated that prolapse was equally uncommon among other institutions treating Bantu women.

In Switzerland, the incidence of genital prolapse among gynecologic admissions was 12 percent at the Kanton Hospital in Zurich, and at the Clinique d'Gynecologie et Obstetrique, Geneva, the incidence was 5.7 percent during the same period of time. In

Hamburg, it was 5.4 percent; in Rome, 6.4 percent. Prolapse was common in India and in North America. Heyns also reported prolapse to be common in Brazil and in Egypt, but less common among Indonesians and Chinese (10).

In summary, it appears that prolapse occurs rather frequently among the white races, the Egyptians, and the women of India. It occurs less frequently among Orientals and African Americans, and is particularly uncommon in the South African Bantu as well as in the black women of West Africa.

The Bantu Woman

The size of the Bantu infant at birth is comparable to that of the European, and the Bantu is often prone to premature bearing down long before full dilatation of the cervix. Grand multiparity is common among the Bantu. In two-thirds of Bantu births, the fetal head is unengaged before the onset of labor. The average age of the Bantu primipara is not much different from that of the European primipara, and retroversion of the uterus is as common in Bantu women as in the European. Early rising after delivery is widely practiced by Bantu women.

Although episiotomy is common in North America, it seems to have been followed by a lesser incidence of prolapse. A routine episiotomy is not performed in the Bantu inasmuch as they are delivered for the most part at home under primitive conditions. The incidence of forceps deliveries is similarly much lower among the Bantu than among Europeans.

As already discussed, the most common single etiologic factor of genital prolapse is parturition, and it may be related to increased intra-abdominal pressure and softening of the pelvic connective tissues and smooth muscle as a result of hormonal influences. The trauma of labor and the increased weight of the uterus during the period of involution may also be contributing factors. The return of the pelvic floor to normal is faster in the Bantu woman than in the European, and subinvolution of the uterus is uncommon in the Bantu.

The Bantu woman differs from her European counterpart in that she makes more frequent use of the squatting position for defecation. However, Bantu women perform about the same hard manual labor as their men, much as do European peasant women. The mesoderm of black women differs in a number of respects from that of the Europeans, as is evidenced by the proliferation of connective tissue. For example, neurofibromatosis is common among black women, keloids develop more rapidly, the corium of the skin is thicker and has more sweat glands, the lips are thicker as a result of more fibroelastic tissue, and uterine leiomyomas are nine times more common than among the Europeans. The same observation seems to apply to the Bantu. Some believe that the woman with a wide, flat pelvis is more liable to develop prolapse, in contrast to the woman with a contracted pelvis, where the bony supports of the pelvic diaphragm are relatively small in comparison to the area of stress and strain. There is little doubt that the Bantu pelvis is comparatively small in relation to that of the European.

Postmenopausal atrophy is difficult to evaluate among the Bantu, considering that the decade from 60 to 70 years of age was the most common period for a patient to be operated upon for genital prolapse at Pretoria General Hospital at the time the Bantu were studied. The European women more frequently reached this age than the Bantu, because the average life expectancy of the former was 63 years. However, those Bantu women who did reach an advanced age did not often show genital prolapse.

Although malnutrition is common among the Bantu and deficiency diseases are frequent, these factors do not appear to predispose these women to genital prolapse. The Bantu woman has more pronounced lordosis than does the European woman.

The Oriental Woman

Zacharin (28) has studied possible causes for the relative infrequency of both genital prolapse and urinary incontinence among Orientals. His dissections of Chinese cadavers at the University of Hong Kong revealed that their primary urethral suspensory mechanism was almost vestigial, in contrast to the magnificent development of the levator ani complex in the usual occidental female. Unanswered, yet, is whether this unique development of the levator ani is an inherited characteristic or one acquired from their traditional way of life lifelong habit of sitting and of defecating in the squatting position.

CONGENITAL PROLAPSE

An occasional case of congenital origin associated with defective musculature or innervation becomes evident in infancy or childhood. Genital prolapse in the newborn has been reported, although it is rare. It may be associated with a congenital pelvic neuropathy affecting the pelvic muscles. Treatment is by manual reduction and, if the prolapse recurs, the wearing of a tiny pessary, the latter made from a rolled and tied l-inch Penrose drain. The pessary, removed only for cleaning, may be worn for several weeks (25). If vaginal and uterine edema is so great as to preclude manual replacement of the prolapse, the latter may be covered with hypertonic saline packs for several days, followed by temporarily sewing together the posterior half of the labia minora and majora (1). The stitches are removed after they have been in place for 2 weeks. Initial treatment by replacement is usually without recurrence if there is no significant associated primary neuropathy.

Stallworthy (26) has pointed out that a small percentage of those persons in the general population with congenital defects of their supporting tissues may marry and later reproduce. The fact that some subsequently develop prolapse does not prove that it was the pregnancy or delivery that caused the prolapse.

NULLIPAROUS GENITAL PROLAPSE

In North America approximately 2 percent of the women who develop prolapse are nullipara. Often nulliparous prolapse will be associated with a lifestyle of heavy physical labor, which produces marked increases in intra-abdominal pressure. When prolapse becomes evident before the menopause, the primary etiology appears to be pathologic elongation of the cardinal and uterosacral ligament complex of the upper suspensory support system, so that such patients typically display a prolapse of the upper vagina and coexistent elongation of the cervix. This may bring with it some traction-produced cystocele and enterocele. In the postmenopausal patient, however, the effects of atrophic changes may be superimposed upon a generalized muscular and connective tissue hypoplasia. This may be predicted by a relative absence of rugal folds, particularly evident in the vaginal epithelium covering the bladder. Local underdevelopment of the pelvic floor is often associated with noticeable hypoplasia of the uterus, occasionally related to and made worse by postmenopausal atrophy. Such a patient, on straining, may still display bulging of the tissues at the outlet even after extensive repair.

PSEUDOPROLAPSE WITH ANESTHESIA

During diagnostic dilatation and curettage, with the patient under general anesthesia, the cervix of a movable uterus can easily be brought to the vaginal outlet, but this may or may not represent observation of genuine prolapse. There is significant difference in the findings suggesting prolapse when the evaluation involves an anesthetized patient. Under anesthesia, the levator ani is in effect paralyzed, the patient is not straining but is recumbent and relaxed, and there is no increased intra-abdominal pressure. However, direct traction on the cervix is an abnormal pull in an abnormal direction. Under such circumstances the pulled-upon cervix acts as a driving wedge through the levator hiatus, which has already partly been separated by the speculum distending the introitus and retracting the pelvic floor (20). A patient evaluated in this way may have no genuine genital prolapse, particularly when pelvic relationships are being evaluated with the tone of the muscular and connective tissue supports paralyzed by anesthesia. The best assessment of the true degree of genital prolapse and the weakness of support can be determined with certainty by examination of the unanesthetized patient, first recumbent and then standing, using neither speculum nor tenaculum. It is helpful to ask the patient to bear down in order to see which organ appears first, since this will provide a reliable suggestion as to the site of primary damage. Insertion of speculum and traction with a tenaculum will provide reliable help in determining the technical features of a planned repair.

ELONGATION OF THE CERVIX

Elongation of the cervix is most commonly seen in association with anterior segment damage and was characterized by Paramore (18) as "expansion of the escaped cervix." The apparent enlargement of the cervix is secondary to congestion within the tissues of the cervix under circumstances in which the cervix has dropped anterior to the genital hiatus. Although unable to maintain support of the cervix, the levator plate still exists as a supporting tissue posterior to the cervix. The edge of the genital hiatus in that circumstance acts as a mechanical barrier to the return circulation of the cervix, favoring venous stasis and apparent hypertrophy of the cervix itself. Persisting constriction causes not only edema and lymphangiectasia but later fibrosis, and the circulatory changes may at times result in ulceration of the surface of the cervix.

SEGMENTAL DAMAGE

There are certain natural cleavage planes (also noted in Chapter 1) about the female pelvic organ systems that, under certain stressful situations, permit segmental avulsion and pathologic sliding of one or more organ systems upon another. These concepts are of the utmost practical significance and, for clinical purposes, may be summarized as follows:

1. A retropubic plane between the pubis and urethra is brought into clinical significance when the pubourethral ligament portion of the urogenital diaphragm has become avulsed or stretched, permitting the proximal urethra to rotate from its usual situation with consequent "wheeling" and rotational descent of the bladder neck (see Fig. 1.29). This is usually the result of the shearing trauma of the descending fetal head beneath a wide-angled gynecoid pubic arch (see Fig. 2.3). An equally undesirably close fit of the fetal head may also be due to a relatively small fetal head or to a short precipitous labor or arrest in the second stage.

2. The posterior vaginal plane of cleavage exists between the posterior vaginal wall and the anterior wall of the rectum, that is, in the rectovaginal space. The organ systems anterior to this space are to a large extent interconnected by common attachments, especially in the upper two-thirds of the vagina. The cul-de-sac of Douglas, which of itself has both flexibility and mobility, along with the rectovaginal space, forms a more or less frictionless midline plane down which the structures anterior to the rectovaginal space can sometimes slide without disturbing those primarily rectal structures posterior to the rectovaginal space (Fig. 5.4). Therefore, prolapse of the upper vagina may permit the entire uterus and much of the bladder to protrude outside the introitus (see Fig. 5.3), with coexistent enterocele (sliding hernia), frequently without accompanying rectocele (22). Such a condition, especially involving the bladder, may be called primary anterior segment damage, and often results from chronically increased intraperitoneal pressure or from damage sustained during the first stage of labor as a result of bearing down or attempting delivery before the cervix is fully dilated. Anterior segment damage, per se, does not include damage to the levator ani or its sheath.

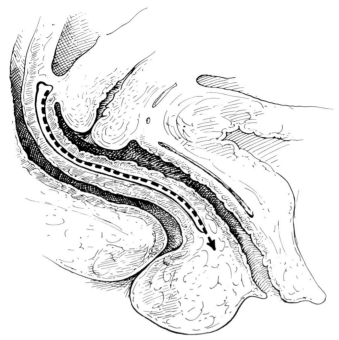

Figure 5.4. Sagittal section of the pelvis showing the rectovaginal space. Significant increases in intra-abdominal pressure may force the cervix and the posterior vaginal wall along this natural cleavage plane (*dotted line*).

3. The perineal and anterior rectal segments reflect damage to the support and attachments of the perineum, and to the posterior structures of the rectovaginal space, including the anterior wall of the rectum and its fascial envelopment. Perineal segmental damage is commonly associated with avulsion of the vaginal and perineal attachments to the levator ani (fibers of Luschka) as a result of unrecognized or unrepaired obstetric trauma to these attachments during the second stage of labor. The central portion of the rectovaginal septum (the fascia of Denonvilliers) can be traumatically detached from the cranial margin of the perineal body to which it is attached (27). The damage will be evident as a mid- and lower vaginal rectocele and can be expected when there is a narrow pubic arch. This type of relaxation will often be seen without significant degree of cystocele, uterine prolapse, or enterocele, because the latter structures may all be adequately supported in their normal and usual relationships.
4. The lower or retrorectal segment is, fortunately, the least common site of damage but, when present, is usually associated either with acquired major damage to the levator ani or to its innervation. Occasional congenital neuropathy may be coexistent with a spina bifida. Defects in the lower perineal segment permit perineal prolapse or descent of the anus so that the patient with a flat perineum may actually sit upon her anus, a most distressing situation.

PROLAPSE OF THE RECTUM

This occurs predominantly in women who are thin and elderly and is more common in nulliparous than multiparous patients (14). It is probable that aging has produced a diminished tone of the pelvic muscles, and chronic constipation and laxative abuse are seen. There is sometimes a coincident uterine prolapse (13, 24) (Fig. 5.5).

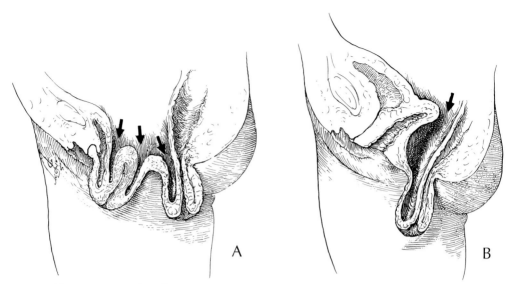

Figure 5.5. Rectal prolapse associated with enterocele. **A.** Rectal prolapse coincident with genital procidentia. **B.** Rectal prolapse posterior to the vagina, which is not involved. (From Nichols DH. Types of enterocele and principles underlying the choice of operation for repair. Obstet Gynecol 1972;40:257–363; reproduced with permission of Lippincott-Raven.)

The symptoms are primarily those of rectal protrusion with straining or lifting, incomplete bowel movements, and rectal incontinence. As the condition becomes more advanced and the prolapsed rectum remains outside a greater portion of the time, bleeding develops. The physical examination of the patient at rest is often clear, but when the patient strains as by a Valsalva maneuver the bowel protrudes. Its walls are thick, especially anteriorly, and there usually is an enterocele sac containing small bowel. The anus is usually patulous up to 3 or 4 finger breadths in diameter, and the condition is surprisingly painless.

True rectal prolapse must be differentiated from rectal mucosal prolapse and from hemorrhoids, since the treatment of each is different. Examination of hemorrhoids shows them to be lobular, with a visible succus between the masses of tissue. Prolapsing mucous membrane, being a single layer, is thinner to palpation than is the multiple-layered thickness of a true rectal prolapse. The mucosal folds of a mucosal prolapse are found to be radial in their direction, in contrast to those of rectal prolapse, which are arranged concentrically.

Rectal prolapse is probably the result of a rectorectal intussusception, rather than a sliding hernia. The anatomic abnormalities that are noted are probably the result and not the cause of the prolapse.

Of the treatments for rectal prolapse that have been offered, the most successful are transabdominal (15). Others are transperineal, and some are combined. Simple obliteration of the cul-de-sac on the assumption that the prolapse represents a sliding hernia has not been consistently effective, there being a 63 percent recurrence rate (15). Intraabdominal and transperineal plication of the levator muscles has been employed, but the greatest lasting successes have been reported on transabdominal rectal and sigmoid suspension operations with or without the use of foreign materials. Retrorectal levatorplasty (see Chapter 14) may be used for the early stages, and for the elderly or poor-risk patient, perineal anal encirclement as by the Thiersch technique has been recommended; however, this does involve inserting a foreign body around the anus, and there is a resultant small anal diameter and risk of ulceration. Mucosal prolapse is treated by mucosal resection, and hemorrhoids are treated by resection, obliteration, or injection.

Because rectal prolapse is often associated with anal incontinence, a knowledge of the causes and treatments of rectal prolapse requires some thoughtful appreciation of the normal mechanisms of lower bowel function and some consideration as to how this may be pathologically altered.

Levator Ani Function in Defecation

Bowel function is to a large extent the product of habit. Defecation of sigmoid colon content is achieved by first voluntarily relaxing the pelvic diaphragm, unlocking the colic valve, and relaxing the external anal sphincter. Modest increases in intra-abdominal pressure, as by bearing down, then force the stool content downward. Rectal filling opens the internal sphincter. The gastrocolic reflex pattern regularly assists by promoting intestinal peristalsis. A disorder of any of these steps predisposes to or causes constipation. Regular and excessive bearing down may stretch the anatomic integrity of the pudendal nerve and consequently weaken the muscles it innervates, occasionally resulting in a permanent loss of muscle tone in the now denervated pelvic diaphragm and external anal sphincter. The neuropathic loss of the tone of the anal sphincter permits it to relax at inopportune times, producing rectal incontinence that may be most difficult to treat surgically. The Parks group has suggested that this loss of voluntary muscle tone within the pelvic diaphragm may be associated with coincident urinary stress incontinence as well (9).

Rectal Continence

The levator ani and the external anal sphincter differ from other striated muscles of the body in that they maintain a constant state of tone inversely proportional to the quantity of the rectal content. Because intestinal peristalsis continues around the clock, although at apparently various degrees of intensity, this aforementioned tone is responsible for our normal rectal continence when we are both awake and asleep. Were it not for the effectiveness of this tone, we would regularly soil ourselves during sleep when the rest of our voluntary muscle system is relaxed.

Contraction of the levator ani and puborectalis muscles exerts pull upon the genital hiatus toward the pubis, creating an angle in rectal inclination that seems to function effectively as a valve, according to the observations of Parks (19), and there is reflex reciprocity with the tone of the external anal sphincter. These muscles are innervated by the pudendal nerve and its accessory branches, and they function in synergism. The innervation of the puborectalis is less certain, possibly coming from a sacral plexus component.

Neuromuscular pressure receptors within the intrinsic striated muscular content of the levatores ani are responsible for mediating this tone and apparently communicate with the central nervous system by way of the pudendal nerve on each side of the body, which arises generally from S3 and S4. Either congenital or acquired pathology of the pudendal nerve can alter the efficiency of its work and thus influence the ability and efficiency of these neuromuscular receptors to influence pressure and maintain this responsive muscular tone. Acquired damage may result from the trauma of stretching of the pelvic floor during childbirth and quite possibly from the chronic habit of excessive straining at stool.

Constipation, then, is *not* necessarily caused by the presence of *rectocele*, although it may coexist. The primary symptoms of rectocele are aching after a bowel movement and incomplete bowel movements often requiring manual splinting or expression to achieve evacuation. Effective posterior colporrhaphy should relieve these primary symptoms but will not necessarily relieve constipation other than that produced by stool being caught in a pocket of rectal wall precluding complete emptying of the bowel. There are many women with rectocele who are not constipated, and there are many more constipated women without rectocele.

In the patient with perineal descent, constipation may appear as an early symptom caused by loss of integrity of an intact pelvic diaphragm, which produces levator funneling during bearing down. As this phenomenon of bearing down becomes more regular and intense, the pudendal nerve may be further damaged by stretching. This disturbs the innervation of both the pelvic diaphragm and the external anal sphincter, with resultant partial paralysis and atrophy of these muscles, contributing to anal *incontinence* as a later symptom.

Henry (8) has suggested the following relationship between rectal prolapse and anal incontinence:

I think the primary pathology is one of neuropathy affecting the pelvic floor—in many patients a consequence of damage to the pudendal nerve; damage inflicted by traumatic childbirth. Incontinence may not develop initially if the internal anal sphincter is functioning normally. Pelvic floor denervation initiates rectal prolapse because of disruption of the anorectal flap valve. The prolapse starts with descent of the anterior rectal wall and at a later stage a circumferential complete prolapse intussuscepts through the anus. The dilatation of the internal anal sphincter caused by the prolapsing rectum then destroys the only mechanism protecting anorectal continence and a major functional problem results. Because the internal sphincter recovers, many patients recover a reasonable degree of control after successful repair of the prolapse. If continence is not recovered within six months we will offer the patient a transperineal post-anal repair (of the puborectalis and the pelvic diaphragm).*

Few types of segmental relaxation develop independently. More frequently the patient presents combinations of segmental damage. With the exception of severe generalized prolapse developing in postmenopausal years, the degree of damage of one particular segment is usually more evident than is the damage to other segments. Most of the reconstructive effort should be directed to the primary site of the most significant damage.

When a perineal defect suggesting injury of the retrorectal segment is accompanied by a high residual urine volume, particularly in the nulliparous patient, a urethrocystometrogram and neurologic evaluation should be considered to evaluate the possibility of defective pelvic innervation and resulting incompetence of the levator ani. There may be a coexistent spina bifida occulta, or a low spinal disc syndrome producing constipation and difficulty in emptying the bladder.

High rectocele is associated with pathologic overstretching of the vaginal and rectal supporting tissues, and there is often coexistent enterocele that must be identified and repaired. Reconstruction that will ensure restoration of a horizontal axis to the upper posterior vagina will lessen the chances of recurrence. Jeffcoate (11) recognized his posterior colporrhaphy as a frequent cause of dyspareunia or apareunia among Liverpool patients and stated that the need for posterior colporrhaphy in a particular patient should be determined by examining the *unanesthetized* patient. Only if the examination shows a need for posterior vaginal repair should the procedure be included in a particular patient's surgical reconstruction.

Although various cleavage planes may be developed within the pelvis that suggest the lines along which genital prolapse has developed, the most significant is clearly that provided between the interfaces of the rectovaginal space. Significant increases in intra-abdominal pressure that are exerted on tissues anterior to the rectovaginal space may result in a prolapse of the upper vagina and elongation of the cardinal-uterosacral ligament complex. Because of the attachment of the base of the bladder to the upper vagina and cervix by the supravaginal septum, descent of the cervix is likely to be accompanied by a traction descent of the bladder. The same findings may be observed after obstetric damage to the upper suspensory structures of the birth canal. In this situation, the descent of the cervix brings the anterior wall of the pouch of Douglas with it, and a traction type of enterocele is produced (Chapter 15). Traction to a tenaculum applied to the posterior lip of the cervix permits demonstration of the length of the cervix, the location and width of the posterior cul-de-sac, and the length and strength of the usually hypertrophic uterosacral ligaments (Fig. 5.6). The posterior peritoneal wall of such an enterocele is attached to the anterior

*Personal correspondence with author.

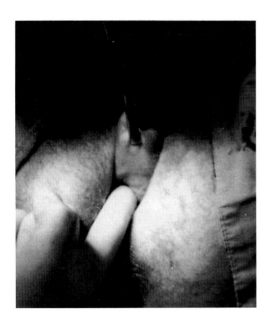

Figure 5.6. Palpation of the cul-de-sac of Douglas. The length and strength of the uterosacral ligaments as well as the location of the lowermost tip of the cul-de-sac of Douglas are determined by applying traction to a vulsellum applied to the posterior lip of the cervix. The elongated cervix and the long, strong uterosacral ligaments are shown. The lowermost extent of the cul-de-sac of Douglas is seen as the transverse shadow above the index finger.

surface of the rectum, which usually does not become involved in this type of prolapse. Because the uterine cervix and anterior vaginal wall function and are supported as a unit, weakness and subsequent hypertrophy of the connective tissue in this area are the greatest. Elements of the cardinal-uterosacral ligament complex are long and hypertrophic. Enterocele is (as stated) invariably present, whereas rectocele may be absent or of a minor degree (Figs. 5.7 and 5.8). This type of traction enterocele occurs not only as a result of traction upon the anterior wall of the cul-de-sac of Douglas but may also follow damage to the subperitoneal fibromuscular connective tissues, from whatever cause.

It is essential for the surgeon evaluating a patient with prolapse of the vaginal vault to determine which of these two fundamentally different types is present, since the successful treatment for one is significantly dissimilar from that of the other (as discussed in Chapters 9 and 16).

With prolapse of the vagina and its consequent vaginal telescoping, the depth of the vagina is shortened and the width of the anterior vaginal wall is often increased, depending upon the duration of the problem.

With eversion, the length and the width of the vaginal wall increase, and appropriate modification of the techniques of colporrhaphy may be required (Chapters 10 and 11).

It would be helpful to abandon once and for all the concept of a single cause of genital prolapse. Rather, we should recognize that there are many different causes that may be more or less evident, acting singly or, more commonly, in almost any combination to account for a particular clinical situation and its solution.

PROLAPSE AND OTHER LESIONS OF THE URETHRA

Distinction must be made between urethral prolapse, urethral caruncle, and urethral carcinoma. The first represents a telescoping of the urethra coincident with prolapse of other pelvic organs. It is a symmetrical, circumferential, red and soft intussusception of benign urethral mucosa. It is seen occasionally in the postmenopausal or premenarchal patient. If symptomatic, as by bleeding, a simple resection is advised. The urethral caruncle is a granular protrusion of postmenopausal urethral mucosa that bleeds readily on contact. If it is painful or bleeding, local estrogen therapy may be tried. Failing this, the treatment may be by local resection (12). Urethral carcinoma, in contrast, has a granular and red appearance, bleeds readily upon contact, and is firm or hard to the touch. It

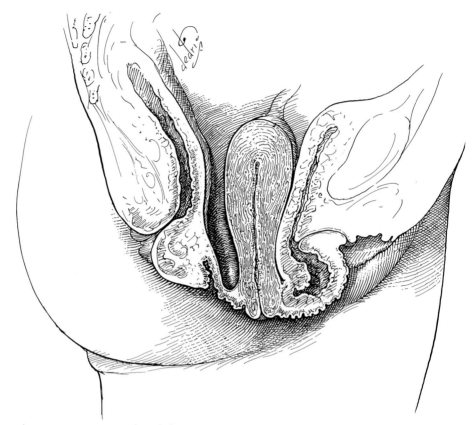

Figure 5.7. Uterovaginal or sliding prolapse. There is enterocele but no rectocele present. The uterosacral ligaments are long and strong. Note the position of the uninvolved anterior rectal wall. (From Halban and Tandler, 7.)

should be studied first by confirmatory biopsy and staging, and then treated aggressively by surgery or radiation by one experienced in this care.

SUMMARY AND CONCLUSIONS

Genital prolapse is usually a manifestation of either prolapse of the upper vagina or eversion of the lower vagina. Although these are phenomena of different etiologies and prognoses, they may occur separately or in combination. The surgeon must recognize and differentiate primary sites of weakness from resulting secondary changes, for the optimal results of treatment will depend upon adequate repair of the primary damage. Progression of residual prolapse as a result of unrecognized and unrepaired weakness can be expected when a repair has failed to correct the primary problem.

It is possible that genital prolapse is more common among clinical diabetic patients because of weakness induced by high glycosylation of connective tissues coincident with hyperglycemia. This attractive thesis is discussed further in Chapter 24.

When symptomatic genital prolapse and massive rectal prolapse coexist, each should be treated, although by different surgical procedures. The genital prolapse should be treated, in most instances, by transvaginal colpopexy and colporrhaphy. The rectal prolapse generally should be treated by transabdominal rectopexy with resection of pathologically elongated large bowel as necessary.

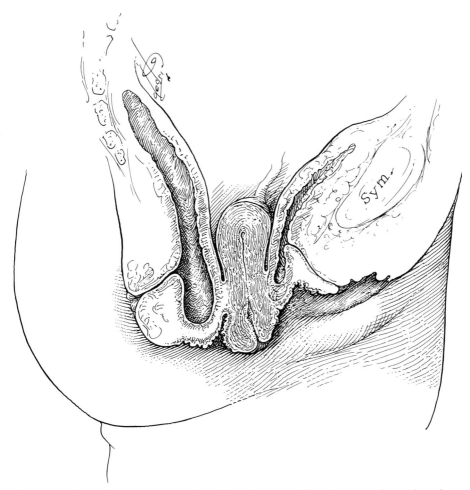

Figure 5.8. General postmenopausal genital prolapse resulting from atrophy and weakening of all of the endopelvic supporting tissues. A rectocele is present but no enterocele. The uterosacral ligaments are weak and hard to define by palpation. Note the defect in the support of the anterior rectal wall. (From Halban and Tandler, 7.)

For discussion of the specific types of cystocele, rectocele, perineal prolapse, and enterocele, the reader is referred to Chapters 10, 11, 14, and 15, respectively. Postpartum chronic eversion of the uterus is discussed in Chapter 24.

References

1. Ajabor LN, Okojie SE. Genital prolapse in the newborn. Int Surg 1976;61:496–497.
2. Beecham CT. Classification of vaginal relaxation. Am J Obstet Gynecol 1980;136:957.
3. Bonney V. The sustentacular apparatus of the female genital canal, the displacements that result from the yielding of its several components, and their appropriate treatment. J Obstet Gynaecol Br Emp 1914;45: 328–344.
4. Cooper S. Dictionary of practical surgery. 2nd ed. 1813 (cited by Ricci).
5. Geldenhuys FG. Genitale prolapse by die Bantoe. S Afr Med J 1950;24:749–751.
6. Geldenhuys FG. On the etiology of genital prolapse. MD thesis, South Africa, University of Pretoria, 1951.
7. Halban J, Tandler J. Anatomie und Ätiologic der Genitalprolapse beim Weibe. Vienna: Braumüller, 1907.
8. Henry MM. Personal communication, September 2, 1987.

9. Henry MM, Swash M, eds. Coloproctology and the pelvic floor. 2nd ed. London: Butterworths, 1992.

10. Heyns OS. Genital prolapse. In: Charlewood GP, ed. Bantu gynaecology. Johannesburg: Witwatersrand University Press, 1956.

11. Jeffcoate TNA. Posterior colporrhaphy. Am J Obstet Gynecol 1959;77:490.

12. Kaufman RH, Friedrich EG Jr, Gardner HL. Benign diseases of the vulva and vagina. 3rd ed. Chicago: Year Book, 1989:224–228.

13. Keighley M, Madoff RD, Watts JD, Rothenberger DA, Goldberg SM. Rectal prolapse. In: Henry MM, Swash M, eds. Coloproctology and the pelvic floor. 2nd ed. Oxford: Butterworth-Heinemann, 1992:316–350.

14. Küpfer CA, Goligher JC. One hundred consecutive cases of complete prolapse of the rectum treated by operation. Brit J Surg 1970;57:481–487.

15. Madoff RD, Watts JD, Rothenberger DA, Goldberg SM. Rectal prolapse—treatment. In: Henry MM, Swash M, eds. Coloproctology and the pelvic floor. Oxford: Butterworth-Heinemann, 1992:308–339.

16. Magdi I. Obstetric injuries of the perineum. J Obstet Gynaecol Br Commonw 1942;49:687–700.

17. Malpas P. The choice of operation for genital prolapse. In: Meigs JV, Sturgis SH, eds. Progress in gynecology. New York: Grune & Stratton, 1957;3.

18. Paramore RH. The statics of the female pelvic viscera. London: HK Lewis, 1925;2:273.

19. Parks AG. Anorectal incontinence. Proc Roy Soc Med 1975;68:681–690.

20. Porges RF. A practical system of diagnosis and classification of pelvic relaxations. Surg Gynecol Obstet 1963;117:769–773.

21. Ricci JV. One hundred years of gynecology. Philadelphia: Blakiston, 1945:272.

22. Ricci JV, Thom CH, Kron WL. Cleavage planes in reconstructive vaginal plastic surgery. Am J Surg 1948;76:354–363.

23. Sabatier RB. Mémoirs de l'Acad. de Chir. de Paris, 1757;3:361 (cited by Ricci).

24. Schoetz DJ Jr, Veidenheimer MC. Rectal prolapse: pathogenesis and clinical features. In: Henry MM, Swash M, eds. Coloproctology and the pelvic floor. London: Butterworths, 1985:303–307.

25. Shuwarger D, Young RL. Management of neonatal genital prolapse: case reports and historic review. Obstet Gynecol 1985;66:615–635.

26. Stallworthy J. Personal communication.

27. Tobin CE, Benjamin JA. Anatomical and surgical restudy of Denonvilliers' fascia. Surg Gynecol Obstet 1945;80:373–388.

28. Zacharin RG. A Chinese anatomy: the pelvic supporting tissues of the Chinese and Occidental female compared and contrasted. Aust N Z J Obstet Gynaecol 1977;17:11.

CHAPTER 6

Choice of Operation for Genital Prolapse

For the patient for whom nonemergent gynecologic surgery is recommended, a careful physical examination and work-up must precede the recommendation passed on to the patient. The patient must then be given adequate time to think about it and express any questions or concerns that she may have. This is sometimes best done at a revisit. If the patient has questions or difficulty about accepting a recommendation, a second opinion can be offered. The patient must also be told that her questions and concerns can be addressed again not only preoperatively but also during the hospital postoperative phase and full convalescence. It is helpful for the surgeon to anticipate the usual questions that a patient may have regarding a particular procedure and, lest they be forgotten, answer them before they have been asked. These might include considerations as to her future sex life, her future fertility, and her views concerning the retention or removal of her ovaries.

The surgeon should identify in each case the site, etiology, and extent of damage to the supporting tissues of the birth canal in order to define the objectives and to select the procedure necessary to ensure a satisfactory repair. Questions relevant to decision making include (*a*) What are the symptoms and do they correlate with the anatomic damage? (*b*) Has there been demonstrable progression of the prolapse? (*c*) What are the chances of restoring a vagina to normal with minimal chance of recurrence of prolapse? In large teaching centers, sophisticated study can be part of an ongoing research protocol. Dynamic analysis and evaluation of patients before and after surgical repair can be performed by magnetic resonance imaging (MRI) of the pelvic floor. The technical difficulty with MRI is that the patients must be evaluated while they are recumbent rather than standing, for it is in the latter position that gravity may add a significant contribution (13). Dynamic pelvic floor fluoroscopy may be helpful in the clinical evaluation of patients with prolapse because opacifying the small bowel with ingested barium sulfate will accurately identify enterocele. The procedure provides information about the emptying function of the rectocele as well (7).

Every operation must be tailored to the needs of each individual, taking into consideration the patient's reproductive potential, her marital state, age, habits, occupation, work, and activities, as well as the effect of any incidental diseases that may be present. If there is a desire for future pregnancy, it is usually better to postpone reconstructive surgery until childbearing has been completed.

For those who cannot wait, the surgical treatment of symptomatic genital prolapse requires some resourcefulness for the patient who cannot retain a pessary and wishes to have more children. If there is marked elongation of the cervix, cervical amputation with the Manchester-type repair (see Chapter 9) can be useful; in this procedure, that portion of the cardinal ligament that has been separated from the amputated portion of the cervix can be crossed in front of the remaining cervix (Fig. 6.1). For the patient without cervical elongation, a transabdominal sacrocervical colpopexy, using fascia lata or a synthetic

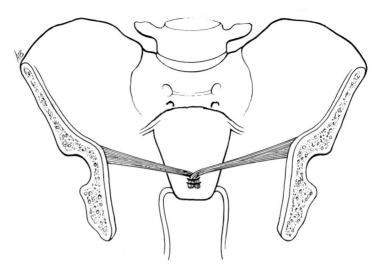

Figure 6.1. Amputation of the elongated cervix. The cervix, if long, has been amputated, and the now shortened cardinal-uterosacral ligament complex has been crossed and sewn to the anterior surface of the remaining cervix and lower uterine segment.

plastic fabric, is useful (1, 28, 29, 41). However, significant relaxation of the anterior vaginal wall may develop following subsequent obstetric delivery, especially in the patient with a history of coincident bladder exstrophy (10). Transvaginal sacrospinous cervicopexy can be employed successfully in the premenopausal patient who is anxious to preserve her fertility (20, 35). Any symptomatic defect of the anterior vaginal wall should be repaired to lessen the possibility of postoperative urinary stress incontinence. Kovac and Cruikshank have reported successful sacrospinous fixation of the uterosacral ligaments in 19 patients, 5 of whom have since delivered vaginally. Most of these procedures were bilateral. One or two additional sutures plicated the uterosacral ligaments in the midline to close off the cul-de-sac at the time of coincident repair of any enterocele that was present (20).

Coital interest must be respected. It is important to avoid excessively shortening or narrowing the vagina of a sexually active patient. Planned massive weight loss should be accomplished preoperatively, because the removal of ischiorectal fat from beneath the pelvic diaphragm may decrease the effectiveness of its support.

An individual with chronic respiratory disease, such as asthma, hay fever, chronic bronchitis, or a smoker's chronic cough, usually has subjected her pelvic supporting tissues to major and pathologic surges of increased intra-abdominal pressure. These will continue after any type of surgical reconstruction, predisposing her to an early recurrence of the prolapse. The type of activities and work to which the patient has been accustomed must be considered; for instance, increased intra-abdominal pressure from frequent heavy lifting has considerable influence on the strains to which the pelvic supporting tissues are subjected after an indicated repair. Errors in posture, such as chronic slouching, tend to rotate the pelvis forward so that the forces of gravity may direct the weight of the pelvic contents through the movable, vulnerable soft tissues of the pelvis instead of the back of the unyielding, rigid pubic bone, as when the patient holds her shoulders back and the bony pelvis is in its normal position.

It is paradoxical that, although the symptoms of various components of genital prolapse are generally associated with specific and demonstrable anatomic weakness, the anatomic defects do not always produce symptoms. Whether this indicates a stage in the evolution of the weakness or to some extent represents accommodation and forbearance on the part of the patient is unknown. It is unlikely that elective surgery can make an asymptomatic patient feel better, however. Conversely, the surgeon should be equally cautious in recommending surgery to a patient who has symptoms without substantiating pathology. An asymptomatic cystocele and/or rectocele should be repaired under the following circumstances:

1. When it protrudes through the vulva when the patient strains
2. When it is clearly progressive
3. When it contributes to an abnormal vaginal axis in a patient in whom other reconstructive pelvic surgery has been recommended
4. When vaginal hysterectomy is being performed as the primary procedure

EVALUATION OF GENITAL PROLAPSE

Keeping in mind that most forms of symptomatic genital prolapse are progressive, one must determine which damage is primary and which is secondary, because, unless the primary cause is identified and corrected (or, as Bonney wrote, "necessarily overcorrected" [5, 6]), recurrence and progression are to be expected. We believe it unwise to evaluate a genital prolapse for repair while the tissues of a postpartum patient are still undergoing involution. Postponing such an evaluation for another 3 to 6 months, until involution is complete, will ensure a more reliable appraisal.

The convenient but simplistic concept of thinking of genital prolapse in terms of the position of the cervix in relation to the introitus fails to take into account the significant differences in the etiology of each component of an individual's genital prolapse. For example, pathologically increased intra-abdominal pressure may not only have produced damage but may directly influence the incidence of recurrence. This is most obvious in the patient with chronic ascites or in the pateint who is undergoing long-term peritoneal dialysis. The weight of intra-abdominal fluid favors rapid recurrence of pelvic prolapse, thus ruling out the "standard" repair operations for those patients, unless the excessive peritoneal fluid is removed. Because the uterus is but passively involved, the primary defect with prolapse will be found in the uterovaginal supporting tissues, and it is to these supporting tissues that appropriate repair must be directed (Fig. 6.2). In many instances, it is appropriate to perform a vaginal removal of a prolapsed but otherwise normal uterus in order to mobilize the supporting tissues of the cervix and uterus adequately for use in the vaginal vault reconstruction (Fig. 6.3).

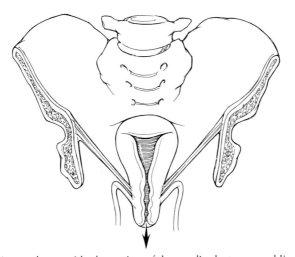

Figure 6.2. Uterine prolapse with elongation of the cardinal-uterosacral ligament complex.

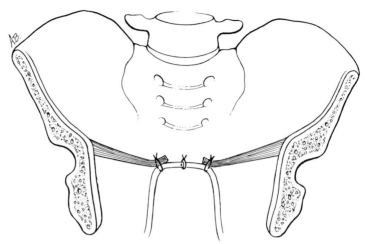

Figure 6.3. Hysterectomy, showing the now shortened cardinal-uterosacral ligament complex fixed to the vaginal vault on either side.

The quality of the paracolpium is critical in the support of the uterus following hysterectomy, providing it is effectively reattached to the vault of the vagina. If it is strong and the reattachment is strong after the hysterectomy, cystocele and rectocele will not regularly be accompanied by prolapse of the vaginal vault (9). It is the authors' view that human fascia can either stretch or rupture. As to the stretching phenomenon, witness the behavior of the anterior abdominal wall during pregnancy. Although eversion of the vaginal vault can occur uncommonly as a consequence of an isolated deficiency in genital support, that is, with an attenuated vaginal portion of the cardinal-uterosacral ligament complex, it is far more frequently seen as the consequence of damage to the several levels of pelvic support (5, 6). In order to achieve a more perfect reconstruction, the observant surgeon will have gone to some lengths to determine preoperatively the sites of damage and to reaffirm them by examination under anesthesia preceding hysterectomy and repair. The results of surgical correction of these meaningful observations will determine the extent and long-term success of the patient's surgery.

Pelvic versus Orthopedic Origin of Symptoms: Diagnostic Use of Pessaries

The place of the vaginal pessary in presurgical evaluation is principally to determine whether a patient's symptoms of backache and falling out are of pelvic or orthopedic origin. If there is question as to which of these factors accounts for the complaint, a properly fitted vaginal pessary should be inserted as a therapeutic test and observation made as to whether the patient's symptoms are relieved. The pessary should be removed after a few weeks and the patient observed for another few weeks to determine whether the symptoms recur.

In addition to their usefulness as a nonsurgical treatment of uterine retroversion or prolapse, pessaries can assist in the diagnostic differentiation of a gynecologic versus an orthopedic etiology for backache. A low backache arising from genital relaxation is usually absent on arising, but comes on and gets worse as the day progresses. A backache of orthopedic origin will often be worse when relaxed muscles allow for greater joint instability in the morning, but will improve as the day progresses. If a patient's backache has both gynecologic and orthopedic components, one may wish to predict the degree of relief she could expect from surgery to correct her genital relaxation. Insertion of a properly fitting pessary that restores the pelvic viscera to their normal relationships can help make this determination. If the patient experiences relief from wearing the pessary 2 to 4 weeks, it is then removed to see if symptoms return.

If the symptoms are significantly relieved while the patient is wearing the pessary and recur after its removal, the patient's complaints probably are of intrapelvic origin and correctable by appropriate reconstructive gynecologic surgery. If the symptoms are unrelieved by the pessary and unaffected by its removal, they are probably due to problems unrelated to weakness of pelvic connective tissues, in which case therapy should be directed more appropriately toward proper orthopaedic and hygienic measures.

Although pessaries are not a definitive solution for genital relaxation, they are very useful for temporizing until future surgical reconstruction or for relieving a patient who is not a surgical candidate. Preoperative use of a pessary in advanced degrees of prolapse may aid in decongesting the mucosa by improving circulation and reestablishing vaginal tonicity, especially if combined with vaginal estrogen therapy in the postmenopausal patient. Symptomatic women who wish to complete childbearing before having a surgical repair may also be candidates for a pessary.

Pessaries useful in symptomatic uterine retroversion include the Smith, Hodge, and Risser pessaries. The Gehrung pessary is useful in cystocele, rectocele, and some procidentias. Pessaries helpful in uterine prolapse or vaginal vault eversion include the ring, Gellhorn, cube, and inflatable doughnut pessaries. The ring and Gehrung pessaries as well as the Smith, Hodge, and Risser will permit coitus; those pessaries that fill the vaginal canal will not.

A pessary should be checked by the physician during the first week after its insertion and quarterly for as long as it is in use. Preferably, the patient or her caretaker should be able to remove the pessary at bedtime and reinsert it upon arising in the morning. If not, she should be seen monthly to remove and cleanse the pessary and to check the vagina for irritation or ulceration. Since the vagina will tend to enlarge with time to accommodate the pessary, the patient may need to be fitted in the future with a larger size.

A differential point in the history of such patients is that a backache that is present on arising and tends to improve as the day goes on is likely to be a symptom of orthopedic weakness, whereas a backache that comes on after the patient is on her feet for a time and is rather promptly relieved when lying down is the type of complaint probably related to genital prolapse. As a diagnostic aid, this characteristic discomfort may be reproduced at examination by traction upon the cervix, which will stretch the retroperitoneal pelvic nerve supply contained in the uterosacral ligaments.

When symptoms are relieved by the use of the pessary, the gynecologist should be prepared to resist the patient's request for reinsertion of the pessary as a substitute for the indicated surgery. She should be advised that the pessary is only palliative, not curative, and acts by continuing a stretch in the opposite direction of tissues that have already been pathologically elongated. Silent progression of the prolapse and widening of the levator hiatus usually will continue until a pessary can no longer be retained. At that time, the now older patient will be a less favorable operative risk, and with fewer remaining years in which to enjoy the comfort that surgery should provide.

Types of Genital Damage

Although genital damages may appear superficially similar, various combinations of possible etiologies may be present. These distinctive differences are of great importance, since they have to do not only with the rate and likelihood of progression of the disease but also with the prognosis for surgical success. Variations in the technique of repair are indicated when significant damages have been produced by (*a*) "normal" supporting tissue that has been stretched or attenuated by chronically increased intra-abdominal pressure; (*b*) congenitally attenuated supporting tissues but with normal intra-abdominal pressure; (*c*) congenitally attenuated supporting tissues coexistent with chronically increased intra-abdominal pressure; and (*d*) any of the above to which may be added the postmenopausal degenerative changes in pelvic supportive tissues. The surgeon must take such factors into consideration if operative results are to be uniformly good. Thus there should be no standard technique for all repairs because there is no standard damage to the supporting tissues.

Bonney (5, 6) suggested that three levels of damage to pelvic supports should be considered; these might have occurred singly or in any combination (Fig. 6.4A). There is obvious need to develop skill in three-dimensional thinking in the assessment of pelvic damage. Successful surgical reconstruction requires identification of each level of damage with appropriate repair.

1. Damage to the upper steadying apparatus (Fig. 6.4B), the round and broad ligaments, may result in excessive mobility of the uterine fundus and is commonly associated with retroversion. Uncomplicated damage to this level of support is usually nonprogressive and asymptomatic and does not, of itself, indicate surgery.
2. Damage to the middle holding group (Fig. 6.4C), the cardinal-uterosacral ligament complex, results in a gradual but progressive eversion of the upper vagina, often with coincident elongation of the cervix. If the upper supports are strong or the fundus is pathologically adherent, the uterine body may remain in its usual intra-abdominal location while the cervix elongates and descends. The cervix and anterior vagina often function as a single unit, however, and often share in the response to damage by the development of cervical elongation, a cystocele, and enterocele. These changes are basically due to obstetric trauma, are slowly progressive, and together constitute the most common type and appearance of prolapse. Because the pelvic diaphragm is usually intact in this situation, rectocele does not characteristically accompany this type of prolapse. Extensive posterior colporrhaphy is not often necessary. Satisfactory treatment includes vaginal hysterectomy, excision of any enterocele, and shortening and reattachment of the transected cardinal-uterosacral ligament complex to the posterior vaginal vault. To preserve length, the vaginal

---

Figure 6.4. Some frequent types of genital damage. The three levels of normal genital support (upper, middle, lower) are indicated by *thick short arrows. Thin long arrows* indicate weakened support. **A.** Sagittal section through normal female pelvis shows good support of all levels. The upper level contains round and broad ligaments. Uterosacral and cardinal ligaments are contained in the middle level. The lower supporting group includes the pelvic and urogenital diaphragms, and the perineum and muscles contained therein. The uterine fundus is situated anteriorly. The vagina is not everted. **B.** Damage is to the upper supports with consequent retroversion of the uterus. The positions of the vagina, bladder, and rectum are normal. **C.** Damage is to the middle supporting group alone. Because the intra-abdominal position of the uterine fundus is maintained by strong upper-level support, the upper vagina becomes everted with descent and elongation of the cervix. Strong lower support resists formation of cystocele or rectocele, but middle support damage is often accompanied by enterocele. **D.** Loss of lower supports. The lower vagina is everted with cystocele and rectocele, but normal upper and middle supports hold the upper vagina and uterus in position for the present. **E.** Defective middle and upper supports, retroversion and descent of the uterus, and inversion of the upper vagina. Strong lower supports resist eversion, and true cystocele and rectocele are not present. **F.** Defective middle and lower supports, eversion of the upper vagina, descent of the cervix, and eversion of the lower vagina with cystocele and rectocele. Strong upper supports retain the uterine fundus in its usual position, permitting elongation of the cervix. **G.** Damage to the upper and lower, but not the middle, supports. There is retroversion of the uterus and eversion of the lower vagina with cystocele and rectocele but no eversion of the upper vagina or descent of the cervix. **H.** Damage to all three levels of support. The vagina is turned inside out and the entire uterus lies outside the pelvis. Eversion is complete. (From Nichols DH. The choice of operation for genital prolapse. Postgrad Med 1970;47:163–167. Used with permission.)

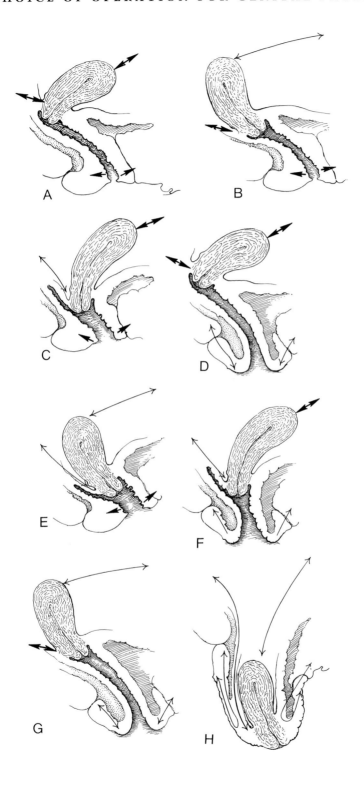

vault may be approximated in the sagittal plane (i.e., the 6 to 12 o'clock positions), and a noticeably widened posterior fornix should be narrowed by appropriate wedging or resection.

3. Damage to the lower group of supporting tissues (Fig. 6.4D), the pelvic and urogenital diaphragms, the perineum, and the muscles contained therein, usually results in eversion of the vagina with development of a cystocele and a low or middle rectocele, both of which should be corrected by appropriate anterior and posterior colporrhaphy.

4. Actual damage to the upper and middle, but not lower, supports (Fig. 6.4E) is quite frequent, however, and the resulting eversion of the upper vagina often develops with descent of a normal-sized, usually retroverted uterus but with no eversion of the lower vagina. Effective treatment would include vaginal hysterectomy with shortening of the uterosacral ligaments and excision of any enterocele, as in number 2 above.

5. Damage to the genital supports of the middle and lower but not to the upper (broad ligament and fundus) vagina is also often seen (Fig. 6.4F). This produces simultaneous elongation of the cervix with eversion of both upper and lower vagina and development of both cystocele and rectocele. Because the uterine fundus remains supported at a normal intra-abdominal level, the cervix will elongate until it protrudes beyond the vulvar orifice. A uterine sound introduced into such a uterus will reveal a surprising depth of the uterine cavity, largely accounted for by the length of the cervical canal. The gynecologic surgeon should anticipate technical changes peculiar to the increased length of the cervix.

6. The treatment of damage to the lower vaginal and upper uterine, but not the middle, supports (Fig. 6.4G) is usually the same as for number 3, essentially an anterior and posterior colporrhaphy, although the presence of uterine pathology might indicate either vaginal or abdominal hysterectomy.

7. The result of damage at all three levels of support is likely to be a vagina turned completely inside out (Fig. 6.4H). Most women with procidentia are unable to retain a vaginal pessary for an extended period of time because of the damage to and the relaxation of the pelvic diaphragm. As a result, the treatment of choice will usually be vaginal hysterectomy and extensive colporrhaphy, with corresponding reduction in vaginal width and depth.

PRINCIPLES OF GENITAL PROLAPSE REPAIR

A genital prolapse should be repaired when it is significantly progressive or sufficiently distressing for the patient to have complained of it to the gynecologist (43). It is important to examine each site of pelvic damage, for if any one site is to be repaired, all should be corrected, lest the risk of such uncorrected elements will continue to progress in the future, quite possibly necessitating reoperation. To repair less than all the demonstrable weakness is analogous to repairing all but a portion of an incisional hernia, for, in a sense, genital prolapse is comparable to other types of hernia. For purposes of comparison, let us imagine that the damaged vagina has been opened along each lateral wall and displayed in a linear fashion (Fig. 6.5). Suppose that we liken such a segment to a ventral or incisional hernia. Would it make good sense to repair only one-third or two-thirds of a hernia and not the remainder? Would not the unrepaired segment remain still a hernia, reduced to a weak spot of concentrated weakness that must now bear the full brunt of changes in intra-abdominal pressure and, as a result, tend to enlarge even faster? All genital thirds, or segments, if demonstrably weakened, should be repaired at the same operation so that the entire hernia is corrected. Anterior colporrhaphy generally should reconstruct the full length of the anterior vaginal wall, including the urogenital diaphragm and all supports of the urethra and vesicourethral junction. Since a dropped uterus is the result and not the cause of a genital prolapse, hysterectomy for prolapse but without repair is an exercise in futility.

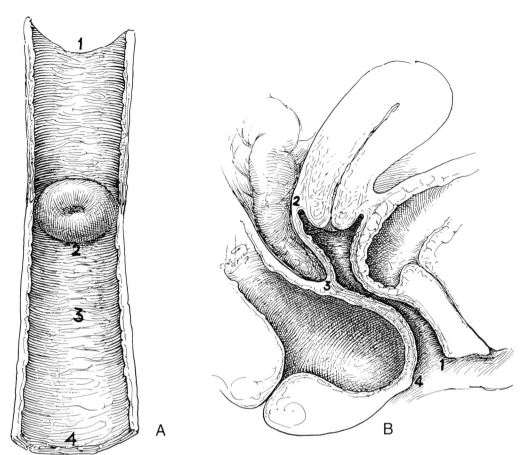

Figure 6.5. Comparison of prolapse to ventral hernia. **A.** Sagittal section of a pelvis shows segmental relaxation. The anterior vaginal segment is indicated between *1* and *2*, the superior between *2* and *3*, and the posterior between *3* and *4*. **B.** The damaged vagina has been imaginatively opened and displayed in a linear fashion. The numbers correspond to the sites of segmental damage.

Because the anterior vagina sits upon and derives considerable support from an adequate posterior wall, anterior colporrhaphy should be followed by repair of any demonstrable damage to the posterior wall. Failure to repair obvious cystocele often requires reoperation in later years. If a surgeon's patients experience a noticeable incidence of dyspareunia or apareunia due to vaginal narrowing, ridges, or an overly tightened perineum caused by careless "routine" posterior colporrhaphy, the surgeon should change his or her technique. In his classic paper indicting posterior colporrhaphy as a cause of dyspareunia and apareunia, Jeffcoate (19) stated that the need for posterior colporrhaphy in a particular patient should be determined by examining the unanesthetized patient. If this examination shows a need for posterior vaginal repair, the procedure should be included in the surgical reconstruction.

Anterior Colporrhaphy

Every parous woman as she grows older will develop some degree of pelvic relaxation including cystocele and rectocele. There may be some coincident nocturia, frequency, and urinary urgency. Only if the symptoms are sufficiently annoying to the patient to warrant surgery is this option offered to them. The postmenopausal woman is placed on weekly, preliminary intravaginal estrogen replacement for at least 2 months preoperatively. The symptoms are then reevaluated prior to an operation. If the symptoms are relieved, the surgery is cancelled, and the estrogen replacement becomes a permanent recommendation. The needs of the whole person must be respected.

Urodynamic testing should be performed on women with severe genital prolapse to identify those at risk for postoperative urinary incontinence that has been masked by the prolapse itself (37). It is particularly valuable in patients over 65 and is essential in continent patients with prolapse who develop incontinence of urine when the prolapse has been reduced, as by a pessary or manual elevation of the vault of the vagina. This is particularly frequent in the patients who are postmenopausal. Many will be shown to have a clinical urinary stress incontinence, others will show uninhibited detrusor contractions, and some will demonstrate a low urethral closure pressure (less than 20 cm of water) that might strongly suggest the addition of a suprapubic anti-incontinence procedure such as the vesicourethral sling coincident with the prolapse repair.

Patients with severe genital prolapse (the organs protruding beyond the introitus) should be studied by urodynamic assessment after the prolapse has been relieved with a properly fitting pessary. In about half the cases "occult" urinary problems will be discovered that may influence and modify the choice of surgical procedure (37).

Simple office cystometry may demonstrate apparent detrusor instability by retroflow from a simple catheter into an asepto-syringe from a bladder filled by retrograde instillations of saline. If negative in the lithotomy position, the test should be repeated when the patient is standing. If retrograde flow is seen, the patient may be given a few days of an anticholinergic and the test repeated. If it is still positive, the patient should have a more thorough urodynamic screening and testing. If the patient is cured, further testing is unnecessary and corrective surgery is probably not indicated. The patient should begin a course of bladder training and retraining without delay in anticipation of a long-term or lifelong reeducation process.

Urodynamic evaluation should also be strongly recommended for incontinent prolapse patients above the age of 65. Many of these patients will demonstrate an unexpected detrusor instability or a low-pressure urethra, either of which may significantly affect the recommendations for treatment of their incontinence; the former by bladder retraining and anticholinergics, the latter by specific surgical steps to increase urethral tone and pressure.

Testing for stress incontinence should be performed before and after reduction of the genital prolapse by pessary or manual support so that the surgical repair will correct all significant and potential defects and surgically correctable symptoms in the urogenital tract (16).

When the vaginal rugae covering the bladder are flattened more than those preserved in the lateral vaginal walls or when there is demonstrable progression in the size of the cystoceles, anterior colporrhaphy is indicated. Anterior repair is indicated if there is bladder symptomatology, a bearing-down sensation, urinary incontinence, urinary stress incontinence, high residual urine with frequent episodes of cystitis, or overflow incontinence in the absence of a nonreversible neuropathy (as may be produced by multiple sclerosis, diabetes, or advanced lues). The technique of colporrhaphy varies according to whether the prolapse is uterovaginal or general and whether the urogenital diaphragm has been damaged. The common midline defects should be repaired. If there is demonstrable lateral detachment of the supports of the vagina from the arcus tendineus, they should be reunited, preferably transvaginally (see Chapter 10). This can be determined at the preliminary physical examination if a lateral wall defect that comes down when the patient strains does not go back when she contracts or "holds" the muscles of her pelvic diaphragm (2).

One should differentiate between rotational descent of the bladder neck (anterior pseudocystocele) and true or posterior cystocele. The presence of vaginal rugal folds helps considerably in making the differential diagnosis, and any coexistent descent of the vaginal vault is important. When rugal folds are absent with cystocele and there is a significant midline defect, the full length of the vaginal wall should be reconstructed, including the support of the vesicourethral junction. The presence of rugae and rotational descent of the bladder neck indicates that support of the vesicourethral junction should be a primary objective of a repair. The work of Green (15) has called attention to the posterior urethrovesical angle and urethral inclination. Demonstrable urethral funneling should be corrected, but the most important goal is to reelevate the vesicourethral junction. The junction should be elevated so that it is once again within the influence of changes in intra-abdominal pressure and no longer is the most dependent portion of the bladder.

Ball (3) has emphasized the significance of urethral funneling: an anatomic defect that physiologically "shortens" the effective urethral length by permitting the transmission of bladder pressure directly to the urine inside the funnel. If the effective vesicourethral junction (i.e., the point at which the distal neck of the funnel joins the remaining urethra) is caudal to the area responsive to changes in intra-abdominal pressure, the increase would be transmitted only to the bladder, and if intravesical pressure exceeds intraurethral pressure, urinary stress incontinence will result.

When does one plicate the urogenital diaphragm? If a rotational descent of the bladder neck is found during anterior colporrhaphy, this is evidence of damage to the urogenital diaphragm, which should be surgically restored even if the patient is continent, lest correction of the cystocele alone flattens the posterior urethrovesical angle, inviting stress incontinence (42).

Dislocation cystocele coincident with vaginal eversion results from damage to lateral connective tissue supports. Under such circumstances there may be preservation of vaginal rugae in the premenopausal patient. This finding is in contrast to the cystocele produced by overdistention with destruction of the fibromuscular elasticity in the vaginal wall itself, often with an increase in the total length and width of the vaginal wall and fornices. The former condition is corrected primarily by restoration of vaginal depth, axis, and support; the latter is corrected primarily by reduction of vaginal width by excision of an appropriately shaped wedge of vaginal mucosa that includes the area of maximum thinning, usually midvaginal.

In perhaps one-quarter of instances of symptomatic genital prolapse, eversion of the vault coexists with that of the lower vagina, and the surgeon must take each of these etiologic differences into account in planning the technique of repair, which will differ from one patient to another.

The surgical repair of coexistent cystocele and urethral detachment is necessarily quite different from that of cystocele alone. Symmonds and Jordan (42) have called attention to the importance of a history of previous stress incontinence, now relieved, in certain patients presenting with an enlarging cystocele. The stress incontinence disappeared because, as the cystocele became larger and the bladder dropped more than the urethra, a posterior urethrovesical angle reappeared. The surgeon must accomplish a reconstruction that will provide adequate support of both the urethra and the bladder neck. Failure to restore urethral support may result in a return of the stress incontinence.

When the middle and lower genital supports have been damaged, the surgical technique should be modified to take into account the higher lateral attachment of the uterosacral and cardinal ligaments, as well as the higher reflections of the anterior and posterior peritoneal folds. The incision circumscribing the cervix is made appropriately further away from the external cervical os. Although good vaginal depth may be obtained in this circumstance by cervical amputation plus an anterior and posterior colporrhaphy (Manchester procedure), the incidence of subsequent uterine disease has made vaginal hysterectomy with repair the treatment of choice when the fundus is freely movable and the patient has completed her family, and when the surgeon is experienced and comfortable with the techniques of vaginal hysterectomy for the uterus which, though movable, is not prolapsed. In fact, most reconstructive surgery is deferred until after the period of desired childbearing. Because vaginal hysterectomy involves opening the cul-de-sac, any coexistent enterocele is readily evaluated and treated.

Posterior Colporrhaphy

Rectocele, of course, may occur at various levels of the vagina, and the entire defect should be repaired whenever an anterior colporrhaphy has been performed. A posterior vaginal repair is particularly indicated if the rectocele is associated with incomplete bowel movements that require digital manipulation for completion or when the patient complains of a sensation of postevacuation rectal pressure or fullness.

If a symptomatic rectocele enlarges progressively during a period of observation, is large enough to alter the normal vaginal axis, or is associated with enterocele, a repair is indicated. Repair should also usually be considered when the patient herself requests it.

Because the strength of the pubovaginalis muscle varies, apparently being better developed among black peoples than among caucasians, the need for so-called levator stitches as a feature of perineorrhaphy is subject to wide variation. In the reconstruction of a torn or defective perineal body, the levator fascia of each side (pubococcygeus-pubovaginalis component) may be approximated at the apex of the proposed perineal body reconstruction some 2 to 2½ inches above the hymenal margin. If these stitches, when necessary, are properly placed, they should constitute a first step in the reconstruction of a wedge or plane of perineum and should not result in a palpable ridge beneath the posterior vaginal wall. Indeed, after each stitch is placed and before it is tied, the operator should apply traction to the ends of the crossed sutures, and, if a ridge is found, the suture should be removed and replaced less deeply and closer to the rectum. If permitted to remain, it may become a subject of distress for the patient, her husband, and her surgeon, for it may represent a cause of future dyspareunia or apareunia, as emphasized by Jeffcoate (19).

Stitches should be tied only as tightly as is necessary to approximate the tissue. Stitches that are too snug will probably strangulate the tissue, with the destruction of basic substrate and replacement by tender areas of rigid inelastic fibrosis. Because the perineal body is composed of a number of different structures, whose strength may vary from one individual to another, there are a variety of deficiencies that can develop.

In the patient without laceration of the external anal sphincter, rectal incontinence as evidenced by chronic soiling and often preceded by loss of sensory discrimination between solid, liquid, and gaseous rectal content may identify the patient who is at increased risk for future rectal prolapse. Careful examination may disclose a perineal descent syndrome with elongation of the levator ani. If voluntary contractions of the pubococcygei and external anal sphincter are of poor quality, a pudendal neuropathy may be related (18, 32, 33). In this circumstance, the internal anal sphincter may be all that provides the remaining degree of continence. When this final vulnerable protective function is gone, the patient's rectum may become totally incontinent. Specific symptoms include obstipation, diminished diameter of passed stool, and often, chronic rectal soiling. If perineal descent is symptomatic or visibly progressive, it should be strongly considered for repair either by retrorectal levatorplasty (30) or by the Parks postanal repair (32).

In the event that rectal prolapse coexists with genital prolapse, the surgery and repair for the genital prolapse should be accomplished as the first of a two-stage single operation, to be followed by a transabdominal Ripstein-type suspension of the rectum (24). In a patient with symptomatic perineal descent, the transvaginal reconstruction should precede the retrorectal levatorplasty.

Prolapse of the rectum may occur coincident with genital prolapse (see Chapter 5). The etiology is different for each of these conditions, as is the surgical cure. Successful surgical treatment for either of these conditions is independent of the surgical treatment of the other, although it may be to the patient's advantage if the conditions are treated sequentially as parts of the same operation (36). Since the conditions appear to have a separate etiology, it is wishful thinking to presume that the correction of one prolapse will automatically avoid the necessity of correcting the other. In fact, correction of one will probably make the other worse if it is untreated.

The Ripstein rectal sling procedure has been used successfully to treat rectal prolapse for over three decades. Any tendency for postoperative fecal impaction created by pulling the sling too tight has been avoided by placing the sling posteriorly, leaving the anterior rectal wall free to distend (24).

Vaginal Hysterectomy

Krige (21) has written:

The choice of a case for vaginal hysterectomy may be easy if the chief indication for operation is definite second or later degree of prolapse. The more enterprising surgeon has learned from experience that certain cases prove to be deceptively difficult, consequently he exercises great care in picking his cases. There are times when a case of large cystocele and rectocele well outside the introitus calls for treatment from below, but excision of the uterus may be a real trial and struggle for the surgeon. However, with increasing experience the surgeon learns to assess the laxity of the vault, mobility of the cervix and viability of the uterus, by manual and speculum examination. A significant bulge in the posterior fornix may indicate high rectocele or potential enterocele and calls for vaginal hysterectomy with repair. Confidence in technique enables one to tackle a different case knowingly. It is a peculiar fact that the struggle in a really difficult vaginal hysterectomy is often not reflected in the patient's uneventful recovery. The surgeon's list of indications not only reveals his or her mental attitude toward the operation, but also confidence or lack thereof in personal operative ability and technique. If training has been inadequate, the correct decision on the indicated operation becomes a problem. There are times when he or she feels the patient should have a vaginal hysterectomy, but courage fails and giving in to the doubt created, the surgeon falls back on archaic abdomino-vaginal operations. Justification for this failure is found in the tradition and conservatism of senior gynecologists and their apparent satisfaction with such procedures, an attitude that has depressingly retarded developments. Under present conditions, the young surgeon has few opportunities to improve personal technique. With proper instruction, vaginal hysterectomy becomes a safe and simple operation.*

Of 1393 vaginal hysterectomies performed by Krige, 90 percent involved simultaneous anterior and posterior colporrhaphy (21). Of 889 vaginal hysterectomies by Navratil (26) for benign disease of the uterus, 73 percent included simultaneous vaginal repair. Gray (14) reported 97 percent repair in 1410 cases, and Hawksworth and Roux (17) reported 90 percent repair in 1000 vaginal hysterectomies.

Richter (36) reported 3468 hysterectomies between 1956 and 1971, of which 2611, or 75 percent, were done vaginally. More than 87 percent (87.4 percent) of the vaginal hysterectomies were combined with a pelvic floor repair. In such experienced hands, vaginal hysterectomy has clearly replaced abdominal hysterectomy in all cases in which a vaginal repair is indicated.

The configuration of the patient's pelvis is a determining factor in whether the uterus can be removed safely from below by the experienced operator. In the examination preceding surgery, the operator should be able to insert his or her fist gently between the ischial spines when palpating the perineum (Fig. 6.6). Helpful information can also be obtained from the vulvar slant, which will help distinguish between the ample measurements of the gynecoid pelvis and the restricted size of the pelvic outlet as identified with the android pelvis (Fig. 6.7).

---

*From Krige CF. The repair of genital prolapse combined with vaginal hysterectomy. J Obstet Gynaecol Br Commonw 1962;69:570–583. Used with permission.

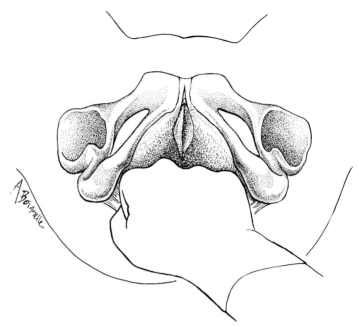

Figure 6.6. Method for determining the configuration of the patient's pelvis. The operator's fist can be inserted comfortably between the ischial tuberosities in the gynecoid pelvis, indicating adequacy of the bony pelvis for transvaginal surgical exposure.

For the patient requiring an abdominal hysterectomy who has a poorly supported vault, it is particularly important to preserve the identity of the cardinal-uterosacral ligament complex so that these structures, now shortened with hysterectomy, are incorporated in the support of the vaginal vault postoperatively. This may be easier to accomplish by using an endofascial hysterectomy than an exofascial hysterectomy. The exofascial hysterectomy, however, is probably safer than its endofascial counterpart, and is associated with less blood loss and weakness. The cardinal-uterosacral ligament complex is harder to define and mobilize with transabdominal hysterectomy than it is with vaginal hysterectomy (9). Total vaginal hysterectomy on the patient without prolapse is more likely to be of the exofascial type, whereas for the prolapse patient the endofascial dissection may make it possible to mobilize more effectively the cardinal-uterosacral ligament complex for incorporation in the support of the vault after hysterectomy.

When vaginal hysterectomy is performed on a patient with an asymptomatic cystocele and rectocele, it is our view that these latter abnormalities should be repaired at the same time to correct an abnormal vaginal depth and axis. This step will significantly diminish the opportunity for future vaginal eversion.

INDICATIONS AND CONTRAINDICATIONS

Primary indications for vaginal hysterectomy are symptomatic or progressive genital prolapse and uterine abnormality, either dysfunction or neoplasia. Inclusion of hysterectomy of a prolapsed uterus in an indicated vaginal repair can be considered if the cul-de-sac of Douglas is free, not obliterated by inflammatory adhesions or endometriosis, and the uterus is movable and not too large. As long as the uterus is freely movable and not too large, it can usually be removed safely by the vaginal route. When there is no prolapse, the anatomic relationships are remarkably similar in all cases, making the technical details of hysterectomy often easier than in the patient with advanced

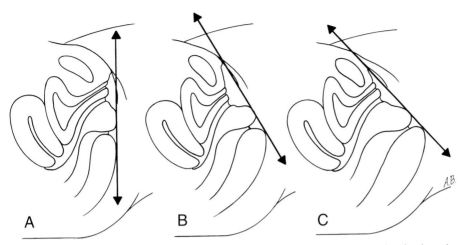

Figure 6.7. Vulvar slant as an indication of type of pelvis. **A.** With a narrow android pelvis, the soft tissue slant of the vulva is perpendicular to the long axis of the body. **B.** A more favorable vulvar slant is present in the roomy gynecoid pelvis. **C.** The axis of the platypelloid pelvis.

prolapse. When hysterectomy is required in the obese patient, the vaginal route is usually accomplished by less morbidity than the abdominal route (31, 34).

The indications for abdominal hysterectomy are those that represent the contraindications for vaginal hysterectomy. Relative contraindications that merit consideration are adnexal disease, inflammatory or neoplastic; conditions producing obliteration of the cul-de-sac; unusually large size of the uterus; and certain types of invasive malignant disease, such as advanced carcinoma of the cervix or the higher stages of adeno-carcinoma of the corpus. Very few surgeons who have once mastered a safe vaginal hysterectomy technique will later abandon it in favor of the abdominal route. As the operator's confidence and experience in vaginal hysterectomy increase, his or her indications for the operation will become more liberal.

The indication for hysterectomy coincident with vaginal reconstruction relates to the degree of the patient's discomfort and inconvenience. When there is a history of prolonged bleeding and one finds a significantly lowered blood count, and other reasons for anemia have been excluded, the chronic blood loss itself, although it may be acceptable to the patient, may well indicate a hysterectomy.

PRINCIPLES OF VAGINAL HYSTERECTOMY

With uterovaginal prolapse, the fundus, of course, may occupy a relatively normal position within the pelvis, although the cervix may be markedly elongated. The operator should have experience performing vaginal hysterectomy upon the nonprolapsed uterus before choosing to treat prolapse of the cervix by hysterectomy instead of a Manchester procedure (see Chapter 9). When the uterus is not prolapsed, ventral fixation or uterine suspension is of no value as treatment for an elongated prolapsing cervix. When the fundus of the uterus has remained at a normal position, removing it or fixing it anteriorly will not remove an elongated cervix from the vagina. The following are some principles of vaginal hysterectomy and repair:

1. Relieve the patient's symptoms.
2. Understand that the goal is to return pelvic anatomy and physiology to normal.
3. Infiltrate paracervical tissue with the "liquid tourniquet" (no more than 50 ml of 1:200,000 epinephrine in 0.5% lidocaine solution).

4. Use a circumscribing incision through the full thickness of the vagina.
5. Open the posterior cul-de-sac under direct vision, shorten the uterosacral ligaments, and attach them to the posterolateral edge of the vagina.
6. Sharply dissect the bladder from the cervix and lower uterine segment.
7. Open the anterior cul-de-sac under direct vision.
8. Clamp, cut, and tie remaining attachments and remove the uterus.
9. Perform an oophorectomy, if desirable.
10. Excise enterocele or redundant peritoneum.
11. Perform culdeplasty if necessary.
12. Repair the full length of the anterior vaginal wall, including adequate elevation and support of the vesicourethral junction.
13. Perform a posterior repair to a point cranial to the rectocele.
14. Perform a perineorrhaphy if indicated.
15. Ensure adequate postoperative vaginal depth, axis, and width.

Because abdominal wall relaxation is not required for transvaginal surgery, the depth and duration of anesthesia are decreased. Postoperative respiratory excursions are more adequate because the abdomen is not immobilized by incisional tenderness and pain, and the attendant complications of atelectasis and pneumonia are decreased. There is no risk of abdominal wound infection or incisional hernia. There will be less postoperative ileus and less need for postoperative parenteral feeding because of minimal handling of bowel. Ambulation is more comfortable because of the absence of abdominal incisional pain. Most important, unsuspected enterocele can be diagnosed and corrected as part of the primary surgical process, along with any symptomatic or progressive vaginal relaxation. All can be corrected during the same operative procedure, without the delay of repositioning and redraping the patient.

Obesity adds little risk to the vaginal surgical patient. The vaginal approach to hysterectomy is preferred in obese women as well as in thin women (31, 34).

Pelvic examination under anesthesia should immediately precede hysterectomy. This confirms the uterine size and mobility, the location of the posterior cul-de-sac, and the length and strength of the cardinal-uterosacral ligament complex. Any question as to the condition of the adnexal or other intra-abdominal pelvic pathology may be resolved by coincident preliminary laparoscopy. If there is some uncertainty about the feasibility of the vaginal route for hysterectomy, the operator can still begin the operation. If progress proves unexpectedly difficult or the operator is unable to find and open either cul-de-sac, vaginal efforts to remove the uterus can be discontinued. Vaginal reconstruction can be completed while a new surgical set-up is being prepared so that the hysterectomy can be completed abdominally.

When hysterectomy is performed because of intrinsic pathology within the uterus itself, the operation is fundamentally destructive, and, as long as it has been accomplished safely, it makes very little difference whether the uterus is removed upside down, sideways, or inside out, as long as removal is safe and without damage to adjacent organs. But when the operation of hysterectomy is part of a reconstruction, the principles pertinent to the two approaches are entirely different. In extirpation for primary uterine disease, the specific technique is unimportant as long as the uterus is removed safely. But when hysterectomy is part of a planned reconstruction, each step must be planned, purposeful, and in accord with the primary objective of using, preserving, and strengthening pelvic support tissues.

Vaginal hysterectomy may be essentially extrafascial and, being less disruptive than abdominal hysterectomy therefore, can be safely employed as the treatment by hysterectomy in a patient with adenocarcinoma of the endometrium if it is of low grade and stage and particularly if the patient is obese or elderly. Coincident transvaginal salpingo-oophorectomy is desirable (14). If postoperative examination of the hysterectomy specimen shows unexpected tumor involvement of the middle or outer third of the myometrium, postoperative external radiation therapy can be planned.

All things being equal, the choice of an abdominal over a vaginal route for hysterectomy might be a little like taking tonsils out through an incision in the side of the neck, an analogy suggested by some in discussing the choice of approach for the repair of vesicovaginal fistula.

Vaginal oophorectomy may also be performed if the ovaries are found surgically accessible or low in the pelvis. Occasionally, the appendix will be found in the operative field and may be removed, unless a valid reason exists for not performing appendectomy. When vaginal appendectomy has been accomplished, the operator must remember to inform the patient so that the absence of an abdominal scar will not mislead those responsible for her future medical care.

LAPAROSCOPIC-ASSISTED VAGINAL HYSTERECTOMY

"Never add the risk of laparoscopy to a surgical procedure unless the benefits of doing the procedure endoscopically outweigh the risks."

Alan Johns

Laparoscopic-assisted vaginal hysterectomy is not a substitute for vaginal hysterectomy but may be a substitution for a total abdominal hysterectomy when the condition and removability of the adnexa are uncertain. The infundibulopelvic ligament or ovarian ligament (if ovarian conservation is elected) may be translaparoscopically transected and secured along with the round ligament and upper broad ligament.

This sequence of combined operation is just as was described in 1897 but uses preliminary laparotomy "for freeing the uterus and adnexa from adhesions under direct visual control, making the organs mobile for the vaginal extirpation" (22). Alternatively, the sequence of laparoscopic-assisted vaginal hysterectomy may be reversed whereby the vaginal hysterectomy is accomplished first, and a coincident laparoscopy is performed only if the pelvic adhesions cannot be freed or the adnexa removed transvaginally. In the majority of instances, the experienced vaginal surgeon will be able to accomplish these goals transvaginally, saving the patient the expense, operating time, and discomfort of laparoscopy.

A significant complication rate exists for many advanced endoscopic procedures relating to operator inexperience with new techniques and instruments (39). At the present time, the overall costs of disposable laparoscopic equipment and increased operating time are significant. They exceed the costs of either vaginal hysterectomy or of total abdominal hysterectomy (4). These excessive costs are significantly reduced, however, when bipolar electrocoagulation with the carbon dioxide laser and reusable instruments replace staplers and disposables (27). Ideally, the well-trained gynecologic surgeon should be comfortable with the techniques of transvaginal total hysterectomy, laparoscopically assisted vaginal total hysterectomy, and transabdominal total hysterectomy. The surgeon should be aware that the technique employed in each instance will be that which best answers the need of the particular patient, and the surgeon should not just use the sole operative route with which he or she is familiar.

Repair of Vaginal Eversion

When all three levels of pelvic support are damaged and the vagina is completely everted, the success of the surgery will depend on all the technical virtuosity, skill, and good fortune a surgeon can summon, but the prognosis for a usable vagina is guarded unless sacrospinous colpopexy or sacrocolpopexy is employed (40, 44). Coincident hysterectomy, if indicated, can be employed without additional risk (11). Enterocele, when present, must always be resected, even in those uncommon instances when the surgeon feels obliged to resort to vaginectomy or colpocleisis.

There are two principal types of colpectomy, subtotal and total. The subtotal operation is especially useful if the uterus is present and atrophic in size, there is no elongation of the cervix, and one desires not to open the peritoneal cavity. The total colpectomy is more advisable when these conditions are not present.

When eversion of a vagina coexists with congenital enterocele, it is essential that the operator open the peritoneal cavity and resect or occlude the necessary enterocele sac to eliminate a residual postoperative enterocele. Such "recurrence" will often be progressive, continuing to dissect between the obliterated vagina and the rectum until it appears as a symptomatic bulge in the perineum. This carries with it all the symptoms of falling out that were present with the original vault eversion, and it is now technically more formidable to repair.

Malpas (23) points out that only the anterior wall of the enterocele descends with the uterus in uterovaginal or sliding prolapse. This kind of enterocele, is, in his opinion, incidental to the prolapse but not the prime anatomic feature, the latter being the elongated cardinal-uterosacral ligament complex. It is, of course, desirable to excise the sac and then perform a high ligation of the neck of the sac along with a culdeplasty in order to minimize the risk of postmenopausal reoperation (see Chapters 9 and 15).

An enterocele may sometimes coexist with general prolapse, but more commonly there is with this type a descent of the cul-de-sac without dissection or formation of a sac between the rectum and the vagina. There is equal descent of both anterior and posterior walls of the cul-de-sac, the latter bringing with it the anterior wall of the rectum. It is essential to mobilize the peritoneum laterally as well as anteriorly and posteriorly and to excise the entire sac, since it is often a prominent anatomic feature of the prolapse itself. If strong cardinal-uterosacral ligaments are not available or even palpable, as is so often the case, an alternative method of supporting the vault must be incorporated as part of the initial procedure. Sacrospinous colpopexy is an example of such a method. Removal of the peritoneal sac is best accomplished after the hysterectomy.

SACROSPINOUS COLPOPEXY

Transvaginal sacrospinous colpopexy with colporrhaphy (see Chapter 16) permits simultaneous correction of vault eversion and coincident cystocele and rectocele through the same operative exposure. About 5 percent of postoperative sacrospinous colpopexy patients will report recurrent symptomatic pelvic relaxation, of which recurrent cystocele is most common. A similar percentage will report new-onset postoperative urinary stress incontinence if appropriate urodynamic testing and an effective remedy were not worked out ahead of time. Comfortable coital function will be restored in the majority of patients (25).

SACROCOLPOPEXY

The surgeon should be familiar with the technique and indications for transabdominal sacrocolpopexy or sacrocervicopexy so that the procedure may be chosen that is best suited to the needs of a particular patient. The following are indications:

1. If there is some other reason for opening the abdomen, such as an adnexal mass, etc.
2. If the patient has sustained a previous operation of support of the vesicourethral junction by anterior colpopexy (Marshall-Marchatti-Kranz (MMK) or Burch) that has permanently altered the axis of the vagina, especially of the anterior wall.
3. If there is recurrence of vault prolapse following a sacrospinous colpopexy that appeared to have been performed correctly.
4. If a patient with uterine procidentia wishes to preserve her potential for fertility, we will occasionally do a sacrocervicopexy using the same principles. The response to subsequent pregnancy has generally been favorable and uneventful, though any

coincident cystocele and rectocele are not repaired at the same time but put off until childbearing has been completed.

5. If a surgeon is uncomfortable with the transvaginal sacrospinous colpopexy technique, the surgeon should do that technique with which he or she may be more comfortable, i.e., transabdominal sacrocolpopexy.

Although uncomplicated uterine retroversion often precedes prolapse, there is no reason to conclude that retroversion causes genital prolapse. Because prolapse and retroversion may coexist, the surgical correction of one should be recognized as having no influence on the cure or progression of the other.

Consequently, uterine suspension or fixation is not a treatment directed to the primary cause of coexistent or eventual prolapse. The progressive development of prolapse will be only temporarily slowed as a result of uterine suspension, and apparent improvement will have been accomplished at the expense of increasing the complexity and difficulty of subsequent definitive repair. In the management of most instances of early progressive genital prolapse, vaginal hysterectomy and repair should be performed rather than uterine suspension and tubal ligation.

SUMMARY

The surgeon should think of prolapse in terms of the sites of damage to the musculoconnective tissue supports of the birth canal rather than give sole consideration to the positions of the uterus and cervix relative to the vulvar outlet. The primary site of damage should be identified and emphasized in the repair, and an effort made to preserve an adequate vagina whenever possible. One must be ever mindful of the importance of the patient's posture and the effects of asthma, bronchitis, hay fever, tight girdles, and corsets as factors increasing intra-abdominal pressure and stress on pelvic supporting tissues. The patient with genital prolapse who manifests any of these additional symptoms and findings is a good candidate for postoperative recurrence. Whenever possible, the surgical intent should be to overcorrect the primary site of damage while making every effort to preserve vaginal length and a normal vaginal axis. A wide vaginal vault should be narrowed.

Generally speaking, the more severe the prolapse, the more difficult the operation, but the greater will be the patient's appreciation. There is no other field in surgery in which the gratitude of the patient and her husband for a good result is so genuine and the surgeon's efforts so truly appreciated.

The surgeon should have and exhibit enthusiasm, knowledge, and confidence about the specific procedure that is planned. Although a surgeon may have performed countless surgical reconstructions, to each particular patient her own surgery is the most important operation of all. It is the surgeon's obligation to choose the operation carefully, explain it thoroughly to the patient, and perform it well. The surgeon's thoughtful and unhurried daily rounds during the postoperative hospital stay add immeasurably to the patient's recovery, both physiologically and psychologically.

As TeLinde (43) has emphasized, there is much to be gained when the gynecologic surgeon follows the results of his or her surgery with periodic pelvic examinations over a number of years, correlating any recurrent disease, and especially late recurrence, with the choice of operation and the surgical technique employed for a particular patient. Such evidence is objective, positive, and purposeful and will help influence one's future choice of procedure, either by reinforcement or change, as circumstances require. Equally significant analysis is practically impossible in a clinic or short-term practice where the patient is not actually followed for a long period of time by the surgeon who was responsible for the choice and technique of repair.

References

1. Aboulghar MA, El-Kateb Y. Treatment of uterine prolapse in young women: sacral cervicopexy by polyvinyl alcohol sponge. J Egypt Med Assoc 1978;61:127–134.
2. Baden WF, Walker TA. Evaluation of the stress incontinent patient. In Cantor EB, ed. Female urinary stress incontinence. Springfield, IL: Charles C Thomas, 1979.
3. Ball TL. Anterior and posterior cystocele: cystocele revisited; of some antifacialists and facialists as I knew them. Clin Obstet Gynecol 1964;9:1062–1069.
4. Boike GM, et al. Laparoscopically assisted vaginal hysterectomy in a university hospital: report of 82 cases and comparison with abdominal and vaginal hysterectomy. Am J Obstet Gynecol 1993; 168:1690–1701.
5. Bonney V. The principles that should underlie all operations for prolapse. J Obstet Gynaecol Br Emp 1934;41:669–683.
6. Bonney V. The sustentacular apparatus of the female genital canal, the displacements that result from the yielding of its several components, and their appropriate treatment. J Obstet Gynaecol Br Commonw 1914;45:328–344.
7. Brubaker L, Retzky S, Smith C, Saclarides T. Pelvic floor evaluation with dynamic fluoroscopy. Obstet Gynecol 1993;82:863–868.
8. Creighton SM, Pearce JM, Stanton SL. Perineal video-ultrasonography in the assessment of vaginal prolapse: early observations. Br J Obstet Gynaecol 1992;99:310–313.
9. DeLancey JOL. Anatomic aspects of vaginal eversion after hysterectomy. Am J Obstet Gynecol 1992;166:1717–1728.
10. Dewhurst J, Tolpis PJ, Shepherd JH. Ivalon sponge hysterosacropexy for genital prolapse in patients with bladder exstrophy. Br J Obstet Gynaecol 1980;87:67–69.
11. Fedorkow DM, Kalbfleisch RE. Total abdominal hysterectomy at abdominal sacrovaginopexy: a comparative study. Am J Obstet Gynecol 1993;169:641–643.
12. Ferrari A, Frigerio L, Guaruerio P, et al. Il muscolo pubo-rettale nel prolasso genitale femminile: modificazione istochimiche. Ginecologia e Ostetricia 1986;2:73–77.
13. Goodrich MA, Webb MJ, King BF, et al. Magnetic resonance imaging of pelvic floor relaxation: dynamic analysis and evaluation of patients before and after surgical repair. Obstet Gynecol 1993;82:883–891.
14. Gray LA. Vaginal hysterectomy. 3rd ed. Springfield, IL: Charles C Thomas, 1983.
15. Green TH. Development of a plan for the diagnosis and treatment of urinary stress incontinence. Am J Obstet Gynecol 1961;83:632–648.
16. Harris TA, Bent AE. Genital prolapse with and without urinary incontinence. J Reprod Med 1990;35:792–798.
17. Hawksworth W, Roux JP. Vaginal hysterectomy. J Obstet Gynaecol Br Commonw 1958;63:214–228.
18. Henry MM, Swash M: Colphoproctology and the pelvic floor. London: Butterworths, 1985.
19. Jeffcoate TNA. Posterior colporrhaphy. Am J Obstet Gynecol 1959;77:490.
20. Kovak RS, Cruikshank SH. Successful pregnancies and vaginal deliveries after sacrospinous uterosacral fixation in five of nineteen patients. Am J Obstet Gynecol 1993;168:1778–1786.
21. Krige CF. The repair of genital prolapse combined with vaginal hysterectomy. J Obstet Gynaecol Br Commonw 1962;69:570–583.
22. Landau L, Landau T. The history and technique of the vaginal radical operation (translated by Eastman BL, Giles AE). New York: Wm Wood, 1897:161–164.
23. Malpas P. Genital prolapse in allied condition. New York: Grune & Stratton, 1955.
24. McMahan JD, Ripstein CB. Rectal prolapse. Am Surg 1087;53:37–40.
25. Mouk BJ, Ramp JL, Montz PJ, Lebherz TB. Sacrospinous ligament fixation for vaginal vault prolapse: complications and results. J Gynecol Surg 1991;7:87–92.
26. Navratil E. The place of vaginal hysterectomy. J Obstet Gynaecol Br Commonw 1965;72:841–846.
27. Nezhat C, Bess O, Admon D, et al. Hospital cost comparison between abdominal, vaginal, and laparoscopy-assisted vaginal hysterectomies. Obstet Gynecol 1994;83:713–716.
28. Nichols DH. Fertility retention in the patient with genital prolapse. Am J Obstet Gynecol 1991;164:1155–1158.
29. Nichols DH, ed. Gynecologic and obstetric surgery. St. Louis: Mosby-Yearbook, 1993:463–464.
30. Nichols DH. Retrorectal levatorplasty for anal and perineal prolapse. Surg Gynecol Obstet 1982;154:251–254.
31. Nichols DH, Randall CL. Techniques to decrease morbidity in the obese patient. In: Ludwig H, Thomsen K, eds. Gynecology and obstetrics. Berlin: Springer-Verlag, 1986:619–620.
32. Parks AG. Anorectal incontinence. Proc Roy Soc Med 1975;68:681–690.
33. Parks AG, Swash M, Urich H. Sphincter denervation in anorectal incontinence and rectal prolapse. J Br Soc Gastroenterol 1977;18:656.
34. Pratt JH, Daikoku NH. Obesity and vaginal hysterectomy. J Reprod Med 1990;35:945–949.
35. Richardson DA, Scotti RJ, Ostergard DR. Surgical management of uterine prolapse in young women. J Reprod Med 1989;34:388–392.

36. Richter K. Ekrankungen der Vagina. In: Schwalm Doderlein: Klinic der Frauenheilkunde und Geburtshilfe. Munchen: Urban & Schwarzenberg, 1971;8.
37. Rosenzweig BA, Pushkin S, Blumenfeld D, Bhatia NN. Prevalence of abnormal urodynamic test results in continent women with severe genitourinary prolapse. Obstet Gynecol 1992;79:535–542.
38. Sand PK, Bowen LW, Panganiban R, et al. The low pressure urethra as a factor in failed retropubic urethropexy. Obstet Gynecol 1987;69:399.
39. Smith DC, Donohue LR, Waszak SJ. A hospital review of advanced gynecologic endoscopic procedures. Am J Obstet Gynecol 1994;170:1635–1642.
40. Snyder TE, Krantz KE. Abdominal-retroperitoneal sacral colpopexy for the correction of vaginal prolapse. Obstet Gynecol 1991;77:944–949.
41. Stoesser FG. Construction of a sacrocervical ligament for uterine suspension. Surg Gynecol Obstet 1955;101:638–641.
42. Symmonds RE, Jordan LT. Iatrogenic stress incontinence of urine. Am J Obstet Gynecol 1961;82:1231.
43. TeLinde RW. Prolapse of the uterus and allied conditions. Am J Obstet Gynecol 1966;93:444.
44. Van Lindert ACM, Groendijk AG, Scholten PC, Heintz APM. Surgical support and suspension of genital prolapse including the Goretex soft tissue patch. Eur J Obstet Gynecol Reprod Biol 1993;50:133–139.

CHAPTER 7

Preoperative Care

The gynecologic surgeon should always be mindful of the whole patient, particularly during preoperative evaluation of the individual and her problem. Despite the inevitable concentration of interest in the pelvis and related reproductive capacity, the gynecologic surgeon must know about the overall characteristics of the patient's physical and mental health, including her past and current medical (as well as gynecologic) history, and be considerate as well of any current systemic problem, particularly any cardiac, blood pressure, or endocrine abnormality.

EVALUATION OF THE WOMAN AS A SURGICAL CANDIDATE

Individuals over 65 years of age account for 21 percent of the total number of inpatient operative procedure and 38.4 percent of total hospital days. As the population continues to age, these percentages will increase in the United States. At current rates of growth the number of people in the world who are over age 60 will triple to 1.4 billion by the year 2030, and will comprise 16 percent of the world's population. This group will consume an increasingly larger percentage of the health dollar. According to the Bureau of Census, the total number of 25.2 million women in the United States in 1990 who are between the ages of 45 and 65 is expected to increase in number to 41.8 million by 2010. By 2050 there will be 80 million Americans over age 65 (1 in 5 compared with 1 in 8 today).

Pulmonary function and renal and hepatic blood flow are reduced in the elderly, in part becaue of reduced cardiac output. Since hepatic metabolic systems are reduced, drugs dependent on hepatic metabolism will have a longer half-life, leading to a prolonged duration of action. Careful attention to the predictable changes can safely eliminate chronologic age alone as a deterrent to anesthesia and surgery. Very elderly patients (those over 90) having elective surgery tend to fare far better in terms of operative morbidity and mortality than those of the same age having emergency operation. Cardiac and respiratory diseases have little impact on short-term morbidity or mortality, but a preexistent deficit of the central nervous system is the most powerful predictor of poor outcome and survival, partly because of late referral for surgery and decreased and late diagnostic services and evaluation (16, 17).

When it was thought that patients in their eighties had a limited life span, they were often encouraged not to proceed with elective surgery, but were supported with less than optimal medical care. Today it is fully recognized that a 70- or 75-year-old woman has a life expectancy of at least another 10 to 15 years, and therefore age per se is no reason not to proceed with surgical intervention when it is indicated in otherwise healthy patients.

A decline in short-term memory, hearing, and other senses such as vision make it somewhat more difficult for the patient to clearly understand options as well as preoperative and postoperative instructions. Dementia can be a major risk factor (5).

It can no longer be assumed that the elderly patient is sexually inactive. For that reason care must be taken in vaginal support and reconstructive operations not to reduce the caliber of the vagina beyond a normal coital size. Although the vagina of the young, estrogen-stimulated woman is somewhat elastic, this is less true of those in the post-menopausal age group, and a relatively small amount of postoperative scarring and contraction may produce marked and unexpected dyspareunia in those older patients with a smaller vagina.

A positive family history including gynecologic disorders as well as systemic maladies should be determined. A history or evidence of pulmonary disease, asthma, emphysema, or excessive smoking would be significant. If the patient has emphysema or significant respiratory symptoms, spirometry and a study of blood gases are advisable. We would urge a preoperative patient to decrease or stop smoking for days or preferably weeks before scheduled surgery. Investigation should include evaluation of any history or "suspicion" of diabetes or phlebitis, any "tendency" to abnormality in bleeding, or any probability of an excessive use of alcohol. Preoperative communication with the patient's internist or her family doctor is mandatory when there is a history of heart disease, angina, or arrhythmia, or if the patient has been taking antihypertensive medication or has a history of rheumatism. A current consultation is equally important if the patient is diabetic, in which case the duration, severity, and current management of the disease should be known to the surgeon. An invitation should be extended to her internist or family doctor to participate in the management of the medical aspects of her postoperative care. Medications the patient has taken within the preceding year should be reviewed and their present effect evaluated. The effects of anticonvulsant drugs and diuretics should be recognized, and, in connection with the latter, any potassium or chloride depletion should be recognized and corrected preoperatively. It is important that the use of oral contraceptives be known so that they may be discontinued at least a month before surgery in order to minimize the chance of pulmonary, coronary, or cerebral thrombosis and embolism. The presence of any disease not under current control, including upper respiratory infections, a history of myocardial infarction, or a history of an increasingly progressive angina in which more symptoms are occurring in spite of reduced activity, should warrant reevaluation and reconfirmation of the indications and benefits for the scheduled surgery. Medical consultation and clearance for surgery are often desirable in such cases. It is equally important to be aware of a history of mental instability or any adverse experience with previous surgery or anesthesia. It is well to inquire whether the patient remembers an allergy or hypersensitivity to drugs taken previously, sometimes long ago. Allergies, particularly to medications, should be made known to both the surgeon and the anesthesiologist, including a history of allergies all but forgotten. Current or regularly used drugs the patient may have become accustomed to taking may have become such a habit that, unless asked, the patient may forget to bring them to the surgeon's attention. As the medical history is developed, the frequent or regular use of aspirin, tranquilizers, antihypertensive agents, antibiotics, birth control pills, or steroids used in the treatment of acne, arthritis, or rheumatism are examples of drugs frequently thought to be of insufficient significance to mention, but each should be reported to the surgeon.

The genitourinary system should have been investigated preoperatively with as much thoroughness as the patient's history and symptoms indicate. The surgical dictation of any previous pelvic surgery should be requested and reviewed. If the cervix is still present, preoperative evaluation should include the report of a Papanicolaou smear taken and evaluated within the year preceding surgery. An adequate evaluation of any recently abnormal uterine bleeding is necessary. Preoperative time should be invested to obtain a truly informed consent to surgery. The surgeon should clearly list the possible complications of all surgery—hemorrhage, infection, damage to nearby organs—but need not specify every conceivable complication which might unnecessarily alarm or frighten the patient. Postmenopausal patients with genital atrophy should take a course of twice weekly intravaginal estrogen administration coincident with pelvic floor exercises preoperatively. This regimen is continued postoperatively, starting the evening of the first postoperative day, using 1 g of estrogen cream in an application. One should expect there to be less postoperative cystitis and faster wound healing secondary to the improvement in vaginal blood supply (9).

Obesity is no contraindication to vaginal surgery per se, and providing the tissues are accessible and the indication for vaginal surgery is clear, the patients do remarkably well. Obesity causes few problems during or after vaginal surgery (24, 25, 28).

PREOPERATIVE LABORATORY STUDY

A preoperative chest x-ray is desirable for the patient over age 60. When the patient is over 50, or if there is any suspicion of cardiac abnormality, an electrocardiogram is advisable, not only for the information it can supply preoperatively, but also as a baseline for comparison with any postoperative study that might be required. Preoperative laboratory screening should include a complete blood count, coagulation studies, biochemical profile, and a blood type and screening determination. The reports of all of these procedures should be recorded on the patient's chart and reviewed before she is taken to the operating room. The patient should be carefully and conscientiously examined for any contraindication to what is usually elective surgery. The life expectancy of the patient and the longevity of her ancestors should always be taken into consideration, for to ignore the patient's overall welfare may precipitate avoidable problems that may ultimately discredit both the surgeon and the procedure performed. Abnormal findings should always be personally evaluated and discussed without placing reliance on the previous opinions of others.

An interesting report by Narr, Hansen, and Warner (23) of the Department of Anesthesia at the Mayo Clinic concerns preoperative screening laboratory tests in asymptomatic healthy patients who underwent elective surgical procedures at the Mayo Clinic in 1988. A total of 3782 patients were studied; routine preoperative screening tests included a complete blood count and tests for levels of creatinine, electrolytes, aspartate aminotransferase, and glucose. Substantially abnormal results were found in 160 of these patients, in 30 of whom the results were predictable on the basis of the history or physical examination. The abnormal test results prompted further assessment in 47 patients. No surgical procedure was delayed, and no association was noted between adverse outcome and any preoperative abnormality. (The anesthesia department at the Mayo Clinic no longer requires preoperative laboratory screening for most patients under 40.) These are *these* anesthesiologists guidelines but are not mandatory for other departments at the Mayo Clinic (yet). Their guidelines for patients of all ages are listed in Table 7.1. All patients have a preoperative review by a staff anesthesiologist of medications, an assessment of allergic and systemic disorders or symptoms, and a physical examination with emphasis on cardiopulmonary status performed 1 to 2 days before the scheduled surgical procedure.

Most institutions require each elective surgical patient to have a preoperative review and consultation with a staff anesthesiologist (29) and may wish to examine their policies in regard to preoperative laboratory testing to see if significant savings might not be effected by elimination of some routine but apparently superfluous preoperative testing of healthy patients under the age of 40.

Blood Transfusion

Of 35 deaths per year nationally from transfusion reaction, one-half are the consequence of clerical error (including provider errors, wrong sample being tested, technical errors in the laboratory, and administration of the wrong blood) and are therefore presumably preventable. The incidence of transfusion reaction is as follows: 1 recipient in 100 may develop chills, fever, or urticaria; 1 in 6000 may develop a hemolytic reaction; and 1 in 100,000 may develop a fatal hemolytic reaction. In addition, there is the chance for the development of infection as a consequence of transfusion, specifically hepatitis, HIV, cytomegalic virus infection, and Howan T-cell lymphotropic virus infection. It

Table 7.1
Minimal Suggested Preoperative Preanesthetic Test Requirements
at the Mayo Clinic[a]

AGE (yr)	TESTS REQUIRED
<40	None
40–59	Electrocardiography, measurement of creatinine and glucose
≥60	Complete blood cell count, electrocardiography, chest roentgenography, measurement of creatinine and glucose

From Narr BJ, Hansen TR, Warner MA. Pre-operative laboratory screening in healthy Mayo patients: cost effective elimination of tests and unchanged outcomes. Mayo Clin Proc 1991;66:155–159. Used with permission.
[a]In addition, the following guidelines apply:
   A complete blood cell count is indicated in all patients who undergo blood typing and who are screened or cross-matched.
   Measurement of potassium is indicated in patients taking diuretics or undergoing bowel preparation.
   Chest roentgenography is indicated in patients with a history of cardiac or pulmonary disease or with recent respiratory symptoms.
   A history of cigarette smoking in patients older than 40 years of age who are scheduled for an upper abdominal or thoracic surgical procedure is an indication for spirometry (forced vital capacity).

should be remembered that transfusion does tend to suppress temporarily the body's immune system, compromising to some small extent the patient's ability to respond to the challenge of postoperative infection and physiologic stress. This potential risk can be eliminated if unnecessary transfusion is avoided.

Homologous Transfusion: Banked Blood

One need not encourage patients to bank 1 pint of their own blood against transfusion during their coming surgery unless a major blood loss (>1000 ml) is anticipated. Likely as not a 1-unit (pint) transfusion will not be used and will then not be given back to the patient, and she will have compromised her own iron storage. Also, if she has bled enough to require transfusion, more than 1 unit will be needed, in which case her own unit of blood will not be adequate to meet her needs. It is better for the surgeon to develop a system of precise anatomic dissection and hemostasis for which blood loss does not require transfusion.

Because transfusion even of the patient's own blood carries a small but definable risk, it should not be employed without significant indication. Single-unit transfusion is rarely indicated. Nonprogressive iron deficiency anemia can be effectively remedied by iron therapy using the oral route.

Platelet Transfusion

When platelets are less than $100,000/ml^3$, the patient's bleeding time should be tested. When preoperative estimate of blood platelets is less than $50,000/ml^3$, platelet transfusion is indicated prior to major surgery. The therapeutic dose of platelets is 1 unit/ 10 kg of body weight. Six units are generally adequate to achieve hemostasis in the adult. The use of a standard 170m filter is recommended for the administration of platelets. Infections that may be transmitted by platelet transfusion are similar to those associated with the use of other blood products.

Routine Intravenous Pyelogram

If each of the 650,000 hysterectomy patients for each year were given a preoperative intravenous pyelogram (IVP) for a nominal charge of $100 each, the cost would be

$65,000,000. One out of 40,000 of these patients would develop a reaction to the intravenous medication, and 16 women per year would die of the reaction. If each patient who had a preoperative pyelogram was to have a postoperative one as well to check on "silent" injury, it would cost the public an additional $65,000,000, or a total of $130,000,000 per year. Routine IVP is not recommended.

MECHANICAL PREPARATION OF THE LOWER BOWEL

Major pelvic surgery will be facilitated if the large intestine is reasonably empty of its usual content during the operation. Placing the patient on a diet of clear liquids the day before admission to the hospital is worthwhile. The frequency with which patients are admitted the same day as surgery is to be performed requires that the patient take an active role in her preoperative mechanical bowel preparation. This preparation effectively reduces the number of bacteria within the bowel and its content but does not sterilize the intestinal tract.

Ingestion of a polyethylene glycol-electrolyte lavage solution (GoLYTELY, NuLYTELY, CoLyte) is most effective for this purpose (10). The powder is mixed with water and refrigerated the night before it is to be taken. Starting at 8:00 a.m. the day before the surgery, it is consumed as a drink at the rate of 1 liter per hour until it is gone. Two tablets of bisacodyl (Dulcolax) are taken at 6:00 p.m. the evening before surgery.

For those patients for whom this routine is unacceptable or impossible, an alternative is for the patient to give herself or be given an enema at bedtime the night before surgery and another early on the morning of surgery if time permits. Disposable enema units are effective and may be more convenient.

PREOPERATIVE HAIR REMOVAL

We believe that preoperative shaving of the vulvar surgical site offers no advantage to the patient and by abrading the skin may precipitate an increased incidence of wound infection (1). Our patients are no longer shaved routinely, but long hairs may be clipped, if desired, to keep them out of the surgical field. Unshaven patients are much more comfortable in the later postoperative recovery phase.

PREVENTIVE OR PROPHYLACTIC ANTIBIOTICS

Postoperative wound infections affect at least 920,000 of the 23 million patients who undergo surgery each year in the United States (this does not include the postoperative evaluation of the vast number of patients having their surgery in outpatient settings)(12). Among inpatients, wound infections are thought to double the expected postoperative stay, with an enormous increase in costs of hospitalization.

Considering the vagina as a site for surgery, one must be mindful that it is inhabited or chronically "contaminated" by multiple bacteria. The bacteriology of the vaginal canal of each woman varies, both in bacterial types and numbers. Variations are related to the time of life, the patient's environment and sexual activity, and, in premenopausal patients, even the time of the month (11). The desirable effects of preoperative cleansing by douching and scrubbing with antibacterial soaps, such as those containing povidone-iodine (Betadine) or chlorhexidine gluconate (Hibiclens), will ensure a significant reduction in bacterial quantity, but this procedure in itself does not "sterilize" the vagina.

There seems to be a significant risk of postoperative infection when an operative procedure combines surgical manipulation and dissection of the vagina with a large opening of the peritoneal cavity and, at its conclusion, leaves areas of surgically traumatized and devascularized tissue crushed by forceps and tied into pedicles. This clinical risk can be reduced considerably if an appropriate broad-spectrum antibiotic is present at the time of surgery in the tissue being operated upon, as suggested by Burke (3). Such protection is especially desirable when the surgical procedure carries an appreciable risk of clinical infection. Ledger et al. (20) and others (7, 15, 21, 27, 34, 35) have found this to be especially likely in premenopausal patients subjected to vaginal hysterectomy and have formulated a useful set of guidelines for antibiotic prophylaxis in gynecology, which include Burke's recommendation that the "antibiotic must be circulating in the patient's tissue before the operation begins and should be promptly discontinued if there is no specific reason for continuing it after the patient recovers normal physiology." Burke emphasized, however, that

Preoperative preventive antibiotics will not eliminate all postoperative septic complications. There will be situations in which the level of bacterial resistance, extent of trauma, size of inoculum of bacteria, or combination will be such that antibiotics will be of little use. Antibiotics are but an adjunct to the natural resistance to bacterial invasion. They by no means replace it.*

We are in accord with this thinking and, in addition, firmly believe that there is no substitute for meticulous precision and efficiency in technique and hemostasis to minimize tissue trauma.

Preventive antibiotics are thus particularly useful in curbing morbidity when major vaginal surgery is performed and especially when local hemostasis has been augmented by preliminary infiltration of tissue with a vasoconstrictor. An initial intramuscular injection of an antibiotic 1 hour before the start of surgery "on call to the operating room" seems to provide an effective tissue level when needed; but because there is often an unpredictable time variable of 1/2 to 3 hours between "on call to the operating room" and the actual initial incision, it appears that a proper level of antibiotic can be delivered to the tissues for surgery if it is given intravenously in the operating room immediately before the onset of anesthesia. Initial intravenous administration of prophylactic antibiotics during anesthesia is not recommended (32) because of possibly masked, irreversible, and lethal anaphylaxis, though the risk is small. The antibiotic probably will reach an effective tissue level within 20 to 30 minutes of the time of intravenous administration. If the operation is to be of less than 2 hours total duration, a single dose of antibiotic is desirable. If the operative time is longer than 2 hours duration, the intravenous dose should be repeated 2 hours from the beginning of the operation. Our first choice of antibiotic is 2 g of a first-generation cephalosporin such as cefazolin (Ancef or Kefzol), which has a half-life of 80 minutes; if a second dose is given 2 hours after the first, the half-life totals 120 minutes.

The decreased febrile morbidity has been impressive and noteworthy and, by shortening the patient's hospital stay, cost-effective. Although, in general, cephalosporins are contraindicated for the patient with a history of "penicillin allergy," a single preoperative dose may occasionally be used if the surgeon feels that the indication is warranted and the risk-benefit ratio is favorable and if the allergic manifestation after penicillin injection was of the nature of a mild skin rash. If, on the other hand, the patient had a previous anaphylactic reaction to penicillin, this must be thoroughly respected and an alternate such as minocycline, metronidazole (19), or clindamycin and gentamicin chosen. There has been much speculation as to why reduced postoperative morbidity has been demonstrated using antibiotics to which anaerobic organisms are not sensitive. Perhaps the antibiotics suppress the aerobic flora, permitting the body to concentrate its defensive energy on the surviving anaerobes even though the latter were not sensitive to the antibiotic. Another possibility relates to possible interdependence of an anaerobic infection on a coincident aerobic colonization. The reverse of this situation might explain the similar effectiveness of preoperative metronidazole (Flagyl) (13, 19).

---

* From Burke JF. Use of preventive antibiotics in clinical surgery. Am Surg 1973;39:6–11. Used with permission.

We believe it advisable to apply elastic stockings, of graduated compression if available, from the feet to the midthigh preoperatively, particularly if the patient has appreciable varices or a history of previous phlebitis or thrombosis. Alternately, they may be applied at the conclusion of an operation when the patient has been in the lithotomy or a marked Trendelenburg position, before the legs are lowered and the head is raised. Whether this practice reduces the risk of embolism is debatable, but it effectively reduces the incidence of thrombosis (33) and the size of the venous bed into which blood will pool as soon as the patient's body is leveled or her feet have been taken down from the stirrups. Under such circumstances the prophylactic use of elastic stockings will appreciably reduce the degree of postoperative hypotension, which will predispose some patients to cardiac or cerebral thrombosis or might at least confuse the initial recovery room phase of the patient's postoperative course.

We do not recommend the use of subcutaneous minidoses of heparin (5000 IU of calcium heparin, subcutaneously 2 hours before surgery and twice a day for 5 days (4, 6, 36)), or dihydroergotamine (DHE)-heparin 5000 IU 2 hours before surgery and every 12 hours thereafter for 5 days (30, 31), other than in the patient with a history of phlebitis, fearing an insufficient effectiveness in reducing the incidence of embolization to offset the risk of a significant increase in intraoperative and postoperative bleeding (2). Intermittent pneumatic calf compression is a good substitute (22).

STEROIDS

When a patient is taking cortisone or prednisone, it should, if possible, be stopped 10 days before surgery and not resumed until after the first 4 or 5 days postoperatively. In such patients the surgeon should strongly consider the use of nonabsorbable suture in buried tissue layers subject to tension. If temporary suspension of the drug cannot be safely accomplished, massive doses of vitamin A (50,000 to 100,000 units daily) or anabolic steroids may reverse the unwelcome inhibition of collagen formation and inflammatory reaction (18).

PREOPERATIVE PSYCHOLOGICAL PREPARATION

In addition to the usual physiologic and anatomic preparations for surgery, there should be an appropriate psychologic evaluation of the patient by the surgeon. It is always good to encourage the patient's expression of her questions and possible fears. Such adequate preparation will add immeasurably to the patient's expectations of a successful outcome, and she will be less dismayed by postoperative discomforts and the time required for complete recovery. It is as important for the surgeon to understand the manner in which the patient conceives of her problem and its treatment (14) as it is for her to understand how her surgeon views her condition and the surgery recommended. The most desirable one-to-one relationship requires a considerate surgeon and an informed, confident patient.

The implications of hysterectomy to the individual patient's psychology should be understood by the physician as he or she considers how a particular patient perceives of her problem and the results of the recommended surgery. These considerations were well summarized by Polivy (26). For some women, an escape from the concerns regarding conception may be entirely offset by the fear that the operation will mean a loss of femininity. Being freed of the inconveniences of menometrorrhagia and dysmenorrhea spares many patients predictable and undesirable disabilities. The gynecologist should make certain the patient also understands that the quality of her response to her husband will likely be enhanced by her freedom from the fear of pregnancy.

Hysterectomy in the absence of demonstrable significant pelvic pathology seems more likely to be followed by subsequent emotional depression or milder instability. There are several helpful points to aid in the recognition of a candidate disposed to postoperative psychological difficulties. The surgery addict, often a hysterical neurotic with the scars of many operations, will usually report intense but ill-defined pains and often harbors a need to suffer. The surprisingly indifferent woman should also be a warning, however, because indifference often serves as a simple facade behind which there exists an immature refusal to even think about the operation. Predictably, this degree of rejection is likely to be followed by an almost infantile type of emotional response to all postoperative discomforts and dysfunctions. When noted preoperatively, apparent indifference should be considered a mask, repressing anxiety and a denial of the trauma to come. In sharp contrast, the overanxious patient evidences worry about technical details, the site and size of her incision, the type of anesthesia, and the postoperative visiting hours. It would be expedient to recognize such concerns as evidence of good candidacy for postoperative unhappiness and perhaps severe emotional instability. Still another problem is the would-be seductive patient, whose fantasies in regard to her doctor-patient relationships may readily transcend the usual bounds of professional responsibility. The desirable degree of insight into the probabilities of the patient's mental and emotional stability after surgery may usually be gained, but only as a result of discussing with the patient before surgery her feelings about the loss of her uterus and her expectations following surgery, as well as her concepts related to previous operations and her reactions to those experiences.

Predisposing factors to postoperative psychiatric disturbances that may prolong the period of disability should be suspected when an operation proves the absence of demonstrable pelvic disease, when there is a history of previous psychiatric care, especially depression, or when there are evidences of marital discord, particularly in a younger patient. An attempt should be made to recognize and assess such factors and to place them in proper perspective ahead of time. When accomplished, both the patient and her surgeon will be spared hours of postoperative apprehension, indecision, and lack of progress. When a distinct need for professional psychiatric help is suspected, it will be most effective if such support is made available well ahead of time so that the psychiatrist, too, may have developed a desirable degree of rapport with the patient before the strain of postoperative discomfort is added to any preexisting psychiatric needs.

Patients who seem neurotic preoperatively are certain to be manifestly neurotic postoperatively. In such instances the surgeon will be well advised to search for and dispel myths and fears that may well exist and have long been repressed and to reassure the patient particularly of the preservation of her femininity, giving due consideration to possible ethnic attitudes and customs. Often the latter may have traditionally clear-cut and deeply ingrained concepts about the occurrence of menstruation and the importance of preserving the uterus. Including psychological aspects in a preoperative evaluation of the patient will help avoid what might otherwise become a medically unexpected and surgically unwarranted complication, which all too frequently can make a surgical experience a most unhappy and unsatisfactory memory for all concerned.

When developed preoperatively, the patient's understanding and confidence will ensure cooperation, an improved postoperative course, and a more optimistic long-term evaluation of her result. Although both patient and surgeon are aware that the surgeon has accompanied many other patients down the same surgical pathway, to each individual patient her operation is the all-important one, and her surgeon can do no less than to keep her point of view constantly in mind. This is the poorest of times to appear impatient, hurried, or indifferent, or to suggest the importance of anything other than this patient's current problem throughout pre- and postoperative periods. Advice and restrictions in postoperative activities should not be detailed without a knowledge and appreciation of the individual's home situation. A quiet personal conversation will do much to dispel the fear of being abandoned during the stay in an unfamiliar hospital room. The surgeon should emphasize the intention of seeing the patient each day throughout her period of hospitalization. No matter how busy one's daily schedule, time must be found to answer any of the patient's questions carefully and in an unhurried manner in order to dispel her unnecessary fears. Knowledge of a chronically ill child or parent, a husband's current employment crisis, or the pressing problems of other members of the patient's immediate family will enable the surgeon to understand some patients' apparently unreasonable anxiety. Some appreciation of the patient's relationships with her family and her husband is usually very important. If a genuine neurosis is present, the surgeon must clearly understand and honestly question whether his operative measures will bring about the desired gynecological cure for any coincident symptoms of neurotic or hysterical origin. In such tragic situations, surgery too often provides only an excuse for the patient to blame her marital disharmony upon the effects of her surgery. With continued failure to recognize the shortcomings in her own relationship with her husband, an operative procedure that was indicated and satisfactorily performed may be blamed for having made her worse.

A considerate preoperative conversation with the patient in the hospital is of inestimable value in providing her with a chance to bring to light any last-minute questions or problems that may have been troubling her and to relate herself more closely with her surgeon. Certainly, at some time before the day of the operation, if the surgeon knows he or she may be away or unavailable during a portion of the patient's postoperative stay, such an explanation should be clearly given to the patient, in order to dispel thoughts of postoperative abandonment. Such an explanation should describe the arrangements that have been made for her care during the absence, clearly indicating who will be responsible, how this individual can be reached, and when the surgeon expects to return to resume personal supervision of her care.

PHYSICAL AND PSYCHOLOGICAL PREPARATION OF THE SURGEON

Copenhaver (8) observed the importance of appropriate preoperative physical and psychological preparation of the surgeon in influencing a good surgical outcome:

Too little attention has been given to the environmental and inner tensions that influence the outcome of a surgical procedure. Pressures created by an unrealistic schedule, by nervous or unhappy associates, and by preoccupations of the surgeon with other problems may result in poor or hasty judgment at the operating table. A serene operating room and competent surgical nurse have much to do with the quality of surgery.

Speed at the operating table too often has been equated with surgical skill. When such speed reflects a masterful organization of surgical techniques, it may be an asset. However, too often such speed reflects the need to meet a later appointment, a desire to impress younger physicians and nurses, or just the inner restlessness of the surgeon. It is believed that uncontrolled speed at the operating table is the foremost cause of surgical complications.

Fatigue of the surgeon and major surgery are a bad combination. If a surgeon has been obliged to go without rest for a long time, it may be wise to defer an operation. If an extensive, radical, or tedious operation is to be performed, it is better to start such a procedure early in the morning when the operating team is physically and mentally alert.

A depressed or anxious or emotionally unstable person breeds disaster in the operating room. Psychologic well-being of the operating room team and good surgery go hand in hand.
Preoperative and postoperative evaluation and care . . . involve liberal use of medical consultants, for it is better to prevent a medical or surgical complication than to manage one.*

ANESTHESIA

The authors' route of choice for anesthesia is intrathecal, if the patient is willing, and the surgeon is confident that the operation will be completed within 2½ hours before

---

* From Copenhaver EH. Surgery of the vulva and vagina. Philadelphia: WB Saunders, 1981, p.5. Used with permission.

the anesthetic effect has worn off. There is less variation in the patient's blood pressure during surgery, which makes the operation safer for the frail and aged or those with serious medical problems. There is less atelectasis, coughing, and nausea postoperatively. A well-balanced, well-monitored general anesthesia is a satisfactory alternative choice, however, and some surgery can be accomplished under local infiltration anesthesia. If muscle or striated sphincter plication is planned, the anesthesiologist should be requested to refrain from using curarelike agents lest intraoperative identification by stimulated muscle contraction be inhibited.

CONCLUSION

Before a woman can be assured of a good surgical result, the gynecologist must make certain of the patient's physical as well as psychological readiness for surgery by correcting any factor likely to delay either her recovery from the operation or her resumption of normal activities. The success of gynecologic surgery depends as much on the adequacy of the preoperative appraisal and preparation of the patient as on the technical skill and clinical judgments of the gynecologist.

References

1. Alexander JW, Fischer JE, Boyajian M, et al. The influence of hair removal methods on wound infections. Arch Surg 1983;118:347–352.
2. Bonnar J. Venous thromboembolism and gynecologic surgery. Clin Obstet Gynecol 1985;28(2):432–446.
3. Burke JF. Use of preventive antibiotics in clinical surgery. Am Surg 1973;39:6–11.
4. Butterman GJ, et al. Optimization of postoperative prophylaxis of thrombosis in gynecology. Geburtshilfe Frauenheilkd 1978;38:98.
5. Capen CV. Gynecologic surgery: pre-operative evaluation. Clin Obstet Gynecol 1988;31:673–685.
6. Clarke-Pearson DL, Synan IS, Dodge R, et al. A randomized trial of low-dose heparin and intermittent pneumatic calf compression for the prevention of deep venous thrombosis after gynecologic oncology surgery. Am J Obstet Gynecol 1993;168:1146–1154.
7. Classen DC, et al. The timing of prophylactic administration of antibiotics and the risk of surgical-wound infection. N Engl J Med 1992;326:281–286.
8. Copenhaver EH. Surgery of the vulva and vagina. Philadelphia: WB Saunders, 1981, pp. 3–5.
9. Felding C, Mikkelsen AL, Clausen HV, Loft A, Larsen LG. Preoperative treatment with estradiol in women scheduled for vaginal operation for genital prolapse: a randomized, double-blind trial. Maturitas 1992;15:241–249.
10. Fleites RA, et al. The efficacy of polyethylene glycol-electrolyte lavage solution versus traditional mechanical bowel preparation for elective colonic surgery. Surgery 1985;98:708–715.
11. Galask RP, Larsen B, Ohm MJ. Vaginal flora and its role in disease entities. Clin Obstet Gynecol 1976;19:61–81.
12. Haley RW, et al. Identifying patients at high risk of surgical wound infection. Am J Epidemiol 1985;121:206–215.
13. Hamod KA, Spence MR, Rosenshein NB, et al. Single-dose and multidose prophylaxis in vaginal hysterectomy. Am J Obstet Gynecol 1980;136:976–979.
14. Harwood A. The hot-cold theory of disease. JAMA 1971;216:1153–1158.
15. Hemsell DL, Cunningham FG, Kappus S, et al. Cefoxitin for prophylaxis in premenopausal women undergoing vaginal hysterectomy. Obstet Gynecol 1980;56:629–634.
16. Hosking MP, et al. Outcomes of surgery in patients 90 years of age and older. JAMA 1989;261:1909–1915.
17. Hosking MP, Warner MA. Preoperative evaluation and prognosis after surgery in elder patients. Geriat Med Today 1990;9:19–26.
18. Hunt TK, Ehrlich HP, Garcia JA, et al. Effect of vitamin A on reversing the inhibitory effect of cortisone on healing of open wounds in animals and man. Ann Surg 1969;170:633–640.
19. Jackson P, Ridley WJ. Simplified antibiotic prophylaxis for vaginal hysterectomy. Aust N Z J Obstet Gynaecol 1979;19:225–227.
20. Ledger WL, Gee C, Lewis WF. Guidelines for antibiotic prophylaxis in gynecology. Am J Obstet Gynecol 1975;121:1038–1045.
21. Mickal A, Curole D, Lewis C. Cefoxitin sodium: double-blind vaginal hysterectomy prophylaxis in premenopausal patients. Obstet Gynecol 1980;56:222–225.
22. Morrow CP. Discussion of paper by Roberts. In: Mishell Dr, Kirschbaum TH, Morrow CP, eds. Yearbook of obstetrics and gynecology. St. Louis: Mosby–Year Book, 1989:241.

23. Narr BJ, Hansen TR, Warner MA. Pre-operative laboratory screening in healthy Mayo patients: cost effective elimination of tests and unchanged outcomes. Mayo Clin Proc 1991;66:155–159.
24. Nichols DH, Randall CL. Techniques to decrease morbidity in the obese patient. In: Ludwig H, Thomsen K, eds. Gynecology and obstetrics. Berlin: Springer-Verlag, 1986:619–620.
25. Pitkin RM. Vaginal hysterectomy in obese women. Obstet Gynecol 1977;49:567.
26. Polivy J. Psychological reactions to hysterectomy: a critical review. Am J Obstet Gynecol 1974; 118:417–426.
27. Polk BF, Shapiro M, Goldstein P, et al. Randomized clinical trial of perioperative cefazolin in preventing infection after hysterectomy. Lancet 1980;1:437–440.
28. Pratt JH, Daikoku NH. Obesity and vaginal hysterectomy. J Reprod Med 1990;35:945–949.
29. Roizen MF, et al. The relative roles of the history and physical examination, and laboratory testing in preoperative evaluation for outpatient surgery: the "Starling" curve of preoperative laboratory testing. Anesth Clin North Am 1987;5:15–34.
30. Sasahara AA, DiSerio FJ, et al. Dihydroergotamine-heparin prophylaxis of postoperative deep vein thrombosis: a multicenter trial. JAMA 1984;251:2960.
31. Sasahara AA, Koppenhagen K, Haring R, et al. Low molecular weight heparin plus dihydroergotamine for prophylaxis of postoperative deep vein thrombosis. Br J Surg 1986;73:697.
32. Spruill FG, Minette L J, Sturner WQ. Two surgical deaths in association with cephalothin. JAMA 1974;229:440–441.
33. Turner GM, Cole SE, Brooks JH. The efficacy of graduated compression stockings in the prevention of deep vein thrombosis after major gynecological surgery. Br J Obstet Gynaecol 1984;91:588–591.
34. Wenzel RP. Preoperative antibiotic prophylaxis. N Engl J Med 1992;326:337–339.
35. Whelton A, Blanco LJ, Carter GG, et al. Therapeutic implications of doxycycline and cephalothin concentrations in the female genital tract. Obstet Gynecol 1980;55:28–32.
36. Wille-Jørgensen P, et al. Prophylaxis of deep venous thrombosis after acute abdominal operation. Surg Gynecol Obstet 1991;172:44–48.

CHAPTER 8

Vaginal Hysterectomy

In the selection and recommendation of an operative procedure for hysterectomy, there is no place for surgical histrionics or dogmatic pronouncements. It should be the intention of the gynecologist to gain by personal experience equal confidence in his or her abilities and the results that can be expected by both the transabdominal and transvaginal operations. In this course of evaluating each patient's problem, he or she should choose the approach that seems clearly in the best interests of that individual.

INDICATIONS FOR VAGINAL HYSTERECTOMY

Ultimately, the indications for abdominal hysterectomy may become the contraindications for vaginal hysterectomy, for instance, the presence of a suspicious adnexal mass, uterine immobility, invasive cancer, very large uterine leiomyomas, or lack of operator experience, enthusiasm, and confidence (24, 62, 80, 81). Indications relating to the choice of operative routes are listed in Table 8.1.

A patient with prolapse may complain of a significant leukorrhea, and a discharge coming from the cervix suggests a coincident pyometra. When pyometra is discovered and there is no obvious cause, a barium enema may help differentiate the diagnosis of coincident sigmoid-uterine fistula from coexistent diverticulosis-diverticulitis. In this instance one must carefully plan for coincident dissection of the apparent sigmoid loop from the back of the uterus, and for safe closure of the sigmoid defect. This will often require laparotomy.

The Leiomyomatous Uterus

There is no medical necessity to perform hysterectomy by any route upon an asymptomatic woman with a myomatous uterus less than 12 gestational weeks in size (22). Because fibroids generally stabilize or regress after menopause, hysterectomy for the asymptomatic fibroid is rarely indicated. Sudden growths of the leiomyomas in a postmenopausal patient not taking estrogen may be an indication for definitive therapy as well as demonstration of a silent ureteral obstruction secondary to uterine compression. The latter is rare, but in patients with fibroids larger than 12 weeks gestational size, can be easily evaluated by renal ultrasound (11).

The symptomatic leiomyomatous uterus of between 14 and 18 weeks gestational size may be decreased in size considerably by the preoperative use of a gonadotropin-releasing hormone agonist (68, 76). This will permit one to benefit from the advantages of vaginal hysterectomy, including decreased operative blood loss and shorter hospital stay and convalescence.

SHRINKING A FIBROID PREOPERATIVELY TO PERMIT VAGINAL HYSTERECTOMY

One can give depot leuprolide acetate (Lupron) intramuscularly, 3.75 mg per month, for 3 months. This will probably induce a temporary state of amenorrhea, and when

Table 8.1.

Vaginal versus Laparoscopic Assisted versus Abdominal Approach to Possible Hysterectomy

Indication	Approach		
	Vaginal	Laparoscopically Assisted Vaginal Hysterectomy	Abdominal
Myomata uteri	Occasionally	Occasionally	Usually
Pelvic inflammatory disease	Rarely	Occasionally	Always, except for posterior colpotomy
Recurrent dysfunctional uterine bleeding	Usually	Rarely	Occasionally
Endometriosis	Rarely	Occasionally	Usually
Adenomyosis	Usually	Occasionally	Occasionally
Symptomatic pelvic relaxation	Usually	Rarely	Occasionally
Adnexal mass	Rarely	Occasionally	Usually
Pelvic pain	Rarely	Occasionally	Usually
Cancer of cervix			
Stage O and Ia	Usually	Rarely	Occasionally
Stage IA, IB, IIA	Occasionally	Rarely	Usually
Cancer corpus	Occasionally	Occasionally	Usually

Modified from Thompsom JD: *Clin Obstet Gynecol* 24:1255, 1981.

accompanied by thrice daily administration of ferrous sulfate, permitting a significant rise in depressed preoperative hemoglobin and hematocrit levels, it reduces the risks of transfusion. Friedman (21) reported three cases of unexpected heavy vaginal bleeding during leuprolide acetate treatment in patients with degenerating submucous leiomyomas, requiring transfusion and emergency myomectomy. A rare case of angina myocardial infarction has been reported in a woman undergoing treatment with depot leuprolide acetate (52), which suggests that one should be cautious in its use in a patient with a strong family history of coronary heart disease.

Since estrogen administration enlarges uterine tissue, growth factors are likely to act as local mediators of estrogen activity. Flaumenhaft (20) observes that

insulin-like growth factor I (IGF-I) mRNA synthesis by rat and pig uteri is induced by estrogens. Inappropriate expression of growth factors, such as IGFs, may be involved in the pathophysiology of leiomyomatous disease. In fact, levels of IGF-II mRNA (79) and receptor for IGF-I (12) are increased in leiomyomatous tissue compared with normal myometrium. Inhibiting such expression might potentially aid in controlling the disease process. Interestingly, treatment of women with leiomyomas with the gonadotropin-releasing hormone agonist, leuprolide acetate, resulted in decreased secretion of IGF-I and IGF-II from leiomyoma explant cultures from untreated women (68). Treatments interfering directly with growth factor activity in fibroids may someday help control their growth.*

* From Flaumenhaft R. Growth factors. Prim Care Update Ob/Gyn 1994;1:171–172. Used with permission.

CONSERVATION OR PROPHYLACTIC REMOVAL OF THE OVARIES

From a theoretical standpoint, the desirability of ovarian removal at the time of hysterectomy should be considered by the vaginal surgeon by the same criteria as would be observed during an abdominal operation. Because the ovaries are not technically as readily accessible during a vaginal hysterectomy as during abdominal laparotomy, there is a significantly decreased frequency of ovarian removal on a prophylactic basis when hysterectomy is accomplished by the vaginal approach.

When evaluating the indications for castration, the surgeon should consider seriously and critically whether the effects of removing the ovaries justify the relatively small chance that the individual may in the future develop a neoplasm of the ovary if the ovaries are preserved (61). Because estrogen replacement is readily available after castration, many will argue that the usual replacement therapy relieves only the subjective vasomotor symptoms of the menopause and, unless long continued, does not prevent the degenerative changes that may progress in diverse forms after castration. It is essential to remember that estrogen replacement therapy, to be effective, must be given prophylactically. Although the particularly undesirable bony changes are preventable, once developed they apparently are not reversible. Moreover, Robinson et al. (69) pointed out that the standard postmenopausal daily dose of 1.25 mg of conjugated estrogen will be only partially successful in altering postmenopausal blood serum lipid levels, that a dose of 2.5 mg per day is somewhat more effective, but that the optimal effect may require 5 mg per day or more, a dose likely to produce such distressing secondary effects as breast tenderness, fluid retention, and weight gain.

Randall (63) notes that patients for whom estrogen supplementation or replacement had been prescribed after a surgical menopause tended to discontinue the medication after 1 or 2 years. He suggested the reason might be the fact that the more significant of the degenerative effects that may follow estrogen withdrawal may not become symptomatic until long after estrogen effects are no longer demonstrable, and as a result the patient does not associate immediate cause and effect. Mattingly and Huang (50), describing their studies of steroidogenesis in the postmenopausal ovary, have demonstrated that although estrogen production falls precipitously after cessation of menstruation, stromal steroid production persists for a long time after the menopause, for which reason they have emphasized that the postmenopausal ovary continues to have a significant metabolic function. The same authors report a survey of published reports of patients in whom ovaries had been conserved at the time of hysterectomy. In reports totaling 7765 patients followed for varying intervals after hysterectomies, only 12 individuals were known to have developed cancer in the preserved ovaries, an incidence of only 0.15 percent. However, the overall incidence of ovarian malignancy suggests that the *eventual* frequency of ovarian cancer is likely to approximate 1 per 100 patients. Castration should not be routine at any arbitrarily designated age, but so-called prophylactic oophorectomy should be considered after the age of true ovarian senescence, whether that be demonstrable at 40 or 70 years of age. If there are indications for intraperitoneal surgery in a postclimacteric patient with nonfunctioning ovaries, one should certainly consider prophylactic oophorectomy, because the tendency of the ovaries to neoplasia does not disappear when steroidogenesis ceases. The postmenopausal ovary should never be considered too old to develop malignancy, but if the ovaries are still functioning at the time of hysterectomy, the operator should consider the advantages as well as the risks of ovarian preservation. Because there seems no arbitrary age at which all ovaries should be removed, we believe the view of the surgeon who elects not to perform routine oophorectomy is defensible, and that one's philosophy concerning ovarian preservation should determine the procedure recommended, whether surgery involves the transabdominal or the transvaginal route.

Prophylactic Oophorectomy in the Premenopausal Patient

Any benefits of elective oophorectomy on the premenopausal patient presuppose that there will be long-term postoperative estrogen replacement therapy. The benefit of reducing the incidence of ovarian cancer does not outweigh the adverse effects on the bones and cardiovascular system of the patient who does not participate in long-term estrogen therapy (74).

If the patient has a family history positive for ovarian cancer, she might be considered a candidate for prophylactic oophorectomy at the time of vaginal hysterectomy. She should be told that this will reduce her chances of developing carcinoma of the ovary, but should not be offered a guarantee that this possibility is eliminated, since the disease seems to have certain potential general coelomic manifestations. Elective oophorectomy in the premenopausal patient is a preoperative decision in which the patient should be a participant.

Transvaginal removal of the grossly normal ovary might be encouraged in the patient over 55, discouraged in the patient less than 35, and the operator's advice somewhat flexible in between (L Burnett, personal communication, 1987), depending more upon the present degree of ovarian activity than upon the chronologic age of the patient. Castration of the younger patient will accelerate the onset of osteoporosis and other degenerative changes.

Elective oophorectomy at the time of vaginal hysterectomy can be achieved 90 percent of the time with only an extra 10 to 15 minutes addition to the length of the operation (72). Endoloop sutures can be used when the ovaries are high in the pelvis (29). For those in whom oophorectomy is desirable but technically difficult by the transvaginal route, laparoscopic oophorectomy can generally be performed immediately following the vaginal hysterectomy.

In the majority of vaginal hysterectomy patients for whom coincident oophorectomy has been planned, the operation can be successfully implemented transvaginally (7). For the uncommon situation in which the ovaries cannot be safely removed vaginally, vaginal hysterectomy followed by laparoscopic salpingo-oophorectomy or oophorectomy can be offered to the patient. In this event the peritoneum must be closed and the wound made airtight, if necessary, by occluding the vagina temporarily with the inflated 30-ml bulb of a large Foley catheter.

OUTPATIENT ON SHORT STAY VAGINAL HYSTERECTOMY WITHOUT COLPORRHAPHY

A short hospitalization can be considered for patients without prolapse who are candidates for vaginal hysterectomy without repair, provided that there are no coincident severe medical problems, the patient has an operating telephone, has an available support person during the first 48 postoperative hours, and sustains no intraoperative injury.

If the patient agrees to adhere to a protocol of communication and understanding and there is no coincident medical disease and no repair has been performed, he or she can usually be discharged on the first postoperative day. Following stabilization and discharge from the postoperative recovery room, the patient must be ambulatory, must be tolerating a clear liquid diet, and must be successfully voiding. Two postoperative hematocrit measurements at least 4 hours apart must change no more than 3 volume percent. The patient must be able to tolerate a liquid diet, void effectively, and be ambulatory at the time of discharge (75). Following discharge the patient may be asked to record her temperature every 4 hours for 2 days, refrain from heavy lifting, driving, or exercise for a week, drink six glasses of liquid during the first 24 hours, and begin eating solid foods during the next 24 hours. She must also refrain from douching or using intravaginal tampons for 4 weeks, have a support person with her for the first 48 hours, and notify the surgeon if she notices vaginal bleeding heavier than a menstrual period, persistent nausea and vomiting, persistent unrelieved pain, or an oral temperature above 101°F. The patient should be contacted by telephone by a staff member the evening of surgery and for the first 2 postoperative days (75).

Vaginal hysterectomy can even be performed in a free-standing outpatient surgical center. The patient may be discharged the same day within 8 hours of the starting time of the surgery (60).

VAGINAL HYSTERECTOMY FOR THE PATIENT WITHOUT PROLAPSE

The vagina is often the appropriate route for hysterectomy when the uterus is movable and whether it is prolapsed or not. It is the easiest of hysterectomies to perform, since the anatomy of the supports of the uterus is constant and unaltered by disease. Hospitalization can be shortened (40), and the patient often may be home by the second or third postoperative day. Provided the uterus is movable, vaginal hysterectomy upon the markedly obese patient is faster and more comfortable than abdominal hysterectomy (62). Vaginal hysterectomy can be performed easily on the nulligravida patient.

If the uterus is movable, the less the prolapse, the easier the hysterectomy. The greater the prolapse, the more difficult the hysterectomy. This is because the anatomic differences between cases are less in the former and greater and less predictable in the latter. Massive vaginal eversion with procidentia can be among the most challenging of all gynecologic surgical cases, demanding precise surgical judgment with each progressive step and creative resourcefulness. One may perform a hundred such operations and the anatomic challenges, findings, and solutions of no two will be identical.

As the operator's experience in transvaginal surgery increases, it becomes apparent that in general the patient's convalescence is more comfortable after a vaginal than after an abdominal hysterectomy. Moreover, the vaginal operation provides optimal opportunity for the correction of frequently coexistent problems of pelvic relaxation during the same operative procedure.

The gynecoid pelvis provides the most room for successful transvaginal hysterectomy, whereas the android type may compromise exposure. The type of pelvis can often be appreciated by the slant the vulva makes with the body axis. The gynecoid pelvis has the most room, and the vulvar slant is about 45 degrees with the horizontal. The android and anthropoid pelvises are often contracted, and the angle is about 90 degrees, or perpendicular to the horizontal. The platypelloid pelvis, also often contracted, makes a 30-degree angle with the horizontal. The operator can judge the width of an adequate vaginal outlet by the distance between the ischial tuberosities when the operator's closed fist is inserted between them. (See Fig. 6.6.)

Usually a movable uterus can readily be removed from below. Conversely, the uterus that is not movable should rarely be approached transvaginally even when the vaginal operation seems otherwise indicated, as might be the case in an extremely obese patient or one for whom there is evident need for a vaginal or perineal repair.

The phenomenon of pseudoprolapse can demonstrate the degree of uterine mobility; with the pelvic musculature effectively relaxed under anesthesia, if moderate traction brings an ordinarily well-supported cervix nearly to the introitus, the uterus is sufficiently mobile to permit a vaginal hysterectomy. Under such circumstances a vaginal hysterectomy can be readily accomplished even when removal of the uterus is the primary and perhaps the only objective of the operation.

Getting the Postoperative Patient to Void

The ability to resume a normal voiding process may be inhibited by reflex urethral spasm and by local postsurgical edema. Stimulation of the alpha-adrenergic receptors in the urethra, often from associated levator muscle spasm, may produce a degree of contraction of periurethral smooth muscle that prevents spontaneous urination. A temporary blockade of alpha receptors may be induced by administering an alpha blocker at the time of catheter removal. A single 10-mg oral dose of phenoxybenzamine (Dibenzyline) will usually be sufficient to relax the urethra and permit comfortable voiding, and the dose may be repeated in 8 hours if necessary. If the patient is voiding adequate amounts, catheterization for residual urine is unnecessary. When the occasional patient is unable to void satisfactorily with this regimen, she may be taught the technique of self-catheterization, or if unwilling or unable to learn this technique, discharged from the hospital with an indwelling silicon-coated transurethral catheter that is removed at home 2 weeks later.

Manner of Operating

One contemplates the evolution of his or her own technique as a result of personal experience and comparison with the procedures described by other operators. It usually becomes apparent that a surgeon learns to identify and embrace a large group of basic fundamental principles and has not merely memorized a sequence of operative steps. Step 4 need not follow step 3; it may even follow step 6 or 7, or be skipped altogether, depending upon the characteristics of a particular patient's tissues and the operator's development of tissue relationships. The "whys" of doing something are every bit as important as the "whats." Illustrations enhanced by sagittal drawings have helped us visualize important operative details. By adding a third dimensional or spatial geometric concept to the reader's way of surgical thinking, it can be shown that only in cases of advanced prolapse does the surgery start in tissues that actually come out of the pelvis (56).

Initial Procedures

The rectum should have been carefully cleansed by an electrolyte purgative such as GoLYTELY, NuLYTELY, or CoLyte taken the morning before the day of surgery. Alternatively, an enema may be given approximately 8 hours before and not just shortly before surgery. A single dose of a "prophylactic" antibiotic, usually a cephalosporin, is given when the patient is ready for transport to the operating room (27, 28). The patient should have been instructed to void just before coming to the operating room. Only if it is palpably distended must the bladder be catheterized at the beginning of surgery. It is our opinion that the bladder with a little urine in it is easier to identify than one that is empty. If desired, 30 ml of dilute indigo carmine, methylene blue solution, or sterile evaporated milk can be instilled into the bladder preoperatively as a means of ensuring recognition of an unanticipated bladder opening, which will occasionally occur during the course of a gynecologic operative procedure. This is recommended routinely for every patient who has experienced a previous cesarean section.

The techniques to be described have not been used in all cases but have been used in the cases reported in which we consistently have achieved the best results. Obstetrician-gynecologists who prefer to stand doing episiotomy repairs will find advantages to standing during vaginal hysterectomy and repair (Fig. 8.1). This position seems to provide desirable mobility with minimal muscle tension on the part of both operator and assistants. When standing it will be necessary to elevate the operating table almost to its maximal height. Regardless of operative technique, some operators prefer to be seated.

Horizontal light sources are very desirable while working within the pelvis. Because operating room spotlights tend to wander during the course of the procedure, some operators find that a fiberoptic forehead lamp provides a readily directed shadowless illumination in the very depths of the wound and into the hollow of the sacrum. It is important that the operator and all assistants keep their visual attention on the operative field; no one but the anesthesiologist needs to watch the upper half of the patient, and no one needs to watch the nurse, clock, technician, or one another. A retractor held by a disinterested assistant can become a source of injury if allowed to wander, or it may obscure the telltale spurt of a small unsecured artery. When tension upon a pedicle or

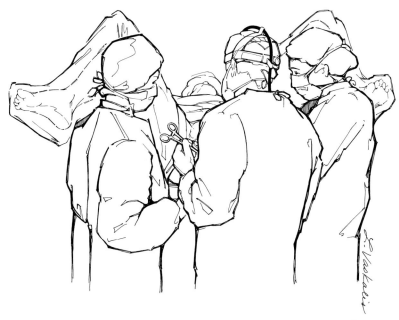

Figure 8.1. The positions of the surgeons, standing, in relation to the patient. The surgeon is at the center, the surgeon's first assistant is to the surgeon's left, and the second assistant to the right. All surgeons in this position are free to move without risking a troublesome back strain.

adjacent structure is relaxed, bleeding from a momentarily exposed vessel may remain undetected because the visual attention of the operator and his or her assistants has not been concentrated upon the operative field.

A careful preoperative bimanual pelvic reexamination under anesthesia should then be performed, for this helps the operator to conclude whether to proceed with the hysterectomy vaginally or abdominally (Fig. 8.2). The size, position, shape, and especially the mobility of the uterus should be carefully determined. The freedom and position of the cul-de-sac should be noted and the thickness and length of the uterosacral ligaments evaluated. Elongation of the cervix should be noted, since this will help identify the point at which incision through the vagina should begin. The direction and depth of the vaginal axis at rest should be noted (36).

When the anus itself seems to be the most dependent portion of the patient's perineum and she literally sits on her anus, this uncommon finding usually correlates with a major defect in the integrity of the levator ani. The latter may be associated with postmenopausal estrogen deficiency and loss of tissue tone, but it is more likely due to major trauma to the levator ani and pelvic diaphragm, an acquired or congenital deficiency of innervation, or degenerative neurologic disease (see Chapter 14).

If there has been any history of abnormal bleeding, a preliminary dilatation and curettage (D&C) should be performed to clarify the cause of the bleeding. The preliminary curettage gives additional information in regard to the size, mobility, consistency, position, and "internal architecture" of the uterus. The position of the uterus is also important. A prolapsed uterus will rarely be found in anteversion, unless there has been a previous suspension or fixation procedure. A retroverted uterus is usually accompanied by pathologic elongation of the infundibulopelvic ligaments, with the ovaries in the cul-de-sac, making them much more accessible to surgical removal through the vaginal incision if the decision is to do so during the course of the operation.

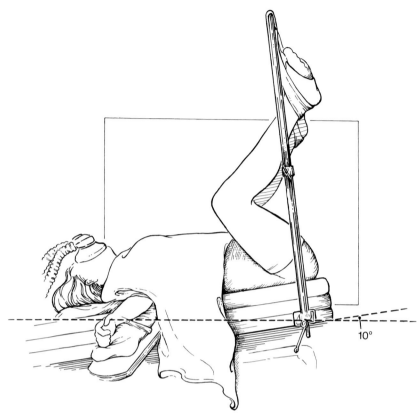

10°

Figure 8.2. Depiction of patient prepared for surgery. The direction and depth of the vaginal axis should be carefully noted. The operating table is then tilted and locked in a 5- to 10-degree Trendelenburg position.

One alternative is to discontinue the vaginal approach to hysterectomy if during the course of the procedure unexpected difficulties are encountered. An interrupted vaginal operation can be completed through a transabdominal approach, but in most instances this sequence should be regarded as evidence of an initial error in surgical judgment.

Following examination under anesthesia and preliminary curettage of the uterus, traction is made by a double-toothed tenaculum applied to the anterior lip of the cervix, and the integrity of the urogenital diaphragm and the anterior vaginal wall in relation to the pubis is identified. This gives the operator considerable insight as to whether coexistent suspension or support of the urethra and lower vagina should accompany the repair, as well as the extent to which restoration of the normal vaginal axis and depth is likely to be achieved by the planned reconstruction. Another tenaculum applied to the posterior lip of the cervix makes it easier to also evaluate the location and size of the cul-de-sac of Douglas as well as the strength and size of the uterosacral ligaments, which become more readily demonstrable as they are placed on a stretch (Fig. 8.3). The attachment of the cul-de-sac to the cervix then usually becomes more obvious, helping to indicate the site for the operator's placement of the initial incision to circumscribe the cervix.

If the labia minora are large enough to interfere with adequate exposure of the vagina, they should be temporarily fixed to the skin lateral to the labia majora by a suture on each side.

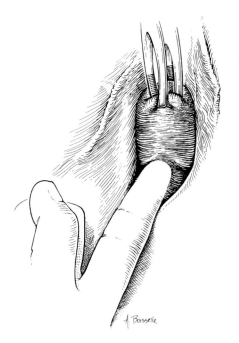

Figure 8.3. Palpation of the cul-de-sac of Douglas. Traction is made to a tenaculum applied to the posterior lip of the cervix and the site of the cul-de-sac of Douglas palpated. The length and strength of the uterosacral ligaments are noted.

The cervix, having been grasped anteriorly and posteriorly with two double-toothed tenacula, is drawn downward as the cervix and upper vagina are adequately exposed by suitable vaginal retractors.

Blood loss during surgery, particularly in premenopausal nonhypertensive women, generally can be lessened considerably by selective paracervical infiltration of not more than 50 ml of 0.5% lidocaine (Xylocaine) in 1:200,000 epinephrine (Adrenalin) solution (25), the so-called liquid tourniquet. Use of this agent has been beneficial to us in three ways: first, it has markedly decreased operative blood loss and the need to consider transfusion; second, it has seemed to lessen anesthesia and the need for postoperative analgesia; and third, it has great helped in identifying the development and separation of cleavage planes. We inform the anesthetist before the injection. Because of the temporary ischemia produced, the immediate resistance to infection could be reduced (19). However, since prophylactic antibiotics have been given preoperatively, a therapeutic concentration should already be disseminated within the pelvic tissues (see Chapter 7). In our hands there has been no demonstrable increase in morbidity. We usually employ this vasoconstrictive solution. When a patient is receiving halothane or cyclopropane anesthesia, has been taking a beta blocker such as propranolol, is unstable, or has severe hypertension or coronary heart disease, we may in such patients substitute infiltration by normal saline solution.

The actual infiltration is most easily accomplished by use of a pressure syringe and a 22-gauge spinal needle (Fig. 8.4). The areas of the bladder pillars are injected, along with the lower cardinal ligaments and the insertions of the uterosacral ligaments. Before injecting the solution, traction is made on the plunger of the syringe to make certain that no blood is obtained, thus avoiding intravenous or intra-arterial injection of the solution. If a bloody aspirate is obtained, the needle is repositioned. The emphasis is placed on injecting the tissues around the cervix into the tissues to which the cervix is attached, rather than injecting the cervical tissue itself. Although employment of the "liquid tourniquet" may reduce blood loss considerably, it is not a substitute for careful dissection and meticulous surgical hemostasis. Although a wait of 15 minutes from the time of completion of the injection until the start of surgery permits wider dissemination of the fluid into the

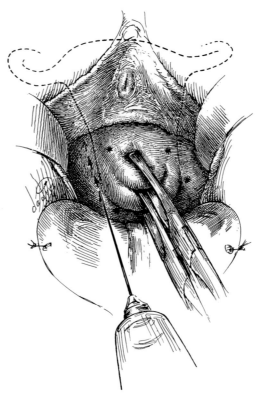

Figure 8.4. Application of the "liquid tourniquet." The cervix is grasped with two double-toothed tenacula, one anterior and one posterior to the external os, and downward traction is made. Vaginal retractors of adequate length and proper design will then provide satisfactory exposure of the cervix and upper vagina. In a premenopausal patient who has received preventive antibiotics, the tissues beneath the vagina along the circumference of the cervix, along a line where a circumcisionlike incision is about to be made, may be first carefully infiltrated with a mixture of 1:200,000 epinephrine (Adrenalin) and 0.5% lidocaine (Xylocaine). This is readily accomplished using a pressure syringe and a long 22-gauge spinal needle so that the full length of the vaginal insertion of the cardinal-uterosacral ligament complex is injected. Before injecting solution at each puncture site, one applies traction on the plunger of the syringe to make certain that no blood is obtained, in order to avoid intravenous or intra-arterial injection of the solution. If a bloody aspirate is obtained, the needle is repositioned. The "bladder pillars," the paracervical portions of the cardinal ligaments, and the cervical insertions of the uterosacral ligaments (*asterisks*) should be the objectives of this infiltration. About 50 ml of this solution, half into either side, and 8 ml at each injection site, will usually provide adequate infiltration.

intercellular connective tissue (54), the time required is a luxury that the hourly cost of an American operating room will not permit.

Operative Technique

Because the anatomic relationship between the bladder and the cervix may be altered by scar tissue in the patient with previous cesarean section, 60 ml of dilute indigocarmine solution may be instilled into the bladder. The dye will stain the bladder mucosa, and its violet hue can be observed during sharp dissection, avoiding an unexpected cystotomy.

The correct spot for circumcision of the vagina before hysterectomy is often at some distance from the external cervical os (23). Decreased rugae mark the upper limits of the vagina, where there is a blending with the epithelial layer of the cervix whose surface shows no rugae. We have found the full thickness of the vaginal wall, because of its mobility, to be more readily identified by dissection with the scissors than with the scalpel. Using either curved Mayo scissors or a scalpel (as one prefers), the vagina is opened by a circumcisionlike incision around the cervix, through the full thickness of the vaginal membrane. This incision should be made along the grooved depression noticeable in the transverse rugae (Fig. 8.5A–C). Posteriorly, the incision opens the tissue exposing the uterosacral ligaments and peritoneum of the cul-de-sac, but the initial incision should not cut the uterosacrals or actually open the peritoneum into the cul-de-sac.

Bandler (3) has pointed out that bleeding tends to be greater the closer the initial incision is made to the external cervical os, in which case more dissection involving the transection of several cervical branches of the uterine blood vessels will be required

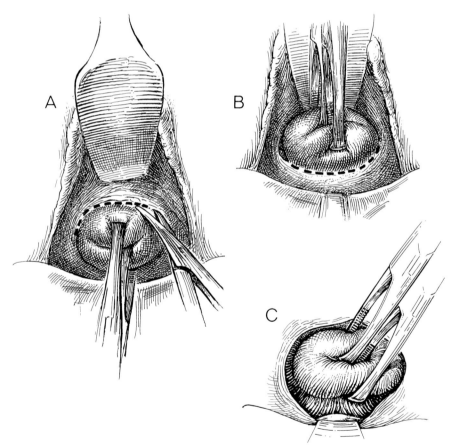

Figure 8.5. Circumcision of the vagina. **A.** The cervix has been circumscribed by an incision that goes through the full thickness of the wall of the vagina along the groovelike depression marking the attachment of the bladder to the cervix. **B.** The path of the incision is shown by the *broken line.* Laterally and posteriorly, this incision should expose in sequence the surface of the bladder pillars, the cardinal and the uterosacral ligaments, and finally the peritoneum of the cul-de-sac, but it should not extend into any of these structures. **C.** The tenacula are repositioned so that their external teeth are in the cut edge of the incision. The cul-de-sac of Douglas is noted as the whitish tissue in the 6 o'clock position.

before reaching the cul-de-sac. Conversely, bleeding will be less when the incision is made further above the external cervical os, but the risk of inadvertently opening into the bladder or rectum is increased. A compromise is usually elected based in large part upon the operator's estimate of the length of the cervix and the palpable level of the peritoneum of the posterior cul-de-sac (Fig. 8.6).

After incision around the cervix, the double-toothed tenacula are removed and re-applied so as to pull the cut edge of the vagina over the lower cervix and external os. It then becomes of great importance for the operator to continue the dissection in the correct cleavage plane, since dissection in the wrong plane will greatly increase the blood loss and, more important, will jeopardize the blood supply of the tissue flaps upon which the success of the repair will depend. The full thickness of the vaginal membrane should virtually be peeled back from all underlying connective tissue, but only for a short distance, unless there has been marked elongation of the uterosacral ligaments, in which case the vagina is "skinned" from the external surfaces of the connective tissue plane covering these ligaments for a considerable distance. This may be accomplished by utilizing the tips of only partially opened scissors in a "cut-and-push" maneuver. If unexpected infection is present in the cervix, one may free it from the surrounding tissues to the level of the internal os and then amputate it from the fundus before opening the peritoneum either anteriorly or posteriorly, thereby reducing the possibility of contamination and postoperative peritonitis. Shortening the cervix in this manner occasionally makes it easier for the operator to hook his or her finger around the fundus of the uterus to facilitate opening the anterior peritoneum.

The cul-de-sac of Douglas is usually readily identified (Fig. 8.7) by putting the subvaginal tissue layer on a stretch with forceps; but if difficulty is encountered and the peritoneum is not evident, the full thickness of the posterior vaginal membrane is undermined and then incised vertically (Fig. 8.8). At the conclusion of the hysterectomy, the edges of the resulting T-shaped incision may be trimmed appropriately and converted to a vault-narrowing V-shaped incision in the upper vagina, which may then be closed from side to side.

Sometimes after circumcising the cervix and stripping back the wall of the vagina, the operator may be unable to identify the posterior peritoneal fold (lining the cul-de-sac of Douglas), if the dissection has been in the wrong plane or the cul-de-sac has been obliterated by adhesions. At this stage of the operation, it is often quite helpful to begin

Figure 8.6. Circumsion of the elongated cervix. Traction to both the anterior and posterior lip of the cervix puts the uterosacral ligament on a stretch where it can be easily identified and palpated and its strength estimated. The inferior margin of the cul-de-sac of Douglas is located at the point where the uterosacral ligaments join the cervix. The circumscribing incision should be made at this point (*dashed line*) to overlie the inferior margin of the cul-de-sac of Douglas. This is the location for the circumscribing incision irrespective of the length of the vaginal portion of the cervix. An elongated cervix is depicted.

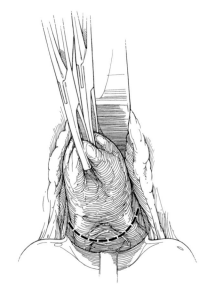

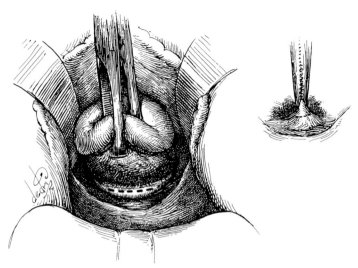

Figure 8.7. Opening the posterior cul-de-sac. With the vaginal membrane of the posterior fornix made taut by traction on the tenaculum on the posterior cervix, the cul-de-sac of Douglas is identified (*left*), held with the forceps (*right*), and opened transversely beneath the cervix with the Mayo scissors (*dashed line*).

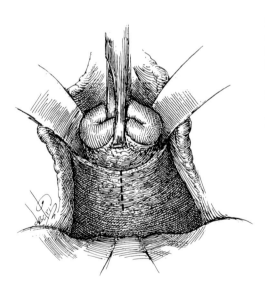

Figure 8.8. When difficulty is experienced identifying the peritoneum. The full thickness of the posterior edge of the vagina is undermined and then incised vertically. At the conclusion of the hysterectomy, the edges of the T-shaped incisions may be trimmed appropriately. Closure of the resulting V-shaped defects anteriorly and posteriorly may be accomplished as circumstances warrant—by excision of four somewhat triangular corners of the vaginal membrane and closure in the midline if the objective is to decrease the caliber and increase the length of the upper vagina.

the hysterectomy in an extraperitoneal fashion by next severing the uterosacral and caudal portions of the cardinal ligaments close to the cervix. Unless abnormally restrained as by adhesions, the uterus will then come noticeably closer to the operator, bringing with it the site of both its posterior and anterior peritoneal attachments. We occasionally employ this maneuver and only later in the procedure identify the peritoneum and open it under direct vision (6, 25, 39). This procedure, the same as the "climb-up" maneuver recommended by Krige (42), is infinitely preferable to stabbing around blindly in the hope of opening into the peritoneum, a rather haphazard technique that involves considerable risk of making an undesirable opening into adherent bowel or the rectum.

The peritoneum is readily opened by the Mayo scissors, but no more than is necessary to admit an examining finger or two (Fig. 8.9) in an effort to reduce unnecessary bleeding and to avoid an incision that could detach a uterosacral ligament from the uterus at this time. The interior intra-abdominal surface of the cul-de-sac is explored with one or two fingers to identify any enterocele or potential enterocele for later excision. Any pathologic adhesions or cul-de-sac irregularity should be noted, and the nature of any intraperitoneal fluid should be observed. The operator's index finger should also sweep superiorly to ensure the freedom of the posterior surface of the uterus, confirm the size of the uterus, and note the position of any fibroids or other pathology that would be encountered later in the operation. Although the uterosacral ligaments should not be included in this preliminary incision into the cul-de-sac of Douglas, their thickness and possible elongation should be noted at this time.

We prefer to purposefully avoid the routine placement of hemostatic interrupted sutures uniting the peritoneum and vaginal cuff at this stage, even when oozing persists, because such sutures so frequently result in an increased risk of future enterocele if later in the operation the operator fails to resect any excess of peritoneum in the cul-de-sac before placing the pursestring closure of peritoneum cranial to these sutures. Any excess of peritoneum should always be excised before the cul-de-sac is closed.

The uterosacral ligaments are clamped and, if elongated and strong, should at this time be shortened (Fig. 8.10), after which they are cut from the uterus. (We believe that double-clamping "for safety" is purely elective, according to the surgeon's preference.) The tip of the clamp should include the uterosacrals and the lower portion of the cardinal ligaments.

When placing a suture around this pedicle, it is important that the flexibility of the operator's wrist provides impetus that follows the needle's curve. The needle should be pushed through the tissues only along the course of its curved direction, and pulled through along the axis of the needle's curve, to avoid the laceration of tissue more likely to occur when the needle is pushed through in a straight line. As the follow-through of the player's golf swing or tennis stroke affects the accuracy of the ball's flight, the swing and flexibility of the surgeon's wrist minimize the size of the opening and the trauma to tissues that can result from each placement of a hemostatic suture around the pedicles.

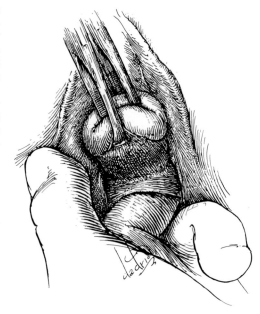

Figure 8.9. Opening the peritoneum. To reduce unnecessary bleeding, the opening in the peritoneum is made no larger than to admit one or two examining fingers. The nature of any intraperitoneal fluid is noted. The uterosacral ligaments should not be detached by this incision, but their thickness and possible elongation and site of attachment to the cervix are noted. The interior of the cul-de-sac should now be explored, and any enterocele or potential enterocele recognized so that it may be excised later in the operation. Any pathologic adhesion or cul-de-sac nodularity should be identified. The operator's exploring index finger sweeps superiorly, identifying the freedom of the posterior surface of the uterus, confirming the size of the uterus, and noting the position of any fibroids or other pathology that will be encountered later in the operation.

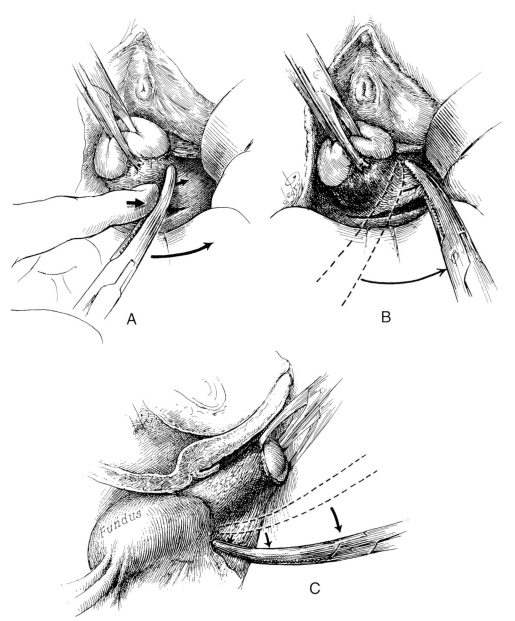

Figure 8.10. Shortening and cutting the uterosacral ligaments. **A.** The uterosacral ligaments are identified and clamped, and if these appear elongated and seem strong, the clamps may be so placed as to ensure some shortening of the ligaments as they are cut from the uterus. The tip of this clamp usually includes the lower portion of the cardinal ligament. Necessary shortening is accomplished by placing the unlocked clamp across the uncut uterosacral ligament. The operator's finger presses the clamp as shown; the heel is moved a further distance than the tip. A lateral retractor, shown, displaces the vaginal wall, previously stripped from the surface of the ligament. **B.** When the desired amount of shortening has been achieved, the jaws of the clamp are locked in the lateral portion of the ligament as shown. **C.** Sagittal section shows shortening of the uterosacral ligament, when desirable, before cutting it.

The uterosacral ligaments are secured by transfixation ligature to the posterolateral surface of the vagina at about the 4 and 8 o'clock positions. This suture should include the full thickness of the vaginal wall so that the ligaments will be firmly and permanently reattached to the vagina at this point (Fig. 8.11). These uterosacral sutures should be held without cutting to facilitate later identification and possible inclusion in the repair.

The operator's attention may now be directed anteriorly where the full thickness of the cut edge of the vagina may be identified between forceps at either side of the 12 o'clock position. The cervix should be steadied in position by the tenacula, but excess traction is to be avoided, for excess traction at this stage may pull the "knee" of the ureter into the operative field and appreciably increase its vulnerability. Using Mayo scissors, with the points directed away from the bladder, a 1-cm snip is made in the midline and the vesicovaginal space is now entered. The opening may be enlarged by spreading the tips of the Mayo scissors, which are then withdrawn without closing them (Fig. 8.12).

The midline incision (Fig. 8.13) is then extended through the full thickness of the upper anterior vaginal wall, which has previously been separated from the bladder by dissection within the vesicovaginal space. The full thickness of the vaginal wall is now separated from the bladder (Fig. 8.14). If the position of the cervix at this point suggests that there is not as much prolapse as the operator suspected, this inverted T incision becomes especially advantageous. If, however, there is as much or more prolapse than the operator expected (increased somewhat because the uterosacral ligaments have been released from their hold upon the uterus), then only a horizontal vaginal incision may be necessary, because in the latter situation the vesicouterine peritoneal fold becomes noticeably closer to the surgeon's hand and vision.

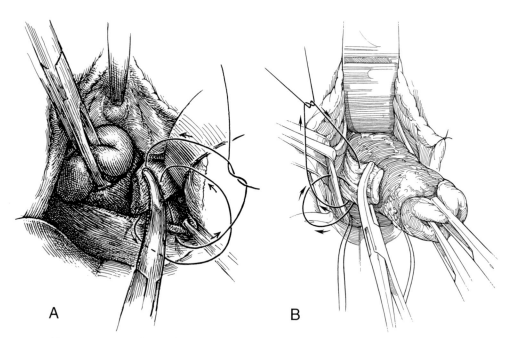

A   B

Figure 8.11. Transfixing the uterosacral ligaments. **A.** The cut ends of the ligaments are secured to the posterolateral surface of the vagina by a transfixion ligature at about the 4 and 8 o'clock positions. These sutures include the full thickness of the vaginal wall, and by this means the ligaments should be firmly and permanently reattached to the vagina at this point. The ends of these uterosacral sutures are left long, however, to facilitate later identification and probable involvement of the ligaments in closure of the repair. **B.** A similar modified Heaney stitch is performed on the opposite side of the pelvis.

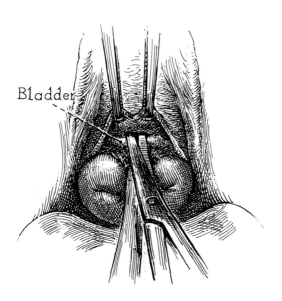

Bladder

Figure 8.12. An incision of the upper vagina into the vesicovaginal space. The operator's attention may now be directed anteriorly where the full thickness of the cut of the vagina is picked up between Kocher hemostats at the 12 o'-clock position. Using Mayo scissors with the points now directed upward and away from the bladder, a 1-cm snip is made in the midline of the anterior vaginal wall, the vesicovaginal space is entered, and the opening is enlarged by spreading the tips of the Mayo scissors.

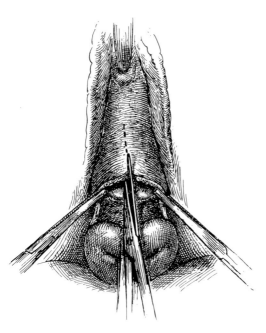

Figure 8.13. A midline incision is often made in the upper 2 inches of the vagina, again through the full thickness of the anterior vaginal wall that has been separated from the bladder by the preceding dissection.

The bladder, readily identified by its looseness, may be picked up in the midline with forceps and placed on some tension. The supravaginal septum is incised and entered in the midline with the points of the curved Mayo scissors pointing downward or posteriorly (Fig. 8.15*A*). The plane of separation follows the line of fusion between the posterior layer of the connective tissue of the anterior vaginal wall as it fuses with the encapsulation of the cervix. The handles of the Mayo scissors should be elevated during this maneuver to ensure that the tips of the scissors are directed away from the undersurface of the bladder (Fig. 8.15*B*). Sharp dissection of the bladder from the cervix is accomplished by meticulously snipping the fine fibers that bind the connective tissue capsule of the bladder to that of the cervix. This is much safer than bluntly stripping the bladder

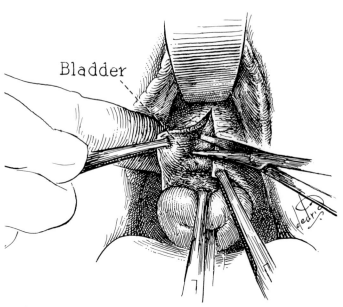

Figure 8.14. Mobilization of the vaginal membrane. Mobilization is accomplished by extension laterally within this opening in the vesicovaginal space, while the full thickness of the vaginal wall is separated or reflected upward and away from the bladder.

away from the cervix with either the finger or a sponge. Laceration of the bladder from blunt stripping commonly occurs in the lowest section of the bladder fundus at some distance from the ureteric orifice (35). As the scissors approach the vesicouterine peritoneal fold, the tissues will usually become readily distinguished, but recognition of the peritoneum can usually be ensured by the following maneuver: While making firm pressure with the closed, curved tips of the Mayo scissors pointing toward the cervix, and while elevating the handles of the scissors above the horizontal, one spreads the tips of the scissors apart and withdraws them while maintaining pressure of the scissor tips against the cervix. In this way, the proper cleavage plane will be entered bloodlessly and safely, after which the opening may be readily enlarged. This dissection is carried upward until the freedom of the anterior vesicouterine peritoneal fold is recognized by its almost frictionless smoothness to palpation, or it may be visualized as the white line of a double fold of peritoneum. Having established the desired opening along the proper cleavage plane, one then places a retractor beneath the bladder to hold it away from the cervix. The anterior vesicouterine peritoneal fold may be opened at this time (Fig. 8.16) and a long-handled retractor inserted. Either immediately before or after this retraction of the bladder superiorly, the "bladder pillars" may be clamped, cut, and ligated near their attachments to the cervix.

The so-called bladder pillars are never as strong as they may appear to be. Figure 8.17 indicates how portions of the cervical capsule will usually be included in this tissue. Surgical utilization of this maneuver provides an appreciable degree of protection to the ureters by ensuring that dissection will be closer to the cervix and relatively away from the ureteral knee.

Although the gauze-covered thumb may readily strip the bladder capsule along a cleavage plane indistinguishable from the supravaginal septum up to the anterior peritoneal fold, there is a risk of tearing the bladder if the correct plane has not been entered. This plane may be obscured by adhesions and fibrosis following previous low cervical cesarean section, and careful sharp dissection will lessen the risk of unwanted bladder

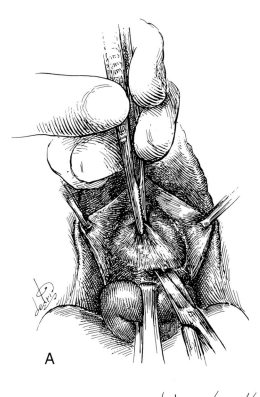

A

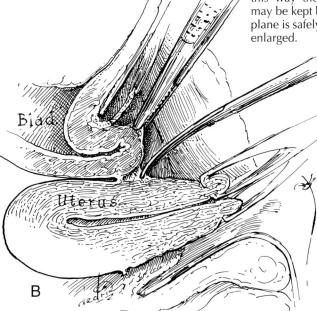

B

Figure 8.15. A. The bladder is identified by its looseness and picked up in the midline by lightly applied forceps. The bladder wall is then placed on slight tension, and the supravaginal septum is identified in the midline and incised with a curved Mayo scissors, the curve and the scissor points directed downward along the anterior cervix, opening through the tissue normally fusing the posterior wall of the bladder to the cervix. **B.** Sagittal drawing shows how the handles of the Mayo scissors should be consciously elevated during this maneuver to aid in pointing the scissor tips away from the undersurface of the bladder. As the scissors approach the vesicouterine peritoneal fold, the tissue can be safely rendered more visible by the following maneuver: Firm pressure is made with the closed but curved tips of the Mayo scissors pointed toward the cervix. While elevating the handles of the scissors above the horizontal, one spreads the tips of the scissors apart and withdraws them, all the while maintaining pressure by the tips against the cervix. In this way the correct cleavage plane may be kept bloodless while this tissue plane is safely entered and the opening enlarged.

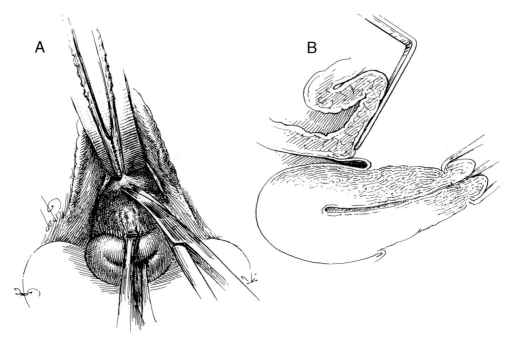

Figure 8.16. Opening the anterior peritoneal fold. **A.** If not opened earlier or adequately, the anterior peritoneal fold, which is readily picked up by a Bonney forceps, may be opened confidently at this time. **B.** Exposure is facilitated at this time by displacing the bladder anteriorly and holding it out of harm's way with a retractor. The anterior vesicouterine peritoneal fold is at this time much easier to observe, and it may be brought closer to the operator after detachment of the cardinal ligaments. Usually it may be identified by the somewhat frictionless sensation that is imparted to the operator's examining finger, or it may appear as a whitish fold of tissue because of the doubled thickness of peritoneum where it folds back upon itself to extend beneath the bladder, the latter held out of harm's way by a retractor, as shown.

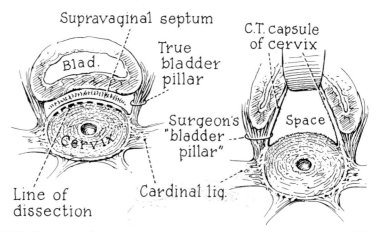

Figure 8.17. Erroneous dissection beneath the connective tissue capsule of the cervix. When the dissection between the cervix and bladder is carried out beneath the connective tissue capsule of the cervix (*dashed line*), there is an apparent increment in the thickness of the "bladder pillar," as indicated in the drawing to the *right*.

penetration. Occasionally the operator's readiness to dissect and desire to stay as far away from the bladder as possible will cause him or her to incise within the connective tissue capsule of the cervix. This is particularly likely to occur if the initial incision around the cervix was too close to the external cervical os. As the operator continues by sharp dissection, he or she may, by not entering the anatomic plane between bladder and cervix, dissect further and beneath the peritoneum covering the anterior uterine segment. The smooth undersurface of the peritoneum may be recognized by palpation but is not readily visualized, and it should not be opened blindly, since it is difficult to be assured of the actual site of its reflection from the superior surface of the bladder unless it is accessible under direct vision. Failure to proceed with caution at this stage is one of the most common reasons for unintentional bladder penetration. Fortunately, if bladder injury does occur at this point, it will be well above the bladder trigone and relatively easy to repair after the uterus has been removed. Bladder injury is usually recognized by the escape of a sudden gush of urine. The indication for and technique of immediate repair is considered in the discussion of operative complications in Chapter 22.

A proper time to open the peritoneum while extending the mobilization and identification of the bladder is soon after the smooth, thin layer of peritoneum has been visualized, usually as a fold or double reflection appearing after the cardinal and uterosacral ligaments and the surgeon's "bladder pillars" have all been separated from the uterus. Cutting all pedicles close to the cervix results in further descent of the uterus, and this descent brings the peritoneum down with it. After the anterior peritoneal fold has been recognized by palpation and visualized but not yet opened, the portion of the bladder pillars closest to the cervix may be included in the clamp (Fig. 8.18) across the adjacent portion of the cardinal ligament. However, a small, rather superficial artery in the bladder pillar will often bleed as the vaginal membrane is reflected from the midline over the cervix. When such bleeding occurs, it is advisable to separately clamp and ligate the vessel and adjacent bladder pillar on each side close to the cervix. Similarly, one should identify the cardinal ligament tissue to each side of the cervix, at which point we believe it advisable to make an effort to clamp, cut, and ligate that structure without picking up the uterine vessels separately.

With vaginal hysterectomy one good clamp at a time (as opposed to "double-clamping") is used on the cardinal ligament. With this approach traction to the cervix brings with it the uterine artery that pulls the ureter down, and a second clamp decreases the distance from the clamp to the ureter, putting the latter at some degree of risk. With a total abdominal hysterectomy, on the other hand, one may use two clamps at a time on each portion of the cardinal ligament detached from the uterus, since upward traction on the uterus pulls the uterine artery away from the ureter.

Occasionally when one encounters an intermediate or advanced degree of uterine prolapse, a clampless technique may be employed, in which uterine pedicles are ligated by primary passage of the needle without preliminary clamping (Fig. 8.19). If using this technique, one should be careful not to cut the pedicle until the first cast of the stitch has been placed and tightened. Then the pedicle of the ligated tissue should be cut, the first cast of the knot tightened again, and the second cast placed and tightened.

If separately identified, the uterine vessels should be safely clamped and ligated with a tie that is cut short so it will not be used for subsequent traction. When there is a large uterus or when an irregular or intraligamentous fibroid has distorted the usual anatomic relationships, it is particularly useful to make such a deliberate attempt to exclude the uterine artery and adjacent veins in the initial clamping across the cardinal ligaments. At this point a cautious push or pull on the clamped tissues should be made in the axis of the ascending branch of the uterine artery (which may tear a small vein that can be readily clamped along with the uterine artery). This cautious but deliberate pull or push on the cardinal ligament tissue caught in the initial clamp will invariably result in enough separation of the anterior and posterior layers of ligament attaching to the lower uterine

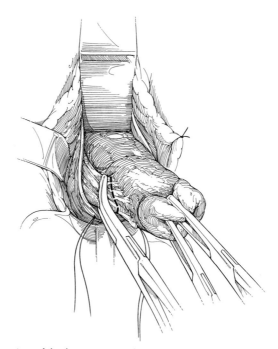

Figure 8.18. Separation of the lower cervical portion of the cardinal ligaments of the uterus. The anterior peritoneum has been palpated or visualized but not yet opened. That portion of the bladder pillars closest to the cervix may be included in the clamp across the remaining lower portion of the cardinal ligament, which should be clamped near the cervix. The cardinal ligament is then cut from the cervix, and the hemostat is replaced with a transfixion Heaney type of ligature. After this has been tied, it may be brought through the vaginal wall at the 3 or 9 o'clock position and tied again, so that the ligament is fixed to the vagina at these points. The clamp on the cardinal ligament often includes the uterine artery and adjacent veins, but if not, they are clamped and tied separately. The fascia of the cardinal ligament is cut from its continuation anterior and posterior to the cervix. During this time, the uterine vessels, as they are released from the fascia encircling and attaching to the cervix, will often stand out conspicuously and can be clamped and tied. The suture should be cut promptly to avoid traction on the ligature of the uterine vessels.

segment to disclose an underlying segment of the uterine vessels, which usually promptly and literally bulge into the operator's view. The uterine vessels can then be clamped (extraperitoneally, without including the peritoneum either anteriorly or posteriorly), cut, and ligated with a minimal amount of ligamentous tissue. After ligation of the vessels, the remaining superior portions of the broad ligament, including adjacent peritoneum both anteriorly and posteriorly, may be clamped and caught in a transfixing ligature without risk of disturbing or jeopardizing the ligation of the uterine vessels.

Safe entry into the peritoneal cavity through the anterior vesicouterine peritoneal fold can be accomplished by a variety of techniques, each best chosen according to plan and correlated with the specific degree and type of prolapse involved. The presence or absence of coexistent cystocele that the operator intends to repair, the size of that cystocele, the extent of cervical descent, the degree of mobility by which the cervix can be brought closer to the operator by traction on the tenaculum, and the length of the cervix are all factors that must be taken into consideration. Often the site of the anterior vesicouterine peritoneal reflection is at the same level as the reflection of the posterior peritoneal reflection (within the cul-de-sac of Douglas) to the uterus.

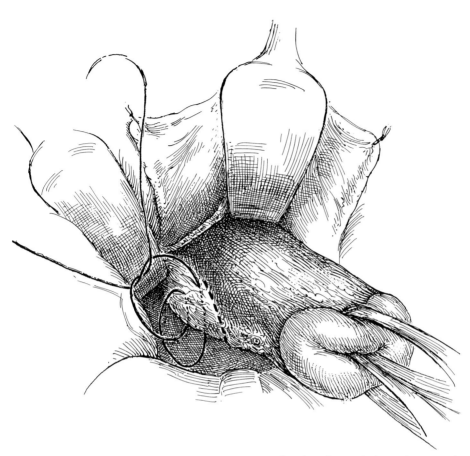

Figure 8.19. Clampless ligation of the paracolpium. In the clampless technique, the suture is placed as in a Heaney stitch and the first cast of the knot tied. Then the pedicle is cut from the uterus and the Heaney stitch is tightened and a second and third cast placed to make it secure.

The anterior peritoneal fold should be opened only under direct vision, never blindly, because the latter procedure could easily damage the bladder unnecessarily. Grasped with forceps, the peritoneum is tented as a vertical fold and may be readily opened with the scissors. The operator's index finger explores the anterior cul-de-sac, noting any pathology or adhesions, while making certain that the incision has properly entered the peritoneal cavity anteriorly. The operator may then insert both index fingers into this anterior peritoneal opening, enlarging it by spreading the fingers laterally. A long-handled Heaney or Deaver retractor may then be inserted (Fig. 8.20) as a means of keeping the bladder up and out of the operative field. The relationship of the ureter to the uterine artery during hysterectomy is shown in Figure 8.21.

Had the operator been unable to identify the anterior peritoneal plication with certainty, further attempts at an anterior opening into the peritoneal cavity should have been delayed until a point of safe opening could be positively identified by either longitudinal section of the cervix or by inserting the first and second left fingertips through the posterior peritoneal opening over the fundus of the uterus (39) and spreading them beneath the vesicouterine peritoneal fold, making it both palpable and visible (Fig. 8.22). To facilitate later identification of the edges of the peritoneum, it is permissible to tag the midline of both the anterior and the posterior edges with a suture left long so as to be readily retrievable when the operator is ready to close the peritoneum.

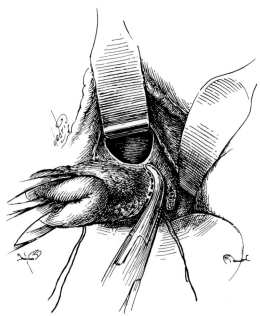

Figure 8.20. Clamping, cutting, and ligating the upper cardinal and lower broad ligaments. Maintaining somewhat lessened traction on the cervix and uterus, the upper portions of the cardinal and lower broad ligaments are now clamped, cut, and ligated. With each application of these clamps, the tips of the hemostats should be so placed as to be visible within the peritoneal cavity, both anteriorly and posteriorly, thus ensuring that the broad ligaments will be sealed off by bringing together the anterior and posterior peritoneal leaves of the broad ligament between the jaws of the hemostats. This step should effectively prevent extension of any tendency toward laceration of the tissues thinly supporting the very vascular venous plexuses usually located within the layers of the broad ligament. A single correctly placed ligature securely tied and promptly cut (leaving ends not less than 3 nor more than 5 mm long) will ensure reliable ligation of the uterine vessels. A second ligation suture "to make sure" doubles the risk of the suture-placing needle entering a uterine vessel and also doubles the risk of the needle puncturing or fixing a ureter; unless the second tie is squarely and simply atop the first one, the two-ties-per-side technique appreciably increases the amount of tissue devitalized by the ligatures, which must be absorbed during convalescence. Considering all of the possible consequences, we have long believed that one properly placed ligature is the better technique.

When the anterior cul-de-sac is particularly difficult to identify, as in the patient with previous cesarean section, a Sims uterine sound bent in the shape of a U may be inserted through the posterior peritoneal opening and over the uterine fundus. The tip can be palpated, and dissection beneath the tip will expose the peritoneum of the anterior cul-de-sac, which can be safely opened.

With the peritoneum opened both posterior and anterior to the uterine fundus, the upper cardinal and lower broad ligaments are then clamped, cut, and ligated. During application of these clamps, from the cornual angles downward, the tips of the hemostats should be so placed that each is within the peritoneal cavity, both anteriorly and posteriorly. This placement serves to seal off the broad ligament by compressing both anterior and posterior peritoneal leaves of the broad ligament between the jaws of the hemostat (Fig. 8.23). This step effectively prevents extension of any laceration into the very vascular venous plexus located within layers of the broad ligaments. These hemostats should be immediately replaced by transfixing ligatures.

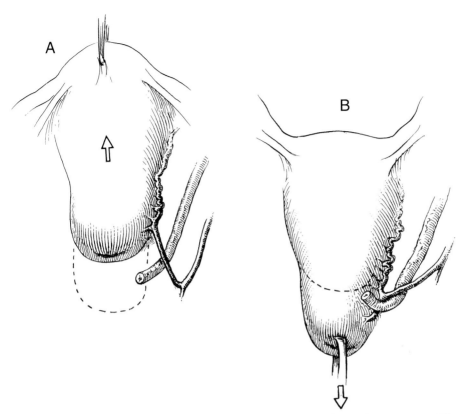

Figure 8.21. The relationship of the ureter to the uterine artery during hysterectomy. The *dotted line* represents a usual position of the uterus. **A.** The relationship between the uterine artery and the ureter when upward traction is applied to the uterine fundus as in abdominal hysterectomy. **B.** The change in this relationship when downward traction is applied as during vaginal hysterectomy.

During the course of the procedure after the cardinal and uterosacral ligament complex has been ligated and both anterior and posterior cul-de-sac opened, it may become apparent that traction applied to the cervix fails to move the uterus any further in a downward direction. One or more of several factors may be interfering with the delivery of the uterus, for under normal circumstances the broad ligament and its contents, including both round and ovarian ligaments, offer little resistance to downward traction. At this point, one should suspect and determine with certainty whether the patient has had a previous ventral fixation or Gilliam type of uterine suspension or whether there are adhesions binding the uterus to other intra-abdominal organs. Any one or more of the following conditions also could be arresting descent of the uterus: (*a*) parametrial and broad ligament fibrosis from previous or chronic infection, or radiation therapy, (*b*) pelvic endometriosis, (*c*) undiagnosed pelvic carcinoma, extending from either the uterus or an extrauterine site.

Another possibility that should not be overlooked in one's preoperative assessment is a mechanical obstruction to further descent of the uterus by a large fibroid uterus with leiomyomas so situated as to interfere with delivery of the uterus. The operator is then faced with a choice among several alternate procedures. The first is to abandon the vaginal approach to hysterectomy at this point and finish the operation through a transabdominal incision. Allen's caution (1), with which we concur, was as follows:

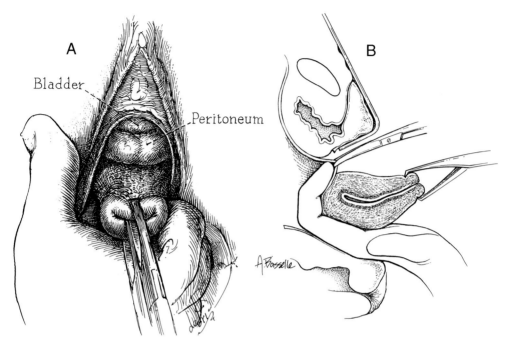

Figure 8.22. Alternate method of opening the anterior peritoneal fold. **A.** The first and second fingers of the operator's left hand have been inserted through the opening of the posterior cul-de-sac and flexed above the uterine fundus. The anterior vesicouterine peritoneal fold, now identified and distended by the tips of the operator's fingers as shown, may be opened safely under direct vision. At this point the midpoint in the anterior peritoneum may be tagged by a single suture and left long to facilitate identification of the edge of the peritoneal opening. A long-handled Heaney or Deaver retractor may then be inserted to hold the bladder anteriorly while the uterus is removed. **B.** Sagittal section shows flexing of the operator's fingers over the fundus of the uterus to visualize the anterior vesicouterine peritoneal fold.

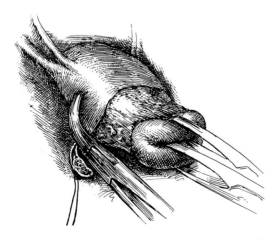

Figure 8.23. Clamping, cutting, and ligation of the middle broad ligament. Traction is continued on the cervix, drawing it closer to the operator. This maneuver also makes apparent any tissues to which the remainder of the uterus may still be attached. Any remaining portions of the middle broad ligaments are clamped, cut, and ligated, again taking care to make certain that both anterior and posterior leaves of the broad ligament and covering peritoneum are compressed within the grasp of the forceps.

I do not believe that large tumors should be attacked through the vagina. How large a tumor one should attack depends on one's experience and skill, but also on the location of the tumor in the uterus. Relatively small tumors immediately beneath the bladder or extending out into the broad ligament, where the uterine blood supply is reached with difficulty, are much more important as contraindications than large tumors if they are in the fundus. Once the lower blood supply is secured, these upper tumors can be reached and morcellated with, shall I say, impunity.*

The alternative would be to consider the possibility of amputating the cervix and morcellating any fibroid tumors of the uterus (Fig. 8.24), providing they could be grasped safely through the vagina. Werner and Sederl (81) and others have recommended bisection of the noncancerous uterus with sequential removal of one side of the hysterectomy specimen and then the other (Fig. 8.25). The option chosen by the operator should be one that reflects both the patient's own best interests at that time and the confidence, experience, and technical ability of the operator.

MORCELLATION TECHNIQUES

Vaginal hysterectomy by morcellation is a safe and effective alternative to abdominal hysterectomy or removal of the moderately enlarged uterus and offers cosmesis and smoother recuperation. In addition, any coincident cystocele and rectocele can be repaired through the same operative exposure (30). Anterior vaginal wall defects should be repaired at the time of the original surgery to lessen the likelihood that unrepaired defects will progress postoperatively, requiring a second operation (73).

The bladder and ureters must be freed completely from the cervix and lower uterine segment and the uterine arteries secured and transected before beginning the morcellation. The urinary organs must be guarded most carefully by retractors, and only after the anterior peritoneum is opened can this vigilance be relaxed (43). The danger of hemorrhage only occurs when one is working too close to the lateral portions of the uterus or if one fails to maintain traction to one uterine vulsella that has been placed on the edges of the wound.

In opening the uterus for bisection, the initial incision is usually made in the midline of the anterior wall (43). Vulsellas are applied to the cut edges in a sequential fashion to provide better exposure. Hemorrhage is prevented by downward and outward traction upon the forceps. If the uterus, even though "unrolled" and flattened, is still so large that it cannot yet be delivered, its transverse diameter can be made smaller by the excision of longitudinal strips from the whole length and thickness of the anterior wall. Alternatively, and when the hypertrophy is concentrated in the fundus, a series of rhomboid-shaped wedges may be excised. When the uterus is still fixed in position, but its anterior wall has been removed to create more space, a finger can be passed over the fundus, adhesions broken up, the appendages liberated, and all the parts delivered. If, however, the posterior wall is free from adhesions, it too can be bisected and each half of the uterus removed separately.

Traction is continued on the cervix to draw it closer to the operator. The middle portion of the broad ligament may then need to be separately clamped, cut, and ligated, with care again being taken to make certain that both anterior and posterior leaves of the broad ligament peritoneum are included within the grasp of the hemostat on either side. Transfixion ligatures should by now have secured the blood supply to the uterus (including both the ascending and descending branches of the uterine artery), and the operator has determined that the uterus is not held by any previously unsuspected adhesions.

When it is low in the pelvis, the fundus of the uterus may be delivered through either an anterior or posterior peritoneal opening (Fig. 8.26A); but when the fundus is freely

---

* From Allen E. Discussion. Am J Obstet Gynecol 1951;61A(Suppl):219. Used with permission.

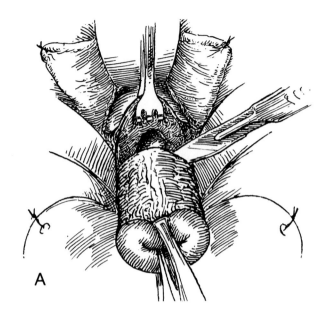

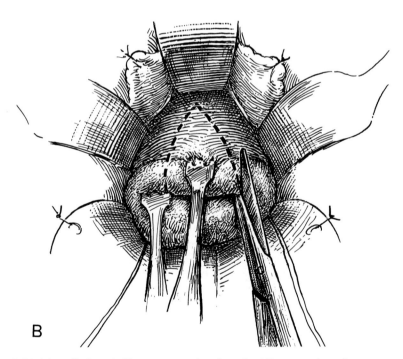

Figure 8.24. Morcellation. **A.** The uterosacral and cardinal ligaments have been cut and ligated and the cervix amputated. **B.** The myometrium is firmly grasped by Palpated clamps, and the first of several wedges of anterior or posterior uterine wall may be excised in the midline, gradually reducing the size of the uterus. (*Continues on following page.*)

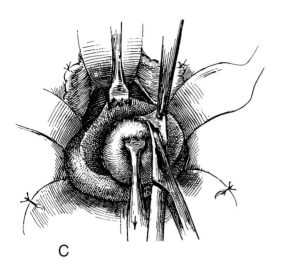

C

Figure 8.24 continued. Morcellation. **C.** Piecemeal excision in the direction of the closest fibroid is continued until its pseudocapsule is reached and opened. The fibroid is grasped with a tenaculum, traction is applied, and almost bloodless dissection continues in the plane of the pseudocapsule as shown until the fibroid can be removed either intact or piecemeal, depending upon its size.

movable and can be readily visualized, one can deliver it without flipping it (Fig. 8.26B). Hemostats are applied to the cornual angle of the uterus on either side, and the uterus is removed. The uterus should always be opened in the operating room as soon as it has been removed to determine whether there is any unexpected uterine neoplasm, which might influence operative therapy.

The technique of delivering the uterus without flipping it decreases the potential risk of contaminating peritoneal surfaces as a result of contact with a bacteriologically dirty cervix. Recognizing that the frequency with which retroperitoneal infection in the cellular tissues as compared to the infrequency of peritonitis accounts for posthysterectomy morbidity, prophylactic amputation of the external cervix may be indicated whenever uterine size or relative immobility of the uterus seems likely to result in more than the usual manipulation of the uterus as the fundus is being freed up and removed.

If at this point the body of the uterus is movable but too large to permit comfortable delivery by "flipping" the fundus through either the anterior or posterior peritoneal opening and morcellation is not desired, the myometrium can be incised circumferentially (Fig. 8.27A). Incision for this purpose should be placed parallel to the axis of the uterine cavity and parallel with the serosal covering of the uterus (Fig. 8.27, B and C). It frees the uterus much as a banana is peeled by turning the skin inside out, bringing the cervix still closer to the operator, but without violating the integrity of the endometrial cavity (Fig. 8.27C). The incision is carried symmetrically around the full circumference of the uterus through the myometrium just beneath the serosa (Fig. 8.27D). Incision of the lateral portions of myometrium medial to the remaining attachment of the broad ligament results in considerable additional descent of the uterus and greatly increases the mobility of the as yet unremoved fundus (Fig. 8.28).

Our sustained enthusiasm for this maneuver has permitted the delivery of unexpected, moderately enlarged uteri, often containing adenomyosis, without resorting to laparotomy. Others have shared our enthusiasm (41).

The cornual angle hemostats are, in turn, replaced by transfixion ligatures (Fig. 8.29). After these are tied, an additional bite is taken through the round ligament on each side, and the suture is tied again (Fig. 8.30). This will permit traction on the adnexal pedicles, to be borne principally by the round ligament (which has been ligated higher than the infundibulopelvic ligament by virtue of the extra bite). It is important not to pull the ligature off the pedicle of an ovarian artery within the ovarian ligament.

Figure 8.25. Bisection of the uterus when it is enlarged or fixed in position. **A.** The uterus can be bisected and removed one-half at a time. The cardinal ligament and uterine artery are clamped, cut, and ligated, and a clamp has been placed on the lower portion of the broad ligament. The cervix may be split in the midline, as shown, and the hemisection of the uterine corpus made along the path indicated by the *dotted line*. **B.** When the cardinal and uterosacral ligaments have been secured, but the uterus cannot be delivered into the wound because of adhesions around the adnexa or anterior uterine wall, the uterus can be incised posteriorly (*dashed line*). This improves uterine mobility considerably and provides direct access to the adherent adnexal areas. After these have been freed from the uterus, the incision can be carried around the circumference of the uterus, if necessary, and each half removed separately.

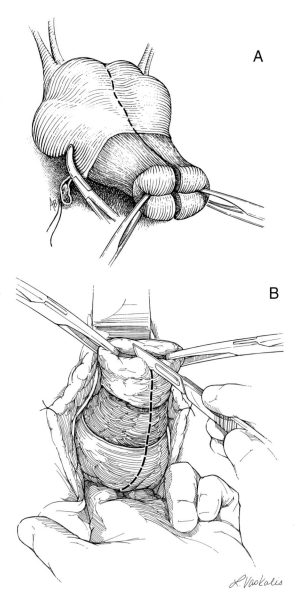

At this time the adnexa should be carefully inspected on each side, and, if removal is desired, it should be accomplished with particular care to ensure ligation of the ovarian vessels (7, 57, 72) (Figs. 8.31 and 8.32).

When vaginal oophorectomy of an obviously benign ovarian tumor is to be performed, one should first clamp and cut the mesovarium and then remove the ovary, using the clamp on the mesovarium as a handle so as not to fill the vagina with the ovarian tumor and obstruct one's vision of its pedicle.

If the operator has decided upon castration and the uterus is being removed, one may remove the ovaries alone, sparing the tube and mesosalpinx, which may aid appreciably in subsequent peritonealization by covering the intraperitoneal mesovarium stump. Should the operator prefer to preserve the tube, care must be taken when ligat-

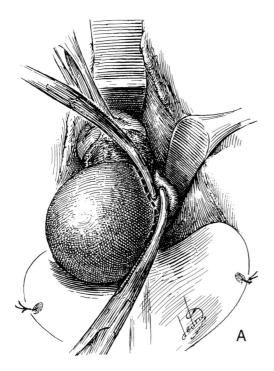

Figure 8.26. Delivery of the uterine fundus. **A.** The fundus of the uterus may be delivered by way of either anterior or posterior peritoneal opening, and hemostats may be applied to the cornual angles as shown. After both sides have been clamped, the uterus is cut away. **B.** When the fundus is freely movable and descends without undue traction, the uterus may be freed and delivered without "flipping" the fundus either anteriorly or posteriorly. Hemostats are applied to the cornual angles of the uterus on either side, after which the uterus is cut away from these hemostats and the cut ends are securely ligated.

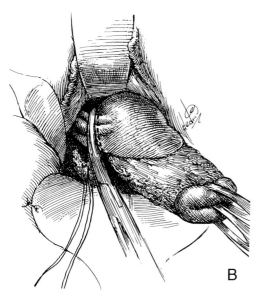

ing the ovarian pedicle to preserve the mesosalpinx and tubal blood supply. When the tube also is to be removed, the slanted Deschamps ligature carrier with its blunt point is good for ligation of the infundibulopelvic ligament. After the cornual angle stitches have been tied, the uncut ends of the sutures can be secured in a clamp and held long for use later in the procedure. If adhesions are great, the leaves of the broad ligament may be spread by funneling with the scissor tips for mobilization of the components ligated separately (6).

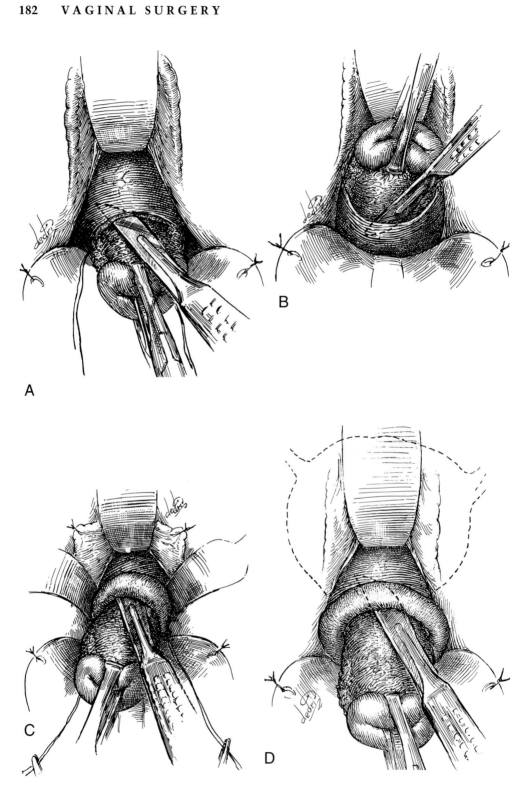

A

B

C

D

The surgeon should attempt to hook a finger separately into both the anterior and the posterior peritoneal cul-de-sac. If a "pocket" can be demonstrated, one has identified an enterocele, enterocele sac, or potential enterocele (Fig. 8.33). At times it will be helpful to pack the interior of the sac with a moistened gauze sponge to facilitate identification and to aid dissection. Because the patient should already be in a 5- or 10-degree Trendelenburg position (see Fig. 8.2), the contents of the abdomen can usually be readily packed away from the operative field by relatively little gauze packing. The excess peritoneum or an enterocele sac can be easily separated from the surrounding connective tissue by alternating sharp and blunt dissection as far down as the anterior surface of the rectum, which is identified by the small condensations of fat adherent to the peritoneum and by the noticeably longitudinal muscle layer of the outer rectal wall. As the anterior or vesicouterine peritoneum is inspected, any excess of redundant peritoneum left after the opening and dissection of the anterior peritoneal cul-de-sac should be excised at this time to lessen the possibility of a postoperative anterior enterocele. The bladder, if at all distended, should now be emptied of urine by catheter, since this will often seem to facilitate reperitonealization by making the anterior cut edge of the peritoneum more readily visible and accessible. Should difficulty be encountered in locating the anterior peritoneum, tissues inferior to the anterior peritoneum may be lightly grasped with successive gentle bites of two unlocked hemostats in such fashion as to "walk up" or roll these tissues toward the operator until the anterior peritoneal edge is identified. When unmistakably visible, the peritoneal edge is grasped by a hemostat while sutures are being placed to close the peritoneal opening.

Traction is made on the previously clamped and held transfixion ligature of the uterosacral ligament (Fig. 8.34). By pulling on this suture, one can readily identify the ligament on tension. Peritoneal closure is begun using a full length of absorbable, synthetic, size 0 suture, usually a single strand of polyglycolic or polydiaxanone suture. Beginning with a stitch through the peritoneal surface and into the left uterosacral ligament, the posterior peritoneum is then reefed in a linear fashion by a series of bites until the same level on the opposite uterosacral ligament location is reached (Fig. 8.35). This posterior peritoneal reefing should be along the level of the reflection of peritoneum from the anterior wall of the rectum. The operator should not place reefing sutures higher than this level, for to do so would displace an undesirably excessive amount of rectum into vaginal space.

The pursestring sutures to close the peritoneum and any suture placed for the purpose of bringing the uterosacral and/or the infundibulopelvic and round ligaments together should be carefully placed above or proximal to the ligature on the pedicles. The purpose of the suture that brings the ligamentous structures together is twofold: to pro-

---

Figure 8.27. A Lash incision into the myometrium. **A.** The inferior and major blood supply of the uterus (the ascending and descending branches of the uterine artery) have already been secured by transfixion ligature and the operator has determined that the uterus is not deviated or fixed by any previously unsuspected adhesions. If it is now determined that the body of the uterus is too big to permit delivery, the outer superficial myometrium can be incised circumferentially. **B.** Both anterior and posterior myometrial incisions should be kept parallel to the axis of the uterine cavity and should completely traverse the outer myometrial layer of the uterus. **C.** If the circumferential incision has been properly placed, this will permit enucleation of the bulk of the uterus without transgressing the endocervical or endometrial cavity, much in the manner of peeling a banana as its skin turns inside out. The large, bulky uterus is thereby increased in length and decreased in width, which in essence "makes the cork smaller than the neck of the bottle." **D.** The large but movable uterine corpus (*dashed line*) is shown in relationship to the myometrial incision.

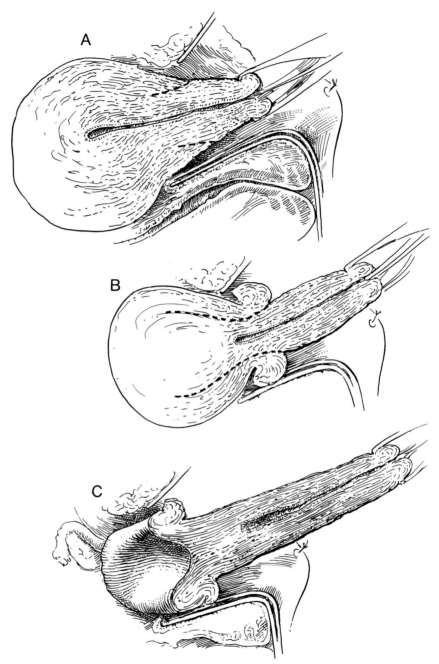

Figure 8.28. A. Sagittal drawing of a large, bulky uterus. The cardinal and uterosacral ligaments have been separated from the sides of the uterus, but delivery of the body is difficult because of its size. The pathway for incision into the myometrium parallel to the axis of the uterus is identified by the *broken line*. **B.** The incision has been deepened, as traction further exteriorizes the cervix. The myometrial incision will be extended further as indicated by the *broken line*. **C.** The uterus can now be delivered outside the pelvis. The length has increased as the diameter has been decreased, as shown. The cornual angle can now be clamped under direct visualization and the uterus cut free.

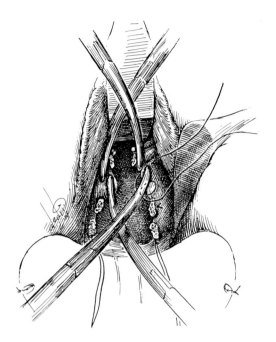

Figure 8.29. Ligation of the adnexal pedicle. Each hemostat is then replaced by transfixion ligature as shown.

mote a firm tissue union, and to ensure that all ligated pedicles will be extraperitonealized. The ligatures on the uterine vessels will not be caught up on an approximating suture. Although the vessels will retract into the parametria, their ligated pedicles also remain extraperitonealized.

After the peritoneal closure stitch has been passed through the uterosacral ligament and adjacent peritoneum, first on the patient's left and later similarly on the right side, traction on the previously held uterosacral transfixing ligatures is relaxed. The homolateral adnexal pedicle suture on the patient's right side is then grasped, and gentle traction is again made to bring the round ligament into view. The peritoneal closure stitch is passed through the round ligament proximal and medial to the previously placed pedicle ligation. The round ligaments do not support the vagina; they are incorporated in the pursestring stitch only to better peritonealize the pelvis. The anterior peritoneum is then identified, and any excess is excised and reefed by a series of bites that continue to and through the left round ligament, at which point the stitch has been continued in clockwise fashion entirely around the peritoneal opening and through the round and uterosacral ligaments on each side. Peritoneal closure following vaginal hysterectomy is done primarily to incorporate the strength of the subperitoneal connective tissue retinaculum into a firm scar at the bottom of the pelvis that will resist increases in intra-abdominal pressure. The mesothelial lining of the peritoneal cavity per se has little supportive value.

Care must be taken to remove all intra-abdominal intraperitoneal packing, after which all slack in this pursestring type of peritoneal suture is taken up by reefing the tissues fairly snugly along the suture both anteriorly and posteriorly. Only after such reefing should the pursestring suture closing the peritoneum be tied. To be effective, all reefing should be accomplished before, not as, this stitch is tied. This plication of tissues at the bases of the uterosacral ligaments actually draws the pubococcygei and their fasciae together (45, 46), narrowing the genital hiatus. After the pursestring peritoneal closure stitch has been tied, both ends of the stitch should be left long without cutting and held for later use. Because the uterosacral ligaments are relatively fixed in position, the movable round ligaments that are also included in the pursestring suture will be brought to

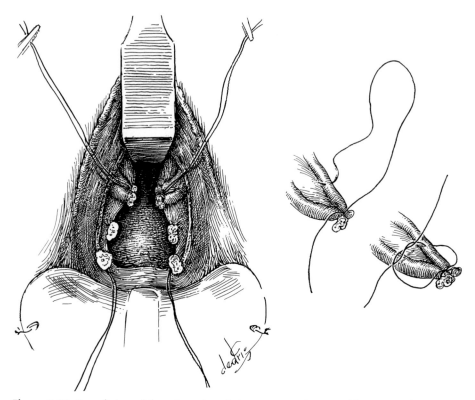

Figure 8.30. Transfixion of the adnexal pedicle sutures to the round ligament. The sutures are tied, after which an additional suture bite is placed in the round ligament on either side, to which the pedicle is again tied as shown on the *right*. This maneuver ensures that later traction on the adnexal or the cornual angle pedicle will, in fact, be exerted on the round ligament that has been ligated more proximal than the infundibulopelvic ligament by virtue of the extra ligature. This technique reduces the risk that a tie that has secured the ovarian artery within the pedicle of the ovarian ligament may be pulled off the pedicle during only moderate traction. Because of this risk, the ovarian pedicles as well as the adnexa should be carefully reinspected on each side just before the peritoneum is closed. When the cornual angle stitches have been secured, the ends of these sutures should be tagged long enough to be readily identified when the adnexa and ovarian pedicles are to be reinspected later in the procedure.

the semifixed uterosacral ligaments, rather than the other way around, fixing the peritonealization in a posterolateral direction over the levator plate, tending to reestablish the horizontal axis of the upper vagina, and appreciably lessening the chances of the postoperative development of an enterocele.

The round ligament pedicle stitches may be tied together beneath the base of the bladder, providing for additional safety as auxiliary support to the intra-abdominal contents should the peritoneal sutures be broken or become untied. The retracting sutures in the labia minora may now be cut and the vagina prepared for closure. If no colporrhaphy is to be done, to preserve maximal vaginal depth, the inverted T-shaped incision in the anterior vaginal wall is trimmed to an inverted V (Fig. 8.36) and the vagina closed in a sagittal direction.

After completion of the anterior colporrhaphy, as closure of the anterior vaginal wall begins, the needle on one end of the preserved peritoneal closure stitch is passed through

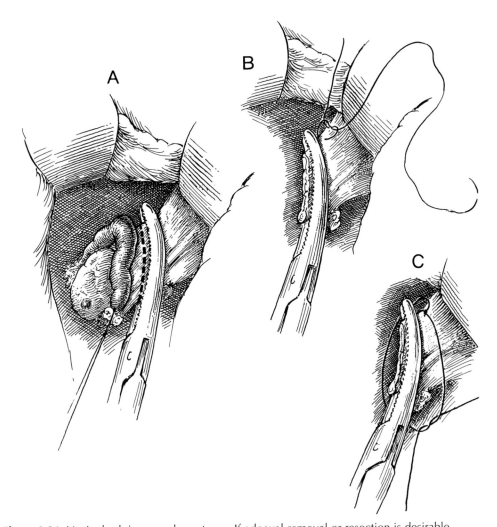

Figure 8.31. Vaginal salpingo-oophorectomy. If adnexal removal or resection is desirable, it should be performed at this time. Vaginal salpingo-oophorectomy may be accomplished as follows. **A.** Downward traction is applied to the round ligament suture. The ovary may be grasped in a sponge holder and a forceps applied across the infundibulopelvic ligament. **B.** The ovary and tube are excised, and a transfixion suture of medium thickness is placed. **C.** The tie is completed as the forceps is removed.

each side of the uppermost portion of the anterior vaginal wall, from the inside out on one side and outside in on the other, at precisely the level at the vault that will correspond to the previous attachments in the cardinal ligaments, and held for tying later. The end of the peritoneal closure stitch sewn beneath the anterior vaginal wall at its apex as noted above is then tied to its other held end (of the previously tied peritoneal pursestring suture), taking care, as when previously preparing to tie the peritoneal pursestring suture, to reef the tissues to be tied rather snugly together before seating and tying the knot (Fig. 8.37). This suture fixes the anterior vault to the edge and level of the peritoneal pursestring, effectively lengthening the anterior vaginal wall and aiding in the support of the vaginal vault.

Figure 8.32. Transvaginal oophorectomy when the infundibulopelvic ligament is short. The mesovarium has been clamped and the ovary removed. There is a single penetration of the mesovarium at its midpoint, and each end of the suture is passed around the distal tip of the hemostat and tied beneath the heel of the clamp.

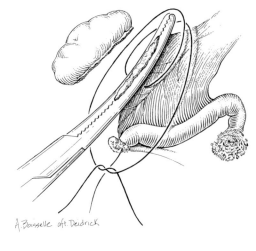

A. Boisselle aft. Deidrick

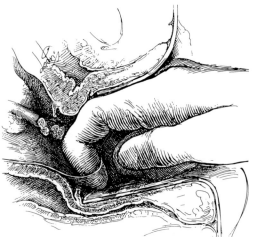

Figure 8.33. Sagittal section showing exploration of the cul-de-sac. The importance of recognizing evidence of a potential enterocele or the demonstration of an existing enterocele sac always warrants careful exploration of the cul-de-sac by the operator's fingers. For demonstration or identification purposes, a suspected sac can be packed with a gauze sponge to facilitate demonstration of excess peritoneal connective tissue by both sharp and blunt dissection down to a point where the excision of excess peritoneum will extend across the anterior surface of the rectum. Any fat that is present belongs on the rectal side of the dissection. Rectum should be recognized promptly during this dissection either by the characteristic condensations of fat or by the longitudinal muscle fibers of the outer layer of rectal wall. In the same manner, the anterior peritoneum should be inspected. If there is excessive redundant peritoneum anteriorly, it should be excised at this time, lessening the postoperative possibility of an anterior enterocele.

Tying the held end of the peritoneal closure stitch to an uppermost stitch in the anterior vaginal wall with a bite or two to either side of the midline and the uterosacral ligaments also effectively unites the anterior connective tissue capsule of the vagina to the area in which the uterosacral ligaments have been brought together as a result of the placement of the peritoneal stitch. Because each uterosacral ligament has in effect been united to the posterolateral surface of the vaginal wall, this has the effect of uniting the tissue capsule of the anterior vaginal wall to that of the posterior vaginal wall (36).

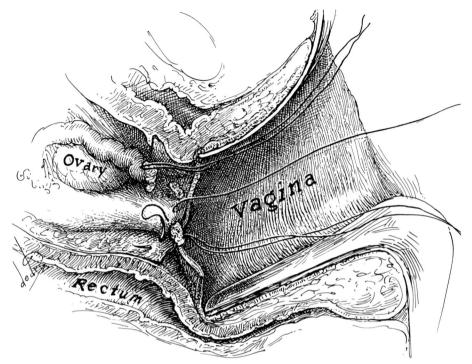

Figure 8.34. The beginning of the high peritoneal closure stitch through the peritoneal surface of the uterosacral ligament, and then through the posterior peritoneum just above its cut edge.

The anterior vaginal wall is closed by either running or interrupted subcuticular sutures. A subcuticular closure ensures a more exact and smooth approximation of the epithelial layers. This alignment effectively reduces the development of postoperative loci of granulation tissue in the suture line, and in virtually doing so, it reduces the opportunity for future development of an enterocele and appreciably strengthens the vault (6, 58).

By having closed the vagina from side to side in a longitudinal direction (Fig. 8.38) rather than front to back, one will have developed an additional 2 or 3 cm of vaginal length, which at times may mean the difference between a depth that may contain the patient's sexual partner and a shorter depth that may not (Fig. 8.39).

CULDEPLASTY

When there are strong uterosacral-cardinal ligaments, as usually seen with uterovaginal prolapse, with obvious shortening or telescoping of the vagina, the operator can confidently gain additional vaginal depth by fixing the vagina posterior to this ligament complex. One method of doing this is to use the McCall culdeplasty (51) or a modification of it.

In our modification most of the peritoneum of any coexistent enterocele is excised first, before the polyglycolic acid-type culdeplasty stitches are placed, eliminating the enterocele while reducing the size of the subsequent cul-de-sac (Fig. 8.40A). An appropriate wedge should be removed from an unusually wide vault (Fig. 8.40B) and the edges approximated. The culdeplasty stitches should be tied under direct vision, eliminating the chance that the now buried proximal end of a fallopian tube will prolapse postoperatively into the line of vaginal incision.

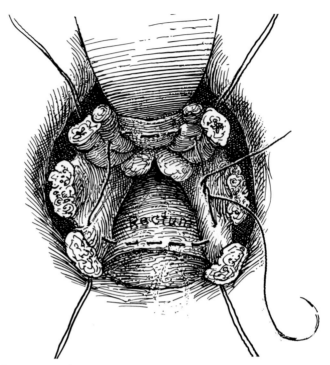

Figure 8.35. Purse-string closure of peritoneum. If a marking suture has not been placed and difficulty is experienced in locating the anterior peritoneum, the tissue caudal to the anterior peritoneum is lightly grasped with successive gentle bites of an unlocked hemostat, in such fashion as to "walk up" this area until the anterior peritoneum is recognized and grasped in a forceps. Peritonealization is accomplished using a full length of absorbable 0 or 2/0 suture, held in a light hemostat for identification later. We prefer to begin this stitch on the peritoneal side of the left uterosacral ligament. Traction is made on the previously clamped and held transfixion ligature of the uterosacral ligament; by putting the ligament on tension, one can readily identify it. The posterior peritoneum is reefed by a series of bites until the opposite uterosacral ligament location is reached. The suture passes through the right round ligament, the anterior peritoneum, and the left round ligament and is ready to be tied.

If the posterior vault is wide, as after an enterocele repair, a V-shaped wedge of excess vaginal membrane may be dissected free and removed. This maneuver also serves to bring the vaginal attachments of the uterosacral ligaments still closer together toward the midline. Tying the pursestring peritonealization stitch under direct visualization avoids the possibility of trapping any intra-abdominal structure, such as an ovary, a knuckle of tube, or bowel, into the stitch.

The performance of this step is entirely consistent with the pursestring peritonealization described, as well as surgical narrowing or V-shaped wedging of a voluminous vaginal vault also as described.

Uncommonly (but usually in a patient with procidentia), one may be unable to demonstrate palpable usable uterosacral ligament strength, and alternate methods of fixing and stabilizing the vaginal vault must be found, lest the unfixed vault should later telescope and evert. In such an instance, and after the peritoneal cavity has been closed, the vault may be sewn to the fascia of the pelvic diaphragm (34) or the sacrospinous or sacrotuberous ligament (see Chapter 16).

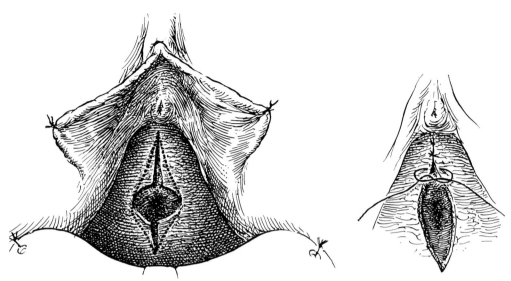

Figure 8.36. Narrowing of a wide vaginal vault. Before the vault of the vagina is closed in a longitudinal direction, it can be narrowed, when desired, by excision of small wedges of tissue of a size as indicated by the *dotted lines*, thus converting the T-shaped incisions to a V shape. One trims only enough vaginal wall as to leave vaginal flaps that can be closed with subepithelial sutures without tension, everting the edges to avoid irregular overlapping or pockets of inverted epithelium.

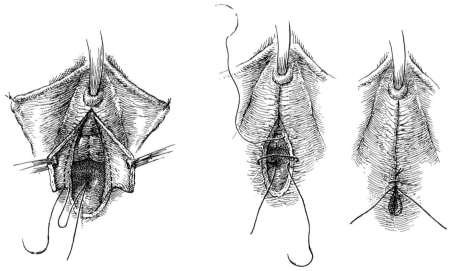

Figure 8.37. Elongating the anterior vaginal wall. The amount of vagina to be removed by anterior colporrhaphy is shown by the *dotted lines*. One end of the tied peritoneal closure stitch is passed through each side of the vault of the anterior vaginal wall as shown. The anterior colporrhaphy is completed, and the peritoneal closure stitch end is tied, bringing the anterior vaginal wall to the site of the previous peritoneal closure and lengthening the anterior vaginal wall.

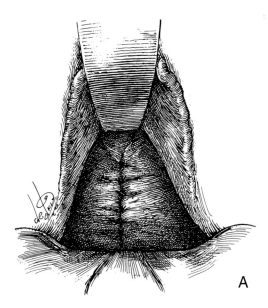

Figure 8.38. Closing the vaginal wall.
A. The objective is to bring the cut-across edges of the vaginal membrane together to facilitate union in a smooth suture line with as little irregularity as can be achieved. Placement of subcuticular sutures in the vaginal membrane requires the use of fine needles and smaller sizes of suture material and favors accurate placement of each suture, which accounts for our preference for this technique using 00 polyglycolic acid-type suture (Dexon or Vicryl). It takes time and care and results in a vaginal closure that is a fitting completion of a skillfully performed operation.

A

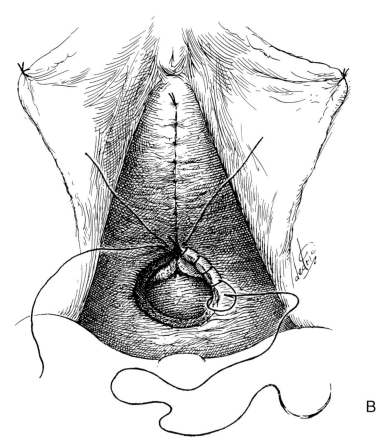

B

Figure 8.38 continued. Closing the vaginal wall. **B.** An important step in preserving vaginal depth when such is the goal is the side-to-side approximation of vaginal tissues anterior to the site at which the uterosacral ligaments have been transfixed to the wall of the vagina. Posterior to this point the vault may be left open for drainage and the full thickness of the vaginal wall between the uterosacral ligaments oversewn by a running locked hemostatic stitch from one uterosacral fixation site to the other.

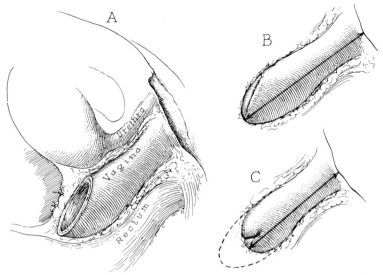

Figure 8.39. The advantage of side-to-side closure. **A.** The unclosed vagina. **B.** The increase in vaginal depth obtained by longitudinal side-to-side closure of the vaginal vault. **C.** Transverse front-to-back closure, which results in a shorter vagina.

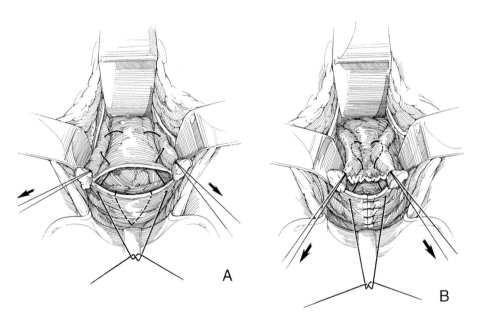

Figure 8.40. The modified McCall culdeplasty. **A.** Any enterocele sac has been resected, and using a long-lasting polyglycolic acid suture, the stitches are placed through the vaginal wall, through the cut edge of the peritoneum, and high on the medial surface of the uterosacral ligament, and a bite is taken in the peritoneum overlying the anterior surface of the rectum. The same structures are stitched in reverse order on the opposite side. When using a monofilament suture, it is wise to place a second McCall stitch approximately 1 cm cranial to the first. In the event of unexpected breakage of one of the sutures during the tying process, there will still be one unbroken suture left to support the vault of the vagina. A very wide posterior vault may be narrowed by excising an appropriately sized wedge as shown by the *dashed line.* **B.** The sides of the V-shaped wound in the posterior vaginal wall are closed with interrupted polyglycolic acid sutures. This closure not only narrows the vault but also brings the uterosacral ligaments that are fixed to the vault closer together. After the peritoneum is closed, the McCall stitches are tied. (*Continues on the following page.*)

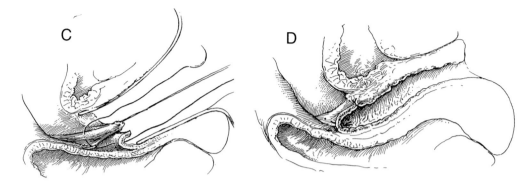

Figure 8.40 continued. The modified McCall culdeplasty. **C.** The first half of the modified culdeplasty stitch is shown in sagittal section before tying and closure of the peritoneal cavity and vaginal vault. **D.** The stitch is shown after tying and subsequent closure of the peritoneal cavity and vaginal vault. The apex of the vagina is now cranial and posterior to the new peritoneal cul-de-sac.

CONFIRMING URETERAL PATENCY

If at the conclusion of surgery there is any question as to ureteral patency, the issue may be quickly resolved by administering an intravenous dose of indigo carmine. Ten minutes later the bladder is distended by 300 ml of normal saline, and the patient is cystoscoped to observe the efflux of violet-colored urine from each ureteral orifice.

After surgery the vaginal cavity may be lightly packed for 24 hours with 2-inch plain or iodoform gauze, and a silicone-coated transurethral Foley catheter may be inserted. We do not routinely pack the vagina. Packing, when used, provides not just a hemostatic pressure to obliterate potential spaces, but also serves as a bolster to protect the new sutures in the vaginal vault and as a blotter to soak up secretion in the vaginal vault, removing blood serum and preventing pooling (16). It has not been our practice to insert an indwelling transurethral catheter routinely if no colporrhaphy has been done because we believe the incidence of subsequent cystitis is much less if the patient is able to void by herself. The presence of vaginal packing, however, does make it difficult for some to initiate voiding, and a transurethral Foley catheter would be inserted if vaginal packing had been used. The packing and the catheter are removed the morning of the first postoperative day. Before the operation is completed, a rectal examination is performed to check for anal stricture and to confirm rectal integrity. If a stitch through the rectal mucosa is noted, it should be visualized on the rectal side, cut, and the ends permitted to retract into the perirectal tissues.

VAGINAL HYSTERECTOMY AND PARTIAL VAGINECTOMY

Experience has demonstrated certain advantages to employing a vaginal hysterectomy with partial vaginectomy for the definitive treatment of in situ carcinoma of the uterine cervix in cases where there is extension of the disease onto the vagina (77). In the hands of an experienced vaginal surgeon, this approach seems to offer the advantages of specific preoperative and intraoperative delineation of the lesion to be removed, not found in other techniques.

This operation, consisting of vaginal hysterectomy and removal of a predetermined amount of vaginal cuff, is useful as the definitive treatment of intraepithelial carcinoma of the cervix with extension to or involvement of the vagina as determined by preoperative colposcopically directed biopsy. As part of the preparation at surgery, the vagina can be lightly painted with tincture of iodine or freshly prepared Schiller solution. Failure of any area to take up the iodine stain establishes clearly all non-glycogen-containing areas of the cervix and vagina. The multicentric origin of the disease can be appreciated and all nonstaining areas of the cervix and vagina visualized. This enables the operator to determine the level at which the cuff along with a comfortable margin of uninvolved tissue should be amputated, a decision that can only be estimated or surmised during an abdominal hysterectomy.

The amount of vagina being removed is easier to measure during a vaginal hysterectomy than by an abdominal approach, because in the vaginal operation the cardinal ligament support system is cut from the uterus after the vagina has been "measured and cut" and the vagina is much less stretched, whereas during an abdominal hysterectomy the stretch of the vagina is greater, because by traction on the uterus, the cardinal ligaments are cut before the vagina is stretched and cut. That which appeared to have been a 1-inch cuff of (stretched) vagina with a uterus removed abdominally may, as the previously stretched tissue contracts, proves to be only 1/3 or 1/2 inch of vagina.

By doing an essentially extrafascial vaginal hysterectomy, one may develop additional mobilization of the parametrium, being mindful of the location of the ureters, and more tissue in an appropriate amount can be removed with the operative specimen than by the standard intrafascial total abdominal hysterectomy. This may be of particular advantage if the pathology report discloses superficial unsuspected microinvasion of less than 3-mm depth (which by probability has not yet progressed to the point of lymphatic extension).

Finally, the patient having vaginal surgery has a distinctly less complicated, usually more simple, and certainly more comfortable postoperative course, unimpeded by the greater likelihood of ileus, intestinal obstruction, and the abdominal discomforts seen more frequently after abdominal total hysterectomy. The patient's rehabilitation is usually shorter following vaginal surgery since there is no painful abdominal incision with which to contend.

The operation can be performed by an experienced vaginal surgeon upon a patient without uterine prolapse, but if any coexistent prolapse and/or vaginal relaxation is present, it can be repaired at the same time as the hysterectomy.

Schuchardt Perineal Incision

This incision is used when transvaginal exposure is awkward and accessibility seems limited, and it may be of value either for hysterectomy or to provide exposure for fistula repair. It usually appears desirable for the right-handed operator to make the incision on the patient's left side. The tissues to be incised may be infiltrated thoroughly by 0.5% lidocaine (Xylocaine) and 1:200,000 epinephrine (Adrenalin) in a fanlike fashion, using a 22-gauge spinal needle (Fig. 8.41). The needle is inserted through the skin of the perineum midway between the anus and the left ischial tuberosity (54). To further reduce blood loss, the incision may be made with the electrosurgical scalpel. The skin incision follows a curved line from the 4 o'clock position at the hymenal margin to a point halfway between the anus and the ischial tuberosity (Fig. 8.42). To protect the nearby rectum from damage during this incision, the operator may insert the index finger of the left hand into the vagina, depressing the perineum and rectum, while at the same time the assistant on the surgeon's right inserts an index finger into the vagina, providing pressure in an anterolateral direction to keep the tissues on tension. The incision is started immediately behind the site of the hymenal margin and is continued posterolaterally in a gentle curve around the anus to end at a point midway between the anus and the left ischial tuberosity. The surgeon and the assistant introduce their index fingers more deeply into the vagina, maintaining tension, and the vaginal portion of the incision is continued in a posterolateral direction as high as is necessary to provide the desired exposure of the

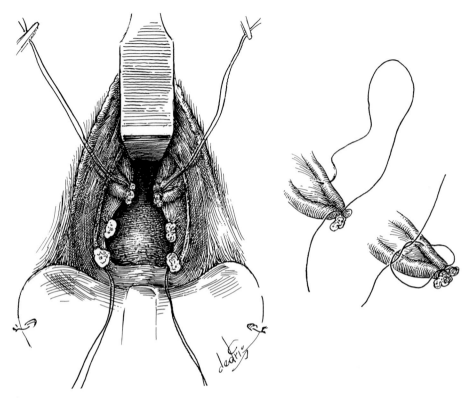

Figure 8.41. Perineal infiltration by a "liquid tourniquet." From a point midway between the anus and the ischial tuberosity, and using a no. 22 spinal needle, the tissues are thoroughly infiltrated by a solution of dilute epinephrine (1:200,000) in 0.5% lidocaine along the pathways shown by the *arrows.* The site of the Schuchardt incision is shown by the path of the *heavy broken line.* (From Nichols, DH, ed. Gynecologic and obstetric surgery. St. Louis: Mosby-Year Book, 1993. Used with permission.)

vaginal vault. The lowermost fatty tissue of the ischiorectal fossa will have been divided. In the depths of the wound the medial portion of the pubococcygeus muscle will become visible, and a portion of this may be divided if necessary. Bleeding points are clamped and coagulated with the electrosurgical unit as they are encountered, care being taken not to coagulate the surface of the rectum, since it tends to remain prominently in the wound. At the conclusion of the operation the Schuchardt incision is closed in layers. The vaginal stitches may include and unite the severed portions of the pubococcygeus muscle, bringing them together beneath the edges of the vaginal incision.

When the case is difficult or the operator not yet experienced in this procedure, instillation of 60 ml of sterile evaporated milk, infant formula, or a solution of methylene blue into the bladder will permit prompt recognition of any unexpected bladder penetration.

If an incision of this depth is not required, a classical mediolateral type of episiotomy incision may be made on one or both sides, which should be carefully closed by reapproximation of all incised tissue layers.

PROCEDURE

Iodine is applied to the cervix and upper half of the vagina, and areas are noted that do not take the stain. A rim of colpohemostats is applied to a fold of the vagina at least 1½ inches away from the lateral margin of the cervix and lateral to any nonstained tissue

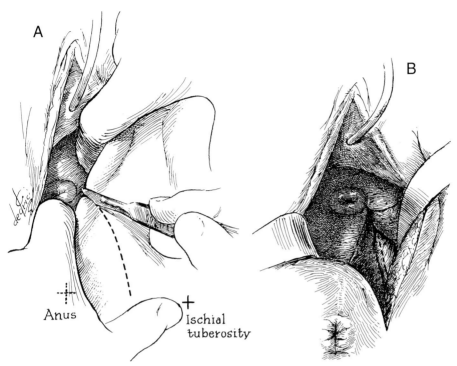

A

B

Anus

Ischial
tuberosity

Figure 8.42. The Schuchardt perineal incision. **A.** The Schuchardt incision is started immediately behind the site of the hymenal margin and continued posterolaterally in a gentle curve around the anus to end at a point midway between the anus and the left ischial tuberosity. The surgeon and the assistant introduce their index fingers deeper into the vagina, maintaining tension, and the vaginal portion of the incision is continued in a posterolateral direction as high as is necessary to provide the desired exposure of the vaginal vault. **B.** The lowermost fat tissue of the ischiorectal fossa has been divided, and in the depths of the wound the medial portion of the pubococcygeus muscle is visible. A portion of this may be divided if necessary, as shown by the *dotted line*. Bleeding points are clamped as they are encountered and coagulated with the electrosurgical unit, care being taken not to coagulate the surface of the rectum should it be visible within the wound. At the conclusion of the operation, the Schuchardt incision is closed in layers.

within the vagina (Fig. 8.43). The cervix is tucked into this fold and an incision made through the full thickness of the vagina with Mayo scissors or the electrosurgical scalpel (Fig. 8.44). Counterpressure from anterior, posterior, and lateral retractors permits the bladder and its fascia to recede promptly from the point at which the vagina was held by the colpohemostats. The vaginal flap is established circumferentially and, being mindful of the position of the ureters, the lateral fascial bundles are clamped, cut, and ligated on either side. By gentle dissection the rectum is separated from the tissues to be removed, the posterior cul-de-sac is identified, and an opening is made into it, after which the posterior and lateral portions of the uterosacral ligaments are clamped, cut, and ligated.

The fundus of the uterus can be brought through either the anterior or posterior colpotomy, and the adnexa inspected and removed if desired. Hemostats are applied over the cornual angles of the uterus, and the uterus, cervix, and parametrial tissues are removed en masse. The hemostats are replaced by transfixion ligatures. Areas of venous oozing around the base of the bladder may be identified, but no active bleeding is to be expected. The vaginal vault can then be closed with an absorbable suture on each side

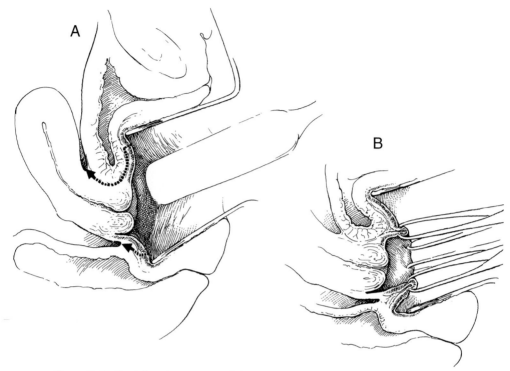

Figure 8.43. Partial vaginectomy with hysterectomy. The vagina and cervix are carefully exposed and thoroughly examined, and the amount of vagina to be removed with the specimen is determined with precision. **A.** Sagittal drawing shows the lines of proposed dissection. Infiltration here by 1:200,000 adrenaline in 0.5% Xylocaine solution aids hemostasis and the later identification of the connective tissue planes and spaces. **B.** Distal to this point the vagina is grasped circumferentially by a series of single-toothed tenacula.

that goes through the anterior vault, round ligament, and anterior peritoneum on each side. A second set of sutures goes through the posterolateral vault, uterosacral ligament pedicle, posterior peritoneum, and the same structures on the opposite side. (Fig. 8.45).

When the vagina after hysterectomy seems too short for marital comfort, anterior and/or posterior colporrhaphy can be performed if required and the Schuchardt incision closed. A sheath of mobilized peritoneum can be sewn to the distal cut edge of the vagina and the peritoneal cavity closed cranially (Fig. 8.46). An obturator should be worn postoperatively during the period of vaginal reepithelialization. Distal length can be added by using the Williams vulvovaginoplasty (see Chapter 20), or a perineorrhaphy (see Chapter 11) if the perineum is deficient.

THE SCHAUTA RADICAL VAGINAL HYSTERECTOMY

Despite the interest and efforts of enthusiastic American exponents (McCall, Barclay, Smale, Hatch, and Crisp), the Schauta-Amreich radical vaginal hysterectomy is not often performed in most American clinics. As a result few are teaching this interesting operation. In Europe many of those accomplished in its technique are no longer in practice (Bastiaanse, Amreich, Mitra, Ingiulla, Navratil, and Tapfer). The operation has been kept alive, however, by Novak (57) of Yugoslavia, Reiffenstuhl (67) of Austria, Massi (47–49), Carenza, and Villani (8–10) of Italy, and Dargent (16) of France, among others.

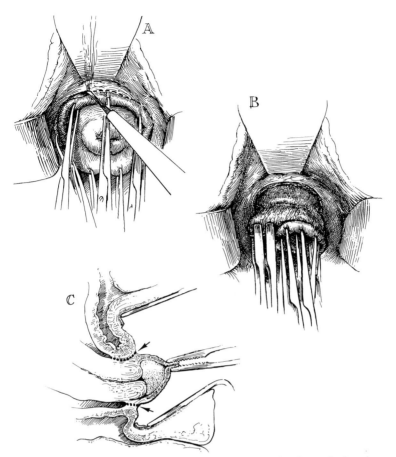

Figure 8.44. Partial vaginectomy with hysterectomy. **A.** Traction is applied to the tenacula and against countertraction supplied by the retractors. An incision is made by electrosurgical knife, scissors, or scalpel through the full thickness of the vagina. **B.** The vagina is inverted as a sleeve over the cervix. An alcohol-soaked sponge is applied against the face of the cervix, the single-toothed tenacula are removed, and the anterior and posterior walls of the vagina are brought together by a series of Krobach mouse-toothed clamps, straight Kocher hemostats, or heavy sutures. **C.** Sagittal section further illustrates the line of sharp dissection to be followed to gain both anterior and posterior entry to the peritoneal cavity.

Carenza considered the operation of benefit to individuals with earlier stages of invasive squamous cell carcinoma of the cervix (IA, IB, IIA) with negative lymphography. We occasionally find the operation suitable for the young patient in whom it is desirable to preserve ovarian function, for the very obese patient in whom exposure to the radical abdominal hysterectomy might be difficult, for the patient at high medical risk who cannot take a prolonged or deep general anesthetic, and for the patient with genital prolapse and a large and symptomatic cystocele and rectocele. In situ carcinomas of the cervix are better treated, when hysterectomy is desired, by simple total abdominal or vaginal hysterectomy, with the removal of an appropriate cuff of vagina if there is vaginal involvement by the tumor.

Radical vaginal hysterectomy is limited to those patients in whom careful preoperative study of biopsy or conization material indicates no evidence of lymphatic or vascular invasion. No matter how small the primary lesion, the likelihood of metastases

Figure 8.45. When there has been no coincident prolapse of the vaginal vault, depth may be preserved by closure from side to side as suggested by Durfee. A stitch of polyglycolic acid-type suture is passed through the full thickness of the lateral vaginal wall, the round ligament portion of the adnexal pedicle, a reefing of the anterior peritoneum, and the same structures in reverse order on the opposite side. A second stitch is placed through the full thickness of the posterolateral vaginal wall, the uterosacral ligament stump, a reefing of the posterior peritoneum, and the same structures in reverse order on the opposite side. Any gaps in the vaginal wall may be closed by interrupted sutures.

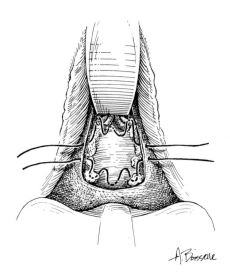

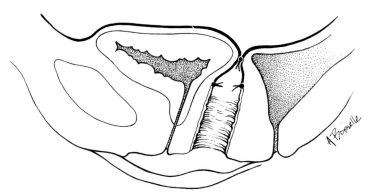

Figure 8.46. Lengthening the vagina. Proximal length can be added to a shortened vagina by attaching its cut edges to the margins of previously freed peritoneal flaps (7). The peritoneal cavity is securely closed by a separate cranially placed suture, as shown.

should be inferred in those persons showing evidence of vascular or lymphatic invasion or penetration.

Evidence of actual or potential vascular involvement requires transabdominal lymphadenectomy as part of the initial surgical procedure. Negative preoperative lymphadenography is helpful, and detailed microscopic examination of the hysterectomy specimen postoperatively should include specific attention to recognition of any previously undisclosed evidences of lymphatic or vascular penetration. Should this be found, the patient must be given surgical pelvic lymphadenectomy or appropriate deep x-ray therapy to the pelvic lymph nodes. Postoperative endolymphatic therapy with radioactive isotopes is an attractive consideration but is of unproven value. Nodes whose lymphatic pathways are totally obstructed by tumor might fail to receive the necessary radiation, although it is quite likely that an adequate cancerocidal dosage can be delivered by this route to nodes partially infiltrated by metastatic disease and, quite possibly, to similarly involved lymph nodes that are surgically inaccessible.

Controversy concerning the importance of lymphadenectomy persists, although generally held present opinion favors lymphadenectomy. The possibility remains, however, that even when involved with early metastases the lymphatic system may play a protective role in the body's immunologic defense and the patient's survival against the propagation of a neoplasm. The possible importance of this factor continues to be emphasized by Crisp (15), echoing the convictions of Högler (31) and in 1994 of Massi (48).

The radical vaginal operation makes it possible to remove a greater amount of parametrium than is likely from the abdominal approach, but it is conjectural as to whether this will, in fact, provide a better prognosis. The radical vaginal hysterectomy also permits the removal of a predetermined amount of vagina or vaginal cuff at the time of the original operative procedure and under the direct vision and control of the operator. The exact amount of vagina to be removed should be determined by preoperative colposcopy and colposcopically directed biopsy and further demarcated by staining of the vagina with iodine solution at the time of surgery before the incision is placed in the vagina. In the hands of an experienced gynecologic surgeon the operation appears to be associated with a lower incidence of serious complications, particularly urinary fistulas, than does the abdominal counterpart.

At the present time we believe that for those women in whom vascular or lymphatic penetration has been established preoperatively by biopsy study or lymphography, certain advantages of a combined abdominovaginal hysterocolpectomy, including lymphadenectomy, can be seriously considered. The vaginal portion of the operation permits the widest possible excision of parametrium, rectal pillars, and uterosacral ligaments, and the abdominal lymphadenectomy, either extraperitoneal or intraperitoneal, completes the procedure. It would seem advisable, therefore, to plan an operative procedure that would combine the best features of both the abdominal and the vaginal operations into a single or composite operative procedure, which in the interests of shorter operating time, the patient's safety, and surgical efficiency might be accomplished by the simultaneous use of two operating teams.

There are several advantages of the radical-vaginal portion of the composite operation. Initial staining of the vagina with iodine ensures that all of the vaginal tissues that might be involved will be removed with the cervix. The vaginal approach also ensures vastly improved dissection of the paracolpium, the inferior portion of the horizontal connective tissue ground bundle, the inferior portion of the rectal pillars, and the vesicouterine ligaments. Ureteral exposure and dissection can best be accomplished during the vaginal portion of the operation. Meanwhile, through an appropriate incision, the abdominal team will have begun the bilateral extraperitoneal or intraperitoneal lymphadenectomy, which may be completed while the vaginal team is closing the Schuchardt incision. A combined synchronous operation has been reported by Mitra (53), Navratil (54), Howkins (33), and Vidakovic (78), among others, in various sequential modifications. The combined operation should be of particular value for those in whom vascular or lymphatic penetration has been established preoperatively by biopsy study or lymphography. However, it remains to be seen whether such a combined operation will provide an improved prognosis.

Although coincident extraperitoneal pelvic lymphadenectomy can be performed to obtain information as to possible nodal metastases, laparoscopic pelvic lymphadenectomy can be performed (14, 16).

Radical Trachelectomy

Dargent (personal communication, September 1994) has described his experience with radical trachelectomy, which may provide an important alternative to radical hysterectomy for some women with invasive cervical cancer who wish to have children. In all cases, a laparoscopic pelvic lymphadenectomy preceded the trachelectomy to make certain the women had negative nodes.

Radical trachelectomy is a modification of the Schauta radical hysterectomy in which an appropriate vaginal cuff is removed at the same time as the proximal part of the cardinal ligaments and most of the cervix. But the upper cervical canal and uterus are left intact, and the vaginal mucosa is later reapproximated to the endocervical canal. The operation can be performed in women whose cancers are from stage IA to stage IIA. The inner limit of the tumor must be at the level of the orifice of the cervix, and the cervical canal itself has to be free of cancer.

Several living, normal babies have been delivered to a small number of these patients by cesarean section. This pilot study is an example of a trend toward a more conservative management of invasive cervical cancer, but awaits long-term confirmation of its effectiveness.

The technique of the Schauta-Amreich radical vaginal hysterectomy may be described as follows, including some modifications concerned particularly with the method of exposure of the ureter in the bladder pillar.

Technique of the Radical Vaginal Operation

The perineal tissues to be incised by the Schuchardt approach and the vaginal tissues at the site of vaginal circumcision are thoroughly infiltrated by 0.5% lidocaine (Xylocaine) in 1:200,000 epinephrine (Adrenalin) solution (Fig. 8.47). When this has been thoroughly dispersed in the tissue to be incised, a Schuchardt incision is performed. The vagina is grasped in a circumferential fashion by a series of single-toothed forceps and is circumcised using either the cold scalpel or the electrosurgical unit (Fig. 8.48). The single-toothed tenacula are replaced with Krobach mouse-toothed clamps (Fig. 8.49A). By sharp and blunt dissection both anterior and posterior cul-de-sacs are exposed (Fig. 8.49, B and C). The left paravesical space is entered, and the ureter is palpated (Fig.

Figure 8.47. The Schauta radical vaginal hysterectomy. A Schuchardt incision has been made and a gauze pack temporarily sewn into the incision. The vagina is being infiltrated by 0.5% lidocaine in 1:200,000 epinephrine solution. The *small crosses* mark the site of each needle penetration.

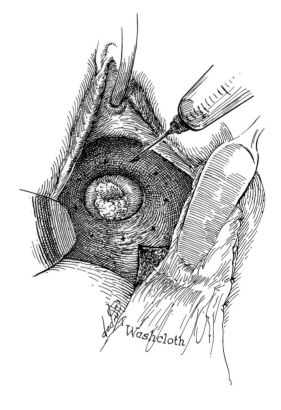

8.50) in the bladder pillar between fingers placed in the paravesical space and a finger inserted in the vesicovaginal space. As Högler (31) has pointed out, the larger any cystocele, the more lateral the location of the ureters.

The "bladder pillar" is incised along its lateral edge, superficial to the ureter (see Fig. 8.50), and the ureter is exposed. The left uterine artery is then skeletonized and ligated (Fig. 8.51). The right paravesical space is developed, followed by identification (Fig. 8.52) and

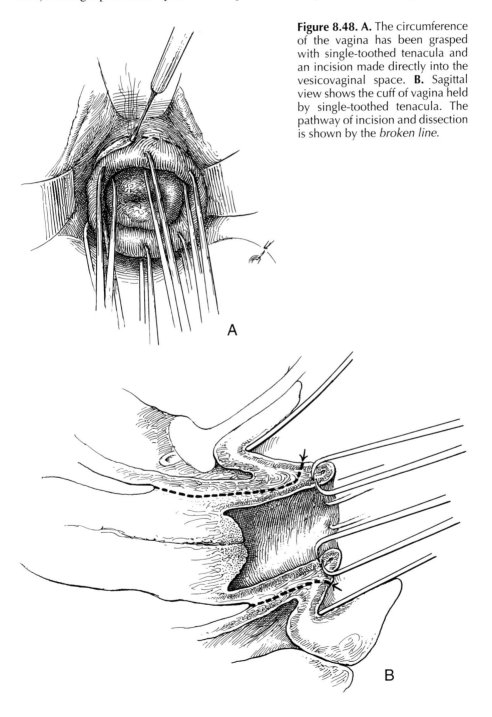

Figure 8.48. A. The circumference of the vagina has been grasped with single-toothed tenacula and an incision made directly into the vesicovaginal space. **B.** Sagittal view shows the cuff of vagina held by single-toothed tenacula. The pathway of incision and dissection is shown by the *broken line.*

A

B

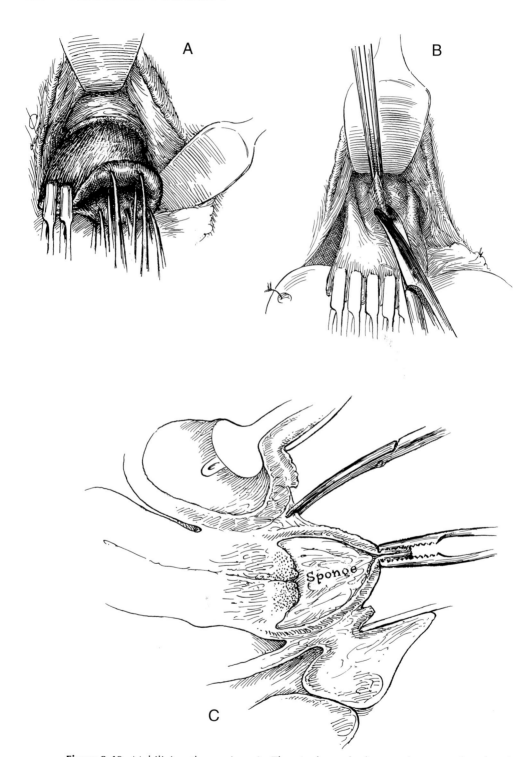

Figure 8.49. Mobilizing the vagina. **A.** The single-toothed tenacula are replaced with Krobach mouse-toothed forceps. **B.** The connective tissue septum between bladder and cervix is cut by sharp dissection. **C.** Sagittal view shows sharp dissection of the connective tissue beneath the bladder and cervix. The handles of the scissors are elevated, directing the incision away from the bladder. (*Continues on following page.*)

D

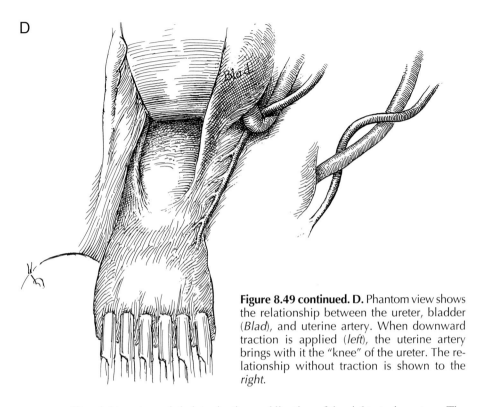

Figure 8.49 continued. D. Phantom view shows the relationship between the ureter, bladder (*Blad*), and uterine artery. When downward traction is applied (*left*), the uterine artery brings with it the "knee" of the ureter. The relationship without traction is shown to the *right*.

exposure of the right ureter and skeletonization and ligation of the right uterine artery. The bladder pillar is cut from the cardinal ligament at an appropriate spot. The cul-de-sac of Douglas is opened and the abdominal contents thoroughly and effectively displaced by an intraperitoneal pack. The peritoneum is carefully dissected from the medial side of the rectal pillar (Fig. 8.53), each rectal pillar is carefully cut from its attachment to the rectum, and each uterosacral ligament is divided. The anterior peritoneal cul-de-sac is opened, and appropriate retractors are inserted. Each cardinal ligament is clamped and cut close to the pelvic sidewall (Fig. 8.54), and the adnexa are examined and excised if necessary. Each broad and round ligament is clamped and cut, and the specimen is removed from the operative field. The peritoneum is closed, and the exposed undersurface of the bladder is reduced in size by raphing or gathering in a series of transversely placed interrupted mattress stitches, the lateral ones of which cover the ureter at the ureterovesical junction, burying this junction in a fold of the bladder wall. If a cystocele is present, the remainder of the anterior vaginal wall is incised in the midline to expose the urethrovesical junction. An anterior colporrhaphy with pubourethrovaginal ligament plication stitches (Chapter 10), with or without Kelly stitches (depending upon the presence of coincident urethral funneling), is performed, and packing is introduced into the pararectal-paravesical spaces on each side. To aid in the preservation of vaginal length postoperatively, the cut edge of the vagina at its new vault may be sewn to the peritoneum by a series of interrupted sutures distal to its closure. The Schuchardt incision is closed.

LAPAROSCOPY AND HYSTERECTOMY

"Never add the risk of laparoscopy to a surgical procedure unless the benefits of doing the procedure endoscopically outweigh the risks." Alan Johns

For the hysterectomy candidate in whom there is uncertainty about the condition of the adnexa, and adnexal or pelvic adhesions that might compromise the ability to safely

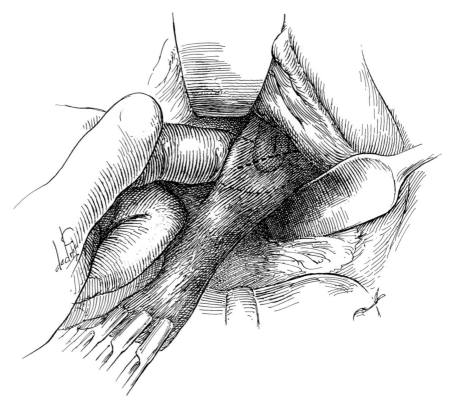

Figure 8.50. Palpation of the ureter. The paravesical and vesicovaginal spaces have been opened, and the ureter is palpated within the bladder pillar on the patient's left. An incision is made in the lateral margin of the bladder pillar along the side of the *broken line*.

perform vaginal hysterectomy, a preliminary diagnostic laparoscopy should clarify whether or not it is safe to perform vaginal hysterectomy with or without oophorectomy. This is a *diagnostic* contribution of *laparoscopy* to the planned hysterectomy surgery.

When troublesome adhesions have been identified before hysterectomy, they can be severed during preliminary laparoscopy and the adnexa freed or removed, thus making vaginal hysterectomy safely possible in this particular patient and permitting surgical attention to support of the vault postoperatively as well as to coincident repair of any other features of pelvic relaxation through the same transvaginal operative exposure. This, then, is *laparoscopic-assisted vaginal hysterectomy*. Portions of the hysterectomy may be added to that which is done laparoscopically (e.g., transection of the round ligaments or broad ligaments, preparation of the bladder flap) (55). On occasion it has been shown that the entire hysterectomy can be done through the laparoscope (66)—the so-called *laparoscopic hysterectomy*, though even then the specimen is usually removed by way of the vagina rather than by morcellation through the laparoscope.

A difficulty with a totally laparoscopic hysterectomy concept is that little or no provision is made for effectively reattaching the transected but damaged ligamentous supports of the uterus to the vagina to aid in vaginal support after hysterectomy. Now that it has been shown that total laparoscopic hysterectomy is possible in the hands of a very experienced laparoscopist, it must be proven that the method is as safe or safer than the traditional approach and that it is cost-effective (56).

Laparoscopically *assisted* vaginal hysterectomy, on the other hand, may increase the numbers of patients who can safely enjoy the reduced pain and shorter hospitalization afforded by vaginal hysterectomy in contrast to abdominal hysterectomy.

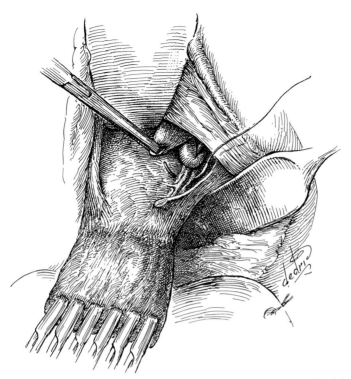

Figure 8.51. Exposure of the ureter. The left ureter has been exposed in the bladder pillar and the uterine artery skeletonized, preparatory to its ligation.

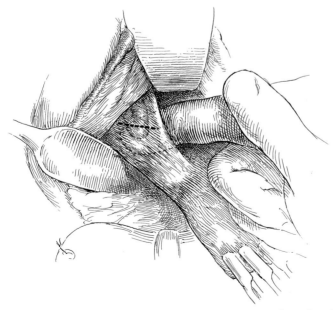

Figure 8.52. Palpation of the opposite ureter. The right ureter is palpated and the bladder pillar will be incised in its lateral margin as shown by the *broken line.*

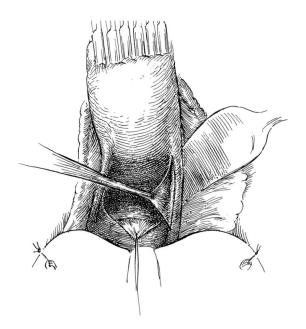

\Figure 8.53. Dissection of the rectal pillars. Both anterior and posterior cul-de-sacs have been opened. The peritoneum medial to the left rectal pillar is dissected free, in preparation for ligation of the pillar close to the rectum.

Laparoscopic-Assisted Vaginal Hysterectomy (LAVH) and Vaginal Hysterectomy Laparoscopically Assisted (VHLA)

If the uterus is movable and of less than 16 weeks gestational size, it can generally be removed transvaginally. It will be found in many such cases that the ovarian tissue can be removed transvaginally, saving the patient the additional discomfort and expense of coincident laparoscopy. But if the infundibulopelvic ligament is short, or the ovaries adherent to the pelvic sidewall, precluding safe transvaginal extirpation, they can be separated from the latter and retrieved by operative laparoscopy *following* the vaginal hysterectomy and closure of the peritoneal cavity (VHLA). When scheduled in surgery as VHLA the operative team will know that the vaginal hysterectomy is to be done *first* and that if a planned oophorectomy can be accomplished transvaginally, as is possible most of the time, the optional laparoscopy can be eliminated, saving operating time and expense as well as patient discomfort and extra equipment charges.

If the laparoscopic operator is experienced, LAVH will require a significantly shorter length of stay than a total abdominal hysterectomy (32). This can decrease the number of patients requiring laparotomy for hysterectomy, but at a much greater cost because of the instrumentation and increased operative time (26). The extra costs for disposable equipment (55) can be reduced dramatically and appreciably by the substitution of reusable for disposable laparoscopic instrumentation (13). Whether this increased cost will be offset by a shorter length of stay has yet to be proven.

Patient preference, which is often influenced by aggressive marketing, will generate pressure to obtain laparoscopic hysterectomy. Although, it has been suggested that the major contribution of LAVH may be to shorten the duration of hospitalization following transvaginal hysterectomy (13, 44), this remains to be proven, as length of stay has been progressively shortened following vaginal hysterectomy without repair (75).

Laparoscopic salpingo-oophorectomy may be combined with vaginal hysterectomy in treating women with advanced endometriosis provided that the operator has acquired advanced laparoscopic surgical skills (17), particularly when the surgeon is experienced in the use of bipolar coagulation (59) and either carbon dioxide laser or endoscopic scissors (46).

The surgeon should be experienced and comfortable with the techniques of vaginal hysterectomy, abdominal hysterectomy, and laparoscopic hysterectomy. The procedure

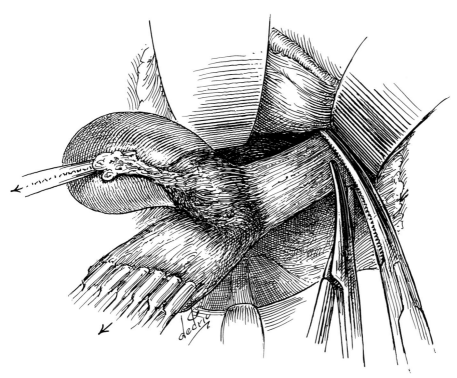

Figure 8.54. Transection of the parametrium close to the pelvic wall. The uterine fundus has been brought through the anterior peritoneal opening and the vaginal cuff and cervix drawn sharply down. The cardinal ligament (parametrium) has been clamped close to the pelvic sidewall and will be cut free, as shown, first on one side and then on the other. The peritoneum will then be approximated and the Schuchardt incision closed.

chosen for a particular patient will be that which best fits the patient's specific needs, and not the only procedure with which the operator is experienced and comfortable.

Boike (4, 5) has pointed out that in most cases transection of upper pedicles, complete freeing of the adnexa, and development of the vesicouterine space are sufficient to allow completion of a successful vaginal hysterectomy. The laparoscopic phase of the surgery should be individualized.

When there has been no coincident repair, most patients following VH, LAVH, or VHLA can be discharged within 24 hours of surgery. However, unless techniques are standardized and experience and credentialing for laparoscopic surgery become generally accepted, the cost of the procedure may outweigh its advantages (37).

Rock and Warshaw (70) note that the majority of laparoscopic techniques and procedures are being performed by surgeons in this country who have not been taught these skills in the controlled setting of a residency or fellowship training program. Pittaway, Takacs, and Bauguess (59) have emphasized that

there are many and perhaps too many courses on advanced laparoscopy, which should be viewed as the necessary first step fore many gynecologists, but a more important aspect of training should be the performance of the surgical technique under the supervision of an experienced advanced laparoscopic surgeon. Unfortunately, the latter requirement in attaining the necessary skills and experience is often not available.*

* From Pettaway DE, Takacs P, Bauguess P. Laparaoscopic adnexectomy. Am J Obstet Gynecol 1994;171:385–391. Used with permission.

Appel (2) has strongly recommended that we develop the new applications of laparoscopic surgery in the surgical laboratories using appropriate models, rather than solely in a clinical operating theater. He suggests that "the best available clinical research techniques should be employed to determine the superiority, or not, of a new laparoscopic procedure when compared to its traditional competition."

Laparoscopic Supracervical (Subtotal) Hysterectomy (LASH)

Donnez and Nisolle (18) have voiced their enthusiasm for laparoscopic supracervical hysterectomy (LASH) for the nonprolapsed uterus, particularly when the indication for hysterectomy is that of recurrent menometrorrhagia following failure of endometrial ablation. Donnez cites a reduced operative time when compared to LAVH, shorter postoperative stay and discomfort, and rapid recovery similar to that observed after laparoscopic surgery for infertility. Because the attachment of the cardinal-uterosacral ligament to the cervix is undisturbed, there should be no additional risk of subsequent eversion of the vaginal vault. The future long-term comparison with the experience of others who have used endometrial ablation as the primary treatment for refractory menometrorrhagia (recurrence rate estimated of 25 percent after 2-year follow-up) will determine the efficacy among the therapeutic options.

Complications of Laparoscopic Hysterectomy

Urinary tract injuries are a particular risk during laparoscopic-assisted hysterectomy (38). They include laser perforation of the urinary bladder, superficial epigastric artery perforation, subcutaneous emphysema, and anesthetic fluid overload regardless of urine output. Incisional herniation may be seen following the use of the large trocar. Periumbilical cellulitis and transient femoral and peroneal neuropathy may be seen. These occur even following subtotal laparoscopic hysterectomy (71).

Ureteral injury may be invited by the use of the endoscopic linear stapler during LAVH. This should be circumvented by the use of electrocautery for coagulation and dissection. Reich (64), noting that the ureter during laparoscopic surgery cannot be palpated as in transabdominal hysterectomy, believes that the ureter must be not only specifically identified during laparoscopic surgery, but often partly mobilized to make laparoscopic surgery safe, and Reich and Buchbinder have described in detail the laparoscopic techniques to identify the ureter (65). They note that ureteral stents are not protective because they frequently cannot be seen in the cardinal ligaments. To demonstrate bilateral ureteral patency, the surgeon can perform a cystoscopy at the end of the hysterectomy and following injection of some intravenous indigo carmine. Postoperatively, early recognition of insult to ureteral integrity is accomplished by obtaining a single-shot infusion intravenous pyelogram (IVP) on anyone reporting lateralized pain of any kind—abdominal, flank, or back.

References

1. Allen E. Discussion. Am J Obstet Gynecol 1951;61A(Suppl):219.
2. Appel MF. Whither laparoscopy? Int Surg 1994;79:376–377.
3. Bandler SW. Vaginal celiotomy. Philadelphia: WB Saunders, 1911.
4. Boike GM. Reply to Chapron et al. Am J Obstet Gynecol 1994;170:1210–1211.
5. Boike GM, Elfstrand EP, DelPriore G, et al. Laparoscopically assisted vaginal hysterectomy in a university hospital: report of 82 cases and comparison with abdominal and vaginal hysterectomy. Am J Obstet Gynecol 1993;168:1690–1701.
6. Candiani GB, Ferrari AG. Isterectomia vaginale. Milano: Masson, 1986.
7. Capen CV, Irwin H, Magrina J, Masterson BJ. Vaginal removal of the ovaries in association with vaginal hysterectomy. J Reprod Med 1983;28:589–591.
8. Carenza L. Attuali indicazioni alla colpoisterectomia allargata nel trattamento del cervico-carcinoma. Patol Clin Obstet Ginecol 1973;1:3–8.
9. Carenza L, Nobili F, Lukic A. The Schauta-Amreich radical vaginal hysterectomy. In: Nichols DH, ed. Gynecologic and obstetric surgery. St. Louis: Mosby-Year Book, 1993:386–403.

10. Carenza L, Villani C. Schauta radical vaginal hysterectomy. Clin Obstet Gynecol 1982;25:913–937.
11. Carlson KJ, Nichols DH, Schiff I. Indications for hysterectomy. N Eng J Med 1993;328:856–860.
12. Chandrasekhar Y, Heiner J, Osuamkpe C, Nagamani M. Insulin-like growth factor I and II binding in human myometrium and leiomyomas. Am J Obstet Gynecol 1992;166:64–69.
13. Chapron C, Dubuisson J-B, Aubert V. Laparoscopic surgery. It is not such an expensive procedure. Am J Obstet Gynecol 1994;170:1210.
14. Childers JM, Hatch KD, Tran Ai-N, Surwit EA. Laparoscopic para-aortic lymphadenectomy in gynecologic malignancies. Obstet Gynecol 1993;82:741–747.
15. Crisp WE. The Schauta operation. Obstet Gynecol 1969;33:453.
16. Dargent D, Arnould P. Percutaneous pelvic lymphadenectomy under laparoscopic guidance. In: Nichols DH, ed. Gynecologic and obstetric surgery. St. Louis: Mosby-Year Book, 1993:583–605.
17. Davis GD, Wolgamott G, Moon J. Laparoscopically assisted vaginal hysterectomy as definitive therapy for stages III and IV endometriosis. J Reprod Med 1993;38:577–581.
18. Donnez J, Nisolle M. Laparoscopic supracervical (subtotal) hysterectomy (LASH). J Gynecol Surg 1993;9:9194.
19. England GT, Randall HW, Graves WL. Impairment of tissue defenses by vasocontrictors in vaginal hysterectomies. Obstet Gynecol 1983;61:271–274.
20. Flaumenhaft R. Growth factors. Prim Care Update Ob/Gyn 1994;1:171–172.
21. Friedman AJ. Vaginal hemorrhage associated with degenerating submucous leiomyomata during leuprolide acetate treatment. Fertil Steril 1989;52:152–154.
22. Friedman AJ, Haas ST. Reply to letter of Fruchter. Am J Obstet Gynecol 1994;170:259.
23. Gitsch E, Palmrich AH. Gynecological operative anatomy. Berlin: Walter de Gruyter, 1977:9.
24. Gitsch G, Berger E, Tatra G. Trends in thirty years of vaginal hysterectomy. Surg Gynecol Obstet 1991;172:207–210.
25. Gray LA. Vaginal hysterectomy. 3rd ed. Springfield, IL: Charles C Thomas, 1983:36–41.
26. Harris MB, Olive DL. Changing hysterectomy patterns after introduction of laparoscopically assisted vaginal hysterectomy. Am J Obstet Gynecol 1994;171:340–344.
27. Hemsell DL, et al. Cephazolin for hysterectomy prophylaxis. Obstet Gynecol 1990;76:603–606.
28. Hemsell DL, et al. Single-dose cephalosporin for prevention of major pelvic infection after vaginal hysterectomy: cephazolin versus cefoxitan versus cefotaxime. Am J Obstet Gynecol 1987;156:1201–1205.
29. Hoffman MS. Transvaginal removal of ovaries with endoloop sutures at the time of vaginal hysterectomy. Am J Obstet Gynecol 1991;165:407–408.
30. Hoffman MS, DeCesare S, Kalter C. Abdominal hysterectomy versus transvaginal morcellation for the removal of enlarged uteri. Am J Obstet Gynecol 1994;171:309–315.
31. Högler H. Schauta-Amreich's radical vaginal operation of cancer of the cervix. Springfield, IL: Charles C Thomas, 1963.
32. Howard FM, Sanchez R. A comparison of laparoscopically assisted vaginal hysterectomy and abdominal hysterectomy. J Gynecol Surg 1993;9:83–89.
33. Howkins J. Synchronous combined abdomino-vaginal hysterocolpectomy for cancer of the cervix—a report of fifty patients. J Obstet Gynaecol Br Emp 1959;66:212–219.
34. Inmon WB. Pelvic relaxation and repair including prolapse of vagina following hysterectomy. South Med J 1963;56:577.
35. Janisch H, Palmrich AH, Pecherstorfer M. Selected urologic operations in gynecology. Berlin: Walter de Gruyter,1979:7.
36. Jaszczak SE, Evans TN. Vaginal morphology following hysterectomy. Int J Gynecol Obstet 1981; 19:41–51.
37. Johns DA. Laparoscopically assisted vaginal hysterectomy. The Female Patient 1994;19:46–58.
38. Kadar N, Lemmerling L. Urinary tract injuries during laparoscopically assisted hysterectomy: causes and prevention. Am J Obstet Gynecol 1994;170:47–48.
39. Käser O, Iklé FA, Hirsch HH. Atlas of gynecologic surgery. 2nd ed. New York: Thieme-Stratton, 1985:1220.
40. Kjerulff KH, Guzinski GM, Langenberg PW, et al. Hysterectomy: an examination of a common surgical procedure. J Wom Health 1992;1:141–147.
41. Kovac SR. Intramyometrial coring as an adjunct to vaginal hysterectomy. Obstet Gynecol 1986; 67:131–136.
42. Krige CF. Vaginal hysterectomy and genital prolapse repair. Johannesburg: Witwatersrand University Press, 1965.
43. Landau L, Landau T. The history and technique of the vaginal radical operation. Eastman BL, Giles AE, trans. New York: Wm. Wood, 1897.
44. Liu CY. Laparoscopic hysterectomy: a review of 72 cases. J Reprod Med 1993;37:351–354.
45. Malpas P. The choice of operation for genital prolapse. In: Meigs JV, Sturgis SH, eds. Progress in gynecology. New York: Grune & Stratton, 1957;3:671
46. Malpas P. Genital prolapse. In: Claye A, Bourne A, eds. British obstetric and gynaecological practice. London: William Heinemann, 1963:655.
47. Massi GB. Alcune riflessioni in tema de radicalita nella churgia vaginale. Riv Ostet Ginecol 1992;4–5:123–129.

48. Massi G, Savino L, Susini T. Reply to letter of Than. Am J Obstet Gynecol 1994;171:287–288.
49. Massi G, Savino L, Susini T. Schauta-Amreich vaginal hysterectomy and Wertheim-Meigs abdominal hysterectomy in the treatment of cervical cancer: a retrospective analysis. Am J Obstet Gynecol 1993;168:928–934.
50. Mattingly RF, Huang WY. Steroidogenesis of the menopausal and postmenopausal ovary. Am J Obstet Gynecol 1969;103:679–693.
51. McCall ML: Posterior culdeplasty: surgical correction of enterocele during vaginal hysterectomy: a preliminary report. Obstet Gynecol 1957;10:595.
52. McCoy MJ. Angina and myocardial infarction with use of leuprolide acetate. Am J Obstet Gynecol 1994;171:275–276.
53. Mitra S. Mitra operation for cancer of the cervix. Springfield, IL: Charles C Thomas, 1960.
54. Navratil E. Radical vaginal hysterectomy (Schauta-Amreich operation). Clin Obstet Gynecol 1965;8:676.
55. Nezhat F, Nezhat C, Gordon S, Wilkins E. Laparoscopic versus abdominal hysterectomy. J Reprod Med 1992;37:247–249.
56. Nichols DH. Vaginal hysterectomy. In Nichols DH, ed. Gynecologic and obstetric surgery. St. Louis: Mosby-Year Book, 1963:297–333.
57. Novak F. Surgical gynecologic techniques. New York: Wiley, 1978.
58. Philipp K. Ergebnisse der routinemassbigen entfernung der Ovarien und/oder Tuben im Rahmen der vaginalen Hysterektomie. Geburtshilfe Frauenheikd 1980;40:159.
59. Pittaway DE, Takacs P, Bauguess P. Laparoscopic adnexectomy. Am J Obstet Gynecol 1994;171:385–391.
60. Powers TW, Goodno JA Jr, Harris VD. The outpatient vaginal hysterectomy. Am J Obstet Gynecol 1993;168:1875–1880.
61. Pratt JH. Technique of vaginal hysterectomy. Clin Obstet Gynecol 1959;2:1125.
62. Pratt JH, Daikoku NH. Obesity and vaginal hysterectomy. J Reprod Med 1990;35:945–949.
63. Randall CL. The risks of gynecologic malignancies in older women. Clin Obstet Gynecol 1964;7:545–557.
64. Reich H. Laparoscopic electrosurgical oophorectomy: risk of using "blanching" as the end point. Am J Obstet Gynecol 1992;167:1150–1151.
65. Reich H, Buchbinder SE. Laparoscopic hysterectomy—ureter transected. In: Nichols DH, DeLancey JOL, eds. Clinical problems, complications and sequelae of gynecologic and obstetric surgery. 3rd ed. Baltimore: Williams & Wilkins, 1995:111–116.
66. Reich H, DeCaprio J, McGlynn F. Laparoscopic hysterectomy. J Gynecol Surg 1989;5:213–216.
67. Reiffenstuhl G, Platzer W. Atlas of vaginal surgery. Philadelphia: WB Saunders, 1975.
68. Rein MS, Friedman AJ, Stuart JM, MacLaughlin DT. Fibroid and myometrial steroid receptors in women treated with gonadotropin-releasing hormone agonist leuprolide acetate. Fertil Steril 1990;53:1018–1023.
69. Robinson RW, Cohen WD, Higano N. Estrogen replacement therapy in women with coronary atherosclerosis. Ann Intern Med 1958;48:95–101.
70. Rock JA, Warshaw JR. The history and future of operative laparoscopy. Am J Obstet Gynecol 1994;170:7–11.
71. Schwartz RO. Complications of laparoscopic hysterectomy. Obstet Gynecol 1993;81:1022–1024.
72. Sheth SS. The place of oophorectomy at vaginal hysterectomy. Br J Obstet Gynaecol 1991;98:662–666.
73. Shull BL, Capen CV, Riggs MW, Kuehl TJ. Preoperative and postoperative analysis of site-specific pelvic support defects in 81 women treated with sacrospinous ligament suspension and pelvic reconstruction. Am J Obstet Gynecol 1992;166:1764–1771.
74. Speroff T, Dawson NV, Speroff L, Haber RJ. A risk-benefit analysis of elective bilateral oophorectomy: effect of changes in compliance with estrogen therapy on outcome. Am J Obstet Gynecol 1991;164:165–174.
75. Stovall TG, Summit RL, Bran DF, Ling FW. Outpatient vaginal hysterectomy: a pilot study. Obstet Gynecol 1992;80:145–149.
76. Stovall TG, Summit RL, Washburn SA, Ling FW. Gonadotropin-releasing hormone agonist use before hysterectomy. Am J Obstet Gynecol 1994;170:1744–1751.
77. Thompson JD, Lyon JB. Vaginal hysterectomy. Clin Obstet Gynecol 1964;9:1033.
78. Vidakovic S. The vagino-abdominal approach to the extended operation. Arch Gynakol 1955;186:420.
79. Vollenhoven BJ, Herington AC, Healy DL. Messenger ribonucleic acid expression of the insulin-like growth factors and their binding proteins in uterine fibroids and myometrium. J Clin Endo Met 1993;76:1106–1110.
80. Welch JS, Randall LM. Vaginal hysterectomy at the Mayo Clinic. Obstet Gynecol 1961;4:199–209.
81. Werner P, Sederl J. Abdominal operations by the vaginal route. Philadelphia: JB Lippincott, 1958.

CHAPTER 9

The Manchester Operation

Occasionally, a symptomatic genital prolapse patient will wish, for any one of various reasons, to retain her uterus. The transabdominal cervicosacropexy or transvaginal sacrospinous fixation described in Chapter 16 may satisfy her needs, but when a major component of the prolapse is cystocele accompanied by marked elongation of the cervix, another surgical choice may be the Manchester (Donald-Fothergill) operation (1, 2, 5, 7–9, 11–13). This procedure was developed long ago in northern England at the site of the wool-processing industry to treat the severe genital prolapses that developed in young working women as a consequence of the heavy lifting that their jobs required.

When there is cystocele, the cervix is elongated and strong cardinal uterosacral ligament support is evident. The Manchester operation, consisting of cervical amputation with mobilization and attachment of the cardinal ligaments anterior to the cervix, followed by appropriate colporrhaphy, will support the vagina (see Chapter 6). One must be mindful, however, that a dropped uterus is the *result* of a genital prolapse and not the cause. The primary corrective attention must be given to remedy the defective or compromised supports of the pelvic organs.

This approach is not as popular in the United States as is vaginal hysterectomy because unwelcome uterine bleeding may occur subsequently and sometimes follows postmenopausal estrogen supplementation. There are also some additional potential difficulties concerning the Manchester operation with which the surgeon must be prepared to contend. If the cardinal-uterosacral ligament complex is of unusually poor quality, it may be inadequate to support the vaginal vault postoperatively. If there is no significant elongation of the cervix, amputation of a normal-sized cervix as a means of mobilizing the cardinal-uterosacral ligaments may disturb the integrity of the internal cervical os, causing the risk of postoperative cervical incompetence. The diminished size or caliber of the vagina following colporrhaphy may interfere with vaginal dilatation during subsequent labor and delivery. This may damage the vaginal repair, which by virtue of the scarring already present from the colporrhaphy will make future re-repair more difficult. Post-Manchester cervical stenosis may lead to mechanical dysmenorrhea and to secondary infertility.

All things considered, the Manchester operation is still a worthy one for the patient who wishes to retain the uterine corpus, but the surgeon who chooses to perform it should be equally adept at vaginal hysterectomy, should the operative change be found necessary during the course of the procedure. Coincident enterocele is often present and should be sought; if found, it should be corrected to lessen the risk of future progression or recurrence of the prolapse.

The technique for the Manchester operation is illustrated and described in Figure 9.1.

TRACHELECTOMY

The cervix remaining after a subtotal or supracervical hysterectomy will occasionally require surgical removal, or trachelectomy. Most frequently this will be required as

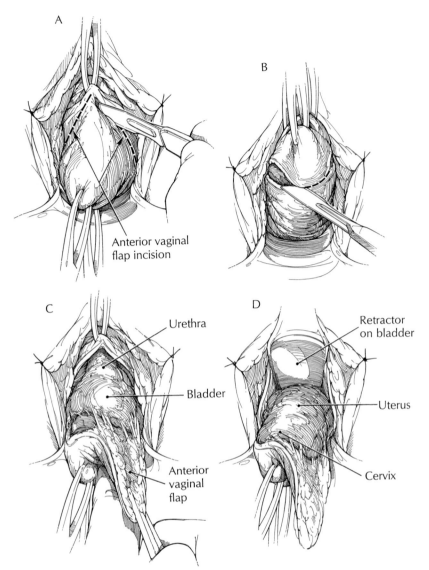

A

Anterior vaginal flap incision

B

C

Urethra

Bladder

Anterior vaginal flap

D

Retractor on bladder

Uterus

Cervix

Figure 9.1. Manchester repair involving an elongated cervix as part of the uterine prolapse and a good-sized cystocele. **A.** The cervix is grasped by tenacula such as Jacobs clamps, and the anterior vaginal wall is picked up with forceps. An inverted V-shaped incision is made through the vaginal wall (*dashed line*). **B.** The cervix is pulled anteriorly and the initial incision continued posteriorly (*dashed line*) until it meets the point at which the incision began. **C.** Downward traction is applied to the entire thickness of the anterior vaginal wall flap, which is dissected from the underlying urethra and bladder. **D.** The bladder may be detached from the uterus by sharp dissection and held out of harm's way by a retractor. **E.** The sidewalls of the vagina are pushed back from the underlying cervix by partly opened scissors to expose the uterosacral ligaments and peritoneum of the cul-de-sac. **F and G.** If an enterocele was present, the cul-de-sac peritoneum is opened (F), the enterocele excised, the peritoneum closed, and the uterosacral ligaments plicated in the midline (G). **H and I.** If the cervix is very long, the uterosacral ligaments can be transected as shown in H and plicated, taking a bite of the underlying posterior wall of the upper portion of the cervix (I). **J.** While traction to the cervix continues, the cardinal ligaments are transected and the hemostats replaced by transfixion ligatures, which are held and not cut. **K.** The elongated cervix is amputated distal to the internal cervical os. **L.** The anterior vaginal wall and cardinal ligaments are fixed to the anterior portion of the cervix by a Fothergill stitch of polyglycolic acid suture. **M.** When this has been tied, the effect is to unite and fix the ligaments in front of the cervix. **N.** Anterior and posterior Sturmdorf stitches are placed over the cervical stump. **O.** The vaginal wall defects in the 3 and 9 o'clock positions overlying the cervix are now brought together with two interrupted stitches. **P.** The anterior vaginal wall is closed from side to side. The shortened cardinal ligaments thus elevate the lower portion of the uterus to which they have been sewn. After the anterior vaginal wall has been closed, a perineorrhaphy and posterior colporrhaphy are performed to repair any demonstrable weakness. (*Continues on pp. 215–217.*)

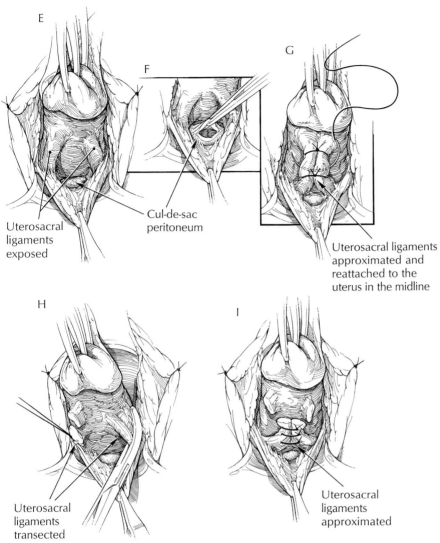

E

F

G

Uterosacral
ligaments
exposed

Cul-de-sac
peritoneum

Uterosacral ligaments
approximated and
reattached to the
uterus in the midline

H

I

Uterosacral
ligaments
transected

Uterosacral
ligaments
approximated

Figure 9.1, E to I continued.

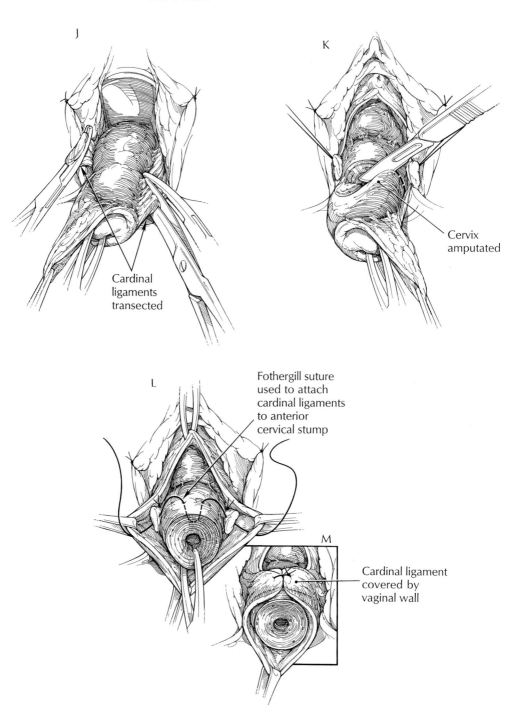

Figure 9.1, J to **M**.

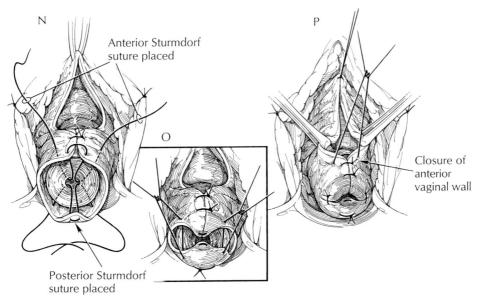

Figure 9.1, N to P.

part of the reparative surgery to relieve a symptomatic prolapse, and because cystocele and rectocele usually coexist, a coincident anterior and posterior colporrhaphy are performed.

Occasionally, the remaining cervix will be the site of severe dysplasia or intraepithelial neoplasia, for which trachelectomy would be an appropriate remedy—with or without coincident colporrhaphy, depending on the presence of cystocele and rectocele. Trachelectomy is most easily accomplished by the transvaginal approach, but there is little indication for "prophylactic" removal of the retained cytologically and anatomically "normal" cervix (10). In any patient with a retained cervix it is most important that it be evaluated regularly, with cytologic study and colposcopy as necessary, since any cervix may harbor future neoplasia.

Ikedife (6) reported a high incidence of primary infertility in women with a long (4- to 6.5-cm) cervix in the absence of uterine or vault prolapse with no other explanation for their lack of fertility.

References

1. Bonney V. An address on genital displacements. Br Med J 1928;431–433.
2. Fothergill WE. Anterior colporrhaphy and amputation of the cervix combined as a single operation for use in the treatment of genital prolapse. Am J Surg 1915;29:161.
3. Fothergill WE. The end results of vaginal operations for genital prolapse. J Obstet Gynaecol Br Emp 1921;28:251.
4. Fothergill WE. A further modification of anterior colporrhaphy combined with amputation of the cervix. J Obstet Gynaecol Br Emp 26:29, 1914.
5. Fothergill WE. Operative treatment of procidentia. J Obstet Gynaecol Br Emp 1911;20:44.
6. Ikedife D. Long vaginal cervix: a clinical entity. J Obstet Gynaecol 1990;10:333–334.
7. Hunter JWA. Conservation of the cervix uteri in operations for prolapse. Br Med J 1939;2:991.
8. Johnston HW. The treatment of uterine prolapse. Surg Gynecol Obstet 1939;69:809–815.
9. Nichols DH, ed. Gynecologic and obstetric surgery. St. Louis: Mosby-Yearbook, 1993;320–322.
10. Pasley WW, Leigh RW. Trachelectomy: a review of fifty-five cases. Am J Obstet Gynecol 1988;159:728–732.
11. Phaneuf LE. Manchester operation of colporrhaphy in the treatment of uterine prolapse. Am J Surg 1951;82:156–162.
12. Shaw WF. Plastic vaginal surgery. In: Kerr JMM, Johnstone RW, Phillips MH, eds. Historical review of British obstetrics and gynecology. Edinburgh: Livingstone, 1954:372–376.
13. Shaw WF. The treatment of prolapsus uteri, with special reference to the Manchester operation of colporrhaphy. Am J Obstet Gynecol 1933;26:667.

CHAPTER 10

Anterior Colporrhaphy

Cystocele is primarily a consequence of damage to the vagina—either its supports or the vaginal wall itself. Bladder damage is secondary to the vaginal defect. The primary site for reconstructive surgery must therefore be directed to the vagina and its supports.

The urethra is maintained in position by two independent anatomic systems that include suspension by the pubourethrovaginal ligament portion of the urogenital diaphragm and support from below by the vaginal wall and its attachments (see Chapter 1). Damage to either or both systems may alter its pelvic location and affect its function.

The bladder itself, on the other hand, is not effectively suspended but is intact, supported by the vagina and its attachments. The supports of the bladder causing cystocele are affected by damage to the vaginal wall itself, to the connective tissue to which the vagina is attached, or both.

When symptoms suggest a surgical remedy, it is the responsibility of the reconstructive surgeon to determine the specific sites and causes of damage for each patient in determining a course of surgical action.

In preoperative patients, evaluation of the presence or absence of urinary stress incontinence generally means damage to the anterior genital segment. Inasmuch as various types of incontinence are often mixed, it is important to determine which particular components apply to a particular patient—whether the problem is primarily one of stress, overflow, urge incontinence, or a combination of these etiologic factors. A proper diagnosis is required for the identification and selection of an appropriate surgical remedy.

TYPES AND ETIOLOGY OF CYSTOCELE

In examining and evaluating the anterior wall (Fig. 10.1), the observer should have in mind that there are distinct types of cystocele that may be present. Cystocele has been described according to whether it is anterior to the interureteric ridge (anterior cystocele) or posterior to it (posterior cystocele) (2). Either or both conditions may exist and must be recognized and corrected if surgery is to be effective.

First, there may be only an anterior cystocele (pseudocystocele or "urethrocele"), in which situation a straining effort results in downward bulging or rotational descent of the urethra with or without a demonstrable tendency of the bladder to herniate behind the vesicourethral junction. The lower third of the anterior vaginal wall underlies the urethra with hypermobility. The urethra may separate from the urogenital diaphragm and the pubourethrovaginal ligament portion of the urogenital diaphragm that binds it to the pubis, or separation of the vaginal sulci from their intermediate connective tissue attachment to the arcus tendineus may permit rotational descent of the urethra with or without actual herniation of the bladder behind the vesicourethral junction. The rotational descent of the vesicourethral junction may be of varying degrees and is often associated with urinary stress incontinence.

With anterior cystocele (pseudocystocele or pseudourethrocele), the diameter of the urethra is unchanged (Fig. 10.2) except at its proximal end, where it may be increased if funneling or vesicalization of the urethra is present (Fig. 10.3). Pathologic dilatation of

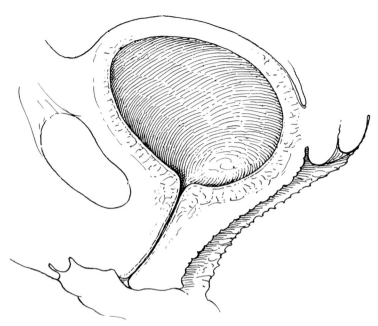

Figure 10.1. Sagittal view of normal vesicourethral relationships. Filling of the normally supported bladder has little or no effect upon the contour of its base.

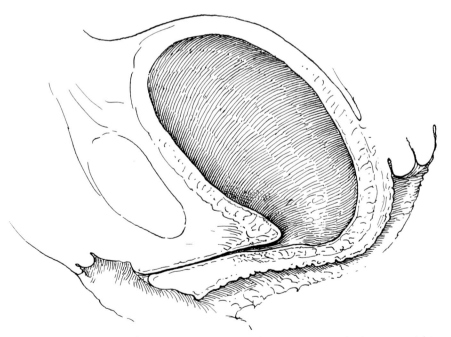

Figure 10.2. Rotational descent of the vesicourethral junction. Note the loss or straightening of the posterior urethrovesical angle.

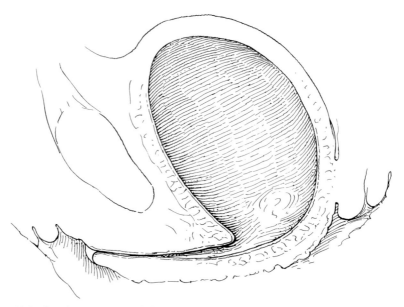

Figure 10.3. Coexistent rotational descent of the vesicourethral junction and funneling of the urethra.

the midportion or distal urethra (true urethrocele) (Fig. 10.4) is quite uncommon, but it could result from pathologic stretching from within the urethra, occasionally digital or manipulative, or rarely from a preexisting infected urethral diverticulum that may increase the urethral caliber after necrosis of its internal wall. A *routine* full-length plication of the normal, undilated urethral wall itself may be followed by later stricture and "postmenopausal stenosis," providing an iatrogenic obstructive uropathy sometimes requiring troublesome periodic urethral dilatation. If the urethra is pathologically dilated, a reduction of luminal diameter to normal can be achieved by placing interrupted mattress plication sutures in its muscular wall.

Distention Cystocele

A true cystocele (Fig. 10.5), almost without exception, is the result of an overstretching of the vaginal wall beyond its ability to involute postpartum, or the consequence of the atrophic changes of aging upon the intrinsic structural components of the vaginal wall with or without earlier damage. Posterior cystocele can coincide with anterior cystocele (Fig. 10.6).

This most common type of cystocele is a late result of an overstretching and subsequent eversion of the wall of the vagina. Rugal folds of the anterior vaginal epithelium are diminished and may disappear as the weakness within the vaginal wall allows the bladder to bulge into the vagina as a result of vaginal overdistention during parturition. The lateral attachments of the vagina and bladder may be relatively undamaged if during labor they are merely compressed against the sidewall of the pelvis as the vagina dilates. Almost without exception, true distention cystocele is the result of the attenuation of the anterior vaginal wall after overdistention of the vagina, possible during even "normal" vaginal delivery, especially in the older parturient. Usually, the cystocele does not become clinically evident until after the menopause. With the postmenopausal loss of estrogen-related elastic tissue and smooth muscle tone, inherently weakened connective tissue support results in increased relaxation and redundancy, with development of a symptomatic and clinically evident cystocele. In such instances the vaginal walls, espe-

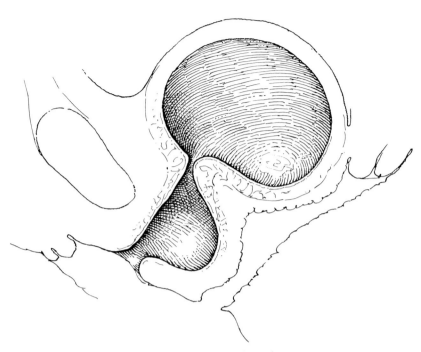

Figure 10.4. Pathologic dilation of the urethra (urethrocele).

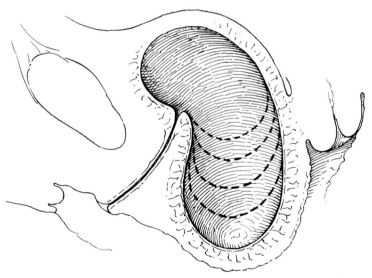

Figure 10.5. Varying degrees of posterior distention-type cystocele (*broken lines*).

cially the anterior and posterior ones, may remain pathologically thinned. Later, as a result of circulatory stasis and chronic hyperemia, they may become hypertrophic in appearance. A basic congenital defect may exist in the elastic tissue and smooth muscle components of some individuals. If surgery is indicated in a patient with greater than average postmenopausal atrophic changes, operation may be preceded and followed by estrogen replacement therapy directed toward reconstitution of the vascularity, elasticity, thickness, and cellular integrity of the vaginal wall.

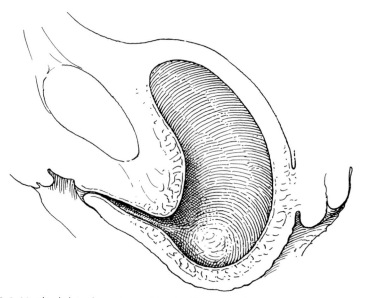

Figure 10.6. Urethral detachment coexistent with cystocele.

Displacement Cystocele

The second major type of cystocele, displacement cystocele, is the result of a primary and pathologic elongation of the lateral or "ligamentous" attachment and support of the vagina and is therefore etiologically quite different from the damage produced by simple overstretching of the connective tissues within a previously normal vaginal wall. Damage to the lateral vaginal supporting tissues may be the result of either of two mechanisms, depending upon whether the cervix was a major participant in the process.

Because the cervix is attached to the upper anterior vaginal wall, the tissues supporting both the vagina and cervix are component parts of the cardinal ligaments and tend to function as an anatomic unit. Displacement of one component is often followed by similar displacement of the other. This may be likened to eversion or prolapse of the upper vagina and may develop rapidly when it is the result of obstetric injury to the cardinal-uterosacral ligament complex, or it may occur more insidiously in older women as a result of long-standing increased intra-abdominal pressure, as with straining and pushing to move the bowel in the patient with chronic constipation.

When lateral support damage has occurred as a consequence of the forces of parturition, disruption of vaginal supporting tissue may have taken place when rapid descent of the presenting part resulted in an inadequately dilated segment of vagina becoming a soft tissue obstruction, slowing the descent of the presenting part until the segment gives way. Under such circumstances the supporting tissues attached to the rolled-up telescoping segment become overstretched and avulsed as the presenting part descends. Because this mechanism may not have damaged the integrity of the vaginal wall itself, eventual repair should shorten the lateral attachments of the vagina and cervix and reestablish the vaginal length. In its pure form this type of cystocele represents an eversion of the vagina with relatively well preserved rugal folds, but sulci disappear to some extent when there is coexistent paravaginal defect.

If one has determined that a cystocele should be repaired, it is essential to determine whether the vaginal vault is partially prolapsed, since this problem can, and generally should, be surgically corrected at the same operative procedure. Examination of the patient while standing and preoperative reexamination in the lithotomy position while under anesthesia (when the pelvic muscles are relaxed and pain is not present) will be confirmatory, and appropriate surgical steps can then be planned to restore vaginal length, for example, with sacrospinous colpopexy (see Chapter 16). One should think especially of coincident and etiologic vaginal vault descent when considering repair of a recurrent cystocele or one seen in a nullipara.

The third frequent type of cystocele results from a combination of the previously mentioned types. The importance of the damage caused by each component may be noticeable at different levels within the vaginal depth. It is essential that the gynecologist contemplating a repair take into consideration which mechanism, or combination of mechanisms, accounts for the pathology demonstrable in the individual patient.

In at least one-fourth of the instances of symptomatic genital prolapse, eversion of both upper and lower vagina coexists. Because the relative significance of these factors differs from patient to patient, the technique of repair must be based upon an appraisal of the relative importance of the etiologic factors that are recognized in each patient.

SYMPTOMS OF CYSTOCELE

Not only is cystocele often asymptomatic, but coincident, socially disabling urinary stress incontinence is infrequent. Feelings of pelvic pressure and "falling out" may be described and are often related to a coexistent uterine or vault prolapse. Descent of the uterus seems to annoy the patient to a degree proportionate to the time during which the condition has developed. Prolapse developing rather rapidly is likely to have come to the patient's immediate attention, resulting in an early request for reconstruction and relief, whereas slowly progressive descensus may have been accepted by the patient without comment or complaint. Consciousness of a mass protruding from the vagina may or may not be associated with a bearing-down sensation, but a sense of pelvic heaviness is usually noticeable after the patient has been standing for a time.

Stress Incontinence with Large Cystoceles

Patients with large cystoceles may have abnormal urinary function without symptoms. For this reason, full-length anterior colporrhaphy is preferred when colporrhaphy is considered necessary (18, 31). Careful and thorough repair of cystocele at the time of colporrhaphy is essential to prevent postoperative progression, often rapid, of an anterior wall defect. Large cystoceles can be associated with an absence of symptomatic stress incontinence, probably consequent to urethral kinking, but total vaginal eversion can be associated with virtually total urinary incontinence (21, 29). A poor urethral continence mechanism can often be protected by a large cystocele, which serves as a pressure-relief system acting to prevent leakage with stress. But unless the surgeon takes deliberate steps to specifically support the vesicourethral junction and to reduce any urethral funneling that may be present, a postoperative urinary incontinence may rapidly develop. When this is related to a low urethral closure pressure, it can be severe and socially disabling.

In some instances, the patient will have learned to employ manual elevation of a large cystocele to facilitate voiding. Surprisingly, only the largest of cystoceles are associated with a significant volume of residual urine. This is most often seen in the patient with a large dumbbell-shaped bladder, often evident with total procidentia. Coincident long-standing bacteriuria may be asymptomatic. This degree of bladder displacement not infrequently gives rise to a degree of persistent urinary stasis that favors both infection and stone formation. Presumptive chronic cystitis is not the inevitable result of supposedly "stagnant urine," a concept all too many observers have concluded without confirming studies. Often women with residual urine will complain that upon standing after apparently emptying their bladders, they quickly become aware of a different set of hydrodynamics than were present in the sitting position. Under such circumstances, although the standing woman has promptly experienced a desire to void again, upon sitting down again she finds that very little additional urine is forthcoming. When the bladder contains a significant volume of residual urine, some overflow incontinence may be seen.

Urinary stress incontinence is not a characteristic or even frequent experience of a majority of the women with cystocele unless there has been a coexistent rotational descent of the bladder neck. Urinary stress incontinence usually requires coincident and specific repair of coexistent damage to the supports of the bladder neck and urethra. A symptom-producing low urethral closure pressure may be demonstrated by urodynamic assessment, particularly in the postmenopausal patient.

ANTERIOR COLPORRHAPHY

Assessment and Objectives

Considering the indications for repair, a well-informed gynecologist will first correlate the anterior vaginal wall damage with the patient's symptoms. He or she must consider the patient's history and carefully check for evidence of coexistent enterocele or prolapse of the uterus, vaginal vault, enterocele, or rectum. Examination of the patient who is standing and bearing down will make this evident. It is also important to take into account a history of previous urinary stress incontinence that may have been relieved as the prolapse progressed, as emphasized by Symmonds and Jordan (45). The supports of the urethra, even though attenuated, may have more strength than those of the bladder because of their continuity with the urogenital diaphragm. Predictably, advanced progression of the bladder descent usually exceeds the accompanying urethral descent, resulting in an angulation or kinking of the urethra at its junction with the bladder. When a large cystocele is present, increases in intra-abdominal and intravesical pressure will be transmitted more to the dependent portion of the cystocele than to the attenuated vesicourethral junction. Hodgkinson (21) observed that within the bladder the hydrostatic pressure is always greater at the bottom of this column of water than midway up or at the top. This tendency, of course, is aggravated in the presence of a coexistent defect of the posterior vaginal wall that is reducing counterpressure. When there is no firm tissue layer beneath the sagging bladder, its elasticity when filling is relatively unrestrained by the absence of adequate posterior vaginal or perineal support.

Choice of Operation

The gynecologist must be mindful of the future functions and strains to which a particular patient's anterior vaginal wall may be subjected—not only coitus, but future pregnancy and parturition, and not infrequently coincident heavy physical work. All of these factors must be correlated with current findings that may themselves be partially the result of earlier attempts at surgical repair. In particular, allowances must also be made for the atrophic changes that have occurred or are to be expected after the patient's menopause.

Recurrent Cystocele

If a cystocele has recurred after an initial repair, the gynecologist contemplating another operation must first try to determine the reason for the unsatisfactory result after the earlier surgery. He or she should review the hospital surgical record of the previous operation and relate the earlier procedure with the current findings and then to the technique and suture choices now under consideration for this particular patient.

Recurrent cystocele may result from a previously undiagnosed vaginal vault eversion, clearly evident only when the patient is examined when she is standing and straining as by a Valsalva maneuver. Very often a postoperatively recurrent cystocele is in fact coincident with a partial eversion of the vaginal vault in which the passage of the vault downwards has brought the anterior vaginal wall and bladder with it, that is, a displacement cystocele. In this circumstance a primary goal of surgical treatment is to resupport the vault of the vagina by colpopexy usually with coloporrhaphy, which will help bring the bladder back into the pelvis.

Recurrent cystocele is the most common complication of colpopexy. Fortunately, the majority of these are asymptomatic, for, as expressed by the late Grandison Royston, "A bladder is as good as it works, not as bad as it looks." The persistent or recurrent effect is nonetheless disquieting to the observant surgeon, who might wish to adjust the technique of anterior colporrhaphy to prevent this development, mindful of the defects for which surgery is being performed, which may be either midline or lateral (paravaginal) or both. Each site of damage should be determined preoperatively and confirmed and remedied intraoperatively. These damages, especially the attenuation of paravaginal supports, differ predictably between patients with no vault eversion, those with partial eversion, and those with total eversion, the last-mentioned involving attenuation of *all* vaginal supportive tissues.

During the physical examination the gynecologist should check the position of the vaginal vault when the patient is standing and bearing down as by a Valsalva maneuver. This will disclose a coincident partial eversion of the vaginal vault, bringing the bladder with it.

When anterior sulci are absent, one should examine the patient for lateral detachment of the urethral paravaginal tissues. Baden and Walker (1) suggest that this can be suspected in a patient with relaxation of the anterior vaginal wall. When such a patient is instructed to tightly squeeze the pelvic muscles, a "holding" position, there is no response producing elevation of the anterior vaginal wall, suggesting that the connective tissue and vascular supports of the anterior vaginal wall have been detached from the arcus tendineus. The vagina is not attached directly to the arcus tendineus (9, 10, 12, 38, 48). The anterior vaginal sulcus is attached to the arcus tendineus by a bridge-like meshwork of intervening connective tissue (see Chapter 1) that may sustain various strains and stretching, or even unilateral or bilateral partial avulsion. This is usually a consequence of trauma from labor and delivery and is therefore seen more likely in parous patients. It may also be related to lifestyle and on occasion follow the pull of massive vaginal eversion, even in the nullipara. Therefore, direct surgical attachment of the vaginal sulcus to the arcus tendineus (12, 41, 54,)(BH Word Jr, HA Montgomery, Paravaginal fascial repair [motion picture], and personal communication) may compensate and to some extent correct the widening of the anterior vaginal wall as seen with certain types of cystocele. Bilateral attachment is generally necessary when stretching or avulsion of the lateral supports is the cause of cystocele, as suggested first by White (54). In our opinion, significant midline defects of the vaginal wall are much more common and will be remedied by the usual midline plications and colporrhaphy as described. Existence or coexistence of the less common lateral defects should be determined preoperatively for appropriate planning of surgical technique. It is essential to determine and surgically remedy any coincident prolapse of the vaginal vault that may be found. One should observe the presence and extent of rugae on the patient's anterior vaginal wall and compare them with those on the lateral vaginal walls. Rugae of comparable size in both sites suggest displacement cystocele, whereas diminished rugae on the anterior wall in the presence of good rugae on the lateral walls suggest distention cystocele. The surgeon must be certain to identify the etiology of recurrent cystocele as from displacement, overdistention, or a combination of the two, with demonstrable defects in either the midline supporting structures, the lateral supporting structures, or both, and note the relationship of the cystocele to the urethrovesical junction or urogenital diaphragm.

Usually, there is little but a surgeon's ego to warrant consideration of repeating the same operative technique. It is probable that the initial repair was technically correct but inappropriately selected. The well-informed and responsible gynecologic surgeon, acquainted with the significant modifications of dependable operative procedures, will choose the best operation for a particular patient's problem. If an adequate operative procedure is completed in a technically correct manner, the operator's knowledge and skill should be rewarded with significantly few instances of postoperative recurrence.

The gynecologic surgeon should ever be alert to the possible correlation between postmenopausal bladder urgency and the probability of an atrophic "urethritis and trigonitis." Postmenopausal atrophic changes result in a significant thinning of the epithelial and subepithelial layers of the urethra and the bladder trigone, with a resultant over-susceptibility to stimulation and irritation. When this can be demonstrated or is even suspected, the patient is likely to benefit at least symptomatically and promptly from adequate estrogen replacement therapy. When a positive response is obtained, further consideration of the need for surgical repair should be deferred for a month or two until the beneficial results and symptomatology have stabilized and can be reevaluated.

Postoperative Urinary Incontinence

Postoperative or recurrent urinary stress incontinence following transvaginal colporrhaphy with colpopexy may be related to a previously undiagnosed low-pressure urethra. Low urethral closure pressure is one of the causes of postoperative urinary incontinence (5). It may be present but unidentified, particularly in the postmenopausal patient, and especially the one who has not had a sophisticated preoperative urodynamic laboratory assessment and has massive eversion of the vagina. A simple method of suspecting this potential in the examining room or the operating room is that of inserting into the bladder a pediatric-sized Foley catheter (no. 8 or 10 with a 3-ml bulb) and partly inflating the bulb with only 0.5 ml of saline, and then applying gentle traction to the catheter to see whether the partly inflated bulb can be drawn easily through the urethra. If the catheter is drawn readily through the full length of the urethra, the latter should be tightened by appropriate plication until the partly inflated bulb can no longer be drawn through. If it can be easily drawn only into the proximal urethra, some pathologic funneling is present. This can be corrected by inserting some Kelly stitches at the vesical neck. Marking the catheter at 1-cm intervals from the bulb will provide a "ruler" to measure urethral length as well as the point of low urethral pressure.

When the urethral closure pressure is less than 10.0 ml of water, this may be remedied by inserting a vesicourethral sling (32, 36), which increases urethral resistance just at the moment during which stress is applied. For the patient without vesicourethral hypermobility, postoperative paraurethral collagen paste injections may help remedy this persistent and interesting problem. A long course of Kegel perineal resistive exercises is worthwhile in most patients (11, 24).

Urinary Incontinence in the Older Woman

Urinary incontinence is common among older women and burdensome. Not only is the condition socially disabling and often a principal factor leading to institutionalization, but also the overall annual cost in health dollars is staggering: estimated at more than 10 billion dollars per year. It is highly treatable and often curable. Resnick (39) has supplied a clear and useful overview of the problem, including its multifaceted medical origins and treatment. He describes the effects of frequently prescribed sedatives, antihypertensives, and cardiac medications upon the suppression of detrusor contractility causing urinary retention and overflow incontinence. He observes, further, that detrusor hyperactivity with impaired contractility is the most common cause of established urinary incontinence in frail, elderly women. Urinary stress incontinence is the second most common cause.

Urinary outlet obstruction may develop as a consequence of urethral kinking coincident with prolapse of the upper vagina, and when this eversion is relieved by repositioning of the vaginal vault in the examination room or by surgical colpopexy or colporrhaphy, an unsuspected latent incontinence may be readily evident.

TREATMENT

A thoughtful medical and surgical history, in addition to a thorough general physical examination, is essential to permit evaluation of all relevant diagnoses and their treatment. Urodynamic laboratory evaluation is desirable and, if available, certainly should precede any surgical reconstructive intervention. If vaginal atrophy is present, twice weekly, long-term doses of 1.0 g of intravaginal estrogen cream are prescribed. Prompted voiding can reduce the incidence of daytime incontinence as much as 50 percent. Anticholinergics may be prescribed when there is evidence of detrusor hyperactivity. Kegel perineal resistive exercises are prescribed with biofeedback or electrical stimulation as indicated along with appropriate behavioral therapy.

When intravaginal pessary use is acceptable, it may be given a trial, and if the effect is satisfactory it will often predict the benefits to be achieved by appropriate reconstructive surgery. Provided that there is no medical contraindication to anesthesia, older patients, including those who are frail, can regularly be brought through a safe surgical experience, for which they are exceedingly grateful.

Asymptomatic Cystocele

There is very little to be said in favor of operating upon an asymptomatic cystocele unless it is coincident with other symptomatic pelvic repair such as rectocele, enterocele, or vault eversion which is sufficiently symptomatic to require repair, in which case all sites of weakness including asymptomatic cystocele should be repaired at the same time, or unless the gynecologist has observed over a period of time an unmistakable evidence of progression in the demonstrable protrusion of the vagina through the vulvar orifice. Within limitations, the more advanced the progression of cystocele, the larger it becomes, the more complicated will be its repair, and the less certain will be the restoration of perfect bladder function, since there may be some permanent impairment of a properly balanced nerve supply. The desirability of appreciating a symptomatic progression is a primary advantage of having the same observer reexamine the patient over a period of years. The individual observer can detect evidence of progression to a degree indicating the need for operative repair and can make that recommendation before the patient's age precludes elective surgery because of increased medical risks. The examiner should record his or her impression of the size of the lesion in a manner permitting reliable comparison with the findings on subsequent reexaminations.

Appraisal of postmenopausal atrophy can often be determined by the degree of vaginal cornification demonstrable on cytologic examination. This index should at least roughly correlate with the persistence or absence of lateral wall rugal folds. If little cornification is present, an estrogen deficiency should be evident. The extent to which this is relevant should be estimated, and thought should be given to the desirability of estrogen replacement.

The gynecologic surgeon should be expected to know in detail the anatomy involved, the techniques of the recommended variations of anterior colporrhaphy, and the indications for possible modifications of one's usual techniques. Only with such information in mind will the operator maintain sufficient technical flexibility to accomplish the objectives recognized before surgery.

Once the gynecologist and patient have decided that the surgery is indicated, a primary objective is the restoration of normal anatomic relationships, with attention to contributing etiologic factors, all in a conscious effort to lessen the chances of recurrence in later years.

TECHNIQUES OF COLPORRHAPHY

Many operations designed to restore a defective posterior urethrovesical angle will elevate the proximal urethra to a position once again responsive to changes in intra-abdominal pressure. It is only when these surgical changes affect the proximal urethra as well as the bladder that a significant aid to continence will have been restored (22).

The techniques used for dissection and repair of the anterior vaginal wall depend on many factors, including the presence of vaginal telescoping or coexistent vault eversion. The patient with a short vagina due to telescoping must be considered a candidate for its surgical lengthening by such an appropriate coincident procedure as vaginal hysterectomy or a Manchester operation, by shortening of the cardinal or uterosacral supports, by a transvaginal sacrospinous colpopexy, or by transabdominal sacrocolpopexy. Restoring vaginal depth by bringing the vagina with bladder back into the pelvis is the essence of surgical treatment for the displacement type of cystocele. In procidentia, as defined by Ricci and Thom (40), the entire uterus is displaced and protrudes outside the pelvis. As a rule, the vagina is completely everted and an enterocele is present, but rectocele may be minimal or secondary. The displacement is greatest and most apparent in relation to the anterior vaginal wall and cervix, because the supporting vaginal and uterine portions of the cardinal ligaments have become markedly elongated and often attenuated. Because the anterior vaginal wall and cervix are attached by continuity to each other and to the pelvic sidewalls, they function as an anatomic unit. With massive prolapse, both suffer severe circulatory changes, not only as a result of stasis due to compression against the sides of the genital hiatus, but also from congestion aggravated by gravity. The resulting degree of chronic congestion apparently stimulates significant lymphangiectasia that, in turn, stimulates considerable fibroblastic proliferation within the anterior vaginal wall. Chronic edema is followed by hypertrophy and fibrosis that thicken the anterior vaginal wall. With advancing years these tissues elongate and "sag" noticeably because they are deficient and defective in other components, especially elastic tissue. The gynecologist will want to mobilize the full thickness of the anterior vaginal wall, including the epithelium and the underlying fibromuscular connective tissue layer, and can enter the desired plane most readily by opening directly into the vesico-vaginal space (44).

The gynecologic surgeon should enter the proper pelvic spaces by sharp dissection. Development of the spaces by blunt dissection is used safely only after they have been entered. If dissection has been initiated in the wrong plane, it takes longer to locate the correct plane than to have found it correctly the first time. This direct approach to the vesicovaginal space is equally useful when initiating anterior colporrhaphy when a cystocele is to be repaired without coincident hysterectomy or cervical amputation, or in a patient in whom there has been previous hysterectomy or cervical amputation. A useful technique was described by Ricci and Thom (40):

The anterior vaginal wall is placed on moderate tension by grasping each lip of the cervix with short tenacula and pulling the prolapsed vagina completely outward and downward. That part of the anterior vaginal wall above the point of fusion above the cervix is rolled or massaged between the index finger and thumb several times to accentuate planes of separation between bladder and cervix and vaginal wall. At the point where the fusion between the vaginal wall and the cervix ends and the avascular space begins, smooth and lacking in rugae, and usually about 3/4 inch above the orifice of the cervix, the reduplicated layers of the entire thickness of the vaginal wall are grasped between two Allis clamps. The full thickness of the vaginal wall is cut between these two instruments with a curved scissors, the tip of the scissors pointing perpendicular to the axis of the cervix, exposing an avascular space and bringing the bladder musculature into view [Fig. 10.7]. The cut surfaces of the vaginal wall are grasped with Allis clamps, and with a straight scissors the vaginal wall is cut upward exactly in midline. This incision is continued to the urethrovaginal junction where the cleavage plane ends. The bladder wall is displaced from both lateral flaps of the incised vaginal wall and cut from the cervix,

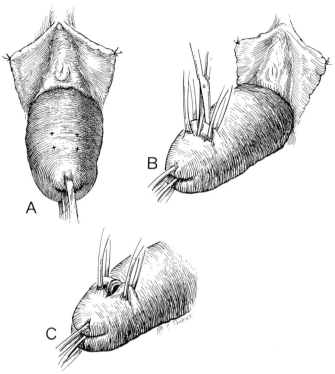

Figure 10.7. Opening the vesicovaginal space. **A.** Procidentia, with the points to be included within the grasp of the Allis clamps noted by *small crosses.* **B.** These points overlie the vesicovaginal space that separates the bladder from the thickened anterior vaginal wall, which is incised by the scissors placed perpendicular to its surface. **C.** The incision opens directly into the vesicovaginal space.

exposing the vesicouterine peritoneal fold, which may be incised, the index finger introduced, and the pelvis explored.*

Cystocele is commonly associated with a degree of uterine prolapse that is less than procidentia. A transurethral Foley catheter is inserted, and the bladder is emptied. Incision into the avascular space through the full thickness of the anterior vaginal wall may be accomplished alternately by an inverted T-shaped incision at the point where the vagina meets the cervix. The midpoint of the anterior vaginal cuff incision is grasped between two forceps and incised exactly in the midline and directly into the avascular vesicovaginal space. The incision is then carried superiorly to the point of fusion of urethra with vagina (Fig. 10.8).

If any resistance to the passage of the catheter is noted, a urethral stricture should be suspected. In such a circumstance one must be careful to avoid urethral plication at this point, making the stricture worse. In fact, one might well dilate such a urethra while the patient is still asleep in the operating room. If the patient is postmenopausal, postoperative vaginal estrogens may be of considerable help in reversing the effects of atrophy.

The remainder of the suburethral anterior vaginal wall is incised in the midline to within 1 or 1.5 cm of the external urethral meatus. The degree of bolstering of the vesicourethral junction will be determined by the extent of the earlier damage to the supports of the vesicourethral junction, the degree of attenuation, and the relative integrity of the tissue available for plication.

---

* From Ricci JV, Thom CH. Uterovaginal extirpation for procidentia. Am J Surg 1952;83:192–200. Used with permission.

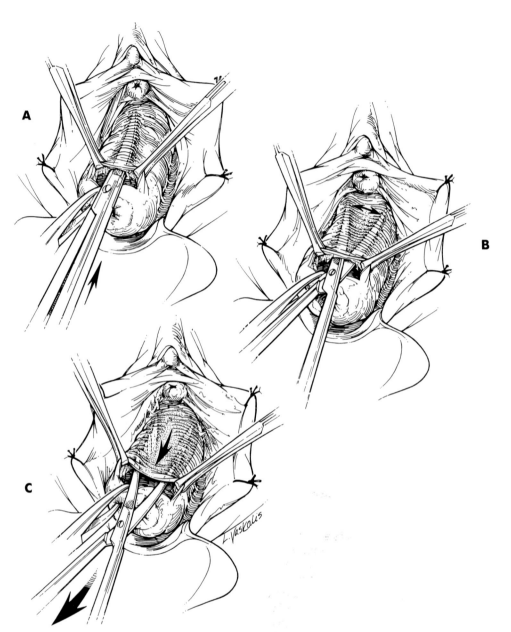

Figure 10.8. The Hilton maneuver in the use of scissors. **A.** To avoid cutting a viscus or unidentified blood vessel, the closed tip of the dissecting scissors may by used to establish a cleavage plane. **B.** Once the scissors have been inserted, the tips may be spread. **C.** The opened scissors are then withdrawn (*arrow*). Thus the connective tissue space is successfully widened without risk to the underlying viscus. (From Nichols DH. Gynecologic and obstetric surgery. St. Louis: Mosby-Year Book, 1993. Used with permission.)

In the performance of anterior colporrhaphy, the surgeon should reconstruct the *full length* of the anterior vaginal wall, including the vesicourethral junction and the supports of the urethra. This reconstruction will involve separating the urogenital diaphragm from the vagina and, after its plication, reattaching it to the vagina. This may be associated occasionally with some temporary postoperative difficulty in voiding. This is far preferable than an occasional iatrogenic urinary stress incontinence from having straightened out the neck of the bladder and obliterated the urethrovesical angle (Fig. 10.9). One must be mindful that the patient is being operated upon in the lithotomy position and under anesthesia. The different tissue relationships that will prevail when the postoperative patient is conscious and standing must be thoughtfully judged. (Vulnerability to urinary continence is greatest when the fully conscious patient is in the standing position.)

Surgical repair of a large hypotonic "decompensated" cystocele probably restores some intravesical pressure, lowering the incontinence. Surgical support of the vesicourethral junction should strengthen the anatomic and physiologic factors favoring postoperative continence. Restoration of vesical tone postoperatively may be a gradual process (39).

By sharp dissection, using either scissors or scalpel according to the preference of the operator, the full thickness of the anterior vaginal wall should be separated from the bladder laterally and anteriorly as far as the lateral limits of the vesicovaginal space, sometimes almost to the pubic rami, in a line of cleavage that preserves the attachment between the subepithelial fibromuscular connective tissue layer and the vaginal epithelium. As the dissection proceeds laterally, it is often possible to free up a possibly incomplete but identifiable musculoconnective tissue between the connective tissue left attached to the vaginal epithelium and independent of the predominantly musculature layer of the bladder wall. Hopefully, such lines of cleavage can be established without compromising the blood supply of these supporting tissues, but greatest care must be taken to open along tissue planes and not simply slice tissue into arbitrary layers at the expense of tissue planes that usually harbor blood supply (Fig. 10.10).

A simpler technique that does not dissect and thereby disturb the vaginal blood supply leaves the entire thickness of the vaginal wall unsplit and retains the attachment of all musculoconnective tissue to the vaginal epithelium. A most carefully measured ovoid or wedge of the redundant full thickness but thinned vaginal wall is excised (44). Unless the entire full thickness of the anterior vaginal wall has been correctly mobilized,

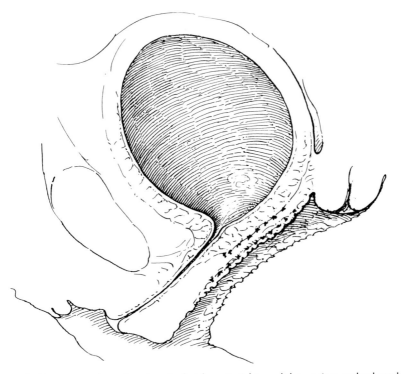

Figure 10.9. Overcorrection of cystocele that has straightened the vesicourethral angle.

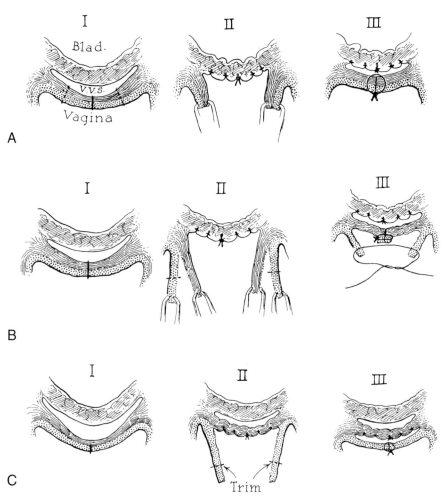

Figure 10.10. Three methods of anterior colporrhaphy. **A.I.** The attenuated anterior vaginal wall to be removed is shown between the *dotted lines.* **II.** The full thickness of this weakened segment has been excised and the fibromuscular bladder capsule has been plicated with some fine absorbable suture, reducing the width of the vesicovaginal space. **III.** The full thickness of the stronger portion of the anterior vaginal walls has been approximated by interrupted subcuticular sutures. **B.I.** A midline incision has been made through the full thickness of the anterior vaginal wall into the vesicovaginal space. **II.** The capsule of the bladder has been plicated, reducing the width of the vesicovaginal space, and the fibromuscular layer of the vagina has been gently dissected from the undersurface of the vaginal skin. **III.** Using a synthetic absorbable or nonabsorbable suture, all of this fibromuscular layer is plicated in the midline without resection. The superficial vaginal membrane is trimmed in the appropriate amount, as noted in II, and approximated from side to side with through-and-through or subcuticular sutures. **C.** Drawings depicting a frequent but rather ineffective colporrhaphy in which the vesicovaginal space is never entered. **I.** A superficial midline incision of the vaginal membrane is made. **II.** This is dissected from the underlying fibromuscular layer of the anterior vaginal wall, which is then plicated. **III.** Excess superficial vaginal membrane is trimmed as indicated and the sides approximated with interrupted through-and-through sutures.

an excision of the superficial epithelial layer alone could be as inadequate an operative procedure as to treat an inguinal hernia by simple excision of an ellipse of overlying skin without having surgically reduced the hernia, nor excised the sac, nor adequately repaired the underlying thinned tissues accounting for the defect.

In most instances the fibromuscular connective tissue capsule of the bladder itself should be narrowed by plication with a running locked 2-0 polydioxanone, polyglyco-nate, on polyglycolic acid-type suture that extends from the connective tissue of the uterosacral ligament at the vault of the vagina all the way to the urogenital diaphragm.

A most common error in the technique of anterior colporrhaphy is illustrated in Figure 10.10C: the vaginal epithelium has been separated from the fibromuscular layer of the vagina, but the vesicovaginal space has not been entered; the fibromuscular tissue is simply plicated in the midline. The vaginal epithelium is then trimmed and closed. This type of inadequate repair can be associated with a high incidence of recurrent cystocele or persistent stress incontinence.

The Gersuny "tobacco pouch" pursestring suture may be employed in reducing the bladder wall size of a very large cystocele (Fig. 10.11), but this stitch per se offers little intrinsic strength. It must, in all instances, be reinforced by a layer of side-to-side plica-tion stitches. If appropriate, reconstruction of the supporting tissues of the posterior vaginal wall is desirable.

Urethrovesical Junction

Recognition of a funneling of the vesical neck is a most important observation, since this development will physiologically shorten the urethra to a degree equal to the length-

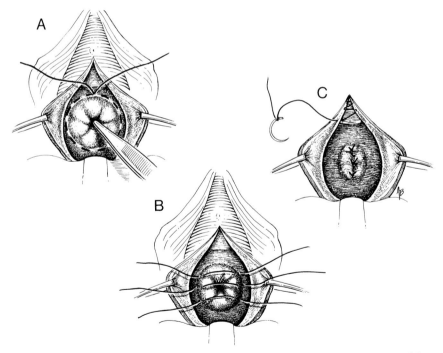

Figure 10.11. The "Gersuny" or tobacco pouch using absorbable suture. **A.** View of the su-ture. **B.** After it has been tied, it must be reinforced by several separate mattress stitches placed in the fibromuscular capsule of the bladder. **C.** A deep layer of sutures is placed on the underside of the anterior vaginal wall. These may be of synthetic absorbable or nonab-sorbable suture material. Excess vaginal wall is trimmed and closed from side to side using absorbable synthetic suture material.

ening of the physiologic bladder neck. In many instances, this effect displaces the physiologically effective vesicourethral junction to a more distal segment of the urethra, where it becomes further removed from and less responsive to changes in intra-abdominal pressure. When this physiologic junction is located below the inferior margin of the pubis, a disturbing tendency toward urinary stress incontinence exists. This should be expected because funneling of the vesical neck usually reflects damage to the supports of both bladder and urethra and contributes markedly toward a functional break in the "bladder base plate" of Hutch and Uhlenhuth (22, 46).

Although the work of Green (19) has called the attention of American gynecologists to both the posterior urethrovesical angle and the significance of urethral inclination, others have emphasized vesicourethral funneling as an anatomic defect that physiologically "shortens" the effective urethral length, thereby favoring the direct hydrostatic transmission of bladder pressure to the urine inside the funnel (Figs. 10.12 and 10.13).

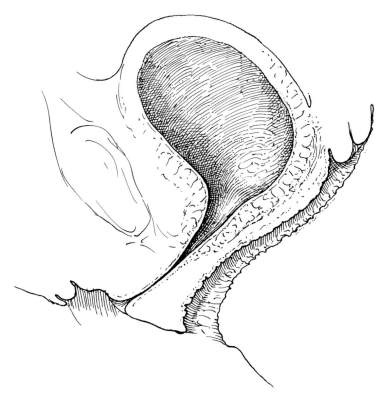

Figure 10.12. Sagittal view of funneling, or vesicalization, of the urethra.

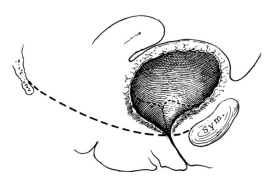

Figure 10.13. Sagittal view of vesicalization of the urethra demonstrating the descent of the "physiologic vesicourethral junction" from a normal level well within the area of response to changes in intra-abdominal pressure, to a lower level at or below the pelvic diaphragm (*lower dashed line*) and beyond the area of equal response with the bladder to changes in intra-abdominal pressure.

When such funneling is demonstrated, it should be corrected by insertion of an appropriate number of vertical mattress Kelly-type sutures, plicating the funnel so as to restore the segment to the normal tone and uniform configuration and caliber of the urethra. Kelly (25) stitches (Fig. 10.14) are subvesical urethral plication stitches that correct funneling and its associated stress incontinence, but they were originally introduced with the intent of strengthening a presumed internal urethral sphincter.

Although the Kelly plication of the vesical neck, designed to correct any funneling that may be present, has a high initial success rate for the relief of urinary stress incontinence, the long-term success rate of having used *only* these sutures falls from 90 to 60 percent over a period of time. This decline is possibly related to gradual postoperative elongation of the smooth muscle into which the sutures were placed (50). The long-term results are significantly better when coincident suburethral plication of the pubourethrovaginal ligaments of the urogenital diaphragm is accomplished, particularly in the patient with urethral hypermobility.

With massive cystocele some elongation of the bladder trigone should be expected, as well as some lateral displacement of the ureterovesical orifices. It is our belief that this condition disturbs the physiology of continence and may be remedied by inserting a U-shaped suture, as shown in Figure 10.15, which is intended not only to shorten the trigone but to narrow it as well. This condition was described by Van Duzen (47) and its remedy was suggested by Royston and Rose (42). It was described more recently by Van Rooyen and Liebenberg (49).

Our studies (30) of the connective tissue supports of the human urethra have convinced us that the urethra is normally suspended from or supported by the pubic bone by bilaterally symmetrical, anterior, posterior, and intermediate pubourethrovaginal ligaments (55, 57). These bands of muscle and connective tissue pass from the pubic bone to the urethra and not the bladder and are thus analogous to the puboprostatic ligaments in the male. Our study established continuity between these ligamentous supports and the urogenital diaphragm. (For further discussion of their histology and anatomy, refer to Chapter 1.) The posterior "ligament" elongates physiologically during the normal voiding process (Fig. 10.16). The important point in the woman is that a defect or injury

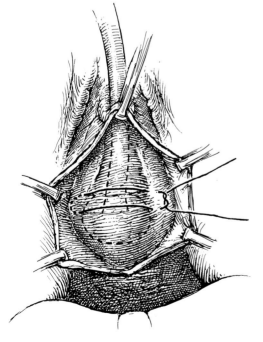

Figure 10.14. The original "Kelly" stitch that was introduced to plicate a presumed internal urethral sphincter.

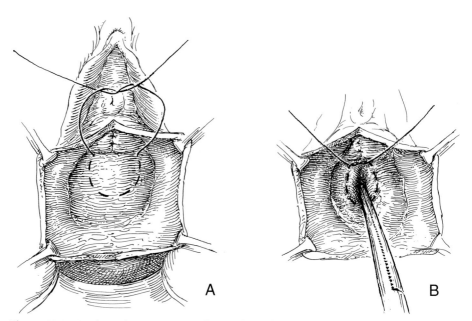

Figure 10.15. U-shaped suture to remedy a widened bladder tirgone. **A.** A U-shaped suture has been placed in the bladder muscularis. **B.** When tied, it will shorten the bladder trigone as well as plicate the vesicourethral junction.

resulting in a loosening or lengthening of the pubourethrovaginal ligaments contributes significantly to the occurrence and persistence of urinary stress incontinence.

We (37) have also demonstrated that the vaginal ends of the pubourethrovaginal ligament portion of the urogenital diaphragm can be identified transvaginally and plicated beneath the vesicourethral junction (Fig. 10.17). The technique we favor may be described as follows: The vagina is incised in the midline and then dissected laterally to the pubic rami, clearly exposing the tissues of the vesicourethral junction. The pubourethrovaginal ligaments can be recognized as paired tissue condensations or thickenings in the sheetlike tissue of the urogenital diaphragm. Because the tissue of these ligaments is continuous with that of the urogenital diaphragm, they are not discrete independent anatomic structures.

Palpation of the inflated bulb of the transurethral Foley catheter will demonstrate the vesicourethral junction; but, as Gardiner (17) has suggested, excess traction on the catheter may, in fact, draw the bulb of the Foley catheter into a pathologically widened and funneled urethra. Forceful catheter traction is not to be recommended. Avoiding traction on the catheter, we apply straight Kocher forceps to the periurethral tissue 1.5 to 2 cm on either side of its fusion to the urethra (Fig. 10.18), as recommended by Gainey (motion picture and personal communication) and Frank (13). After the ligamentous condensations have been identified, the ligaments are further shortened by obtaining a more lateral bite into an often thicker portion of the ligament. If the retropubic attachments of these ligaments are intact and the forceps have been properly placed, downward ventral traction toward the coccyx in the direction in which the fibers of the ligament run to the pubis will actually move the patient a small amount on the operating table. One can usually tell immediately by the degree of resistance to this pull whether there is sufficient ligament strength and length to provide for effective suburethral plication that will elevate the vesicourethral junction. The same procedure of verification and evaluation should be repeated on the opposite side, after which the tips of the forceps may be brought together in the midline without tension, an assuring demonstration that immediate and dramatic elevation of the urethra will result from such plication.

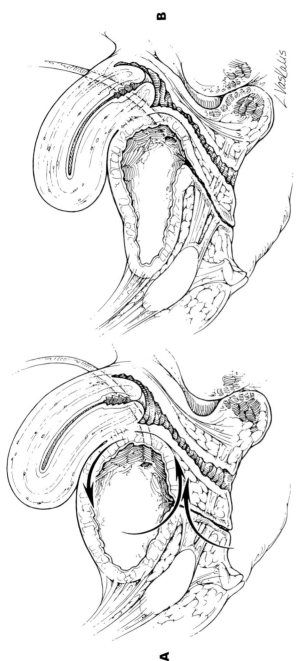

Figure 10.16. Elongation of the posterior "ligament" during the voiding process. **A.** "Wheeling" of the vesicourethral junction occurs physiologically during the normal voiding process to permit temporary flattening of the urethrovesical angle. **B.** When this "wheeling" is present in the patient who is not voiding, the anatomic relationship is pathologic and is conducive to the development of urinary stress incontinence. It can usually be remedied by plicating the pubourethrovaginal ligament portion of the urogenital diaphragm beneath the proximal urethra. Any funneling should be corrected by separate Kelly-type stitches. (From Nichols DH. Gynecologic and obstetric surgery. St. Louis: Mosby-Year Book, 1993. Used with permission.)

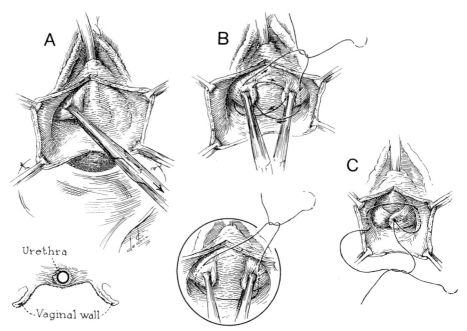

Figure 10.17. Pubourethrovaginal ligament plication. **Lower left.** The small drawing indicates a proper depth of urethral dissection, so as not to overly disturb the ureter's blood supply. **A.** The base of the bladder has been exposed through a midline incision and the paraurethral tissue of the urogenital diaphragm grasped in a Kocher forceps, with only one notch of the ratchet closed. **B.** Traction to the forceps will actually move the patient on the table. A polydioxanone or polyglycolic acid-type suture is passed through each end of the ligament. **Center circle.** An alternate method may be used when synthetic nonabsorbable sutures are applied. **C.** After the ligaments have been plicated, the same suture takes a bite of the vaginal wall, reestablishing fusion.

When a surgeon becomes experienced with the technique of plication of the urogenital diaphragm beneath the vesicourethral junction, as in the use of definitive, pubourethrovaginal ligament plication stitches (3, 4, 22, 37, 36)(HL Gainey, motion picture and personal communication), the long-term results of the transvaginal treatment of stress incontinence in the patient with a hypermobile urethra will be better when a long-lasting absorbable suture such as polydioxanone (PDS) or polyglyconate (Maxon) size 00 is used. If a nonabsorbable suture such as Teflon-coated dacron (Ethabond) or silk is used, the stitch and its knot must be buried beneath an additional layer or two of tissues that are approximated with absorbable suture.

TECHNIQUE OF PUBOURETHROVAGINAL LIGAMENT PLICATION

The size 00 mattress-type synthetic absorbable suture such as polydioxanone (PDS) is placed lateral and medial to the hemostats, as shown in Figures 10.17 to 10.20. With marked degrees of prolapse and with procidentia, we have consistently noted these ligaments to be very much elongated. These structures may at times be found quite far laterally. In most instances we have been able to elevate and satisfactorily support the vesicourethral junction to the desirable restored position behind the pubis. It is essential to effect this retropubic elevation to the most cranial position possible in order to restore relationships that will ensure that sudden increases in intra-abdominal pressure will register in the proximal urethra as well as in the bladder. It is particularly important to

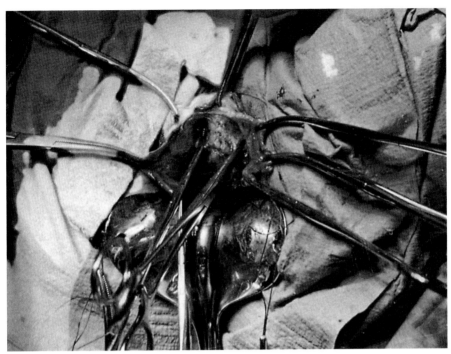

Figure 10.18. Kocher hemostats placed on the pubourethrovaginal ligament portion of the urogenital diaphragm lateral to the urethra.

shorten the pubourethrovaginal ligaments in the patient with massive prolapse, lest the patient suffer a postoperative iatrogenic urinary stress incontinence (45) that may be as distressing and disabling to her as was the prolapse for which she originally sought relief. Should the operator realize that he or she has not raised the vesicourethral junction cranial to the inferior border of the pubis by the essential sutures described, additional pubourethrovaginal ligament stitches should be placed *lateral* to the first until a proper degree of elevation has been achieved. The second stitch also buries and reduces the tension of the initial suture. The last of such buried stitches is *always* sewn to the undersurface of the adjacent vaginal wall, with an appropriate bite, to reestablish a normal site of fusion of the vagina to the urogenital diaphragm (see Fig. 10.17). For these reasons, we believe our periurethral stitches, because they are placed more laterally than urethral plication stitches, can be inserted directly into the urethral attachment of the pubourethrovaginal ligament portion of the urogenital diaphragm and will ensure an even greater degree of successful treatment. Such pubourethrovaginal sutures should always be placed *lateral* to the urethra and not in the urethral wall. After tying they should neither reduce urethral diameter nor produce subsequent stricture, which would be certain to become accentuated after the menopause (Fig. 10.21).

Because relaxation of the muscular component of the pubourethrovaginal ligaments and the urethral attachment to the levator ani (either muscular or fascial or both) is an integral part of the normal or physiologic voiding process, significant surgical plication of these ligaments beneath the vesicourethral junction may inhibit the normal voiding process until healing is well under way and spasm has been relieved. This event is not a function of urethral caliber. Because the extent to which this dropping of the vesicourethral junction can be restored after surgery is widely variable from patient to patient, some disturbance in the postsurgical voiding mechanism may be seen, and temporary inability to void is noted occasionally. Time is very much on the doctor's side, and if one's confidence in the ultimate success of the restorative procedure is shared with

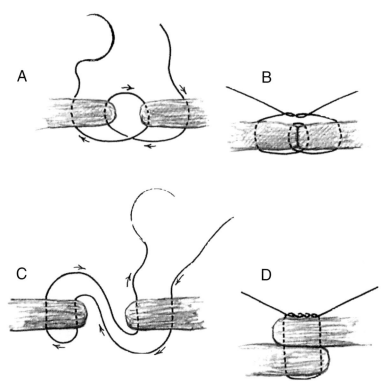

Figure 10.19. Path of ligament plication stiches. **A.** The path of the usual pubourethrovaginal ligament plication stitches is shown by the *arrows*. **B.** The effect of tying. **C.** When the "ligaments" are unusually long, their ends may be overlapped by sutures placed as shown. **D.** The effect after tying.

the patient, even a prolonged period of self-catheterization or catheter drainage can become bearable by both.

Temporary suprapubic cystostomy may be used to advantage in a patient who is considered unlikely to void after anterior colporrhaphy, such as the patient with unusual anxiety or the one with the very large hypotonic bladder. (Suprapubic cystostomy should be used regularly after repair of a fistula at the vesical neck.)

Kelly-type stitches intended to result in urethral plication may be placed deliberately *in* the wall of a pathologically dilated urethra and will indeed reduce the lumen of a dilated or funneled urethra. When Kelly-type plication stitches are placed in the periurethral supporting tissues, they may, in addition to correcting the funneling, unintentionally approximate the paraurethral portions of the posterior pubourethrovaginal ligaments. Pubourethrovaginal ligament sutures, on the other hand, being placed more laterally, are inserted directly into the urethral attachment of the posterior pubourethrovaginal ligament portion of the urogenital diaphragm, as noted by Halban (20) and Martius (28). This placement seems to explain our greater degree of success with this procedure.

Because the optimal place for the use of Kelly plication stitches is in the presence of funneling or vesicalization of the urethra and bladder neck, there are times when one might choose to use pubourethrovaginal plication stitches *and* Kelly plication stitches in a particular clinical situation, such as in rotational descent of the urethrovesical junction coexistent with urethral funneling. The merits of these techniques for each case must be decided individually.

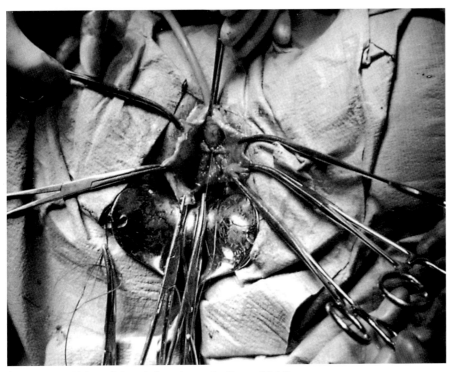

Figure 10.20. Tying of the stitches shown in Figure 10.19.

It is obvious there are other important factors contributing to urinary stress incontinence, including the effects of an attachment of the pubococcygeus to the lateral paraurethral and paravaginal connective tissues, as has been pointed out by Muellner (34). When there is insufficient paraurethral tissue strength demonstrable to indicate success with pubourethrovaginal ligament stitches, supplemental transvaginal methods of support should be considered. Such methods include the bulbocavernosus fat pad transplant where blood supply is needed (see Chapter 19), the pubococcygeus muscle transplant when a strong pubococcygeal muscle is present, or lateral paravaginal reattachment. These alternatives will be described later.

After placement of the pubourethrovaginal ligament sutures, the ends are tied and then held for sewing to the underside of the trimmed anterior vaginal wall later in the procedure. Additional paraurethral plication stitches can be placed in the tissue lateral to the midurethra to provide additional support by plication of attenuated intermediate pubourethrovaginal ligaments without constriction of the urethral lumen, which could result if such stitches were placed directly into the wall of the urethra.

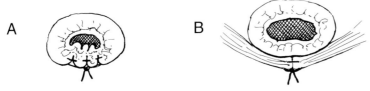

Figure 10.21. Suture plication of the vesicourethral junction. **A.** Suture plication directly into the urethral wall will narrow the urethral lumen. When this has not been a goal of surgery, a urethral stricture may be produced. **B.** By contrast, pubourethrovaginal "ligament" plication may elevate and support the urethra but not permanently alter the size of the lumen. Occasionally both types of stitches will be used.

When the vesicourethral junction has been elevated to a spot cranial to the inferior margin of the pubis, any appreciable funneling of the bladder neck or urethra should be corrected by plication with interrupted sutures of 2-0 long-lasting synthetic absorbable sutures placed directly in the wall of the urethral funnel itself. These can be placed from side to side by the mattress-type suture of Kelly. The stitches of Royston and Rose (42) will shorten a pathologically elongated trigone. When stress incontinence is the sole problem, one may use a buried nonabsorbable suture to plicate the pubourethrovaginal ligaments, being meticulously careful that the suture does not penetrate the lumen of either urethra or bladder lest it form a nidus for future infection or stone.

As a first step in correcting cystocele, the operator may longitudinally plicate the whole length of the connective tissue capsule of the bladder by a series of running or interrupted 2-0 or 3-0 long-lasting synthetic absorbable sutures (Figs. 10.22 and 10.23). After it has been tied but before it is cut, the stitch that has plicated the connective tissue capsule and muscularis of the bladder is sewn to the subvaginal surface of the cardinal-uterosacral ligament complex and, if available, the cut edge of the posterior vaginal wall. This closes a potential space through which the bladder might herniate in the future (6, 26). If vaginal hysterectomy or enterocele closure has immediately preceded the anterior colporrhaphy, the uncut ends of the tied peritoneal closure stitch may be sewn to the upper cut edges of the anterior vaginal wall, effectively lengthening the anterior vaginal wall by pulling it in a cranial direction (see Chapter 8).

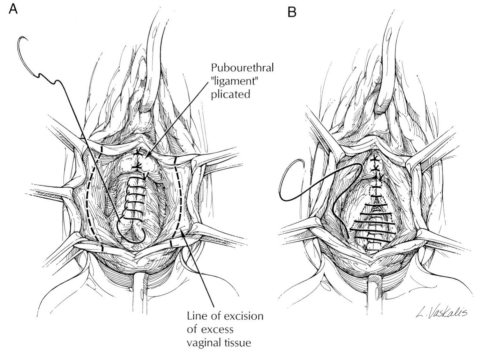

A

B

Pubourethral
"ligament"
plicated

Line of excision
of excess
vaginal tissue

L. Vaskalis

Figure 10.22. Plication of the bladder muscularis. **A.** The pubourethrovaginal ligament portion of the urogenital diaphragm has been plicated, elevating the vesicourethral junction as shown. Any funneling will already have been reduced by Kelly-type sutures. The fibromuscular capsule of the bladder of a patient with cystocele is reduced in width by a running locked, long-lasting synthetic suture placed as shown. Tension on the suture is such that the tissues are approximated but not strangulated. **B.** A second layer of running vertical mattress stitches may be placed as shown, with care taken to not flatten the posterior urethrovesical angle.

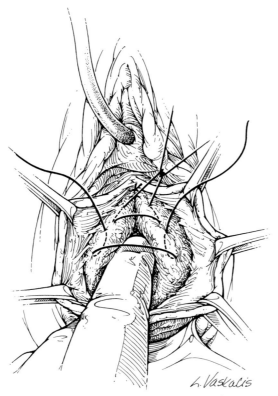

L. Vaskalis

Figure 10.23. Plication of the bladder capsule with interrupted mattress stitches. For the patient with larger cystocele, the operator's index finger depresses the bladder in the midline and the fibromuscular capsule of the bladder is reduced by one or more layers of interrupted long-lasting synthetic mattress sutures placed in a trapezoid configuration. A very large cystocele may receive preliminary reduction by a pursestring suture, the neck of which must be carefully supported by additional side-to-side stitches of absorbable suture material placed in the fibromuscular capsule of the bladder. (From Nichols DH. Gynecologic and obstetric surgery. St. Louis: Mosby-Year Book, 1993, Used with permission.)

When anterior colporrhaphy has been immediately preceded by vaginal hysterectomy, the residual inverted T-shaped flaps of the upper vagina should be carefully trimmed to an inverted V. In removing or trimming the vaginal flaps in a manner designed to provide a desirable contour for the vault of the vagina, one must remember that the greater the amount of anterior wall flap removed, the lesser the amount of posterior flap that can be removed. Otherwise the additional narrowing of the vault with high posterior colporrhaphy will result in a narrowed vagina, and dyspareunia may follow.

It is imperative that the operator judge carefully the amount of vagina to be excised with colporrhaphy to obviate an unexpected and unwanted postoperative or postmenopausal vaginal stenosis. Anterior colporrhaphy should be tailored to correct any coexistent rotational descent of the bladder neck, taking into consideration the possibility of either present or future urinary stress incontinence. One would emphasize again that, although all areas of weakness should be repaired and the supports of the bladder neck adequately reconstructed, it is essential that the operator not *overrepair* the cystocele by flattening the posterior urethrovesical angle, since the patient may be subjected to postoperative urinary stress incontinence (45).

The overenthusiastic or careless excision of too much anterior vaginal wall will simply narrow the vagina without appreciably improving incontinence. When united under any appreciable tension, the vaginal membrane may separate or slough postoperatively, thereby inviting cystocele recurrence. If flap tension is evident, simple longitudinal "relaxing incisions," at the vaginal 3 and 9 o'clock positions that undermine 1 cm of the full thickness of the lateral vaginal walls will release the tension and increase the caliber of a narrowed vagina (see Chapter 20). Such lateral relaxing incisions may be left open and allowed to granulate in, and they usually will be reepithelialized within 2 to 3 weeks. We recognize that in colporrhaphy it is the reapproximation of the subepithelial fibromuscular tissues that will produce the desired repair and not the reapproximation of the superficial vaginal skin.

Sometimes a satisfactory long-term result can be accomplished by separating a thin layer of connective tissue from the vaginal membrane and using mobilization and plication, often with multiple and somewhat incomplete rows of fine synthetic absorbable or nonabsorbable suture. The redundant sling of the fibromuscular tissues is shortened and strengthened by duplication, because the supporting layer of vaginal membrane will be found to fit the newly formed plane of the anterior vaginal wall with much less excision of vaginal membrane than would have been thought necessary.

Aldridge (personal communication) has suggested that full-thickness vaginal wall approximation, after removal of a properly sized, somewhat V-shaped wedge from the vaginal flap beneath the urethra, is more important in supporting the urethra than plication of the urethral wall itself. The suburethral vaginal wall should be closed with running or interrupted 2-0 absorbable stitches, placed subcuticularly if the operator desires, through the full thickness of the underlying fibromuscular layer. The first stitch starts near the urethral meatus. If the repair has been immediately preceded by hysterectomy, the ends of the tied peritoneal closure stitch are sewn to the undersurface of the now trimmed upper vault margins of the anterior vaginal wall near the attachment of the "bladder pillars" to the vaginal wall, thus ensuring maximal elongation of the anterior vaginal wall when these stitches have been tied. Tying is best accomplished by sliding the index finger down the suture strand to a point below the knot while bringing the vaginal wall to the point of peritoneal closure. Because the peritoneal closure stitch, as described, actually includes and has also approximated the uterosacral ligaments, this effectively, even though indirectly, attaches the anterior vaginal wall to the uterosacral ligaments and helps to lengthen the anterior vaginal wall and direct the vaginal axis posteriorly (see Fig. 8.46). As the reconstitution of the anterior vaginal wall continues, subcuticular stitches are placed approximately 1 cm apart. If not previously accomplished, the ends of the pubourethrovaginal ligament suture may be sewn and tied to the undersurface of the vaginal wall at the site of the previous attachment of the vagina to the urogenital diaphragm as indicated in Figure 10.17, thus reestablishing the fusion normally found in this area between the vaginal wall and urethra. The remainder of the full thickness of the vaginal wall beneath the urethra is closed with subcuticularly placed long-lasting absorbable synthetic sutures.

Simultaneous Perineorrhaphy

Because the lower anterior wall rests upon the perineal body for the length of the urethra, it follows that adequate perineal support should also be provided whenever urethral support has been the major objective of any vaginal reconstruction (see Chapter 11). The results of coincident perineorrhaphy will not only reinforce the external genital sphincter system but have improved our long-term results of repair for the cure of urinary stress incontinence.

We do not recommend the Watkins-Wertheim interposition type of operation (51–53) for the treatment of cystocele because of the eventual risk of bleeding from the retained uterus. If pathology develops that would indicate hysterectomy, the operation is made appreciably more difficult as a result of the extensive adhesions to the uterine fundus and the proximity of the lower ureters and the bladder trigone to the adherent fundus. Rarely, transposition using the Ocejo modification (in which the uterus is temporarily split and the entire endometrium is excised) may be used (16) if the vaginal wall is very thin and the uterine cervix is well supported.

Alternate Transvaginal Methods of Support of the Vesicourethral Junction

When traction upon the Kocher hemostat applied to the paraurethral tissue shows no evidence of pubic fixation of the tissue to which the hemostat has been applied (as by its failure to move the patient a small bit), there has either been avulsion or detachment of the paraurethral or paravaginal tissues on one or both sides of the pelvis. Insufficient pubourethrovaginal ligament support for confident reconstruction requires consideration of alternate methods of support. The pubococcygeus muscle transplant may be employed (7, 14, 23).

Pubococcygeus Muscle Transplant of Franz-Ingelman-Sundberg

The finger-thick medial pedicle of the pubococcygeus on each side should be isolated by dissection and transected in the midportion of the vagina at the level of the vesicourethral junction. It is sewn by transfixion suture to the similar pedicle from the opposite side. Such transplanted muscular fibers also provide useful support after repair of a urethrovaginal fistula, especially one occurring at the vesicourethral junction, in which instance, without such transplant, subsequent postoperative urinary stress incontinence would be a probability.

TECHNIQUE

The vagina may be opened in the midline, and the full thickness of the walls is mobilized laterally almost to the pubic rami, through the lateral limits of the vesico-vaginal space if necessary. Palpation of the upper two-thirds of the lateral vaginal wall will permit identification of the medial borders of the pubococcygei, which, with a little dissection, can be visualized. Alternately, an inverted U-shaped incision can be made through the full thickness of the anterior vaginal wall. This will expose the full length of the urethra, most of the bladder, and, laterally, the pubococcygei at the point where they cross the urethra and the vagina.

A finger-sized pubococcygeus is mobilized and separated laterally from the remainder of the muscle (Figs. 10.24 and 10.25). When transected posteriorly, this muscle graft will be suspended by its continuity with the superior extremity of the rest of the muscle. The length of the portion mobilized should be chosen so as to permit the ends of the pedicle of each side to be united snugly but without tension using a series of transfixion sutures placed in a side-to-side fashion beneath the vesicourethral junction.

The free segment of posterior pubococcygeus from which the upper muscle had been cut is now sewn by a mattress suture to the main body of the levator ani on its respective side to prevent its retraction and loss of support; or if a prominent rectocele is present, these fibers may be mobilized and fixed beneath the posterior vaginal wall during the subsequent posterior repair. After assurance of the effectiveness of the transposition, the anterior vaginal wall is closed in the usual manner with fine polyglycolic sutures.

Paravaginal Repair

When midline plication is not an effective answer for the treatment of rotational descent of the vesicourethral junction, another choice is lateral or paravaginal fixation on one or both sides as necessary. Paravaginal defects refer to disturbances in the attachment of the anterior sulcus of the vagina to a connective tissue "bridge" attaching the anterior sulcus to the arcus tendineus. When there are no anterior sulci, the gynecol-

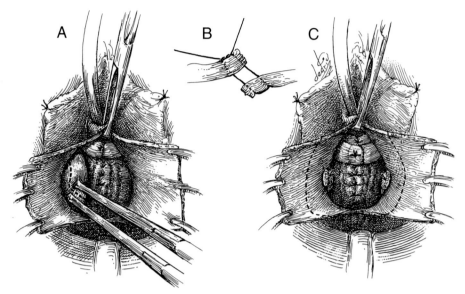

Figure 10.24. Pubococcygeus muscle transplant. **A.** The full thickness of the anterior vaginal wall has been opened for its full extent and reflected laterally as far as the pelvic diaphragm. The pubourethrovaginal "ligaments" have been plicated beneath the vesicourethral junction, and the bladder capsule has been plicated by a series of interrupted mattress sutures. The medial border of the pubococcygeus muscle has been identified and exposed. A finger-thick pedicle has been transected and freed laterally along the *dotted line.* **B** and **C.** A similar step is accomplished on the opposite side, and the muscle bellies are overlapped and approximated by one or more mattress sutures. The transected posterior muscle bundle of pubococcygeus may be fixed to the vaginal wall, and the excess vagina removed as shown by the *dotted line.* The colporrhaphy is completed and the anterior vaginal wall closed from side to side.

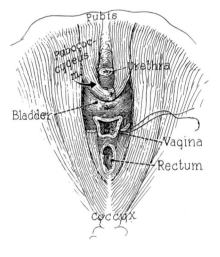

Figure 10.25. Drawing of the important new relationships of the pubococcygeus muscle. The ends of a medial pubococcygeus sling are attached to one another beneath the vesicourethral junction.

ogist should examine the patient for lateral detachment of the urethral paravaginal tissues. According to Baden and Walker (1), such a detachment should be suspected when the anterior vaginal wall is relaxed. If there is no elevation of the anterior vaginal wall when the patient squeezes her pelvic muscles tightly (i.e., in a "holding" position), the connective tissue and vascular supports of the anterior vaginal wall may have been detached from the arcus tendineus.

The vagina itself is not attached directly to the arcus tendineus (9, 12, 38, 48), but the anterior vaginal sulcus is attached to the arcus tendineus by a meshwork of intervening connective tissue that may be subject to various strains and stretching or even partial avulsion. Because this type of strain is usually a consequence of trauma during labor and delivery, detachment of these tissues is more common in parous patients. Although at times it appears that this tissue may be avulsed as a result of trauma, it also can be attenuated and stretched as with massive genital prolapse. Loss of support due to avulsion might be replaced by surgical reattachment, lessening the risk of recurrent cystocele. This damage is in addition to that done to the pubourethrovaginal portion of the urogenital diaphragm, which when concentrated on the posterior pubourethrovaginal ligament can be recognized as a midvaginal or central defect in this support of the vesicourethral junction. This defect results in pathologic rotational descent or "wheeling" of the proximal urethra and should be repaired separately, as described under "Technique of Pubourethrovaginal Ligament Plication."

Detachment or stretching of one or both vaginal sulci from their attachment to the arcus tendineus can be identified both preoperatively and intraoperatively. When present it can be remedied by reattaching the lateral vaginal sulci to the obturator fascia at the site of the arcus tendineus to aid in restoring the support by the vagina of both bladder and urethra. When this is coincident with demonstrable midline weakness, the latter should be repaired simultaneously. It may also be related to lifestyle, however, and may occasionally follow the pull of massive vaginal eversion, even in the nullipara. Therefore, direct surgical attachment of the vaginal sulcus to the arcus tendineus may to some extent correct the widening of the anterior vaginal wall that occurs with certain types of cystocele (12, 41, 54)(BH Word Jr and HA Montgomery, Paravaginal fascial repair [motion picture], and personal communications). Bilateral attachment is generally necessary when stretching or avulsion of the lateral supports has resulted in a cystocele (54). Large midline defects of the vaginal wall are much more common and are remedied by the standard midline plications and colporrhaphy. The existence or coexistence of the less common lateral defects should be determined preoperatively for appropriate planning of surgical technique.

If a patient has a midline vaginal support defect combined with paravaginal defect, she will require both anterior colporrhaphy and paravaginal repair (43). If there is also eversion of the vaginal vault, coincident colpopexy will be required to restore the vagina to a normal depth and axis. If the paravaginal repair can be extended posteriorly all of the way to the origin of the arcus tendineus at the ischial spine, on one or preferably both sides, this may be all that is required to restore a normal vaginal depth and axis. Alternate methods of colpopexy may be transvaginal sacrospinous fixation or transabdominal sacrocolpopexy (see Chapter 16).

If a patient has both a lateral defect and a midline lesion that should have been diagnosed preoperatively, a midline incision in the anterior vaginal wall provides operative exposure for the repair of each of these elements, that is, pubourethrovaginal ligament plication and paravaginal fixation. Attachment of the paraurethral connective tissue to the arcus tendineus on the undersurface of the pubis adjacent to the symphysis has been employed successfully. This is an interesting, effective approach first advocated by others (1, 12, 41, 54)(Word and Montgomery, motion picture and personal communications). A transvaginal technique is shown in Figures 10.26 and 10.27.

TRANSVAGINAL PARAVAGINAL REPAIR TECHNIQUE

1. Insert a transurethral Foley catheter into the bladder.
2. Between two Allis clamps, open directly into the vesicovaginal space.
3. Open the full length of the full thickness of the anterior vaginal wall, including an exposure of the bladder base and urethra.
4. Dissect the full lateral limits of the vesicovaginal space.

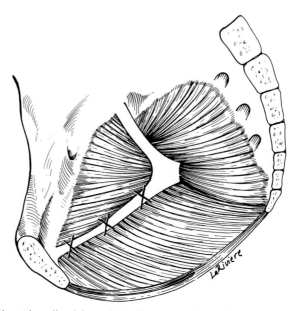

Figure 10.26. The sidewalk of the pelvis. The points along the arcus tendineus or the underlying obturator fascia to which the anterior vaginal fornix may be attached on each side of the pelvis during a bilateral paravaginal repair are indicated by the X's. At least three stitches are placed. The most posterior is near the ischial spine, the most anterior is at the back of the pubis, and the point in between approximates the vesicourethral junction. (From Nichols DH. Gynecologic and obstetric surgery. St. Louis: Mosby-Year Book, 1993. Used with permission.)

5. If there is any funneling present, insert Kelly stitches using polydioxonone (PDS) suture to plicate the pubourethrovaginal ligament portion of the urogenital diaphragm.
6. Plicate the underside of the bladder as necessary using one or more layers of 00 polyglycolic acid mattress stitches.
7. Instill 60 ml of indigo carmine–colored saline into the bladder and clamp.
8. Inject 50 ml of sterile saline between the lateral limits of the vesicovaginal space and the pelvic sidewall.
9. Dissect through the lateral limits of the vesicovaginal space to the space of Retzius and the pelvic sidewall, exposing the obturator fascia, arcus tendineus, and fascia of the pelvic diaphragm.
10. With a Deschamp ligature carrier, place three or four nonabsorbable sutures (such as Ethibond, Prolene, or Surgilene) through the obturator fascia at the site of the arcus tendineus. Put the first stitch at the urethrovesical junction, the second just in front of the ischial spine, and the third halfway to the urethrovesical junction.
11. Hold the vaginal vault in the proper desired postoperative position. Insert a ring forceps into the vagina, open it, and note where the fold of the dissected anterior vaginal wall crosses the edge of the forceps. Using a free end of the suture in the obturator fascia, insert it subcutaneously through the full thickness of the fibromuscular layer of the underside of the anterior vaginal wall flap, and tie the free end there, the opposite end to be used later as a pulley stitch.
12. Perform the same procedure in the opposite side of the pelvis.
13. Tie the lateral (paravaginal) colpopexy stitches first on one side and then on the other, burying the knot.
14. Bring the cut edges of the vagina together in the midline, trimming the excess as necessary to effect a tension-free closure.

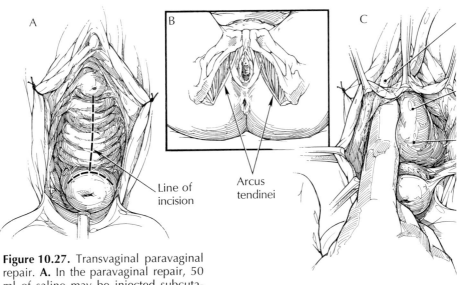

A

B

C

Line of
incision

Arcus
tendinei

Figure 10.27. Transvaginal paravaginal repair. **A.** In the paravaginal repair, 50 ml of saline may be injected subcutaneously along each lateral vaginal sulcus, and an inverted "T" incision made through the full thickness of the anterior vaginal wall along the path of the *dashed line.* **B.** A phantom drawing of the arcus tendinei shows the course of the arcus tendineus from the ischial spines to the back of the pubis. **C.** A Foley catheter has been placed and the full width of the vesicovaginal space developed. The operator's index finger, sweeping the bladder and urethra medially, palpates and by blunt dissection exposes the site of the arcus tendineus. (*Continues on following page.*)

15. Close the anterior vaginal wall with running subcuticular or horizontal mattress stitches.
16. Perform any posterior colporrhaphy and perineorrhaphy that may be necessary.
17. Lightly pack the vagina overnight if desired.

The long-term success of this "White" (54) repair of distention midline cystocele by lateral paravaginal attachment may be compromised because the strength of the anterior vaginal wall has already been damaged. This is in contradistinction to the paravaginal repair of a lateral sulcus defect without midline cystocele in which the damage is primarily to the tissues attaching the sulcus of the vagina to the arcus tendineus (Figs. 10.28 and 10.29). If there are simultaneous lateral paravaginal and midline defects of the anterior vaginal wall and its attachments, both must be recognized and repaired.

The Vaginal Patch

When a large cystocele is associated with an abnormal thinning of the vaginal wall and the surgeon wishes to preserve a coitally adequate vaginal diameter, it is possible to thicken the vaginal wall by subcuticular implantation of a patch of previously resected

D

Lateral pelvic sidewall–
obturator fascia

Sutures passed
through underside
of vaginal wall

E

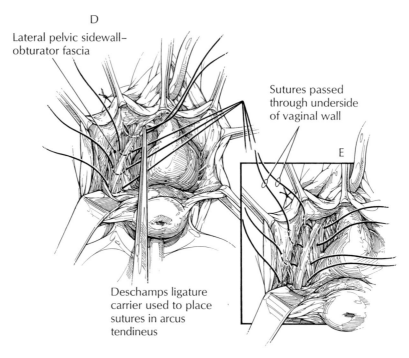

Deschamps ligature
carrier used to place
sutures in arcus
tendineus

Figure 10.27 continued. Transvaginal paravaginal repair. **D.** Starting with a stitch
of nonabsorbable suture in the obturator
fascia at the site of the arcus tendineus
and at the level of the vesicourethral
junction, several additional stitches are
placed, using either the Deschamps ligature carrier or a swaged needle. **E.** Each
of these is sewn to the underside of the
anterior vaginal wall at the site of the sulcus, and on one or both sides as necessary. When all stitches have been placed,
they are tied and the ends cut, so that the
knots are effectively buried. **F.** Any residual midline defect is corrected by colporrhaphy, and the incision closed by
a running subcuticular suture.

F

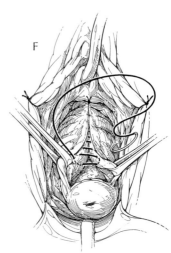

vaginal wall (35, 56). The patch favors reformation of an adequately strong but satisfactorily functional vaginal wall (56).

The patch of resected vaginal wall is sewn into the vesicovaginal space so as to cover
the entire surface of the exposed bladder surface that had previously been in contact with
the anterior vagina. We have used this type of repair only on previously sterilized patients.
The anterior vaginal wall, fixed and infiltrated densely by fibroblastic connective tissue
as occurs after implantation of the patch, probably would not tolerate the stretching and
dilation of labor without avulsion of the patch after disruption of its attachments.

Moore et al. (33) placed a tantalum patch in a similar manner, for the same purpose. Correspondence with Moore has determined, however, that he has abandoned

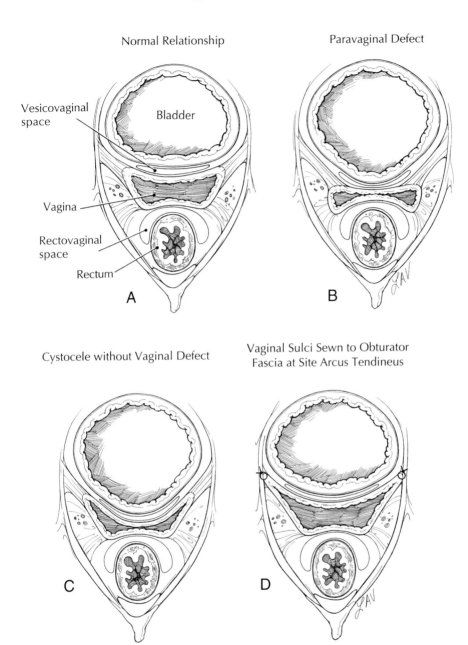

Normal Relationship

Vesicovaginal space

Bladder

Vagina

Rectovaginal space

Rectum

A

Paravaginal Defect

B

Cystocele without Vaginal Defect

C

Vaginal Sulci Sewn to Obturator Fascia at Site Arcus Tendineus

D

Figure 10.28. Coronal drawings of the pelvis. **A.** A normal relationship between bladder and vagina. Note the connective tissue condensation connecting the anterior vaginal sulci to the arcus tendineus along the pelvic sidewall. **B.** A bilateral paravaginal defect. Note the elongation (or avulsion) of the support of the sulci. **C.** Midline cystocele is noted by the sagging of the anterior vaginal wall. Notice that the connective tissue condensations supporting the sulci are undamaged. **D.** When the vaginal sulci have been sewn directly to the sites of the arcus tendinei, the width of the anterior thin vaginal wall is increased, reducing its sagging and demonstrating how paravaginal repair, even without paravaginal defect, will secondarily elevate the bladder to reduce the cystocele.

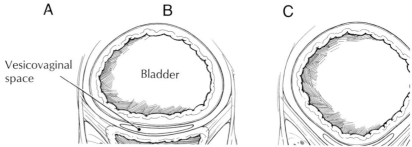

Figure 10.29. Reducing sagging. **A.** The obturator fascia of the pelvic sidewalls is represented by the *standing poles*, the sulci by the *dots and arrows*, and the relaxed anterior vaginal wall (cystocele) by the *sagging line* between the dots and arrows. **B.** This sagging may be reduced by shortening the line at each end (paravaginal repair). **C.** Alternatively, the line in the center may be shortened (anterior colporrhaphy). The effect is similar, and may, in some cases, explain why paravaginal repair may help correct cystocele as well as paravaginal defect.

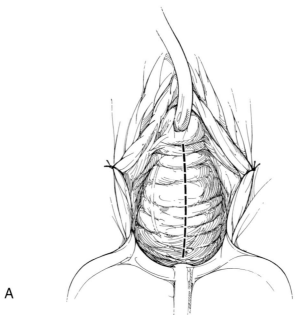

Figure 10.30. **A.** The vaginal patch. The anterior vaginal wall is opened for its full thickness and length along the course of the *dashed line*. (*Continued on following page.*)

the use of tantalum because of fragmentation of this material in an area where it was so susceptible to bending. We have subsequently found the vaginal patch to be most helpful because of its permanence as well as its flexibility. (A somewhat similar but absorbable collagen mesh prothesis was employed successfully by Friedman and Meltzer [15].)

TECHNIQUE

After the vesicovaginal space has been opened (Fig. 10.30*A*) and the full thickness of the anterior vaginal wall has been reflected from the midline laterally for the full extent of the vesicovaginal space, a trapezoid-shaped piece of excised vaginal skin can

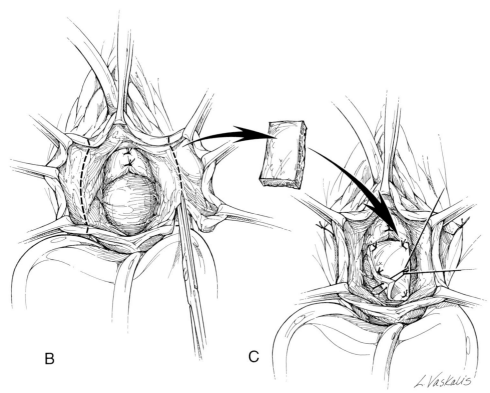

B   C

Figure 10.30 continued. B. The unsplit vaginal wall has been separated from the bladder. After the pubourethral ligament portion of the urogenital diaphragm has been plicated beneath the vesicourethral junction, the excess but pathologically thin anterior vaginal wall is excised along the course of the *dashed lines.* **C.** A full-thickness patch of anterior vaginal wall is harvested from the resected portion, cut to fit the weak spot beneath the bladder, and sewn to the fibromuscular wall of the exposed bladder by a series of interrupted absorbable sutures. (*Continues on following page.*)

be cut (Fig. 10.30*B*). The patch is then tacked to the capsular connective tissue underlying the bladder by three or four sutures on either side along the lateral margins of the vesicovaginal space, from as high in the vaginal vault as can be reached to the area beneath the vesicourethral junction (Fig. 10.30*C*). In unusual cases, one can, if desired, extend the patch anteriorly to reinforce the urethra as well. Sutures should also be placed anteriorly into each pubourethrovaginal ligament. Laterally, the patch can be attached to the firm tissues of the lateral wall of the perivesical spaces, to the obturator fascia, and to the pelvic diaphragm.

Necrosis of the covering vaginal flap could result from ischemia and, for this reason, the cut edges of the vagina must be united without tension. Lateral relaxing incisions may be necessary to reduce the tension on the midline suture line if too much vaginal membrane has been excised.

The preceding technique presumes that the operator wishes to preserve a useful and functional vagina. When this is not the objective, one can make the attenuated vaginal walls effectively support a cystocele repair by deliberately excising much wider flaps of vaginal wall, thereby narrowing the vagina to a finger breadth caliber. The management of postoperative restoration of bladder function is discussed in some detail in Chapter 22.

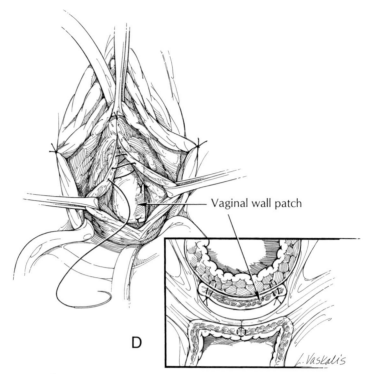

Figure 10.30 continued. D. The cut edges of the remaining anterior vaginal wall are approximated without tension by a running subcuticular stitch, effectively burying the patch as shown and effectively thickening the tissue between the bladder and the vaginal lumen. The patch will probably be converted to collagen within a year, providing permanent reinforcement of the vaginal support to the bladder.

INABILITY TO VOID POSTOPERATIVELY

Relaxation of the muscular component of the pubourethrovaginal ligaments and the urethral attachment to the levator ani (muscular, fascial, or both) is an integral part of the physiologic voiding precess, and significant surgical plication of these ligaments beneath the urethrovesical junction may inhibit the normal voiding process until healing is well under way and spasms have ceased. A temporary suprapubic cystostomy may be helpful if the surgeon suspects that the patient (e.g., a patient with unusual anxiety or with a very large hypotonic bladder) will be unable to void after anterior colporrhaphy. Suprapubic cystostomy should be used routinely after repair of a fistula at the vesical neck.

At the time the silicone-coated no. 16 transurethral Foley catheter is removed, the patient may be given a single dose of an alpha-adrenergic blocker such as phenoxybenzamine (Dibenzyline) (10 mg) to relax urethral spasm. An order is left for the patient to be catheterized only if unable to void. If after a day of unsuccessful trying the patient is still unable to void, she may be taught the technique of self-catheterization, to be used as necessary even after discharge from the hospital. Use of the plastic flexible "Mentor" 14F female catheter facilitates this procedure considerably (Mentor Self-Cath Female Catheter 14 FR, Number 240, Mentor Corporation, Minneapolis, Minnesota 55430). Its use can be discontinued as soon as the patient is able to void adequate amounts spontaneously and there is but little (less than 60 ml) residual urine obtained. A portable ultrasound unit for instantly and accurately measuring residual urine volume is available, significantly reducing the discomfort, inconvenience, and number of bladder invasions by catheter. The following is an example of patient instructions for the use of the Mentor catheter.

Instructions for Intermittent Self-Catheterization

Self-catheterization can be accomplished several times a day, as frequently as you normally void. It is important to be sure that the bladder never holds more than 500 ml (1 pint) of urine at one time. If the bladder is allowed to hold more than 500 ml for any length of time, the urine can stretch the bladder muscle to the point where it will not work as well as it should, and if the bladder becomes too stretched, it cannot receive a proper blood supply, a condition that can precipitate a bladder infection. To avoid these problems, make sure that the bladder is emptied every few hours during the day. Some people do the procedure while standing, some sitting on the toilet, and some lying down. Whichever is the easiest for you is the method you should use.

1. Wash hands and then wash the perineal area. Spread the labia with one hand, and with the other hand wash the opening from where the urine comes, and the surrounding area, from front to back, using a povidone-iodine (Betadine) packet, or a wash-and-wipe disposable towelette. Use one wipe to wash down the left side of the non-hair-bearing inner vaginal lips, another to wipe down the inner surface of the right side, and another to wash down the urethral meatus (the opening from which the urine comes).
2. Hold the labia open with one hand, and grasp the Mentor plastic disposable catheter 2 to 3 inches from the tip, inserting it slowly into the meatus (urethral opening) until the urine begins to drain. Leave it in place until the urine stops coming, and slowly pull the catheter out. If urine begins to drain again, stop and wait until the flow stops before removing the tube. The catheter can be allowed to drain directly into the toilet or container. When the flow of urine is finished, remove the catheter.
3. The catheter should be washed well with soap and water after each use, and then rinsed with clear water.
4. Each day boil the catheters for 3 to 5 minutes, empty the water, and let them dry. They may be stored in a clean towel, an aluminum foil packet, a zip-lock "baggie," or a sterilized jar. You should carry a catheter with you wherever you go. Clearly, the catheters can be reused for an almost indefinite period of time if the above procedure is followed. Should you need a new supply, do not hesitate to request this of your physician, who can prescribe a new supply from a surgical supply house.

References

1. Baden WF, Walker TA. Evaluation of the stress incontinent patient. In: Canton EB, ed. Female urinary stress incontinence, Springfield, IL: Charles C Thomas, 1979:157–158.
2. Ball TL. Anterior and posterior cystocele. Clin Obstet Gynecol 1966;9:1062–1069.
3. Beck RP, McCormick S. Treatment of urinary stress incontinence by anterior colporrhaphy. Obstet Gynecol 1982;59:269–274.
4. Beck RP, McCormick S, Nordstrom L. A 25 year experience with 519 anterior colporrhaphy procedures. Obstet Gynecol 1991;78:1011–1018.
5. Borstad E, Rud T. The risk of developing urinary stress incontinence after vaginal repair in continent women: a clinical and urodynamic follow-up study. Acta Obstet Gynecol Scand 1989;68:545.
6. Boyd ME. Practical gynecologic surgery. Baltimore: Urban & Schwarzenberg, 1990:152–153.
7. Copenhaver EH. Surgery of the vulva and vagina: a practical guide. Philadelphia: WB Saunders, 1981.
8. Delancey JOL. Anatomic aspects of vaginal eversion after hysterectomy. Am J Obstet Gynecol 1992;166:1717.
9. Delancey JOL. Corrective study of paraurethral anatomy. Obstet Gynecol 1986;68:91.
10. Delancey JOL. Structural support of the urethra as it relates to stress urinary incontinence: the hammock hypothesis. Am J Obstet Gynecol 1994;170:1713–1723.
11. Ferguson KL et al. Stress urinary incontinence: effect of pelvic muscle exercise. Obstet Gynecol 1990;75:671.
12. Figuranov KM. Surgical treatment of urinary incontinence in women. Akush Ginekol 1949;6:7–13.
13. Frank RT. Operation for cure of incontinence of urine in the female. Am J Obstet Gynecol 1947;55:618–626.
14. Franz R. Levator plaslik bei relativen Harninkontinenz. Gynakologe 1954;137:393.
15. Friedman EA, Meltzer RN. Collagen mesh prosthesis for repair of endopelvic fascial defect. Am J Obstet Gynecol 1970;106:430–433.
16. Gallo D. Ocejo modification of interposition operation. In: Urologica Ginecologica. Guadalajara: Gallo, 1969.

17. Gardiner SH. Vaginal surgery for stress incontinence. Clin Obstet Gynecol 1963;6:178–194.
18. Gardy M, Kozminski M, DeLancey JOL, Elkins T, McGuire E. Stress incontinence and cystoceles. J Urol 1991;145:1211–1213.
19. Green TH. Development of a plan for the diagnosis and treatment of urinary stress incontinence. Am J Obstet Gynecol 1962;83:632.
20. Halban J. Gynakologische Operation slehre. Berlin-Vienna: Urban & Schwarzenberg, 1932.
21. Hodgkinson CP. Stress urinary incontinence. Am J Obstet Gynecol 1970;108:1141–1168.
22. Hutch JA. A new theory of the anatomy of the internal urinary sphincter and the physiology of micturition. Obstet Gynecol 1967;30:309–317.
23. Ingelman-Sundberg A. Stress incontinence of urine. J Obstet Gynaecol Br Emp 1952;59:699–703.
24. Kegel A. Progressive resistance exercise in the functional restoration of the perineal muscles. Am J Obstet Gynecol 1948;56:238.
25. Kelly HA. Incontinence of urine in women. Urol Cutan Rev 1913;1:291–293.
26. Krige CF. Vaginal hysterectomy and genital prolapse repair. Johannesburg, South Africa: Witwatersrand Press, 1965:62.
27. Lahodny J. Urethrovesikalsuspension mit autologem Fasziengewebe auf rein vaginalem Weg—Kurzarmschlingenoperation. Geburtshilfe Frauenheilkd 1984;44:104–113.
28. Martius H. Martius' gynecological operations. McCall M, Bolten K, trans. Boston: Little, Brown, 1956.
29. McGuire EJ, Gardy M, Elkins T, DeLancey JOL. Treatment of incontinence with pelvic prolapse. Urol Clin North Am 1991;18:349–353.
30. Milley PS, Nichols DH. The relationships between the pubourethrovaginal ligaments and urogenital diaphragm in the human female. Anat Rec 1969;163:433–451.
31. Mishell DR. Discussing paper by Gardy M, et al. In: Yearbook of obstetrics and gynecology. St. Louis: Mosby–Year Book, 1992:227.
32. Moir JC. The gauze-hammock operation. J Obstet Gynaecol Br Commonw 1968;75:1–9.
33. Moore J, Armstrong JT, Wills SH. The use of tantalum mesh in cystocele with critical report of ten cases. Am J Obstet Gynecol 1955;69:1127.
34. Muellner SR. The anatomies of the female urethra. Obstet Gynecol 1959;14:429–434.
35. Nichols DH, ed. Gynecologic and obstetric surgery. St. Louis: Mosby-Year Book, 1993.
36. Nichols DH. The Mersilene mesh gauze-hammock in repair of severe recurrent urinary stress incontinence. In: Taymor ML, Green TH, eds. Progress in gynecology. New York: Grune & Stratton, 1975;6.
37. Nichols DH. Milley PS. Identification of pubourethrovaginal ligaments and their role in transvaginal surgical correction of stress incontinence. Am J Obstet Gynecol 1973;115:123.
38. Reiffenstuhl G. The clinical significance of the connective tissue planes and spaces. Clin Obstet Gynecol 1982;25:811–820.
39. Resnick NM. Urinary incontinence in the older woman. In: Kursh ED, McGuire EJ, eds. Female urology. Philadelphia: JB Lippincott, 1994:475–494.
40. Ricci JV, Thom CH. Uterovaginal extirpation for procidentia. Am J Surg 1952;83:192–200.
41. Richardson AC, Lyons JB, Williams NL. A new look at pelvic relaxation. Am J Obstet Gynecol 1976;126:568.
42. Royston GD, Rose DK. A new operation for cystocele. Am J Obstet Gynecol 1937;33:421–429.
43. Shull BL, Baden WF. A six year experience with paravaginal defect repair for stress urinary incontinence. Am J Obstet Gynecol 1989;160:1432–1440.
44. Sims JM. Clinical notes on uterine surgery. London: Robert Hardwicke, 1866:304–306.
45. Symmonds RE, Jordan LT. Iatrogenic stress incontinence of urine. Am J Obstet Gynecol 1961;82:1231–1237.
46. Uhlenhuth E, Hunter DT. Problems in the anatomy of the pelvis. Philadelphia: JB Lippincott, 1953.
47. Van Duzen RE. The cystoscopic appearance of various types of cystoceles. South Med J 1930;23:580–587.
48. Von Peham H, Amreich J. Operative gynecology. Ferguson LK, trans. Philadelphia: JB Lippincott, 1934.
49. Van Rooyen AJL, Liebenberg HC. Clinical approach to urinary incontinence in females. Obstet Gynecol 1979;53:1–7.
50. Wall LL, Norton PA, DeLancey JOL. Practical urogynecology. Baltimore: Williams & Wilkins, 1993:153–190.
51. Watkins TJ. Treatment of cases of extensive cystocele and uterine prolapse. Surg Gynecol Obstet 1906;2:659–667.
52. Watkins TJ. The treatment of cystocele and uterine prolapse after the menopause. Am Gynecol Obstet J 1899;15:420–423.
53. Wertheim E. Zur plastischen Verwendung des Uterus bei Prolapsen. Centralblat für Gynakologie, 1899;23:369–372.
54. White GR. Cystocele: a radical cure by suturing lateral sulci of vagina to the white line of pelvic fascia. JAMA 1909;53:1707–1709.
55. Zacharin RF. A clinese anatomy: the pelvic supporting tissues of the Chinese and Occidental female compared and contrasted. Aust N Z J Obstet Gynecol 1977;17:11.
56. Zacharin RF. Free full thickness vaginal epithelium graft in correction of recurrent genital prolapse. Aust N Z J Obstet Gynecol 1992;32:146–148.
57. Zacharin RF. The suspensory mechanism of the female urethra. J Anat 1963;97:423–427.

CHAPTER 11

Posterior Colporrhaphy and Perineorrhaphy

Posterior colporrhaphy and perineorrhaphy are separate and distinct operations designed to correct separate and distinct defects. They should be demonstrated preoperatively so that an appropriate surgical plan can be developed ahead of time. Some patients require posterior colporrhaphy alone, some require perineorrhaphy, and some require both (22, 23).

In Chapters 5 and 6, we noted the importance of recognizing specific types of injury to the structures of the posterior vaginal wall or the supporting attachments. Damage may be the result of one or more types of injury. A carefully taken history and a thorough physical examination should be made in the office to clarify the type of injury, since general anesthesia paralyzes the voluntary muscles that largely account for the tone and the soft tissue relationships of the vagina. Examination should identify the site and the degree of damage to all demonstrable components of the posterior vaginal wall. This includes evaluation of vaginal caliber, tone, and support, not only with the patient prone and relaxed on the examining table, but also erect, with and without the addition of voluntary bearing-down effort. Only by considering the findings under all such conditions is it possible to select the operative procedure most likely to restore normal relationships and functions.

There are many women with rectocele who are not constipated, and many constipated women without rectocele. The primary symptoms of rectocele are aching after a bowel movement and incomplete bowel movements that often require manual expression to achieve evacuation. Effective posterior colporrhaphy should relieve these primary symptoms, but will not necessarily relieve constipation other than that produced by stool being caught in a pocket of rectal wall and precluding complete emptying of the bowel.

ANATOMIC TYPES OF RECTOCELE

There are three basic types of damage to be determined, and these occur either singly or in combination with one another.

1. There is stretching and attenuation of the full thickness of the vaginal wall itself, usually after overdistention during childbirth, with permanent loss of some of the intrinsic elasticity of the fibromuscular vaginal tube. The damage is greatest at the sites where the vaginal wall is furthest removed from its anchoring attachments; hence, damage to the anterior and posterior wall will be greater than damage to the lateral vaginal walls, because it is to the lateral vaginal wall that the vagina is fixed or attached. The

vaginal side of rectocele is somewhat similar to its cystocele counterpart, is associated with the flattening of the rugal folds over the site of the rectocele, and is likely to be progressive in its development.

Not only may the attachment of the fascia of Denonvilliers (38) (rectovaginal septum) be avulsed from the perineal body, providing a site of weakness through which a low rectocele may develop, but the fascia may be stretched in direct proportion to the amount by which the vaginal wall to which it is fused has been stretched.

Stretching of the rectal wall in all of its layers increases the size of the rectal reservoir—and although the muscularis may be plicated, increasing the effectiveness of the internal sphincter system, the submucosa may be stretched and thereby attenuated as well. The submucosa is the strongest layer in the wall of the large intestine (19). The feltlike mass of large intestinal collagen is located in the submucosal layer, which can be studied by the electron microscope. A honeycomb pattern of collagen allows blood and lymph vessels to enter and leave the muscularis mucosa and mucosa. The feltlike arrangement explains how a nonelastic fibrous protein in this position can enable the intestinal wall to possess this essential deformation response to stress (19). There is no muscularis mucosa in the anal canal to separate mucosa from submucosa (36).

2. Damage occurs from stretching of the lateral attachments of the vagina to the pelvic sidewall, particularly the vaginal portion of the cardinal ligament. This results from increased intra-abdominal pressure or from pathologic stretching of these attachments during labor, wherein the vagina may have been slow to dilate adequately and a segment has been pushed along as a roll of undilating vaginal wall during the descent of the presenting part, much in the fashion that a coat sleeve may be turned inside out. Vaginal rugae are generally preserved in the redundant vaginal wall involved in such a rectocele.

3. Damage occurs as a result of actual avulsion of these lateral attachments, which have been not only stretched but also torn from the lateral vaginal walls, only to reunite by scarring and fibrosis at a lower level in the pelvis. Because the refusion is often quite dense and fibrous, this is probably the origin of the nonprogressive, postobstetric prolapse described by Malpas (20) (see Chapter 5).

Traumatic detachment of the cranial edge of the perineal body from the subcutaneous rectovaginal septum may provide a site of weakness. Aging and loss of hormone support reduce vaginal elasticity, making damage from overdistention of the vagina more likely. Congenital defects include not only defective supporting tissue but also a congenitally defective nerve supply (31, 37), as might be suspected with a coexistent spina bifida occulta.

All various types of rectocele may coexist in the same patient, producing a combination defect; in addition, they are rather frequently coincident with a defective perineum. The gynecologist must therefore first determine which type of rectocele or combination of etiologic factors is present when planning an appropriate repair.

SITES OF RECTOCELE

Although the majority of rectoceles involve the anterior rectal wall, the posterior rectal wall may be involved, though rarely, and both anterior and posterior rectal walls may be the sites of rectocele (Fig. 11.1).

Posterior Vaginal Wall Weakness

Rectocele, a herniation or ballooning of the rectum and posterior vaginal wall into the lumen of the vagina, may be found to have displaced the posterior vaginal wall at one or several levels and might be described as a low, mid-, or high rectocele. Low rectocele is usually the result of a rather major and inadequately repaired obstetric lacera-

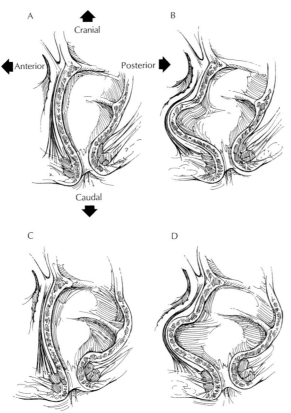

Figure 11.1. Sagittal views of both anterior and posterior rectocele. **A.** Normal rectum; the vagina is to the *left*. **B.** Anterior rectocele displacing the vagina. **C.** The rare posterior rectocele. **D.** Combined anterior and posterior rectoceles.

tion of the perineum, disrupting the attachments of the levator ani (fascia of the pubococcygeus portion) and the bulbocavernosus muscles to the perineal body and lower vagina, and tearing the rectovaginal septum from its attachment to the perineal body (Fig. 11.2). A marked gaping or eversion of the introitus will usually be evident. Although this causes some loss of support to the sides of the urethra, there may be little disturbance of bladder function unless the urogenital diaphragm also has been torn. There may be decreased effectiveness of bearing down during defecation as an associated complaint.

For the most part, a rectocele represents a late effect of the trauma of labor and delivery. There may be congenital underdevelopment of perineal musculature and elastic tissues, often inadequate because of associated abnormal innervation. There may also have been traumatic avulsion of the attachments of the perineal body to the rectovaginal septum, or the perineal body, vagina, and rectum may have been separated from the fibrous attachments of the levator ani–pelvic diaphragm complex. There may have been a laceration of the rectovaginal septum and the "fascia" of Denonvilliers, causing obliteration of the rectovaginal space and fusion of the anterior capsule of the rectum to the capsule of the posterior wall of the vagina. In addition, rectocele may be a result of the traction associated with the progressive procidentia of a general prolapse.

Minor degrees of damage to the rectal wall and its connective tissue supports can be aggravated by the straining efforts associated with chronic constipation. Repeated interference with progress of the focal stream may interfere with normal completeness of

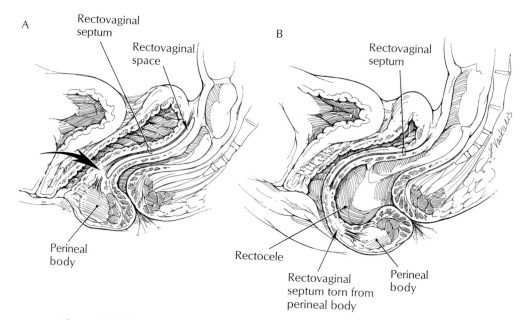

Figure 11.2. The potential effect of rupture of the rectovaginal septum. **A.** During childbirth, and prior to hysterectomy, the rectovaginal septum has been torn from its attachment to the perineal body (*arrow*). **B.** This defect has permitted the development of a large low rectocele between the torn ends, which are now further apart.

defecation, to a degree producing physiologic or functional obstruction as the redundant sacculation of the rectum becomes larger and residual stool stimulates more ineffectual straining. Thus rectocele may be the result of pulsion, or simply the end result of repeatedly increased intra-abdominal pressure, a factor more often evident as atrophic changes decrease the elasticity of the vaginal wall and the integrity of the supporting tissues during a patient's postmenopausal years.

A relaxed perineum may or may not coexist with a demonstrable rectocele. Rarely, a relaxed perineum is due to an inadequate nerve supply to the muscles supporting the two components of the perineal body. More commonly, the defect is the result of overdistention during parturition or, occasionally, the result of inadequately repaired or unrepaired obstetric laceration of the perineum. When this is the sole or major site of damage, virtual absence of the perineal body provides a pathologic degree of exposure of an otherwise normal posterior vaginal wall, accounting for the appearance known as pseudorectocele (Fig. 11.3). When such an explanation is suspected, insertion of the examining finger into the rectum will demonstrate no abnormality in the caliber of the rectum and no irregular distensibility of the anterior rectal wall. Symptoms are usually minimal, and the patient is often considered a candidate for perineal reconstruction or perineorrhaphy only when other surgery is indicated, such as vaginal hysterectomy or anterior colporrhaphy.

Congenital absence of the perineum exposes the posterior vaginal wall, simulating the appearance of rectocele, which need not be present. This condition, too, may be termed a pseudorectocele. Proper treatment requires surgical reconstruction of the defective perineum, using whatever tissues are at hand. When an acquired defect is repaired, the tissues to be reapproximated were previously in apposition, and normal innervation can be expected to be present; there is not the same tissue building that is necessary to repair a congenital defect when connective tissues and muscle must be appropriated from the nearest fibromuscular layers.

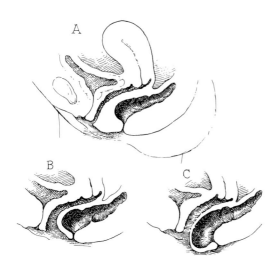

Figure 11.3. Normal and abnormal vaginoperineal relationships. **A.** A normal relationship between vagina, perineum, and rectum. **B.** A major perineal defect; there is no rectocele, but restoration of the perineal body is indicated. **C.** A major perineal defect with rectocele; in this circumstance, perineorrhaphy should be accompanied by an appropriate posterior colporrhaphy.

TRUE LOW RECTOCELE

True low rectocele is usually the result of obstetric forces accounting for a major disruption of the attachments of the levator ani fascia and the bulbocavernosus muscles to the perineal body. Either injury may occur independently without producing a midvaginal or high rectocele, and is most frequently the result of a shearing off of the lower attachments of the rectovaginal septum and the fascia of Denonvilliers from their attachment along the superior portion of the perineal body. When additional etiologic factors are present, such as a defective or absent fascia of Denonvilliers, a coexistent mid- or high vaginal rectocele may develop. Marked gaping and eversion at the introitus will then be noted. Although a relaxed posterior wall removes some support to the sides of the urethra, bladder function will be only slightly disturbed unless the urogenital diaphragm has also been damaged. Any tendency to constipation will be aggravated because of the decreased effectiveness and correspondingly increased bearing-down effort needed during defecation.

MIDVAGINAL RECTOCELE

Midvaginal rectocele, although also due to postobstetric damage, is usually not related to damage involving the levator ani, since the vaginal attachment and effective support of the pelvic diaphragm are below this area of involvement. There may have been pathologic stretching and laceration of the connective tissues between the vagina and rectum, so that not only is this tissue pathologically thin, but also the rectal and vaginal capsules and the rectovaginal septum have often become fused to one another by adhesions. Such fusion tends to deprive both the rectum and the vagina of their desirable capability of independent function. The contour of one must follow the functional contour of the other. A bearing-down sensation, discomfort after a bowel movement, and inability to empty the bowel completely are usual symptoms. Midvaginal rectocele often coexists with high rectocele, and, if one is to be repaired, both should be repaired.

HIGH RECTOCELE

Upper vaginal or high rectocele usually is also the result of a pathologic overstretching of the posterior vaginal wall. Here, the anterolateral attachments of the cardinal ligaments (hypogastric sheath) bind the vagina and cervix together to such an extent that the cervix functions almost as a part or extension of the anterior vaginal wall. The length of the anterior vaginal wall plus the diameter of the cervix normally equals the length of the posterior vaginal wall. The cranial envelope of the rectovaginal space terminates at the most caudal portion of the cul-de-sac of Douglas. This ensures both flexibility and mobility and, with the rectovaginal space, forms a more or less frictionless inclined plane down which the structures anterior to the rectovaginal space can slide without disturbing those primarily rectal structures posterior to the rectovaginal space. Classic procidentia, therefore, although beginning as an eversion of the upper vagina, usually permits the entire uterus and much of the bladder to extend outside the bony pelvis. A coexistent enterocele develops along which the cervix, uterus, and bladder may drop as though in a sliding hernia, and all of this occurs not infrequently without an accompanying rectocele. Such a descensus, noticeably involving the bladder, has been regarded as evidence of primarily anterior segment damage and is usually the result of chronically increased intraperitoneal pressure, but it could be due to damage sustained during the first stage of labor, as when there have been bearing-down efforts or attempts to accomplish delivery before full dilation of the cervix. Therefore, anterior segment damage per se may not be mechanistically related to damage to the levator ani or its sheath.

Etiology of High Rectocele

The peritoneal fusion fascia of Denonvilliers (37) is missing from the posterior vaginal wall covering an enterocele, with consequent loss of support to the anterior rectal wall as well as to the posterior vaginal wall in this area, thus predisposing to high rectocele.

In discussing enterocele, Malpas (20) distinguishes prolapse of the vault of the vagina with an obvious peritoneal sac, the bulge usually containing omentum or a loop of intestine. The posterior wall of the sac is formed by the upper rectum, and high or upper rectocele may coexist. Upper rectocele may also coexist with congenital deepening of the pouch of Douglas, since in this situation, too, there is no fascia of Denonvilliers to provide support to the anterior rectal wall. With uterovaginal or sliding prolapse, on the other hand, the high rectum is not involved, so the peritoneal descent involves only the anterior wall of the cul-de-sac of Douglas, usually without dilatation of the peritoneal sac. Because uterovaginal prolapse may not compromise the integrity of the rectum itself, the major objective of repair will be to shorten the cardinal-uterosacral ligament complex and reattach it to the vault of the vagina, whereas in total vault prolapse, a high posterior colporrhaphy with careful excision of all of the peritoneal pouch is an essential supplement. When cardinal-uterosacral ligament strength is lacking, sacrospinous colpopexy may be used to support the vaginal vault (Chapter 16).

SUMMARY OF LEVELS

Damage may be present in the upper, middle, or lower portions of the posterior vaginal wall in any combination. Damage in the upper vagina may be noted either as an enterocele, a potential enterocele, a high rectocele, or a widened posterior fornix that might be subsequently narrowed. Damage to the midvagina, which has been referred to as the rectal portion of the posterior vaginal wall, is perhaps the most common condition. Not infrequently, this may be the only lesion indicating repair. Reconstruction in this area should be designed to preserve or restore independent movement of the vaginal and the anterior rectal walls. This can be accomplished by the careful identification and preservation of the relatively avascular tissue relationships constituting the rectovaginal space.

If the anterior rectal wall becomes fused to the posterior vaginal wall, either by accident or by design, the possibility for normally independent movement of the walls of these adjacent viscera will be lost. When adhesion occurs, the vaginal wall must not only follow the contour of the rectal wall but must, to some extent, participate in rectal function as well, as mentioned previously. This is likely to result in persistent difficulties with constipation and defecation. Along with Goff (11), we would like to emphasize that it is desirable to preserve the normal independence of these two passageways. Only at the level of the perineal body should the vaginal and rectal walls become fused during the reconstruction of the posterior vaginal wall.

DEFECOGRAPHY AND OTHER STUDIES

Definitive avenues of investigation should be followed on patients who have rectal incontinence. The tests should include manometry, continence tests, and electromyography (4). Colonic transit studies also may be useful. When defecography is employed in the study of patients with defecation disorders, it appears that its main role is to document rectal wall changes during defecation straining as possible causes of evacuation difficulties. Distinct outpocketings of the rectal wall during defecation may be seen along with rectal intussusception, or a combination may be seen (25). Defecography may demonstrate a pathologic inability of the patient to relax the pelvic floor muscles, creating a cause of obstructed defecation. In our present state of knowledge, defecographic measurements cannot be regarded as reliable indicators of the complex physiologic condition of the pelvic floor muscles. Fluoroscopic findings may better demonstrate the ability to evacuate the rectum or retain rectal contents.

When the unanesthetized patient is unable to voluntarily contract her pubococcygei and external anal sphincter during pelvic examination, one should suspect the possibility of causative defective innervation of these muscles. Although this is occasionally of congenital origin (spina bifida occulta), a more likely explanation is an acquired pudendal neuropathy, as from pathologic stretching of the pudendal nerves during labor and delivery with subsequent atrophy of the damaged nerves (31, 32). This pathology can be confirmed by electromyography (37).

Some report good correlation between noninvasive surface electromyography using an intra-anal plug electrode and anal manometry. Parks (24) notes that "defecography demonstrates abnormalities of the rectal wall. These studies complement, but do not replace, good clinical examination and sound professional judgment."

Defecography may provide useful information in patients with rectal incontinence and outlet obstruction constipation symptoms. It has little additive value to anorectal manometry in incontinent patients without such symptoms (27). Defecography is particularly helpful in detecting rectal intussusceptions. However, measurements of anorectal angle and junction in incontinent patients are not significantly different from those in asymptomatic controls. A history of chronic constipation and straining of stool precedes development of fecal incontinence in about half of incontinent patients.

A functional pouch of the posterior rectal wall can be visualized by defecography, and this has been named "posterior rectocele" (6).

Pudendal nerve terminal motor latency can reveal unsuspected neuropathy in traumatic fecal incontinence, and combined with anal endosonography can help in the selection of patients for surgery (10).

The thickness and length of the anterior anal sphincters are substantial, as can be demonstrated by magnetic resonance imaging. This fact has an obvious implication in planning and executing the surgical reconstruction of a sphincter defect (1).

POSTERIOR COLPORRHAPHY
AND THE RECTOVAGINAL SEPTUM

An unexpectedly shortened and persistently uncomfortable vagina after posterior colporrhaphy can result in dyspareunia. To minimize this complication, some years ago we decided to abandon the standard Hegar-Halban levator plication for correction of weakness in the posterior vaginal wall. In selected cases, we now often employ a full-length posterior vaginal wall reconstruction, following the suggestions of Jeffcoate (15) and Porges (26) that the need for and the extent of a posterior vaginal wall repair be determined preoperatively by examination of the unanesthetized patient.

When full-length posterior vaginal reconstruction has been used immediately after vaginal hysterectomy, it has become apparent that, when the operator's finger is inserted into the "avascular rectovaginal space," the progress of such blunt finger dissection is consistently obstructed at the vaginal apex near the cut edge of the vaginal vault by a thin but firm membrane. This membrane usually requires a distinct incision for penetration. The membrane has been studied in more detail to determine whether it has surgical significance.

Tobin and Benjamin (38) had concluded that the tissue described by Denonvilliers in the male included two layers, the ventral peritoneal fusion layer, with which we are at the moment concerned, and a dorsal or posterior layer composed of rectal fascia. A gynecologic contribution to this discussion may be found in the 1957 paper by Uhlenhuth and Nolley (39) written in a rebuttal of a 1954 opinion expressed by Ricci and Thom (28). These provocative studies reached almost diametrically opposed conclusions, which may perhaps be explained by differences in methodology. Ricci's cited evidence, which led him to deny the existence of "fascial tissue" in the integrity of the vaginal walls, was based entirely on the study of hematoxylin- and eosin-stained histologic preparations and involved no correlation with gross anatomic dissections. Uhlenhuth, on the other hand, based his conclusion solely on gross dissection with no attempt at histologic correlation or confirmation. Reconciliation of these controversial reports was the objective of the simultaneous study of both the gross anatomy and related histologic specimens reported with Milley and Nichols in 1968 (21). We believe our studies have demonstrated a rectovaginal septum that can be identified as a distinct and relatively strong connective tissue layer between the vagina and the rectal walls, extending in a curved coronal plane, somewhat in conformity with the curvature of the bony pelvis. This septal structure is attached cranially to the caudal peritoneum and the rectouterine pouch of Douglas, and it extends inferiorly to its caudal fusion with the perineal body. The tissues of this septum are always adherent to the posterior aspect of the vaginal connective tissue but may easily be separated from it by blunt dissection. The demonstrable adherence to "vaginal wall" would seem to explain at least partially why the existence of a septum has, at times, been denied.

In transverse and coronal dissections, this septum was found to curve posterolaterally, paralleling the course of the paracolpium and blending laterally with the parietal layer of the pelvic fascia. It varies in character from a thin, readily perforated, translucent membrane to a tougher layer of almost leathery consistency.

Histologic studies have demonstrated this septum to consist of a fibromuscular elastic tissue, including dense collagen, abundant smooth muscle, and coarse elastic fibers, all readily separable from the fibromuscular elastic tissue recognizable as the posterior vaginal wall. In sections stained by orcein for elastic fibers, the area of the rectovaginal septum contained larger and coarser fibers than were demonstrable in the connective tissue within the vaginal wall proper. It is possible that such differences in elastic tissue fibers give the septum its demonstrable integrity during dissection. Appropriate tissue stains are needed to demonstrate the presence of a septum. We have concluded that the difficulty in demonstrating a rectovaginal septum histologically using standard hematoxylin and eosin staining and the adherence of this septum to the connective tissues of the posterior vaginal wall explain why the existence of this important structure had often been denied.

We believe these observations are of more than academic interest, because the strength and integrity of this membrane is clinically significant and surgically useful. Earlier surgeons attempted to maintain the functional independence of the posterior vaginal and the anterior rectal walls. With one examining finger in the vagina and one in the rectum, the walls of the passageways can normally be shown to move independently, each exhibiting a surprising degree of freedom. The rectovaginal septum normally facilitates the independent mobility of the rectal and vaginal walls and, as a result, ensures their functional independence. The rectovaginal septum also acts as a protective barrier of resistance to the spread of neoplasia or infection between the rectum and the vagina, as was suggested by Uhlenhuth and Nolley (39).

In Chapter 1 it was shown that the rectovaginal septum normally curves posterolaterally as it becomes attached to the fascia overlying the levator ani. Decreasing the vaginal width by approximating the cut edges after excision of a midportion of the septum will therefore increase the pull on the lateral attachments of the septum that tend to direct the vagina posteriorly toward the sacrum. This will tend to restore the original and proper upper horizontal vaginal axis. The excision of the upper vaginal wedge of tissue may help accomplish a similar purpose.

In the repair of obstetric or surgical episiotomy, restoration of the rectovaginal septum as a distinct layer at the apex of the wound will not only permit better support but will ensure better function and increased comfort. This can be readily accomplished by the substitution of the usual through-and-through epithelial stitches with a running subcuticular layer. Not only is the postoperative and postpartum discomfort less, but epithelial inclusion cysts are effectively prevented.

A pathologic thickening of the rectovaginal septum, caused by the development of scarring within the posterior avascular rectovaginal space, can usually be broken down with ease during the preliminary dissection. Its presence can be recognized and is usually demonstrable during a preoperative rectovaginal examination, if the examination is designed to demonstrate limited mobility in terms of the inability of the vaginal wall to be moved independently of the anterior rectal wall. Rupture of the septum, even in the presence of an apparently intact vagina, may result in adhesions and fixation of the vaginal wall to the underlying rectal wall. This injury can lead to the development of midvaginal rectocele. Under such circumstances, uninhibited distention of the rectum must result in distention of the posterior wall of the vagina with consequent high and/or midvaginal rectocele formation and symptomatic interference with function.

If a patient has developed a weakness and thinning throughout the posterior wall of the vagina and the operator elects to repair only the lower part of that weakness by a standard technique of perineorrhaphy without colporrhaphy, the persistence of disturbed function or an early recurrence is predictable, probably with a troublesome exacerbation of symptoms.

Secondary connective tissue hypertrophy of the uterosacral ligaments should often be regarded as one evidence of the body's compensatory response to incipient pelvic floor damage, and full-length posterior colporrhaphy may be desirable whenever this observation has been made. If the full length of the posterior vaginal wall has been opened after vaginal hysterectomy, the vault may be sewn to a uterosacral fixation stitch, and the stitching continued downward, reapproximating side to side the cut edges of the vagina.

The rectovaginal septum appears to have been recognized and carefully restored in the New York Woman's Hospital type of repair as described by Goff (11) and later in Bullard's modification of Goff's technique of posterior colporrhaphy (personal communication). However, a septum as such was not emphasized by Goff as an identifiable or significant structural entity. A possible explanation for this lack of emphasis or recognition is suggested in the following quotation from Uhlenhuth and Nolley (39):

It has been mentioned that the rectovaginal septum adheres closely to the vagina; it is, therefore, probable that the surgeon, in performing a posterior colporrhaphy, does not get into the space between the vaginal fascia and rectovaginal septum, but into the space between the rectovaginal septum and rectal fascia.*

*From Uhlenhuth E, Nolley GW. Vaginal fascia, a myth? Obstet Gynecol 1957;10:349–358. Used with permission.

As the experience of the gynecologic surgeon increases, it becomes apparent that the tissues normally supporting the upper third of the vagina are different from those to which the middle and lower thirds are attached. A low colporrhaphy and perineorrhaphy cannot be expected to provide an anatomically adequate repair of a weakness in the upper third of the vagina.

Harrison and McDonagh (13) wrote that "by far the most commonly neglected step in vaginal plastic procedures is reconstruction of the upper posterior vagina." When high rectocele and enterocele coexist, which is not infrequent, each must be recognized and repaired separately.

Posterior Colporrhaphy without Perineorrhaphy

When the defect to be repaired involves only the perineal body, reflection and mobilization of perineal skin and vaginal membrane should stop at that point, and the gynecologist should proceed to repair only the defective perineum and perineal body. When there is coexistent rectocele of the mid- or upper vagina, however, this herniation also should be approached at this time by extending the reflection of vaginal membrane by dissection into the rectovaginal space to a point above the bulge of the rectocele. Any adhesions binding the anterior wall of the rectum to the full-thickness flap of posterior vaginal wall should be divided by blunt and, when necessary, sharp dissection.

From time to time, an individual who has previously had an otherwise adequate perineorrhaphy demonstrates a symptomatic rectocele that may not have been evident at the time of initial surgery (Fig. 11.4). This may appear to be an enterocele. Under such circumstances, above an adequate perineal body, the operator may simply open the posterior vaginal wall directly into the rectovaginal space through either a transverse or longitudinal incision into the vagina (Fig. 11.5). This can be performed without denuding or opening the perineum.

With lateral traction on sutures or clamps at the hymenal margin, the operator may open the rectovaginal space and establish a line of cleavage between the anterior rectal wall and the connective tissues of the rectovaginal septum, taking care not to open the often attenuated or thinned-out rectal wall. When there is excessive scar tissue resulting from episiotomy repairs, preliminary insertion of the operator's double-gloved finger into the rectum may be advisable for identification and guidance.

Figure 11.4. Perineorrhaphy hiding an unrepaired midvaginal rectocele. Effective repair must always begin proximal to the point of weakness.

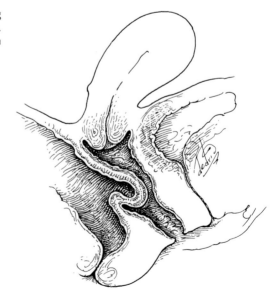

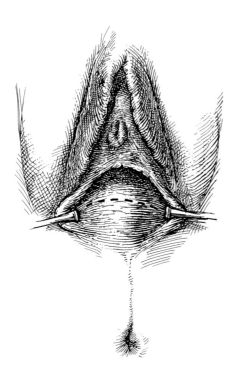

Figure 11.5. An incision for posterior colporrhaphy without perineorrhaphy. When posterior colporrhaphy without perineorrhaphy is desired, the rectovaginal space may be entered through a transverse incision through the posterior vaginal wall proximal to the perineal body.

The dissection freeing the rectum from the posterior vaginal wall and the septal tissues adherent to it should be carried to a level somewhat superior or cranial to any demonstrable rectocele (Fig. 11.6). The amount of vaginal membrane to be removed is determined by estimating the amount of excess vaginal wall; just enough should be excised to permit a normal three finger breadth vaginal introitus and vaginal caliber without demonstrable tightness and stenosis. The amount of vagina removed should take the patient's endocrine age into account, anticipating some future postmenopausal shrinkage and loss of elasticity. DeCosta (8) has called attention to the desirability of leaving the introitus of the older woman a little "loose," anticipating that the rigidity of her husband's erection may not be as firm as in his younger years. It is, in general, better to err on the side of leaving too much vaginal skin when a multilayered repair technique is being used. With this in mind, it is important not to excise any suspected excess of vaginal membrane until the repair is essentially complete, at which time the supposed excess of vaginal epithelium will often fit surprisingly well over the restored rectovaginal septum.

With a high rectocele, the apex of the vaginal incision as well as the identification and mobilization of the connective tissue that is to become the rectovaginal septum should be carried to the very apex of the vagina. It may be necessary to cut through the edge of the vaginal cuff to the attachment of the upper portion of the rectovaginal septum to the cul-de-sac. If the upper margin of the portion of the vaginal wall to be removed proves to be higher than the attachment of the rectovaginal septum to the bottom of the cul-de-sac of Douglas, the latter will likely be opened. This actually is an advantage, however, because it permits identification and facilitates shortening and suturing together the uterosacral ligaments. This can be effected under direct vision, incorporating the ligaments in the top of the posterior colporrhaphy. It provides an opportunity to estimate and excise any excess peritoneum before closing the cul-de-sac. This is particularly appropriate treatment whenever there are relationships, such as excessive width of the vault, suggesting a predisposition to the development of enterocele.

Figure 11.6. Sagittal section demonstrating the initial line of dissection exposing the full perineum and rectocele. Above the perineum the dissection enters the rectovaginal space and continues proximal to the highest point of the rectocele.

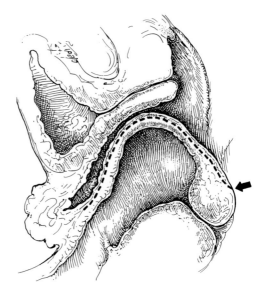

RECTAL PILLARS (DESCENDING RECTAL SEPTA)

The so-called rectal pillars (see Chapter 16) are essentially bilateral concentrations of connective tissue extending alongside the rectum from the lower margin of the uterosacral ligament to the perineal body at the level of its attachment to the levator ani. They separate the rectovaginal space from the pararectal space on either side and contain many elastic fibers within a connective tissue network with both lymphatic and vascular channels.

Enterocele frequently coexists with high rectocele. With enterocele, the posterior vaginal wall has less support from the fascia of Denonvilliers; and under such circumstances, support for the rectovaginal septum often can be developed by approximation of the rectal pillars, bringing them together in the midline anterior to the rectum. If the uterus has not been removed, the uppermost of these approximating sutures may well incorporate the uterosacral ligaments and the posterior aspect of the uterine cervix for additional strength and stability. In performing sacrospinous colpopexy (Chapter 16), it will always be necessary for the operator to penetrate the rectal pillar as he or she proceeds from the rectovaginal space to the pararectal space in the direction of the sacrospinous ligament.

Although ballooning of the anterior rectal wall appears to be the result of rectocele rather than the cause, it may be reduced with one or more layers of running locked 2-0 or 3-0 long-lasting synthetic absorbable suture, which may be continued downward posterior to the level at which the perineal body will be reconstructed (Fig. 11.7). The full thickness of the posterior vaginal wall is closed from side to side, the perineal body is reconstructed, and the perineal skin is closed.

Classical Type of Posterior Colporrhaphy

At about the 3 and 9 o'clock positions, an adequate bite of the hymen and its subcutaneous tissue is picked up by a clamp or suture to provide for lateral traction and expose the vaginal side of the perineal body. Used only for retraction, these lateral sutures or clamps are to be removed during the final steps in reconstruction. A narrow V-shaped or wider U-shaped incision is made through the perineal skin, depending on how large a perineal defect is to be repaired.

After the initial V-shaped opening through the perineal skin, a somewhat triangular segment of skin is dissected from the thus exposed structures of the perineum and peri-

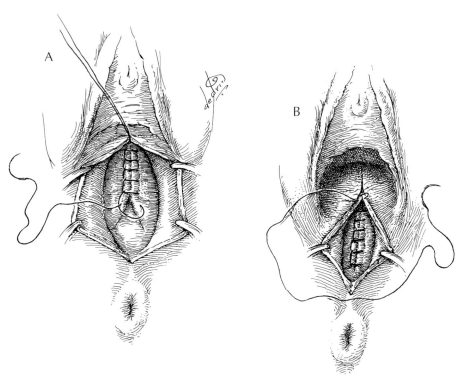

Figure 11.7. Transvaginal plication of the anterior rectal wall. **A.** Any ballooning of the anterior rectal wall may be corrected by one or more layers of running locked, fine absorbable suture commencing proximal to the defect and continuing distally for its full length. Reconstitution may be carried posterior to the site of the new perineal body, yet to be restored. **B.** Side-to-side closure of the full thickness of the posterior vaginal wall is accomplished to the proximal margin of the perineal body and fixed at its cranial margin by suture to the tissue of the rectovaginal septum. In addition, reconstruction of the perineal body may be indicated.

neal body and continued upward by undermining beneath the full thickness of the posterior wall. Adhesions tending to thicken the normal attachments of vaginal membrane may be the result of earlier obstetric damage, and all such attachments should be freed. The vaginal membrane must be freed of all appreciable fixation by scar tissue. In an older patient, when there is atrophy and narrowing of the tissues and skin of the perineum, but when coital ability is to be preserved, only an initial midline skin incision that exposes the subcutaneous tissue of the perineum may be desirable (Fig. 11.8). Occasionally, an inverted T-shaped incision may be made in the posterior vaginal wall to facilitate access to the rectovaginal space. In all repairs of a rectocele it is essential that the vaginal membrane be separated from any and all pathologic adhesions to the perineal body and the rectal wall, to a point well above any demonstrable rectocele. The perineal skin flaps are then undermined and freed up, exposing the surfaces of what is usually a distorted or irregularly deficient perineum, and displaying the defective segments that are to be reconstructed into a more normal perineal body.

After the rectovaginal space is entered as previously described, any anterior ballooning of the rectum may be readily corrected by one or more layers of running locked, fine absorbable sutures placed in the muscularis and connective tissue of the anterior rectal wall, from points both above and below the extent of the area of demonstrable rectocele. The rectal muscularis (and internal anal sphincter) are plicated by a running locked

Figure 11.8. Midline incision for perineorrhaphy. When there is atrophy and narrowing of perineal skin, an initial midline perineal incision may be desirable to expose the base or inferior surface of the perineal body.

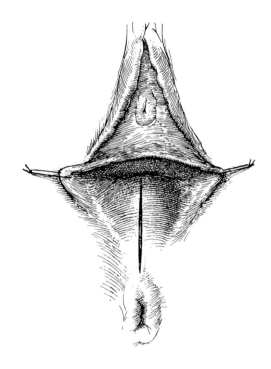

suture as shown in Figure 11.7. Ideally, this should include the submucosal layer, but this is difficult to do without compromising the mucosa, unless it is done with one of the operator's fingers in the rectum to palpate the placement of each suture.

The rectum may be displaced posteriorly by a retractor; and after incision of the estimated excess of vaginal membrane, the cut edges of the full thickness of the posterior vaginal wall, including the still adherent fibers of the rectovaginal septum, are brought together by a running subcuticular suture of 0 or 00 synthetic long-lasting absorbable suture. At the apex, this suture might well include a generous bite of the lateral vaginal connective tissue of the paracolpium, and possibly even the most inferior portion of the uterosacral ligaments (Fig. 11.9) if the incision and dissection have been carried into this area. The running subcuticular suture or sutures should carefully and purposefully avoid attachment to the fascia over the levator ani but should be continued to end in the cranial border of the perineal body. When, on occasion, the vaginal wall seems unusually thin and it may not appear desirable to employ subcuticular suturing, a running locked suture through the full thickness of the posterior vaginal wall, if so placed as to avoid invagination of the cut edges, may be used to reunite the vaginal membrane in the midline. If the vaginal membrane is noticeably thin, as is often seen in a postmenopausal vagina, the stimulus of several weeks of preoperative estrogen therapy may increase blood loss during the operation. However, the resulting vaginal membrane is thicker to close and seems to heal more rapidly. Particularly in the closure of vaginal membrane, it is important, first, that sutures bring the tissues together without tension and, second, that knots not be tied so tightly as to blanch the tissues appreciably. The risk of such strangulation is particularly great when interrupted mattress-type sutures are being tied. This classical type of posterior colporrhaphy was described by Goff (11).

In our modification of the frequently used Goff technique, a wedge or segment of what is estimated to be the proper size and shape is excised from the whole length and full thickness of the posterior vaginal wall, while the septal layer is left attached. It is important to have carefully estimated a sufficient vaginal circumference for satisfactory sexual function. The amount of vaginal wall to be retained, and therefore the size of the

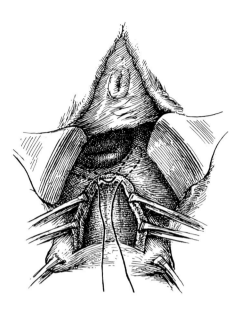

Figure 11.9. Apical suture including the uterosacral ligaments. The suture closing the posterior vaginal wall might, at its apex, include a generous bite of the lateral vaginal connective tissue and, when possible, the uterosacral ligaments.

vagina after colporrhaphy, varies according to the age of the patient, her parity, and the presence or amount of estrogenic hormones.

The lateral cut edges of the vagina, to which the rectovaginal septum has remained fused, are then approximated by intravaginal subcuticular or interrupted sutures (Fig. 11.10), leaving the rectum and its facial investments uninvolved in this suturing and capable of natural independent movement. At the completion of this phase of a posterior repair, the operator should be able to insert a finger between the anterior rectal wall and the reconstituted rectovaginal septum throughout the full length of the repair, demonstrating restoration of the functional independence of the rectal and vaginal walls and the absence of iatrogenic fixation of the rectal wall (Fig. 11.11). The attenuated levator fascia may have been united only in the lower half or third of the vagina, thus permitting a more normal horizontal tilt to the upper vagina. The subvaginal portion of the perineal body is restored by interrupted sutures, and the suture line is continued down the vaginal wall and over the perineal body and back to the hymenal margin.

POSTERIOR COLPORRHAPHY BY LAYERS

The Goff technique of posterior colporrhaphy usually will ensure an anatomically acceptable result, but it may not be as certain to restore the integrity and function of a rectovaginal septum as can be ensured by the layering technique of Bullard. This layering technique essentially consists of (*a*) separation of the septal tissues, first from the anterior rectal wall, and second from the overlying vaginal membrane, and (*b*) thickening of the resulting layer of loosely arranged musculoconnective tissue and restoration of an appreciable layer of septum by several plicating sutures of fine suture.

The dissection and repair should involve the following principles:

1. The posterior vaginal wall should be incised in the midline to a point well above the rectocele, as far as the apex of the vagina when a high rectocele and/or enterocele is present.
2. The rectovaginal space is then identified and the rectal wall separated by blunt dissection from the overlying connective tissue of the rectovaginal septum, usually without difficulty.

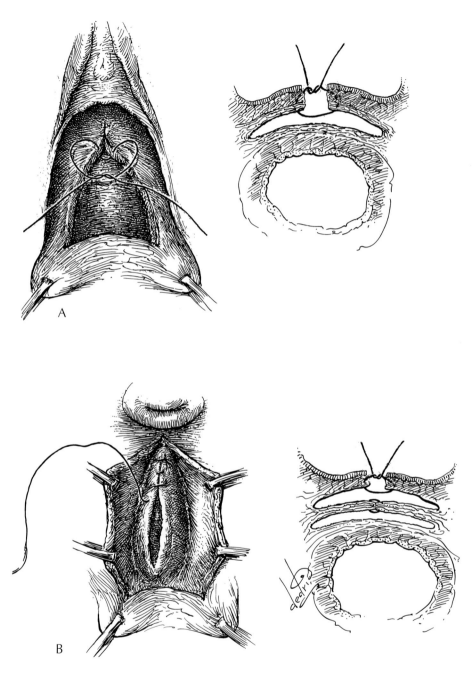

Figure 11.10. Types of closing the vagina with posterior colporrhaphy. **A.** In the Goff method, an appropriate full-thickness wedge of posterior vaginal wall has been excised, and the tissues, including the fused rectovaginal septum, are closed from side to side. A subcuticular suture is preferred. **B.** The Bullard modification. The rectovaginal septum has been dissected from the posterior vaginal wall and closed as a separate layer between rectum and vaginal membrane. When this has been accomplished, excess vaginal membrane is trimmed, and the sides are brought together by interrupted suture. A running subcuticular suture may be used.

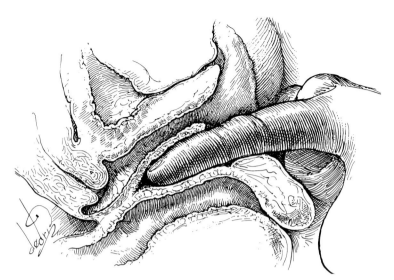

Figure 11.11. Demonstrating preservation of the rectovaginal space. At the completion of the posterior colporrhaphy and before starting the perineorrhaphy, the operator should be able to insert an index finger freely between the posterior vaginal wall to which the rectovaginal septum is attached and the anterior surface of the rectum, demonstrating the desired freedom of the rectovaginal space.

3. Using curved Mayo scissors, by spreading the points in demonstrable planes of cleavage more than by cutting into or through tissue layers, the vaginal membrane may then be reflected anteriorly and away from the connective tissue.

The result is (*a*) a thinned and bulging anterior rectal wall readily identified, (*b*) a loose and somewhat thinned posterior vaginal wall that appears excessive for the caliber of the vagina that is to be restored, and (*c*) a loosely incomplete, somewhat fragmented, and partially detached layer, often only sections of intervening connective tissues, all of which should be carefully preserved and should be incorporated by plication with fine suture material into a restoration of a demonstrably stronger rectovaginal septum.

The tissues of the carefully identified rectovaginal septal layer, throughout a width approximating 3 cm and a length of 5 to 6 cm, are united in the midline. Although thickened by a few plicating sutures, this septum is not attached by suture to either the underlying rectal wall or to the overlying posterior vaginal membrane.

When demonstrating this technique, it was Bullard's habit, after a few sutures had thickened the rectovaginal septum and the edges of the vagina had been trimmed and reunited in the midline (but before suturing to restore the perineal body), to demonstrate the integrity of this rectovaginal septum and its nonattachment to either the vaginal or rectal walls. He would do this by simultaneously inserting two fingers into the space available on either side of the septum, one finger between septum and vaginal wall, the other between the septum and rectal wall. Reduced adhesion between the layers of repair will favor independent mobility of the vagina and the rectum, which we believe should be an important objective of a posterior vaginal repair.

We believe it should be axiomatic that, just as a surgeon might not capriciously discard viable tissue that can be incorporated in the repair of a herniating viscus, the gynecologist need not excise tissue usable in restoring a rectovaginal septum simply because it is adherent to an assumed excess of posterior vaginal wall that will probably be excised. Rather, the gynecologist might carefully identify a line of cleavage that separates connective tissue from the redundant posterior vaginal membrane; after being thickened by fine plicating sutures, this layer may well serve to restore the integrity of a significant rectovaginal septum, which becomes interposed between the anterior rectal wall and the posterior vaginal membrane. Restoration of a recognizable septal layer is an objective and the distinctive characteristic of Bullard's modification of Goff's technique of posterior colporrhaphy.

At the completion of a vaginal repair, there is critical need for an objective evaluation of the result. If the result is not satisfactory and a satisfactory vaginal depth and axis have not been achieved, this is the optimal time for any needed correction or modification. If the patient's condition permits, prolongation of this initial operation is certainly preferable to bringing the patient back for a second operation. A vaginal caliber that is tight at the end of surgery cannot be expected to enlarge after healing is complete. As a matter of fact, if any change occurs, and particularly as the patient grows older, a tight vagina tends to become smaller.

If it is found that, in spite of the operator's intention, the repair has resulted in a vaginal caliber obviously or even suspiciously tight, appropriate relaxing incisions may be made through the thickness of the lateral vaginal walls (see Chapter 20); but when this has been done, the vagina should then be rather tightly packed for 24 hours and the edges of the incision kept apart by nightly wearing of an obturator until the base of the wound is covered by granulation tissue, usually in about 3 weeks. When necessary, full-thickness grafts may be sewn into incisions parallel with the axis of the vagina and made at the point or points of constriction, utilizing vaginal membrane previously resected from either the anterior or the posterior vaginal wall. With this possibility in mind, when portions of the vaginal membrane have been excised, they should be kept wrapped in moist, saline-soaked sponges on the nurse's instrument stand until the conclusion of the operation.

When a suture or sutures are palpated or visualized within the lumen of the rectum, that portion of the suture within the rectal lumen should be immediately cut in order to lessen postoperative pain and the chance of rectovaginal or rectoperineal fistula. The cut ends will promptly retract up and out of the rectal lumen. The effectiveness of the repair should not be jeopardized by the loss of the effect of that single suture.

To minimize oozing and collection of fluid within the spaces between layers, we sometimes pack the vagina lightly with 2-inch plain or iodoform gauze, which we prefer to remove the morning of the day after surgery.

As a result of our studies and experience with these operative techniques, it appears to us that the apparently divergent conclusions of Uhlenhuth and Nolley (39) and Ricci and Thom (28) can now be reconciled. The marked degree of natural fusion of the rectovaginal septum to the posterior vaginal wall makes its histologic demonstration difficult except by special connective tissue staining. During dissection, on the other hand, a septum can be readily identified in a most consistent manner, but only when definite effort to do so has been made. Because for a number of years we have been identifying the septum in the manner described and have been pleased with the results of the technique as described, we recommend these procedures for the consideration of others.

ANATOMY OF THE PERINEUM

Probably the most thorough of contemporary studies of the pelvic outlet and female perineum has been that of Joachimovits (16). He described the connective tissue and smooth muscle system that stems from the os coccyx forward to the urogenital diaphragm and os pubis. Especially in the middle, and in cooperation with the fasciae and transversely striated muscles of this region, this system participates in the creation of a sort of sagittally suspended, supporting carrying strap that represents a protection against descent and prolapse of the pelvic outlet. Therefore, the central tendon of the perineum can be described as a very tightly woven connective tissue structure interspersed with smooth and striated muscle fibers and many elastic fibers, as well as small vessels and nerves. Its distal part reaches to the perineal skin and the upper part to the rectovaginal septum.

The size and attachments of the perineal body are predictably different between the living and the dead, since muscular tonus is absent in the latter. Its strength also appears to be subject to wide individual variation. When well developed, it has the configuration of a pyramid with the base down. It is divided into two distinct parts, a distal fibrous part that is covered by the superficial perineal muscles and that penetrates the border of the urogenital diaphragm, and a cranial part that extends to the rectovaginal septum and contains considerably more smooth and striated fibers. It is connected with the lowermost anterior rectal wall by means of smooth muscle bundles. Some striated prerectal fibers of the levator are found in this part of the perineal body, as well as some fibers of the sphincter ani profundus.

The distal fibrous part of the central tendon of the perineum forms a close union with all the superficial striated perineal muscles. The perineal body is composed of two parts, which can be recognized in its embryology. It comes from two vertical folds of the lateral wall of the cloaca, allowing recognition of ventral and dorsal portions. Growing together in the midline, these folds, together with a crescent-shaped folded mesenchyme covered with epithelium (the urorectal septum), permanently separate the rectum from the urogenital sinus. The lower, usual distal, part arising from mesenchyme located under the skin has only secondarily combined with the larger dorsal part. Subepithelial masses of mesoderm on the distant cloacal part come from both sides to the primitive perineal arrangement. These striated muscle bundles inside the perineal body are derivates of the sphincter of the cloaca. Smooth muscle elements arise from the outer longitudinal muscles of the anterior rectum and the muscle of the posterior vaginal wall.

The superficial or caudal part of the perineal body, which is attached to the superficial perineal muscles, is thus fixed to the ischial tuberosities. It is further fastened by the superficial sphincter ani and ventrally to the bulbocavernosi, although the extent and development of each of these muscles are subject to wide individual variation. Superficially, the perineal body is attached to Colles' fascia.

On the border between the distal and proximal part of the perineal body, the medial margins of the pubococcygei are in contact with the lateral surfaces of the perineal body. Some terminate on the lateral surface of the perineal body (prerectal fibers), but the larger, more lateral bundles pass alongside the rectum to fuse into the levator plate, which extends from the rectum to the coccyx. The existence of these prerectal fibers of the levator muscle can be proven only in man. Joachimovits (16) has described two main bundles on each side, of varying thickness but up to 3 to 4 mm in width, that appear to originate from the pubococcygei at their cranial attachment. The fibers intermingle with those of the deep transverse perinei. When the superficial transverse perinei muscles are missing and the deep transverse perinei poorly developed, one will usually find well-developed prerectal bundles.

The pubovaginalis muscles, closely related to the pubococcygei, pass by the urethra to the connective tissue in the sidewalls near the border of the lower and middle third of the vagina at the level of attachment of the cranial portion of the perineal body to the rectovaginal septum. They form a rather weak muscle sling around the posterior vaginal wall of varying degrees of strength. Occasionally, the entire bundle appears to have been replaced by connective tissue. Because this bundle originates on the pubis, it appears to be more closely related to the puborectalis than to the pubococcygeus.

A small periurethral bundle of levator muscle, heavily mixed with connective tissue elements, attaches to the midportion of the lateral and lower urethral wall. It is superficial to the pubourethrovaginal ligament, but as the muscle and the ligament approach one another on the urethra, there appears to be some blending of their respective fibers. This blending may, in fact, represent portions of terminal fibers from the pubococcygeus that compress the urethra just cranial to its midportion, and probably accounts for the higher intraurethral pressure that is here rather than in either the proximal or distal urethra, as was shown in the normal urethra by Enhorning (9).

The vast majority of muscle fibers that run to the perineum terminate upon the lateral part of the perineal body, though a few fibers may penetrate the perineal body to meet with the opposite side.

The observations of Joachimovits suggest that the prerectal fibers are innervated exclusively by the perineal nerve, whereas the rest of the levator gets its innervation from the pudendal nerve terminating on the pelvic side of the levator ani. He believes that this explains how prerectal muscle bundles can contract independently from the remainder of the levator. The prerectal fibers, genetically much younger than other parts of the levator muscle, testify to their fundamental levator origin by exclusive innervation from this branch of the pudendal nerve.

When the rectococcygeus is present, it may meet its fellow of the opposite side at a point between the rectum and the tip of the coccyx. It may function as a sling that fuses to the outer longitudinal muscle of the rectal wall. Many smooth muscle cells are attached to the medial edges of the levator pillars in the midline, and their clinical significance was investigated by Studdiford (34). The smooth muscle concentration is greater at the dorsal proximal part of the perineal body than at the ventral distal part, to which are attached the aponeurosis and fascia of the deep perineal muscles.

DEFECTS IN THE PERINEUM

An inadequate or defective perineum may result in such an exposure of the midportion of the posterior vaginal wall as to constitute a pseudorectocele (see Fig. 11.3), as noted by Richter (29). Careful digital examination of the rectum will differentiate pseudorectocele from true rectocele. Pseudorectocele is characterized by normal rectal caliber, angulation, and tone, and the posterior vaginal and anterior rectal walls are independent. When a true rectocele has developed, however, the adjacent vaginal and rectal walls will often be joined together with a loss of vaginal rugae over the rectocele and a tendency of the rectum to form a pouch. The pouch can be demonstrated easily when the examiner's finger flexes and extends anteriorly. This ballooning segment can become a pathologic pocket that may trap fecal material, causing incomplete bowel movements as well as postevacuation discomfort.

Defects in the perineum are usually the result of obstetric damage, either from unrepaired or inadequately repaired laceration, or from an ill-timed or incompletely repaired episiotomy. Incomplete repair results in lateral retraction of muscles that are normally attached to the perineal body. Detachment or interruption of the transverse perinei and the bulbocavernosus must be recognized and corrected. Not only will the repair aid in the support of the anterior wall of the rectum, but it will also add considerable support to the anterior wall of the lower vagina and urethra. In this connection, it should be remembered that the length of the perineal body effectively approximates the length of the female urethra, in part because of the passage of the medial portion of the pubococcygeus muscle along the sides of the vagina, urethra, and rectum. This muscle sends slips of connective tissue to fuse with the capsule tissue investing every one of these hollow organs. When indicated, appropriate and adequate perineorrhaphy effectively complements the support of the anterior vaginal wall and the urethra.

In examination of the patient before posterior colporrhaphy, it is important to recognize, as emphasized by Davies (7), that

Any perineal laceration which permits the labia minora to retract laterally and expose a gaping vagina harbors the divided and retracted origin of the bulbocavernosus muscle. Such a lesion lowers the efficiency of the voluntary urethral sphincter and should be considered as an etiologic basis for stress incontinence in the female.*

The operator should also carefully note the position of the patient's anus in relation to the most dependent portion of the buttocks, the tip of the coccyx, and the ischial tuberosities. Posterior displacement of the anus strongly suggests detachment of the anal sphincter from the perineum. This may also be noted with a defect of the levator ani, either because of an intrinsic fault of the muscle or as a result of defective innervation of this voluntary muscle. In either instance, regardless of etiology, straining during defecation may, in effect, produce elongation and funneling of the levator ani, with the anus descending to an even more dependent position. The harder the patient strains, the narrower the stool must become, and the more difficult to defecate. Obstipation is often the result. Barrett (2) proposed that an incision be made posterior to the rectum, and the separated levators attached to each other and to the rectal wall. This technique is considered in the description of retrorectal levatorplasty in Chapter 14.

It should be remembered that, historically, the objective of perineorrhaphy was to improve the patient's ability to retain a pessary. Unfortunately, all too often this concept has been extended to an erroneous comparison to a cork plugging the neck of an inverted bottle. This inadequate and erroneous but popular concept visualizes a good perineal repair as not only preventing progression of upper vaginal prolapse, but also as a factor preventing the development of genital prolapse in general. We disagree with this concept and would refer skeptics to the observation that genital prolapse is uncommon among women with unrepaired third- and fourth-degree obstetric lacerations who have long suffered a complete loss of any support that the perineal body would have offered the uterus, cervix, and upper vagina.

PERINEAL BODY

Because the perineal body in the woman is a structure of considerable anatomic and physiologic importance, the basic objective of perineorrhaphy is to restore an effective perineal body, with realignment of muscles and connective tissues to a degree that will ensure normal relationships and encourage normal, comfortable function.

It must be remembered that the principal portion of the levator ani concerned with support of the lower vagina and birth canal attaches to the sides of the vaginal connective tissue through the fibers of Luschka rather than to the muscular tissues of the posterior vaginal wall itself. Although the levator ani may be lengthened, displaced laterally, and sometimes detached as a result of perineal laceration or other obstetric trauma, damage to the levator ani may also produce only a midvaginal rectocele cranial to the perineal body. When examining such a patient, it is important to note whether external hemorrhoids are present, because weakness of the perineum and anal sphincter may contribute to their development. When there is prolapse of the upper vagina and cervix, however, the distention of the genital hiatus by the protrusion may have lessened the tone of the introitus musculature by much the same mechanism as the dilating wedge of an enterocele in this area may widen the pelvic outlet. Much of the tone of the lateral vaginal walls will be regained after an effective repair, largely as a result of the removal of a major causative factor (the prolapsing cervix, uterus, or enterocele).

Most so-called levator stitches result only in increased approximation of thinned or separated layers of the perineal body and do not usually result in a buildup of the levator itself. If placed far enough laterally to include only the fascia of the pelvic diaphragm, they may reinforce a defective pelvic diaphragm, but if placed directly into the belly of the levator muscle, these sutures may actually destroy portions of the muscle, eventually

---

* From Davies JW. Quoted in Embryology and anatomy. In: Ullery JC, ed. Stress incontinence in the female. New York: Grune & Stratton, 1953:53. Used with permission.

resulting in a shell-like ridge of nonelastic fibrous tissue within the introitus and immediately beneath the posterior vaginal wall. It is preferable to place superficial, side-to-side stitches because they will usually reconstitute the perineal body and draw the fascia of the pubococcygeal muscles closer to the upper lateral sides of the perineal body. This will effectively narrow the widened genital hiatus.

The extent to which reconstruction of a very loose vaginal outlet will contribute to coital satisfaction has been undoubtedly overemphasized. A consensus of the more thoughtful gynecologists recognizes that a noticeable looseness of the vagina is not a common cause of marital incompatibility; therefore, prophylactic "tightening up" of the introitus will not necessarily improve marital relations, which are frayed more often by nonanatomic factors. More realistic considerations of domestic satisfactions must take into account the several factors that are to be involved. However, indicated correction (but not overcorrection) of a damaged or relaxed perineal body can be expected to improve coital satisfaction within an otherwise compatible domestic relationship.

The caliber of the premenopausal or estrogen-maintained vagina with respect to the accommodation of an erect penis has wide limits of compatibility, since vaginal elasticity permits the vagina under normal circumstances to grasp or contain the male organ much as an expansile rubber glove grasps a finger. Thus the normal-sized vagina can adapt comfortably and adequately to a large male organ as well as to a small one. The elasticity of the vagina is therefore important in preserving coital harmony, and unnecessary surgical procedures that tend to result in fibrosis and rigidity should be avoided.

The argument as to which muscle bundles do or do not penetrate the perineal body is, in large part, more academic than practical. The gynecologic surgeon should not regularly attempt to bring muscle bundles into the perineal body that were not there to begin with and should not try to incorporate them in the repair, because such displaced bundles are more likely to be replaced by fibrosis, with a resulting loss of elasticity and persistent tenderness. To understand the objective of repair, we should start with a fairly definite concept of normal fibromuscular attachments and relationships of the perineal body. Making allowance for individual variation, we must also recognize the function of each component and attachment if our effort to restore the more essential relationships is to succeed.

Because the perineal body may be visualized as roughly pyramidal, a repair must restore this body in all three dimensions. The base of the pyramid is situated beneath and parallels the perineal skin. The anterior, posterior, and two lateral surfaces all converge superiorly to the most inferior limit of the rectovaginal space, fusing with the lowermost margin of the rectovaginal septum (Chapter 1).

Although the perineum has been likened to the keystone of an arch, such an analogy is inappropriate. The base of such a keystone would be its widest part, and gravity would pull it down and out of position rather than wedging it more firmly in place, as would be true if the wide part were at the cranial end.

TECHNIQUE OF PERINEORRHAPHY

Reconstruction of the perineal body begins with uncovering the perineal body along its base beneath the perineal skin and on the vaginal (anterosuperior) side. Excess vaginal wall and skin are mobilized, and then the reconstruction is performed. This is often accomplished by side-to-side reapproximation of denuded tissues both deep and superficial. The upper portion of this side-to-side reapproximation of the perineal body should pull the pubococcygei closer without actually including them in the sutures. As a result, the genital hiatus is narrowed. Lower-placed stitches also help to reconstruct the lower portion of the urogenital diaphragm, bringing the transverse perinei together. Similar sutures reattach the bulbocavernosus muscles to the perineal body.

A transverse incision for perineorrhaphy not only carries with it the potential of providing incomplete exposure of the inferior surface of the base of the perineal body, but also adds the additional risk of facilitating creation of a ridgelike, "dashboard perineum" with the probability of associated dyspareunia. This undesirable result is so likely because an inadequate incision directs the surgeon's attention to reconstructing only the anterior and upper portion of the perineal body, because that is the only area he or she has exposed or denuded, leaving the equally important mid- and posteroinferior portions of the perineal body unexposed and not involved in the repair.

For this reason, a "standard" transverse incision is not recommended unless a significant perineal body reconstruction is not planned, and unless the surgeon's intent and efforts are to be directed to the repair of a rectocele well above the perineal body.

After clamps or traction sutures have been applied to the hymenal margin on either side, we prefer to make a V-shaped incision (Fig. 11.12) in the perineal skin layer (U-shaped for especially large perineal defects). The width of the base of this triangle, in relation to the hymenal margin, should be estimated in accordance with the desired size of the resultant vaginal introitus. The greater the amount of epithelium removed, the smaller will be the caliber of the resulting vaginal orifice. A V-shaped incision in the perineal skin will ensure better access to more of the tissues of the perineal body than would be possible with the usual transverse incision along the posterior hymenal margin.

It is important to place the lateral traction sutures or clamps on the hymenal ring and not on the labia minora. This placement prevents obstruction from a superficial transverse ridge or dashboardlike perineum, which may result if the retracting forceps or sutures are too lateral.

All scar tissue is freed by sharp dissection (Fig. 11.13). Reapproximation of the cut vaginal wall is accomplished by a running subcuticular suture. The anterior wall of the freed rectum is imbricated by a running mattress stitch as shown in Figure 11.14. The

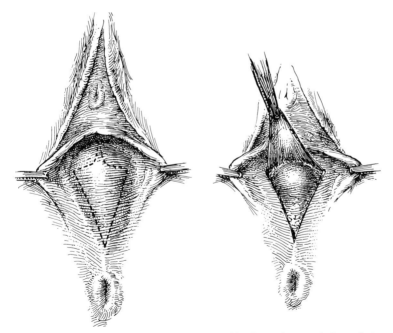

Figure 11.12. Exposing the underside of the perineal body. A diamond-shaped piece of tissue of an appropriate width has been carefully estimated (*left*). The amount of perineal skin to be removed is determined by the quantity of excess tissue; just enough should be excised to permit a normal three-finger breadth vaginal introitus without stenosis. It is better to err on the side of leaving a little too much tissue than too little. The dissection is carried cranially into the vagina, exposing the full site of the future perineal body. If rectocele is present, the rectovaginal space is entered, and the dissection freeing rectum from vagina is carried to a level above any rectocele that is present.

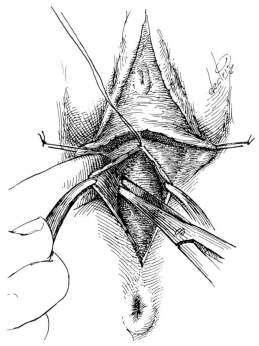

Figure 11.13. Dissection of scar tissue. Scar tissue attached to introital skin is carefully freed by sharp dissection, so that the tissue from which a perineal body will be built can be mobilized readily.

Figure 11.14. Closure of the posterior vaginal wall and imbrication of the rectum. The vaginal walls are approximated by a running subcuticular suture, and the anterior rectal wall imbricated by a running mattress stitch.

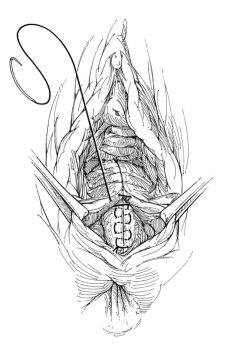

deep tissues of the perineum are united in the midline by a series of interrupted mattress sutures (Fig. 11.15).

It is of utmost importance that any detachment of the connective tissue of the rectovaginal septum from the cranial or uppermost portion of the perineal body be remedied by surgical reattachment that will ensure restoration of normal function, particularly as regards the role of the perineum and its continuity with the rectovaginal septum during the act of defecation. Because considerable scarring from previous trauma may be found in this vulnerable area, dissection through indistinct cleavage planes should proceed with caution to avoid entering the rectum. After this reattachment and restoration by a figure-of-eight suture (Fig. 11.16), incomplete bowel movements may be relieved and a recurrence will be unlikely.

During reconstruction of the lower third of the vagina in advanced cases, when there is little tissue with which to work, it sometimes, though rarely, may be necessary to provide better support to the rectal ampulla (Fig. 11.17) to bring the medial margins of the puborectalis or pubococcygei muscles together by a small series of superficially placed and loosely tied interrupted sutures, which, in turn, may at their insertion be attached to a sagging ampulla. Although at times highly desirable, it is important that such support be accomplished without production of troublesome and inevitably tender ridges beneath the posterior vaginal wall. After each stitch is placed, the ends of the suture should be crossed before they are tied and traction is applied. If a ridge is palpated, the stitch should be promptly removed and replaced, usually closer to the rectum. When perineal surgery is performed under local anesthesia, the voluntary muscle bundles may be more readily identified.

The retracted ends of often long-separated bulbocavernosus muscles should be first identified and then reattached to the perineal body. Separated segments of the transverse perinei should also be reunited if the medial edge of the levator ani and the puborectalis can be identified. For correction of a low rectocele, the adjacent fascia of the pelvic diaphragm is attached to the posterolateral surface of the vagina, duplicating the original attachment of the fibers of Luschka, and fixing and holding the vagina in place. The smooth muscle of the perineal body should then be brought together by a few interrupted mattress sutures to reestablish its integrity (Fig. 11.18).

Although not a common result of perineal injury during childbirth, when posterior displacement of the anus occurs, it is essential that it be repaired. It is necessary to re-

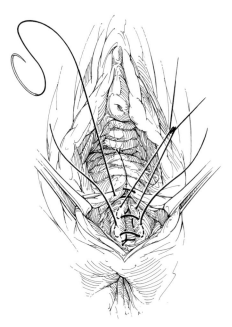

Figure 11.15. Reconstruction of the deep tissues of the perineum. Interrupted mattress stitches bring the perirectal fascia and deeper tissues of the perineum together in the midline.

Figure 11.16. Reattachment of rectovaginal septum to perineal body. The bulging of the anterior rectal wall has been corrected by a running locked suture of polyglycolic acid. The perineal body will be reconstructed in front of this repair. The rectovaginal septum (fascia of Denonvilliers), which is fused to the underside of the posterior vaginal wall, is reattached to the perineal body by a figure-of-eight stitch.

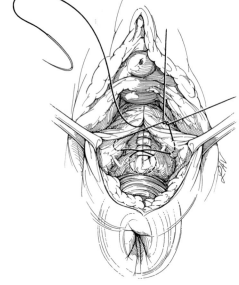

Figure 11.17. Optimal approximation of pubococcygeal fascia. In occasional instances of extreme perineal defect, it may be desirable to bring the fascia of each pubococcygeus together in the midline in front of the rectum; palpable ridges of tissue must be carefully avoided.

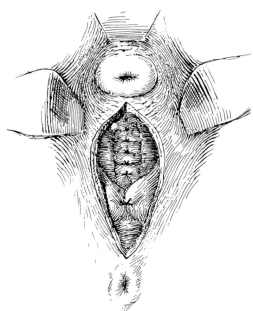

attach the capsule of the external sphincter ani to the perineal body, such as by using a figure-of-eight suture (Fig. 11.19), as described by Kennedy and Campbell (17). This step stabilizes the perineum in a way similar to reattachment of the spokes to the hub of a wheel (perineal body).

Operative compression of the veins communicating with hemorrhoids will often temporarily aggravate hemorrhoids that may have been present; but as postoperative edema subsides, a new tissue equilibrium is usually established after which the hemorrhoids may undergo involution and improvement, especially if any sphincter weakness has been corrected. For this reason, hemorrhoidectomy should not be done at the same time as a posterior colporrhaphy. The need for hemorrhoidectomy can better be evaluated postoperatively after several months.

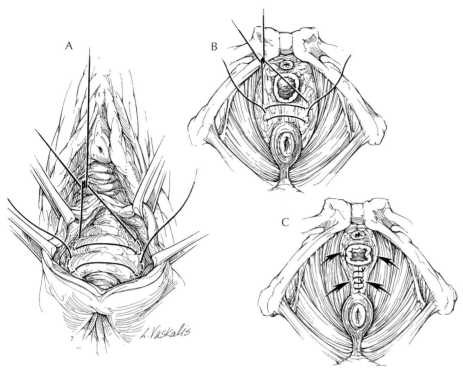

Figure 11.18. Perineal reconstruction without levator plication. **A.** Perineorrhaphy may be accomplished *without* placing stitches directly into the muscle bellies of the pubococcygei, as shown here with a wide genital hiatus. **B.** Phantom drawing of wide hiatus. **C.** When the interrupted stitches in the perineal body have been tied, the lateral attachments of this tissue to the fascia of the pubococcygei will bring the latter closer together (*arrows*), narrowing the genital hiatus to a new and normal position. No stitches have been placed directly into the muscular substance of the pubococcygei.

The superficial perineal fascia may be brought together using running or interrupted sutures, and then the perineal skin may be closed with running or interrupted sutures. Subcuticular sutures should be used in the closure of both the vaginal epithelium and the perineal skin, taking care to avoid irregularities in the approximation of the edges being united or in invaginations of epithelial edges. Irregular bulging or invaginations in the suture line will result in granulations and irregularities in healing that may account for persistent tenderness in the scar.

When a patient's perineum is defective or is absent, Byron Inmon (personal communication, 1981) has shown that the vaginal depth, that is, the length of the posterior vaginal wall, will be increased by perineorrhaphy (Fig. 11.20).

ENDORECTAL REPAIR OF RECTOCELE

Although the primary defect permitting rectocele is in the wall of the vagina and its support, and is therefore remedied by posterior colporrhaphy and perineorrhaphy, a secondary defect may be produced by thinning of the rectal submucosa, the strongest layer of the rectal wall (12), which will increase the size of the rectal reservoir. When the latter exists, and not repairable transvaginally, it may be treated by an endorectal plication using obliterative sutures, which should effectively reduce the pathologically increased size of the rectal reservoir. This should not be done at the same time as transvaginal repair, however, since any infection in the rectovaginal space with a fresh operative

Figure 11.19. Correction of detachment of the anus from the perineal body. Detachment of the anal sphincter from the perineal body may be corrected by a buried figure-of-eight suture placed as shown. This will stabilize both the anus and the perineal body.

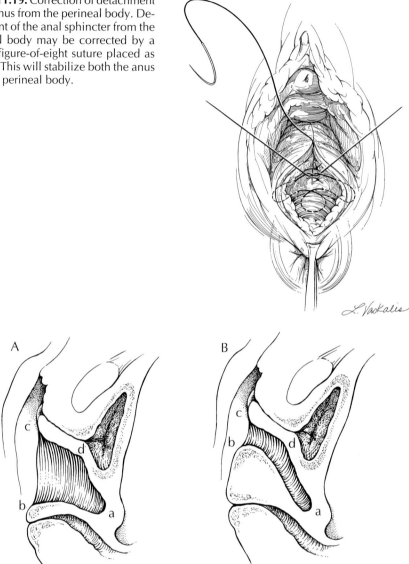

Figure 11.20. The effect of perineorrhaphy upon lengthening the posterior vaginal wall. **A.** Sagittal drawing of the pelvis of a patient with a defective perineum. The anterior vaginal wall (*adc*) is longer than the posterior wall (*ab*). **B.** Lengthening of the posterior vagina (*ab*) after perineorrhaphy. The length of the anterior vaginal wall (*adc*) is unchanged.

wound on both the vaginal and the rectal side would predispose to rectovaginal fistula formation.

In most instances, symptomatic and persistent postoperative ballooning of the anterior rectal wall can be treated by reducing rectal luminal size with transanal, endorectal suture imbrication of the anterior rectal wall using a running, locked stitch placed directly into the perirectal fascial capsule and rectal muscularis. This should restore the rectal reservoir to nearly its former size and relieve the symptom of incomplete bowel movements.

Such imbricating stitches are generally not placed transvaginally in the rectal submucosal layer of tissue because of the proximity to the rectal mucosa. Occasionally, after suture absorption, the resultant scar in the rectal muscularis is insufficient to maintain reduction of the pathologically large size of the rectal reservoir, and the patient's symptom of incomplete evacuation returns even though the vagina and perineum have been restored to a normal anatomic state. This can be remedied by an endorectal reduction in the size of the rectal reservoir using longitudinal plication of the strong rectal submucosal layer beyond its area of pathologic thinning and including the full thickness of the adjacent mucosa and muscularis. The techniques are relatively simple and uncomplicated (22). This is a good therapeutic option for the treatment of a rare posterior rectocele (Fig. 11.21) if it is symptomatic.

Jansen et al. (14) noted the importance of the submucosal layers in intestinal healing; these layers were first described by Halsted (12) as the strongest part of the intestinal wall. Lord et al. (19) demonstrated by scanning electron microscopy that the layers are a honeycomb of collagen fibers forming a strong skeletonlike cylinder through the entire length of the intestine. The cylinder contains a plexus of arterial vascularization (33). Lord et al. determined that surgical anastomosis with inversion of the intestinal layers with good submucosal approximation resulted in primary intestinal healing and rapid restoration of villous epithelium, but bad approximation resulted in secondary healing with a predictably weaker scar.

Sehapayak (30) has emphasized that simultaneous transvaginal posterior repair coincident with endorectal repair of rectocele is contraindicated, since simultaneous interruption of the natural barriers or mucosal lining on each side of the rectovaginal septum may, by the extrasurgical manipulation required, invite infection, abscess formation, and subsequent rectovaginal fistula.

Endorectal repair is a relatively simple operation to correct residual low or midvaginal rectocele and is designed to reduce the size of the luminal rectal reservoir. Sullivan, Leaverton, and Hardwick (35) first described the endorectal repair of rectocele. This repair permitted, after mucosal incision and dissection of flaps, a transanal exposure and plication of the underside of the rectovaginal septum, excision of redundant or prolapsed rectal mucosa, and correction of any coincident anorectal pathology.

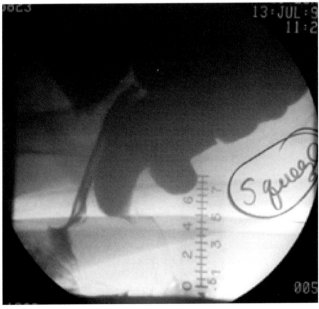

Figure 11.21. Posterior rectocele. The radiologically opacified vagina is noted to the *left* of the photograph, the rectum to the *right*. Notice the rectocele arising from the posterior wall of the rectum. (From Linda Brubaker, M.D., Rush-Presbyterian-St. Luke's Medical Center, Chicago, Illinois. Used with permission.)

As emphasized by Capps (5) and by Khubchandani (18) and associates, the endo-rectal repair can be done under local infiltration anesthesia during a short hospitalization. This approach also permits transrectal reattachment of the puborectalis to the perineal body. These authors report a high rate of success and low incidence of complications. Our patients, however, seem to prefer a short general anesthetic.

Preoperative rectal mechanical cleansing such as by electrolyte solution given the morning before surgery, or enemas until clear, adds little to the total preparatory time. The operation is performed as follows: The rectum is manually dilated to three finger breadths and a Fansler rectal retractor is inserted, the obturator removed, and each quadrant of the rectal mucosa carefully examined. At the site of the rectocele and defect in the submucosa, the anterior rectal wall usually is identified, the full thickness of the weakened rectal wall is grasped by an Allis clamp applied to the distal margins, and a suture of absorbable material—either polyglycolic acid or chromic catgut, size 00—is placed through the full thickness of the rectal wall and tied (Fig. 11.22). All of this ex-

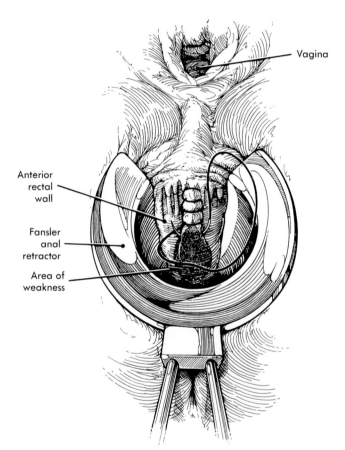

Figure 11.22. Endorectal repair of rectocele. A Fansler rectal retractor has been inserted into the rectum, and the redundant mucosa and submucosa of the weakened anterior rectal wall have been identified. Starting just proximal to the mucocutaneous junction, a running locked obliterative suture has been started. The suture is placed through both mucosal and submucosal layers and includes the rectal muscularis. With each stitch the suture is tightly drawn. No portion of the intact vaginal wall is included in the suture. When the rectal tissue of the rectocele has been obliterated to a point cranial to the low or midvaginal rectocele, the direction of the suture is reversed and a second obliterative layer is placed, reinforcing the initial layer. (From Nichols DH. Gynecologic and obstetric surgery. St. Louis: Mosby-Year Book, 1993:383. Used with permission.)

cess rectal wall is incorporated in a tightly drawn running locked stitch, which closes the weakness in the wall of the rectum in a longitudinal direction. As traction is exerted on each stitch as it is placed, the submucosa is tented toward the surgeon, facilitating placement of the succeeding suture. Although the full thickness of the rectal wall is included in this obliterative suture (Fig. 11.23), digital examination of the vagina during the suturing makes certain that attachment to or penetration of the vagina has not occurred. The suture is carried to a point about 1 cm past the upper edge of the rectocele, then tied and returned as a reinforcing locked stitch to the beginning of the suture line and tied again. Each stitch must be pulled tightly as it is placed to exert a strangulating effect on the tissue contained within the suture. One will occasionally find other areas of weakness within the circumference of the rectum and these can be similarly treated at the same time. The rigid circumference of the Fansler retraction prevents creation of a rectal stricture.

Block (3) describes the obliterative suture as

essentially a tightly drawn running lock-stitch which strangulates and causes to slough the tissues in the grip of each stitch, yet preserves the viability and approximates the tissues at the base of the

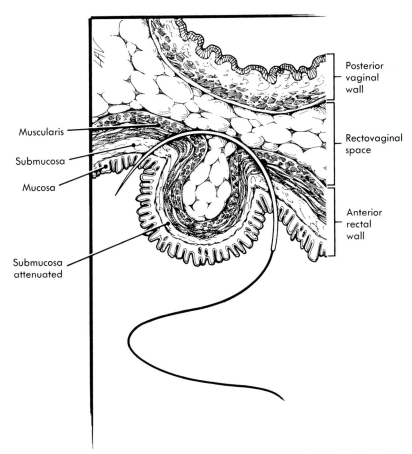

Figure 11.23. Section showing endorectal suture placement. The needle and suture are placed through the full thickness of the rectal wall, including the mucosa, submucosa, and muscularis. The unopened and unsewn vaginal wall is shown. (From Nichols DH. Gynecologic and obstetric surgery. St. Louis: Mosby-Year Book, 1993:384. Used with permission.)

suture. This surgical maneuver is peculiarly adapted to rectal surgery, since it cannot be used anywhere else in the body, but in the rectum it is an amazingly versatile tool for the surgeon.*

Alternatively, in the techniques of Sullivan et al. (35), Capps (5), and Sehapayak (30), the mucosal and submucosal layers are dissected off the underlying rectal muscularis, which is then plicated and the mucosa closed by a separate layer.

At about the 12 o'clock position, the rectal mucosa may be grasped and incised longitudinally from within the rectum, then undermined and reflected laterally. The rectal side of the rectal muscularis is plicated (5, 18, 30, 35), excess mucosa is trimmed, and the edges are sewn or stapled without tension. If desired, a predetermined full thickness of the rectal wall including the muscularis may be excised in its longitudinal axis following endorectal clamping and suturing or stapling (4) (GIA endo 30 or 60). Correction of coincident endorectal pathology, such as excision of symptomatic hemorrhoids or mucosal prolapse or removal of any rectal polyps, can be undertaken simultaneously if within the operator's area of expertise.

Endorectal repair of rectocele as described prevents vaginal stricture, dyspareunia, and rectovaginal fistula.

References

1. Aronson MP, Lee RA, Berquist TH. Anatomy of anal sphincters and related structures in continent women studied with magnetic resonance imaging. Obstet Gynecol 1990;76:846–851.
2. Barrett CW. Hernias through the pelvic floor. Am J Obstet Dis Wom 1909;59:553–569.
3. Block IR. Transrectal repair of rectocele using obliterative suture. Dis Colon Rectum 1986;29:707–711.
4. Bresler L, Rauch P, Denis B, Grillot M, Tortuyaux JM, Regent D, Boissel P, Girosdidier J. Traitement des rectoceles sus-levatoriennes par voie endorectale. J Chir (Paris) 1993;130:304–308.
5. Capps WF. Rectoplasty and perineoplasty for the symptomatic rectocele. Dis Colon Rectum 1975;18:237–244.
6. Cavallo G, Salzano A, Grassi R, DeLillo ML. Functional intraperineal pouch of rectal wall. Dis Colon Rectum 1993;36:179–181.
7. Davies JW. Quoted in Embryology and anatomy. In: Ullery JC, Stress incontinence in the female. New York: Grune & Stratton, 1953:33.
8. DeCosta EJ. After office hours—"dance me loose." Obstet Gynecol 1955;6:120.
9. Enhorning G. Simultaneous recording of intravesical and intraurethral pressure. Acta Chir Scand 1961;276:4–12.
10. Felt-Bersma RJF, Cuesta MA, Koorevaar M, et al. Anal endosonography: relationship with anal manometry and neurophysiologic tests. Dis Colon Rectum 1992;35:944–949.
11. Goff BH. A practical consideration of the damaged pelvic floor with a technique for its secondary reconstruction. Surg Gynecol Obstet 1068;46:866.
12. Halsted WS. Circular suture of the intestine; an experimental study. Am J Med Sci 1887;94:436–461.
13. Harrison JE, McDonagh JE. Hernia of Douglas' pouch and high rectocele. Am J Obstet Gynecol 1950;60:83.
14. Jansen A, et al. The importance of the apposition of the submucosal intestinal layers for primary wound healing of intestinal anastomosis. Surg Gynecol Obstet 1981;152:51–58.
15. Jeffcoate TNA. Posterior colporrhaphy. Am J Obstet Gynecol 1959;77:490.
16. Joachimovits R. Das Beckenausgangsgebiet und Perineum des Weibes. Vienna: Wilhelm Maudrich, 1969.
17. Kennedy JW, Campbell AD. Vaginal hysterectomy. Philadelphia: FA Davis, 1942.
18. Khubchandani IT, Sheets J, Stasik JJ, et al. Endorectal repair of rectocele. Dis Colon Rectum 1983;26:792–796.
19. Lord MG, Valies P, Broughton AC. A morphologic study of submucosa of the large intestine. Surg Gynecol Obstet 1977;145:155–160.
20. Malpas P. The choice of operation for genital prolapse. In: Meigs JV, Sturgis SH, eds. Progress in gynecology vol III. New York: Grune & Stratton, 1957;3.
21. Milley PS, Nichols DH. A corrective investigation of the human rectovaginal septum. Anat Rec 1968;163:433–452.
22. Nichols DH. Gynecologic and obstetric surgery. St. Louis: Mosby–Year Book, 1993:381–384.

---

* From Block IR. Transrectal repair of rectocele using obliterative suture. Dis Colon Rectum 1986;29:707–711. Used with permission.

23. Nichols DH. Posterior colporrhaphy and perineorrhaphy: separate and distinct operations. Am J Obstet Gynecol 1991;164:714–721.

24. Parks TG. The usefulness of tests on anorectal disease. World J Surg 1992;16:804–810.

25. Penninckx F. Fecal incontinence: indications for repairing the anal sphincter. World J Surg 1992;16: 820–825.

26. Porges RF. A practical system of diagnosis and classification of pelvic relaxations. Surg Gynecol Obstet 1963;117:769–773.

27. Rex DK, Lappas JC. Combined anorectal manometry and defecography in 50 consecutive adults with fecal incontinence. Dis Colon Rectum 1992;35:1040–1045.

28. Ricci JV, Thom CH. The myth of a surgically useful fascia in vaginal plastic reconstructions. Obstet Gynecol 1954;7:253–261.

29. Richter K. Erkrankungen der Vagina. In: Schwalm H, Doderlein G, Wulf KH, eds. Klinik der Frauen-heikunde und Geburtshille. Munich: Urban & Schwarzenberg, 1971;8.

30. Schapayak S. Transrectal repair of rectocele: an extended armamentarium of colorectal surgeons. Dis Colon Rectum 1985;28:422–433.

31. Snooks SJ, Burnes PRH, Swash M. Abnormalities of the innervation of the voluntary anal and urethral sphincters in incontinence: an electrophysiological study. J Neurol Neurosurg Psychiatry 1984;47: 1269–1273.

32. Snooks SJ, et al. Risk factors in childbirth causing damage to the pelvic floor innervation. Int J Colorectal Dis 1986;1:20–24.

33. Spjut HJ. Microangiographic study of gastrointestinal lesions. Am J Roentgenol 1974;91:1187.

34. Studdiford WC. The voluntary muscle fibers of the pelvic floor. Am J Obstet 1909;60:23.

35. Sullivan ES, Leaverton GH, Hadwick CE. Transrectal perineal repair: an adjunct to improved function after anorectal surgery. Dis Colon Rectum 1968;11:106–114.

36. Sultan AH, Nicholls RJ, Kamm MA, et al. Anal endosonography and correlation with in vitro and in vivo anatomy. Br J Surg 1993;80:508–511.

37. Swash M. Electromyography in pelvic floor disorders. In: Henry MM, Swash M. eds. Coloproctology and the pelvic floor. 2nd ed. Oxford: Butterworth-Heinemann, 1992.

38. Tobin CE, Benjamin JA. Anatomical and surgical restudy of Denonvilliers' fascia. Surg Gynecol Obstet 1945;80:373–388.

39. Uhlenhuth E, Nolley GW. Vaginal fascia, a myth? Obstet Gynecol 1957;10:349–358.

CHAPTER 12

Rectovaginal Fistula

DIAGNOSIS

Although some rectovaginal fistulas are asymptomatic, the majority are not. The presence of fistula can be suspected from incontinence of rectal gas or of liquid or solid stool even in the presence of an intact perineum and functional external anal sphincter. When these contaminants are passed through the vagina, the bacterial concentration may precipitate a chronic, recurrent vaginitis. There may be dyspareunia when infection and fibrosis are present.

Most cases of rectovaginal or rectoperineal fistula repair should be preceded and accompanied by suitable proctoscopy. Occasionally, the rectal opening of the fistula will be difficult to demonstrate except by gentle probing under anesthesia. When it is still not demonstrable with certainty, traction by an Allis clamp on the external secondary opening, as described by Bacon and Ross (2), will usually produce dimpling at the primary opening, which will often be found in an anal crypt.

When it is difficult to demonstrate a suspected pinhole-sized rectovaginal fistula, its specific site may be determined by filling the vagina of the recumbent patient with warm water or soapy water sufficient to cover the expected site of the fistula, placing a Foley catheter with a 10-ml bulb into the rectum, and instilling air through the catheter. A stream of air bubbles coming through the vaginal water pool indicates the site of the fistula, through which a blunt probe can be placed (Fig. 12.1).

If the vagina will not contain the soapy water, the site of the fistula can be determined by instilling milk or a concentrated solution containing methylene blue or indigo carmine into the rectal Foley catheter and watching where it appears on the posterior vaginal wall. If visualization is still unclear, the surgeon may inject the vaginal side of the fistulous tract with methylene blue using a no. 18, 19, or 20 needle that has been cut off about 1 cm from its hub. Through an anoscope one looks for the blue dye coming through the rectum, and also looks for branches of the fistula (25).

In seeking radiographic demonstration of the tract of a small rectovaginal fistula, one can inject a mixture of barium, mashed potato mix, and water into the rectum using a caulking gun. A lateral radiograph is taken while the patient bears down.

A rectovaginal fistula may occur at any level within the vagina but is most common in the lower third. Most of these fistulas have resulted from obstetric trauma, most often at the apex of an improperly healed repair of a fourth-degree perineal laceration. The patient may give a history of much difficulty expelling the fecal bolus with her first bowel movement, and after much straining probably compromised the repair. Although the tissue may have been properly approximated during the initial repair, a breakdown occurs through the path of least resistance cranial to the perineum, often between the fifth and tenth day after repair. In many instances of fistula it is likely that prophylaxis, including the liberal use of stool softeners and a low-residue diet, might have prevented the complication (7). By these means it is better for the patient to keep her bowel movements on the soft side for a few weeks postoperatively.

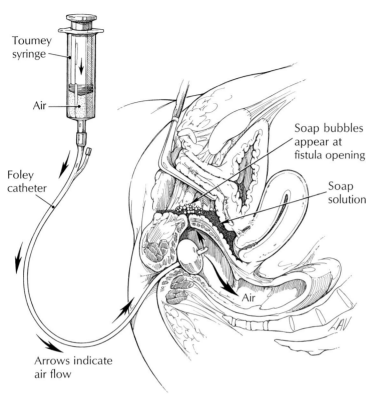

Figure 12.1. Air bubble test for small rectovaginal fistula. The examining table is placed in a Trendelenburg position and a Foley catheter inserted into the rectum. The vagina is filled with mildly soapy water, and air is injected into the catheter. The appearance of soap bubbles in the vagina indicates the presence of a small rectovaginal fistula.

Other causes of rectovaginal fistula are other trauma, suture penetration during episiotomy repair, especially if a long-lasting suture material such as polyglycolic acid (PGA) was used, or perineorrhaphy, Crohn's disease, infection and necrosis of a vaginal hematoma from hysterectomy, perineorrhaphy, posterior colporrhaphy, and pelvic irradiation, and particularly trauma to the vagina in the presence of endarteritis obliterans or the growth of residual or recurrent cancer.

The possibility that a gastrointestinal-vaginal fistula in the upper vagina is arising from the small bowel should be considered if the patient passes liquid stool through the fistula while passing solid stool through the rectum, or if the vagina and vulva are excoriated, as might result from digestion of the skin with digestive enzymes from the small intestine.

Although occasionally congenital in origin (21), the rectovaginal fistula seen today in the developed countries of the world is usually the aftermath of trauma, either unrecognized or unrepaired, or inadequately and unsuccessfully repaired during the initial attempt. Fistulas may be single or multiple, or a single fistula may have several connecting tracts that communicate within the subepithelial tissues with one another, occasionally originating from several openings into the rectal lumen. Less commonly, a single opening in the rectal mucosa may communicate with several fistulous openings in the vagina and perineal skin. The relationship of a fistulous tract or tracts to the external anal sphincter is of paramount importance in planning surgical repair.

Before repair, a relative degree of constipation will permit reasonable fecal continence, but success is not usually achieved in the control of flatus. It is, in fact, the inability to avoid involuntary loss of flatus that usually first makes a fistula known to the patient and equally often accounts for a patient's decision to seek surgical repair. During a period awaiting surgery, there are several things the patient can do to lessen the quantity of flatus, much of which is related to unabsorbed nitrogen from swallowed air. The patient can be advised not to talk while there is food in her mouth, to chew her food well, eating slowly without gulping, and to finish and swallow one mouthful before adding to the food being chewed. Such simple measures will often reduce considerably the amount of air being swallowed and, as a result, the amount of gas that is likely to be expelled. Oral administration of tablets of activated charcoal may absorb the unwanted gas.

When repair of coexistent rectovaginal and vesicovaginal fistulas is being considered, the vesicovaginal fistula should be repaired first, lest postoperative scarring from the rectovaginal fistula repair compromises the operative exposure if re-repair is required.

If the vesicorectovaginal fistula followed pelvic irradiation, usually one should require a preliminary diverting transverse colostomy; followed in 2 or 3 months by repair of the vesicovaginal fistula in the usual manner; then repair of the rectovaginal fistula, which may at times involve a colpocleisis; and then finally, after 2 or 3 additional months, by closure of the colostomy.

PRINCIPLES OF MANAGEMENT

It is important to emphasize certain principles in the management of rectovaginal fistula that, if observed, will increase the probability of successful surgical treatment.

1. A time for fistula repair should be chosen when granulation tissue, infection, and edema are minimal.
2. The repair must interrupt the continuity of the fistula.
3. The repair need not necessarily involve levator plication with its resultant risk of dyspareunia, but a layer of connective tissue should be interposed between the rectal wall sutures and those in the vaginal wall, if possible.
4. The epithelialized fistulous tract must be excised.
5. Closure of the rectal wall in more than one layer is recommended. (A second layer takes much of the tension from the suture line of the first layer.)
6. One should interpose a layer of fresh tissue with an independent blood supply, such as a bulbocavernosus graft, between the layers of repair if necessary, as with postirradiation fistulas.
7. The vaginal side of the fistula may be left open for drainage. When a rubber drain is used, it should be left in place for 2 to 7 days. The time for removal will depend upon the size of the fistula, the amount of drainage present, and whether an abscess was encountered during the procedure.

Hodgkinson (9, 10) favors brief isolation colostomy for obtaining temporary bowel rest, especially for rectovaginal fistulas high in the vagina or those that develop following pelvic irradiation. The required secondary closure is a disadvantage. Sanz and Blank (23) recommend interposition of a Martius graft between the rectal repair and the vagina when the rectovaginal septum is very thin or markedly scarred.

BOWEL PREPARATION

The standard antibiotic erythromycin-neomycin bowel preparation (1 g of each by mouth at 1:00, 2:00, and 11:00 p.m. the day before the operation) is associated with a high incidence of troublesome and annoying gastrointestinal side effects, so we now employ cefoxitin sodium (Mefoxin), which is given 2 g intravenously on call to the operating room and 2 hours later during surgery if necessary, or 2 g in the recovery room if surgery is completed in less than 2 hours from the initial dose, and an additional 2 g the evening of surgery. Hibbard (8) as well as Sanz and Blank (23) have reported increased surgical success when antibiotic coverage is provided.

As Menaker (14) has stated, "systemic antibiotics administered preoperatively and for a short perioperative interval . . . have little effect on intestinal colonization . . . antibiotics are not indicated merely to cover breaks in the operative technique." Only clear liquids by mouth are taken for the 2 days before admission to the hospital, and a half-bottle of citrate of magnesia or two bisacodyl (Dulcolax) tablets are given the afternoon before admission. There should be two Fleet enemas an hour apart the day before surgery, and the morning of surgery plain water or saline enemas until the return is clear. The use of an electrolyte cleanser such as GoLYTELY, NuLYTELY, or CoLYTE consumed the morning of the day before surgery seems to an effective substitute.

The choice one makes out of a number of surgical procedures for a rectovaginal fistula repair is predicated on many things. Foremost among these is the location of the fistula: high, mid-, or low vagina. Second is the etiology of the fistula: trauma, postirradiation, postoperative, postepisiotomy, Crohn disease, active malignant disease, and so forth. An additional consideration is the need for preserving or restoring coital function of the vagina. Another factor is the age of the patient, whether it be at any point in the full-life spectrum from the congenital or traumatic problems of infancy to the effects and influences of advanced years.

TECHNICAL CONSIDERATIONS

A 6-month waiting period can be observed in women with small rectovaginal fistulas caused by obstetric trauma, since some of these will heal spontaneously. During this waiting period the newborn baby has a chance to develop and become less dependent upon its mother, from whom it will have an absence for a few days during hospitalization and repair of the fistula. Others are best closed by an anterior rectal wall advancement technique that provides a tension-free environment for healing (24).

The choice of procedure for repair of rectovaginal septal defects is determined by the etiology and the age of the patient (from infancy to the advanced years), but for the most part by the location of a rectovaginal fistula (low, mid-, or high within the vagina), the presence or absence of a perineal body, and the integrity of the exterior anal sphincter (22). The goals of surgery are as for all reconstructive surgery: to relieve the symptoms and to restore the anatomy and function to normal. The effective combination must be thoughtfully planned and carefully executed for each patient.

It must be remembered that for genital fistulas there is a high-pressure side and a low-pressure side, as noted by Corman (5). In the presence of a symptomatic fistula, the flow of material from a hollow viscus is always from the high-pressure side to the low-pressure side. With rectovaginal fistula, the rectum is the high-pressure side, the vagina the low. Material flows from the rectum into the vagina, not from the vagina into the rectum. (With vesicovaginal fistula, the bladder is the high-pressure side.) Primary attention must be given to closing the high-pressure side, which must be closed securely and effectively. The low-pressure side (i.e., the vagina) will generally close spontaneously, even if unattended, once the continuity of the fistula has been interrupted, the high-pressure side has been effectively closed, and the rectal wound has healed. However, one can make the vaginal continuity over the rectum stronger by excising the epithelium lining the vaginal opening and loosely approximating the sides of the vaginal defect with one or two interrupted stitches, but with the stitches far enough apart to permit postoperative drainage, if there is any.

Repair should be recommended when a fistula has caused troublesome symptoms and when local edema and inflammation have subsided (usually coincident with relief or pain) and should embrace the following technical considerations:

1. The epithelial tract should be excised and the edges inverted into the lumen when possible.
2. The fistula should be closed securely in two layers, usually in a transverse axis, and without tension.
3. Meticulous hemostasis should be accomplished.

Because of the high vascularity of the pelvis, hemostasis in the area of fistula repair is essential to improve wound healing and lessen the chances of hematoma and abscess formation. Infiltration by up to 50 ml of a "liquid tourniquet" such as 0.5% lidocaine in 1:200,000 epinephrine solution is helpful, although phenylephedrine hydrochloride (Neo-Synephrine) solution or saline may be substituted when indicated by the presence of coincident severe hypertension or of coronary heart disease.

OPERATIVE PROCEDURES

The gynecologic surgeon should be familiar with a number of techniques for surgical treatment of a rectovaginal fistula, so that the one chosen will be likely to best fit the specific needs of a particular patient. Following are ten basic operative procedures with which the surgeon should become familiar:

1. Closure in layers without disrupting the perineum
2. Closure in layers following episioproctotomy
3. Transperineal rectal flap transplant dorsal to an intact external sphincter
4. Transperineal transverse repair ventral to an intact external sphincter
5. The transrectal anterior rectal mucosal flap transplant
6. The Noble-Mengert-Fish anterior rectal flap operation
7. The Warren-Miller vaginal flap operation
8. Transabdominal procedures for fistula located in the vault of an immobile vagina; when following irradiation, temporary transverse colostomy might be included
9. Colpocleisis or colpectomy
10. Endorectal repair (see Chapter 24).

The gynecologist should be familiar with all of these techniques so that a choice can be made on the basis of the patient's needs rather than a technique chosen with which the surgeon is comfortable but which may not be universally applicable or suitable to the clinical circumstances.

Autologous fibrin glue has been used in the successful treatment of complex anal fistulas, particularly in those that are recurrent rectovaginal fistulas. Combining autologous fibrinogen in cryoprecipitate with reconstituted bovine thrombin reproduces the final stage of the coagulation process, yielding an occlusive fibrin seal that is replaced with scar formation. The use of an autologous source to prepare the glue eliminates the hypothetical risk of disease transmission (1).

Effect of Fistula Location upon Choice of Operation

The most common postpartum rectal vaginal fistulas are those located in the lower third of the vagina. For these fistulas a sliding rectal flap procedure, such as that described with the Noble-Mengert-Fish operation, mobilizes and then excises a portion of the anterior rectal wall including the fistula and, if the external anal sphincter has been lacerated, permits reunification of its severed ends and construction of a perineal body (see Chapter 13). Corman's modification using a cruciate perineal incision is useful when there is ample perineal skin (5) and it is desirable to narrow the introitus and restore or build up a defective perineum (Fig. 12.2).

If abundant perineal skin is lacking, which is quite common, and one wants to narrow a gaping introitus, the Warren-Miller flap operation (16, 27) is a useful alternative,

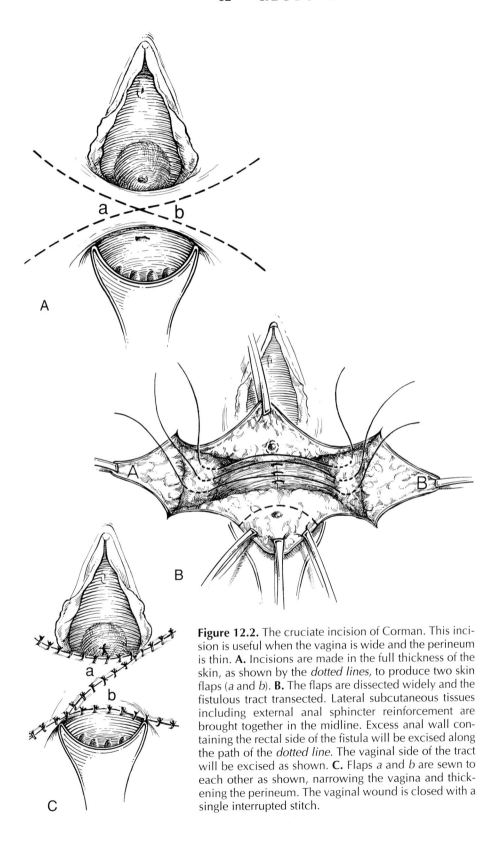

Figure 12.2. The cruciate incision of Corman. This incision is useful when the vagina is wide and the perineum is thin. **A.** Incisions are made in the full thickness of the skin, as shown by the *dotted lines*, to produce two skin flaps (*a* and *b*). **B.** The flaps are dissected widely and the fistulous tract transected. Lateral subcutaneous tissues including external anal sphincter reinforcement are brought together in the midline. Excess anal wall containing the rectal side of the fistula will be excised along the path of the *dotted line*. The vaginal side of the tract will be excised as shown. **C.** Flaps *a* and *b* are sewn to each other as shown, narrowing the vagina and thickening the perineum. The vaginal wound is closed with a single interrupted stitch.

permitting narrowing of the introitus with coincident reconstitution of the integrity of an interrupted external anal sphincter and perineum (see Chapter 13).

When the fistula is in the midvagina and the external anal sphincter and perineal body are intact, a layered closure is useful. The full thickness of the vaginal wall is incised into the rectovaginal space and the rectum and vagina carefully separated from one another. The fistulous tract is transected and the rectal tract excised in its entirety (Fig. 12.3). The rectal wall is closed by two layers of submucosal, interrupted, size 3-0 polyglycolic acid-type mattress sutures placed 2 or 3 mm apart in the rectal wall. These may be placed transversely in the muscular wall of the rectum or longitudinally (13), depending upon available exposure, if the latter will not compromise the rectal lumen. A second layer not only reinforces the first, but also takes some of the tension from the first layer of closure. The epithelialized tract through the wall of the vagina is excised and the opening loosely approximated in a longitudinal direction by interrupted sutures of polyglycolic acid placed no more closely than 1 cm apart, to allow for adequate possible postoperative drainage. Alternately, and after irrigation of the wound, the posterior vaginal vault may be split and a layer of rectovaginal septum interposed from side to side. The edges of the vaginal incision are freshened and made symmetrical, and the vagina is closed with interrupted sutures.

When the operator has determined to use a layered closure after recreating a fresh fourth-degree laceration by excising the epithelialized fistulous tract, and there is little available other tissue to use, the interposition of some "levator" stitches between the rectum and vagina, placed without palpable ridges, will increase the thickness of the perineum and insulate the site of the rectal repair from that of the vaginal side of the fistula (Fig. 12.4).

Rectovaginal fistulas in the pregnant patient resulting from obstetric trauma of a previous delivery may be closed at the time of delivery by episioproctorrhaphy, since the excellent blood supply and laxity of the perineal muscles during pregnancy favor good healing. By a fresh incision an episioproctotomy is performed, "recreating" a fourth-degree laceration. The fistulous tract and scar tissue are excised and the wound repaired as if it were a fresh fourth-degree laceration. Our objection to episioproctorrhaphy in the treatment of rectovaginal fistulas in the nonpregnant patient is that in the event of postoperative infection with abscess formation, the integrity of the perineal body and external anal sphincter may be severely damaged or destroyed. Infection in this area even without tissue destruction seen in abscess formation may initiate chronic painful inflammation, edema, and spasm of the pubococcygeal portion of the levator ani muscle, giving rise to the "levator syndrome" that is so resistant to effective treatment.

Transperineal Rectal Flap–Sliding Operation

For the patient with an intact perineum and intact external anal sphincter in whom the fistula is in the lower third of the vagina, the Noble-Mengert-Fish transperineal rectal flap–sliding operation (15, 18, 20) is our choice, since it does not disturb the perineal body but does permit plication of an intact but lax external anal sphincter, if desired (Fig. 12.5).

It is important that the surgeon slide the full thickness of the anterior rectal wall, including not only mucosa and submucosa, but muscularis as well. In addition, one should sew the muscularis by a few separate interrupted stitches to the underside of the new perineal body and external anal sphincter, taking some of the tension from the anastomosis between the mucosal and submucosal layer of the rectum and the perineal skin (19, 24).

Transperineal Transverse Repair

When the fistula is located in the midvagina and the perineal body and external anal sphincter are intact, the operation of Thompson (25, 28) using a transverse perineal incision is useful. The surgeon should wait for complete resolution of any infection and edema (usually 3 months) and, if spontaneous closure has not taken place, evaluate the

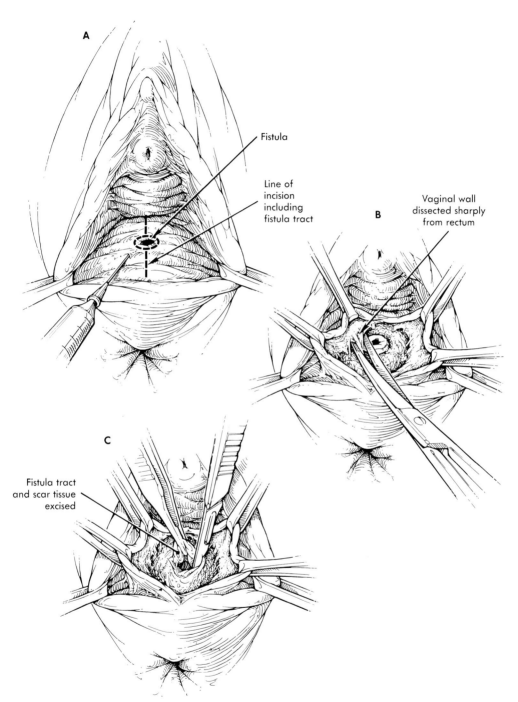

Figure 12.3. Layered closure of a midvaginal rectovaginal fistula. **A.** The tissues around the site of the fistula are thoroughly infiltrated by 1:200,000 epinephrine in 0.5% lidocaine, and an incision is made along the path indicated by the *dashed line*; the incision also circumscribes the tract of the fistula. **B.** The cut edges of the vagina are grasped by Allis clamps and sharply dissected from the anterior rectal wall. **C.** The fistula tract in its entirety is excised along with its surrounding scar tissue. (*Continues on following page.*)

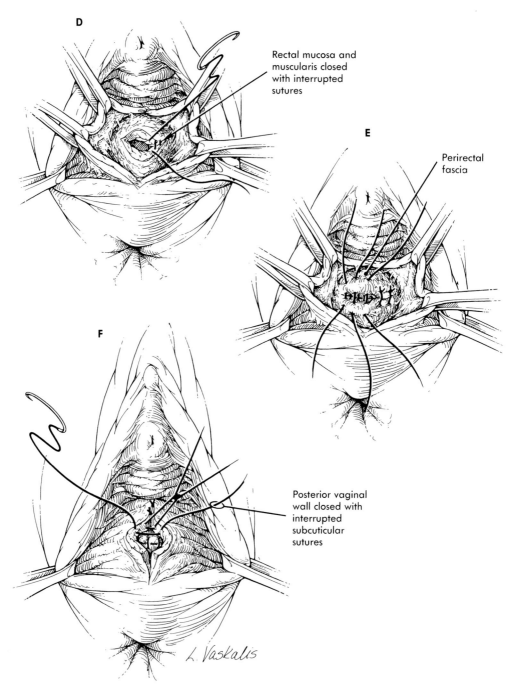

Rectal mucosa and muscularis closed with interrupted sutures

Perirectal fascia

Posterior vaginal wall closed with interrupted subcuticular sutures

L. Vaskalis

Figure 12.3, continued. Layered closure of a midvaginal rectovaginal fistula. **D.** The rectal submucosa and muscularis are closed with interrupted sutures. **E.** This suture line is buried by a second layer of interrupted sutures in the muscularis and perirectal fascia. **F.** The wound may be thoroughly irrigated with sterile saline solution, and the posterior vaginal wall closed longitudinally and at right angles to the repair in the rectal wall using interrupted subcuticular sutures in the fibromuscular wall of the vagina. (From Nichols DH. Gynecologic and obstetric surgery. St. Louis: Mosby–Year Book, 1993. Used with permission.)

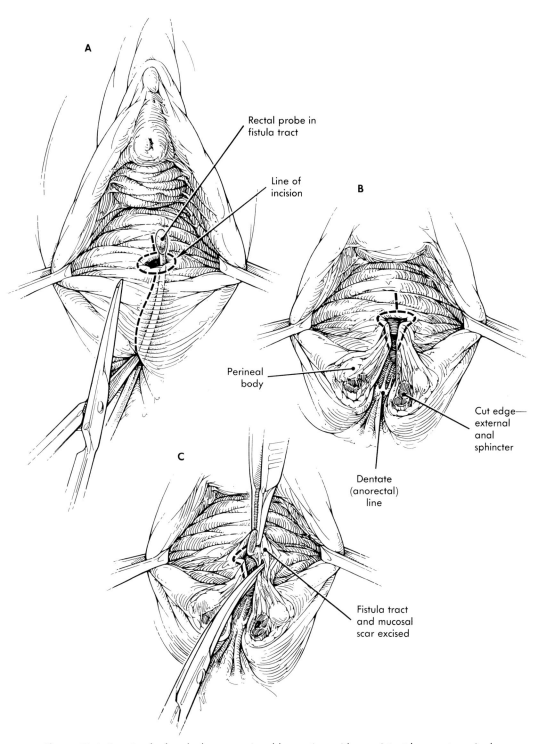

Figure 12.4. Repair of a fourth-degree perineal laceration with coexistent low rectovaginal fistula. **A.** A malleable probe is inserted through the fistula tract. **B.** An incision along this probe exposes the tissue. **C.** The fistula tract is excised along the site of the *dashed line* as shown in B and C. (*Continues on following page.*)

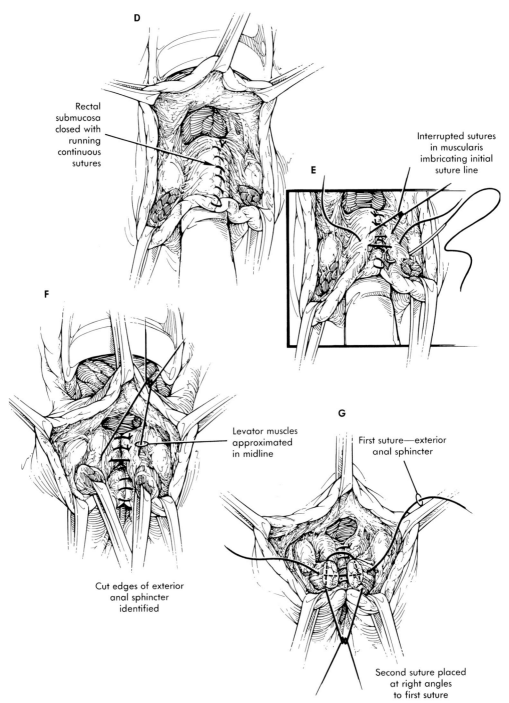

D

Rectal submucosa closed with running continuous sutures

E

Interrupted sutures in muscularis imbricating initial suture line

F

Levator muscles approximated in midline

Cut edges of exterior anal sphincter identified

G

First suture—exterior anal sphincter

Second suture placed at right angles to first suture

Figure 12.4, continued. Repair of a fourth-degree perineal laceration with coexistent low rectovaginal fistula. **D.** The freshened edges of the rectal submucosa are brought together with running continuous sutures placed in the submucosa. **E.** This is covered by a second layer of interrupted sutures in the muscularis of the rectum, imbricating the initial suture line. **F.** The medial surfaces of the levator ani are approximated with interrupted sutures, and the cut edges of the external anal sphincter are identified and grasped with Allis clamps. **G.** The external anal sphincter muscle is reapproximated with two interrupted sutures placed at right angles to each other. (*Continues on following page.*)

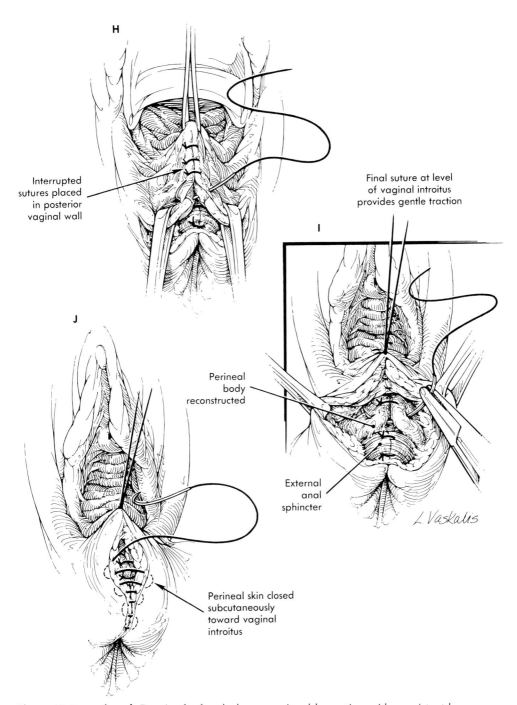

Figure 12.4, continued. Repair of a fourth-degree perineal laceration with coexistent low rectovaginal fistula. **H.** The freshened edges of the posterior vaginal wall are approximated by interrupted sutures. **I.** Upward traction to the lowermost of these sutures in the vaginal wall exposes the tissues from which the perineal body will be constructed; these are approximated with interrupted sutures. This takes much of the tension from the stitches placed within the external anal sphincter. **J.** The wound may be thoroughly irrigated with saline solution, and the perineal skin closed subcutaneously. (From Nichols DH. Gynecologic and obstetric surgery. St. Louis: Mosby–Year Book, 1993. Used with permission.)

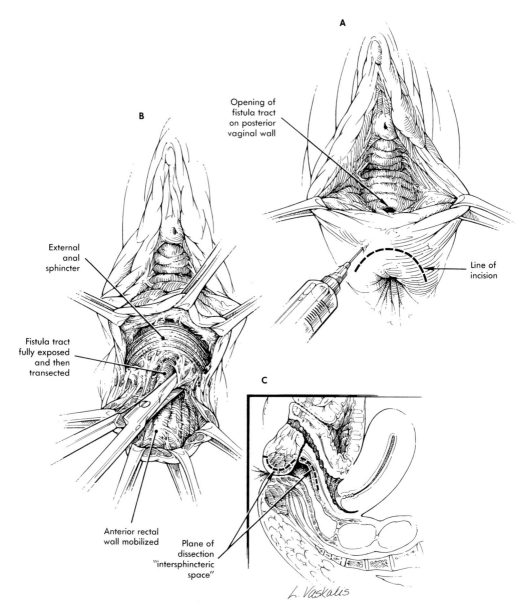

Figure 12.5. Transperineal rectal flap–sliding technique for repair of rectovaginal fistula. **A.** The site of the fistula is noted, and the perineum and perineal body thoroughly infiltrated by 1:200,000 epinephrine in 0.5% lidocaine. A semilunar incision is made around the anus posterior to the external anal sphincter along the course of the *dashed line*. **B.** Allis clamps grasp the edges of the incision, and by gentle traction to those placed on the anterior portion of anus, the dissection proceeds beneath the capsule of the external anal sphincter into the intersphincteric space. The fistula tract is fully exposed as the anterior rectal wall is mobilized, and the tract is then transected. **C.** Sagittal view of the path of dissection beneath the external anal sphincter and into the intersphincteric space. (*Continues on following page.*)

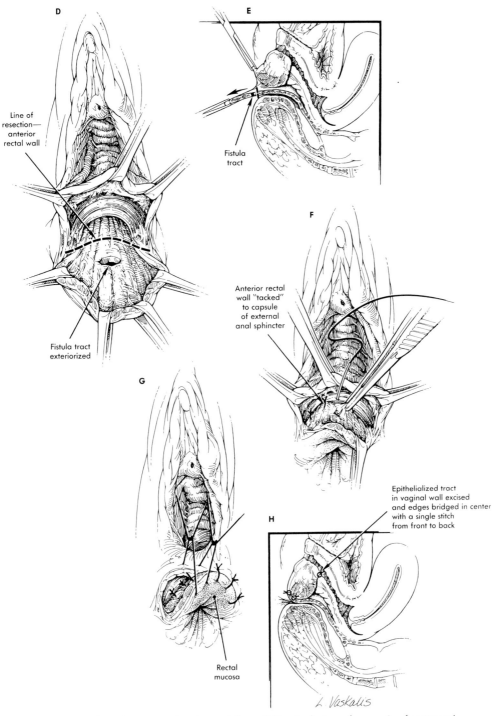

D

Line of
resection—
anterior
rectal wall

Fistula
tract

E

F

Fistula tract
exteriorized

G

Anterior rectal
wall "tacked"
to capsule
of external
anal sphincter

Epithelialized tract
in vaginal wall excised
and edges bridged in center
with a single stitch
from front to back

H

Rectal
mucosa

L. Vaskalis

Figure 12.5, continued. Transperineal rectal flap–sliding technique for repair of rectovaginal fistula. **D.** Continued opening and dissection of the rectovaginal space and gentle traction to the anterior rectal wall exteriorize the fistula. The anterior rectal wall, including the fistula, is excised along the path of the *dashed line*. **E.** Sagittal view of the excision. **F.** The anterior rectal wall is "tacked" to the capsule of the external anal sphincter. **G.** A second layer of interrupted PGA sutures fixes the cut margin of the anterior rectal wall to the skin of the perineum. **H.** Sagittal view showing the placement of these sutures. The epithelialized tract in the posterior vaginal wall is excised and the edges bridged in the center of the opening with a single stitch placed front to back. (From Nichols DH. Gynecologic and obstetric surgery. St. Louis: Mosby–Year Book, 1993. Used with permission.)

external anal sphincter, because if not intact, it too should be repaired. If it is intact, it should not be cut. The transverse perineal incision allows a layered closure without tension. In this operation (Fig. 12.6) a perineal incision is made beneath the posterior vaginal wall ventral (or anterior) to the external anal sphincter, and the rectovaginal space is entered. Identification of the fistula during dissection of the vaginal wall is aided by passage of a malleable probe. After the rectum and vagina have been separated from one another, first laterally, then cranially to the fistula, the fistula is transected at its central portion as noted in Figure 12.6*D*. The epithelialized tract is excised from both rectal and vaginal wall. The rectal defect is closed transversely with two layers, one of interrupted submucosal and the other of intramural sutures, and the vaginal wall closed longitudinally. Interrupted sutures for the vagina may be placed in a single layer, rather widely apart to permit possible postoperative drainage. The perineal skin may be closed transversely, but if it is desired to lengthen the perineal body, the skin and subcutaneous tissue may be approximated in the midline. However, when considerable fibrosis of the perineum is apparent and such a repair as described would result in a reduction in vaginal caliber and size of the perineum and would be certain to cause dyspareunia, an alternate and preferable approach would involve a surgical technique that would preserve the vaginal diameter and the integrity of the external anal sphincter. One such operation is the transrectal sliding mucosal flap operation (6, 11, 12, 19).

Transrectal Sliding Mucosal Flap Transplant

The patient is face down in a jackknife position, with small sandbags elevating the hips. The fistula may then be evident and explored from the rectal side using a small malleable blunt probe until the probe is palpable within the vagina.

With the Smith self-retaining retractor in place, and aided by a Sims retractor providing exposure in the vagina, the rectal circumference of the fistula may be infiltrated by 0.5% lidocaine in 1:200,000 epinephrine solution, and the rectal ostium circumscribed by an incision placed 0.5 to 1 cm from the margins of the tract (Fig. 12.7). This incision is extended distally onto the perineum, where removal of an inverted V-shaped wedge of skin and subcutaneous tissue exposes the anal sphincter. The incision is deepened to identify both internal and external anal sphincters, which may be partially divided sufficiently to remove any tendency toward a postoperative ridge or shelflike effect. The rectovaginal septum is identified close to the posterior wall of the vagina, and the rectovaginal space and anterior rectal wall are mobilized for about 3 cm above the site of the fistula.

A figure-of-eight suture is then placed through the rectal opening of the fistula and tied to the needle eye of the blunt probe. By traction upon the probe from the vaginal side, the fistulous tract is inverted into the vagina and cut off flush with the vaginal skin. A series of interrupted 2-0 absorbable PGA sutures fix the rectal muscularis to the cranial edge of the external anal sphincter, and another layer of sutures sews the mucosal edge of the anterior rectal wall to the posterior surface of the external anal sphincter. A small Malecot or Penrose drain may be placed through the vaginal opening at the site of the previous fistulous tract, where it is sewn in place with a single absorbable suture, and the anal canal is lightly packed with a plug of Vaseline gauze. An indwelling Foley catheter is inserted into the bladder.

Postoperatively, the preliminary antibiotic can be continued for a short time unless a significant diarrhea develops, in which case the antibiotic should be promptly terminated and the diarrhea brought under control. The patient should be kept on a clear liquid diet for 3 days, and when she is passing gas, gradually changed to a low-roughage or bland diet for 3 weeks. Stool softeners should be given, and if there has been no bowel movement by the seventh day, a gentle laxative should be added. The vaginal drain should be removed between the fifth and seventh postoperative days, depending upon the amount of drainage and the stability of the patient's temperature. Sitz baths may

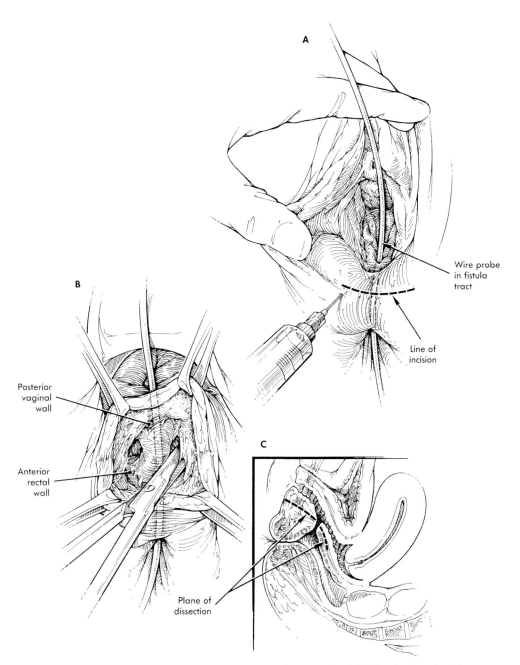

Figure 12.6. Transperineal sphincter-sparing repair of rectovaginal fistula. **A.** A malleable probe has been inserted through the tract of the fistula, and the area to be dissected is thoroughly infiltrated by a solution of 1:200,000 epinephrine in 0.5% lidocaine. The perineum is incised transversely as shown. **B.** The dissection separates the vagina from the perineal body, and by sharp dissection, starting laterally, the entire tract of the fistula is exposed. **C.** Sagittal view showing the path of dissection. (*Continues on following page.*)

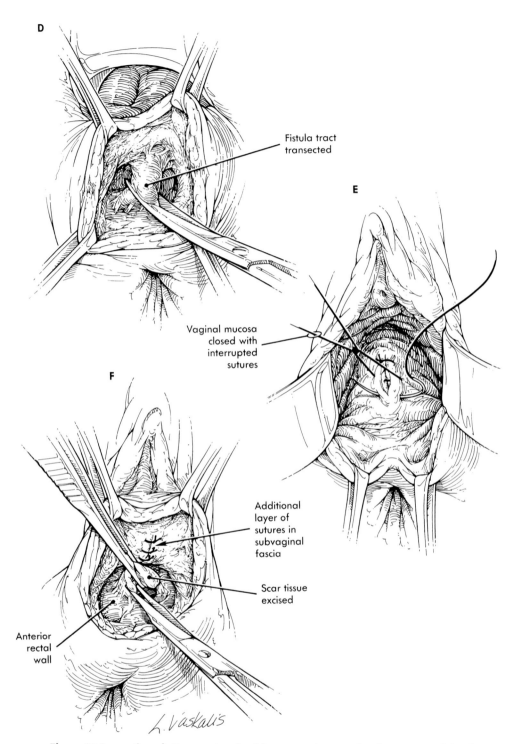

Figure 12.6, continued. Transperineal sphincter-sparing repair of rectovaginal fistula. **D.** After the tract has been isolated from the surrounding tissue, it is transected. **E.** The Allis clamps attached to the vagina are brought posteriorly, exposing the vaginal surface of the posterior vaginal wall. After the epithelialized tract of the vaginal side of the fistula has been excised, the defect is closed with a few interrupted stitches of PGA suture. **F.** The vaginal wall is again retracted anteriorly, and an additional layer of suture is placed in the fibromuscular layer of the vagina on the underside of the posterior vaginal wall. The fistulous tract in the rectum and its surrounding scar tissue are excised. (*Continues on following page.*)

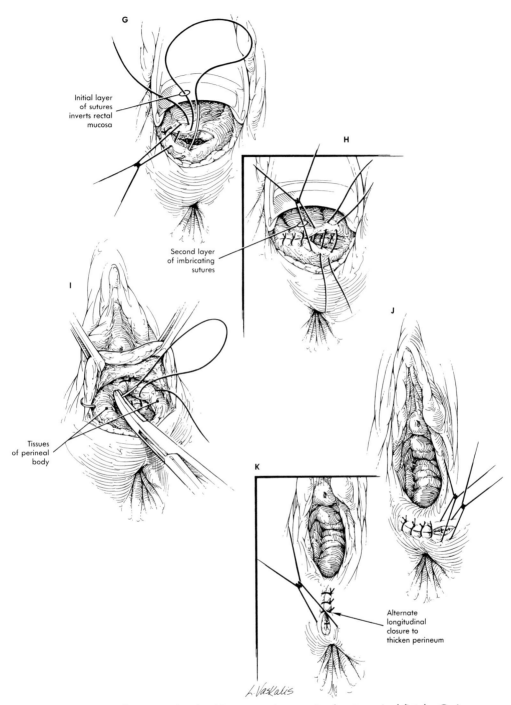

Figure 12.6, continued. Transperineal sphincter-sparing repair of rectovaginal fistula. **G.** A retractor is inserted into the rectovaginal space to better expose the anterior rectal wall. The defect in the anterior rectal wall is closed transversely with a layer of interrupted PGA sutures that inverts the rectal mucosa. **H.** A second layer of imbricating sutures is placed. **I.** The perirectal tissues and tissues of the perineal body are brought together in the midline by an additional layer of sutures. **J.** The edges of the original excision in the perineal skin are brought together by a series of interrupted sutures. **K.** The perineal body can be thickened by closing the incision from side to side, if desired. (From Nichols DH. Gynecologic and obstetric surgery. St. Louis: Mosby–Year Book, 1993. Used with permission.)

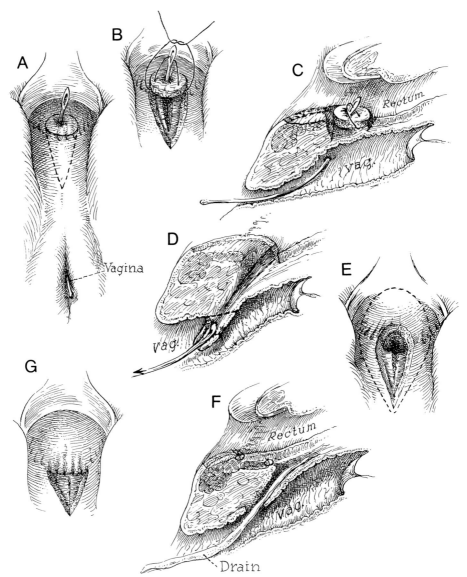

Figure 12.7. The transrectal mucosal flap transplant. **A.** With the patient face down and in a jackknife position, the posterior rectal wall is displaced by a retractor, and the fistula is explored from the rectal side by a small malleable probe. The rectal circumference of the fistula is infiltrated by 0.5% lidocaine in 1:200,000 epinephrine solution and the opening circumscribed by an incision placed 1 cm from the margin. This incision is extended distally onto the perineum, and a V-shaped wedge of epithelium is excised as indicated by the *dashed line*. **B.** Sufficient superficial fibers of the rectal side of the anal sphincter are incised so as to remove this as a postoperative obstruction to the passage of stool and gas, and the mobilized rectal opening of the fistula is sewn to the eye of the malleable probe. **C.** Sagittal view. **D.** Traction on the vaginal end of the probe is made to invert the fistulous tract into the vagina, where it is excised as indicated by the *dashed line*. **E.** The anterior rectal wall is separated from the vagina for about 2 cm. **F.** A series of interrupted sutures fixes the rectal wall to the internal anal sphincter. **G.** Another layer of sutures sews the mucosal edge of the anterior rectal wall to the posterior surface of the external sphincter. A small drain may be placed through the vaginal opening at the site of the previous fistula and fixed in place with a single absorbable stitch.

improve comfort and be given twice daily after the drain has been removed. Coitus is neither advised nor permitted until the end of the third postoperative month.

The Warren flap operation (27) and the Noble-Mengert-Fish operation (15, 19, 20) are useful when there is no functional anal sphincter, since they are often used as very successful surgical procedures to remedy an old fourth-degree laceration and also may be employed when a bridge of tissue not containing significant or functional sphincter muscle connects one side with the other. In the latter condition, the bridge that consists primarily of scar tissue is cut across at the beginning of the operation, and the procedure is essentially the same as that used for reconstructing the vagina after an old healed fourth-degree laceration. They both require approximation of the anal sphincter anterior to the anterior rectal wall. If, rarely, the reconstructed anal sphincter is smaller than one finger breadth, a complementary paradoxical external anal sphincter transection at the 5 o'clock position may be beneficial (16). This will temporarily interrupt the integrity of the sphincter to promote a transient rectal incontinence, but as the tissues between the retracted, cut ends of the sphincter become filled with firm scar tissue to bridge the gap, sphincter integrity and rectal continence will be restored. The patient must be told that this scar tissue formation will require up to 3 postoperative months to heal and stabilize.

Many fresh and unepithelialized fistulas involving the upper third of the vagina, usually after hysterectomy with postoperative pelvic abscess, will close spontaneously if the patient is placed on a no-residue, all-elemental diet with clear liquids for several weeks to inactivate the lower bowel. Several weeks of local estrogen therapy will be beneficial both preoperatively and postoperatively if the patient is postmenopausal. Smaller vault fistulas that do not close spontaneously may be closed transvaginally by a Latzko partial colpocleisis (see Chapter 19), but laparotomy should be considered for those that are large, and only after inflammation and edema have subsided. After bowel preparation, the rectum and upper vagina are separated from each other by sharp dissection. After excision of the epithelialized margins, the rectal opening is closed transversely in two layers and the vaginal opening longitudinally in one layer, interposing or covering each with a layer of mobilized peritoneum and a layer of omentum (26) if the tissues were previously radiated. Complementary defunctioning temporary colostomy is usually not necessary unless there has been a history of prior therapeutic pelvic irradiation.

Postirradiation Rectovaginal Fistula

For those fistulas that occur after therapeutic doses of pelvic irradiation, usually years later consequent to the reduction in blood flow that occurs with endarteritis obliterans, one should first confirm that no active malignant disease exists by biopsy of viable tissue from the fistula margin. If there is no malignant disease, nightly application of intravaginal estrogen cream is prescribed to improve the local blood supply and thicken the genital epithelium. Repair should be delayed for about 1 year from the time this fistula is first noticed to permit adequate stabilization of the blood supply and further confirmation of the absence of recurrent malignancy in this area. Premature repair of this type of fistula, although morphologically correct at the conclusion of the operation but before restabilization or arrest of the vascular obliteration, is prone toward recurrence of the fistula, the size of which may be greater than that of the original and more difficult to repair. For the meticulous and technically precise surgeon, Boronow's operation of partial colpocleisis of the upper vagina is appropriate (4). The somewhat fibrotic vaginal vault fistula is surgically exposed using a Schuchardt incision (see Chapter 8), and the vagina is carefully dissected from the anterior rectal wall for 1 to 2 cm in all directions at the site of the fistula. Meticulous hemostasis is achieved to prevent postoperative hematoma formation, and the defect in the anterior rectal wall is closed transversely without tension by a two-layered interrupted fine polyglycolic acid suture technique, thus closing the high-pressure side of the fistula. A bulbocavernosus fat pad is mobilized, swung beneath the anterior vaginal wall, and sewn in place to cover the site of the fistula repair, and the vagina is closed (Fig. 12.8). A no-residue oral elemental diet is maintained for several weeks, followed by a low-residue diet and stool softeners. Nightly instillation of intravaginal estrogen cream is continued for many weeks until the tissues have healed, followed by long-term weekly dosage.

Rectovaginal Fistula Repair in Crohn's Disease

Because fistulas resulting from Crohn's disease do not characteristically respond to standard surgical techniques, it is essential to recognize the presence of this disorder before a surgical approach can be recommended. Suspicion occurs when there is no known mechanical trauma to explain the origin of the fistula, and the patient may give a history of weight loss and frequent loose bowel movements, often accompanied by intestinal cramping. The fistula is invariably quite painful to touch (especially during the active phases of the disease), even when it has been present for a considerable length of time. Its edge has the roughened red appearance of granulation tissue. Confirmation of this suspicion may be obtained from biopsy, endoscopy, and study of the films of upper and lower gastrointestinal radiography. Repair of the Crohn's disease–induced rectovaginal fistula in the lower vagina may be considered during a phase of temporary remission of the disease, and use of a rectal flap–sliding operation permits excision of bowel wall containing the fistula, but the patient must be made aware of the high risk of surgical failure or of exacerbation of the disease. Provided that the Crohn's disease is in remission, healing following surgical repair can be expected in over 50 percent of patients (17). The rectal flap–sliding operation provides for removal of the rectal component of the fistula. The vaginal tract is excised but can be left open postoperatively for drainage and for healing by secondary intention. Preoperative preparation may include 1 month's administration of metronidazole (Flagyl) (3), 1000 mg daily, along with 20 mg of prednisone daily.

Sigmoid-vaginal fistula is usually the result of perforation of a sigmoid diverticulum coincident with abscess formation from diverticulitis in a usually older patient with diverticulosis. A transabdominal operation often combined with partial colectomy is the proper approach for surgery for this type of fistula.

Colpocleisis is reserved primarily for the large fistula that is sometimes seen after radiation, in which the viability of the adjacent tissue is so poor that good wound healing cannot be optimistically predicted. It, of course, destroys the function of most or all of the vagina, and this must be thoroughly explained to, understood, and agreed upon by the patient.

Transabdominal closure of the fistula is generally reserved for those in the vault of the vagina in which accessibility from below may be limited and repair of the bowel more difficult because of decreased visibility once the two organs have been separated. This is more often seen in the long-standing epithelialized rectovaginal fistula after hysterectomy and pelvic abscess in which local fibrosis and scarring may limit vaginal mobility. When it follows pelvic irradiation, successful closure may require temporary transverse colostomy and bringing into the repair an interposing layer of fresh tissue with an independent blood supply, such as the omentum (26) or the bulbocavernosus fat pad (19, 23). This is because postirradiation fibrosis includes coincident obliteration of local blood vessels with development of endarteritis obliterans, which effectively reduces the blood supply to the irradiated tissues.

Late recurrence of rectovaginal fistula, even 10 or 15 years after the time of an original repair, will occasionally be seen; and for this reason it is desirable for the operator periodically to follow the patient by examination over a long period of time.

Rectouterine Fistula

Unless associated with an invasive neoplasm, rectouterine fistulas are almost invariably the result of coexistent diverticulosis that became adherent to the posterior

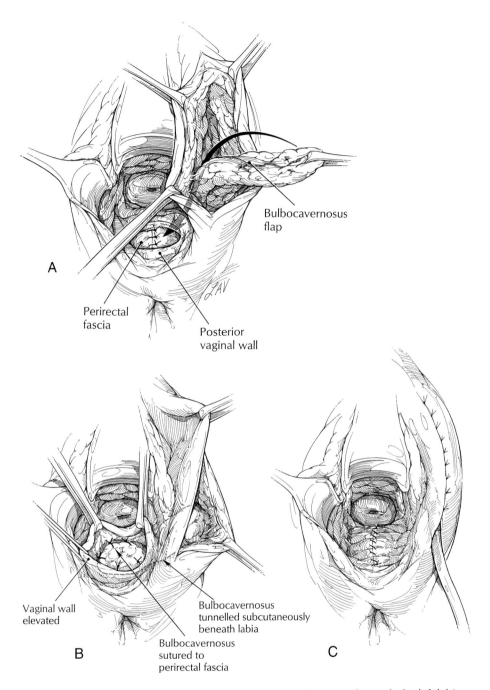

Figure 12.8. The bulbocavernosus fat pad transplant. **A.** The tissue beneath the left labium majora has been infiltrated by a solution of 1:200,000 epinephrine in 0.5% lidocaine, and a longitudinal incision made in the skin as shown. The bulbocavernosus fat pad has been dissected free except at its base, preserving the blood supply. **B.** A tunnel is dissected beneath the lateroposterior vaginal wall; the tip of the fat pad is drawn through the tunnel to cover the repair in the anterior rectal wall. The top of the fat pad is fixed to the perirectal fascia on the opposite side, as shown. **C.** The incisions in the posterior vaginal wall and the labium are closed. A subcutaneous drain has been placed at the site from which the fat pad was harvested.

wall of the uterus, after which an abscess formed and ultimately eroded into the uterine cavity. The condition produces a profuse, cloudy, watery discharge from the cervix that is usually sufficient in amount to require the patient to wear sanitary protection. Early in its course of development the discharge may be intermittent, coinciding with flare-ups of activity within the abscess cavity, and between spells of watery leukorrhea the patient may be relatively comfortable. The diagnosis is readily confirmed by a barium enema and sigmoidoscopy. Treatment is surgical, sometimes requiring a preliminary colostomy, then a bowel resection and hysterectomy 2 or 3 months later, and closure of the colostomy as a tertiary procedure 2 or 3 months after hysterectomy.

Vesicorectal Fistula

This is a rare late complication after hysterectomy and, because of its location high within the vault of the vagina, will usually require a transabdominal approach with dissection followed by separate repair of each organ system. Depending upon the size of the fistula and any previous irradiation, a preliminary diverting colostomy may be desirable. Interposition of omentum between the two fistula closures is desirable.

Anoperineal and Rectoperineal Fistula

A rectoperineal fistula not communicating with the anal sphincter is treated by simple excision of a wide area of surrounding skin, at least 1 cm lateral to each side of the fistula. A probe is placed into the fistulous tract, which is then incised through the full thickness of the overlying skin and subcutaneous tissue. The surrounding skin margin is widely excised, removing the fistulous tract. Any bleeding vessels are tied, and the wound is packed open, to granulate in from the bottom. It is desirable that the skin margins be the last portion of the wound to close. Healing requires a 4- to 6-week period, but the patient remains surprisingly comfortable and there is little disability. If the fistula transgresses the external anal sphincter, a seton may be used to preserve sphincter integrity (18).

Abscess Formation

Fistula repair should be timed to avoid involving an abscess, because the presence of an infection will seriously impede the quality of wound healing. When, at surgery, an unexpected abscess is encountered in the tissues between the rectum and the vagina, the intended procedure must be modified and simply becomes an unroofing operation in which the full thickness of the vaginal wall overlying the abscess is widely excised (Fig. 12.9). This will permit immediate and adequate drainage. Such a wound will also granulate in from its base, and in some instances the communication with the rectum will be closed by the granulation of the base of the wound, in which case no further surgery will be necessary. Alternatively, the rectal side of the fistula may be closed by an endorectal obliterative suture (see Chapter 24).

CARE OF THE PATIENT AFTER FISTULA REPAIR

The following recommendations are made regarding care of the patient after fistula repair:

1. Stool softeners such as docusate sodium (Colace) should be given for 5 weeks. One may give tincture of opium, IO drops in water three times a day for 5 days, if cramps are troublesome.
2. A clear liquid diet is advised postoperatively for 3 days, then a low-residue diet for 3 weeks.

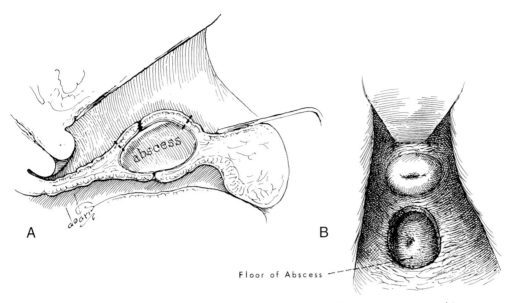

Figure 12.9. An unroofing procedure. **A.** When an unexpected abscess is encountered in the course of the fistulous tract, the cavity is widely exposed by cutting away a generous part of posterior vaginal wall (*dotted lines*). **B.** This exposes the floor of the abscess; the visible central dimple indicates the communication to the rectum. The cavity should be packed and allowed to granulate in.

3. There should be a bowel movement between the fifth and seventh day postoperatively while the patient is still in the hospital. A half-dose of an electrolyte bowel cleanser such as GoLYTELY, NuLYTELY, or COLYTE is preferable to an enema at this time. No coitus is permitted for 2 or 3 months postoperatively.

References

1. Abel ME, Chin YSY, Russell TR, Volpe PA. Autologous fibrin glue in the treatment of rectovaginal and complex fistulas. Dis Colon Rectum 1993;36:447–449.
2. Bacon HE, Ross ST. Atlas of operative technique: anus, rectum, and colon. St Louis: Mosby, 1954:110.
3. Bernstein LH, et al. Healing of perineal Crohn's disease with metronidazole. Gastroenterology 1980;79:357–365.
4. Boronow RC. Management of radiation-induced vaginal fistulas. Am J Obstet Gynecol 1971;1:1–8.
5. Corman ML. Colon and rectal surgery. Philadelphia: JB Lippincott, 1984:108–110.
6. Gallagher DM, Scarborough RA. Repair of low rectovaginal fistula. Dis Colon Rectum 1962;5:193.
7. Hauth JC, et al. Early repair of an external sphincter ani muscle and rectal mucosal dehiscence. Obstet Gynecol 1986;67:806–809.
8. Hibbard LT. Surgical management of rectovaginal fistulas and complete perineal tears. J Obstet Gynecol 1977;130:139.
9. Hodgkinson CP. Correcting failed rectovaginal fistula repair. In: Sanz LE, ed. Gynecologic surgery. Oradell, NJ: Medical Economics Books, 1988:133–139.
10. Hodgkinson CP, Baker RH. Isolation stoma colostomy and radiation-induced rectovaginal fistula. Am J Obstet Gynecol 1966;96:73.
11. Jackman RJ. Rectovaginal and anovaginal fistulas: a surgical procedure for treatment of certain types. J Iowa State Med Soc 1952;42:435–440.
12. Laird DR. Procedures used in the treatment of complicated fistulas. Am J Surg 1948;76:701.
13. Leacher TC, Pratt JH. Vaginal repair of the simple rectovaginal fistula. Surg Gynecol Obstet 1967;124:1317–1321.
14. Menaker GH. The use of antibiotics in surgical treatment of the colon. Surg Gynecol Obstet 1987;164:581–586.
15. Mengert WF, Fish SA. Anterior rectal wall advancement. Obstet Gynecol 1955;5:262.

16. Miller NF, Brown W. The surgical treatment of complete perineal tears in the female. Am J Obstet Gynecol 1937;34:196.
17. Morrison JG, Gathright JB Jr, Ray JE, et al. Results of operation for rectovaginal fistula in Crohn's disease. Dis Colon Rectum 1989;32:497–499.
18. Nichols DH. Recurrent rectal fistula. In: Nichols DH, ed. Reoperative gynecologic surgery. St. Louis: Mosby–Year Book, 1991:211–218.
19. Nichols DH. Repair of rectal fistula and of old complete perineal laceration. In: Nichols DH, ed. Gynecologic and obstetric surgery. St. Louis: Mosby–Yearbook, 1993:472–496.
20. Noble GH. A new operation for complete laceration of the perineum designed for the purpose of eliminating danger of infection from the rectum. Trans Am Gynecol Soc 1902;27:357.
21. Rock JA, Woodruff JD. Surgical correction of a rectovaginal fistula. Int J Gynaecol Obstet 1982;20:413–416.
22. Rosenshein NB, Genadry RR, Woodruff JD. An anatomic classification of rectovaginal sepia/defects. Am J Obstet Gynecol 1980;137:439–442.
23. Sanz LE, Blank K. The Martius graft technique for rectovaginal fistulas. In: Sanz LE, ed. Gynecologic surgery. Oradell, NJ: Medical Economics Books, 1988:125–150.
24. Stern H, Gamliel Z, Ross T, Dreznik Z. Rectovaginal fistula: initial experience. Can J Surg 1988;31:359–362.
25. Thompson JD. Transperineal repair of a rectovaginal fistula. In: Ob-gyn illustrated. New Scotland, NY: Learning Technology Incorporated, 1985.
26. Turner-Warwick R. The abdominal approach repair of simpler and complex urinary fistulas. In: Nichols DH, ed. Gynecologic and obstetric surgery. St. Louis: Mosby–Yearbook, 1993:881–899.
27. Warren JC. A new method of operation for the relief of rupture of the perineum through the sphincter and rectum. Trans Am Gynecol Soc 1882;7:322.
28. Wiskind AK, Thompson JD. Transverse transperineal repair of rectovaginal fistulas in the lower vagina. Am J Obstet Gynecol 1992;167:694–699.

Repair of Old Laceration of the Perineum

Howard Kelly once observed (5) that genital prolapse is rarely observed following complete and unrepaired perineal laceration. Because the principal effectiveness of the pubococcygei and levator ani is exerted lateral and posterior to the rectum, where their fusion forms the levator plate, a midline laceration through the anterior rectum, perineal body, and posterior vagina is not likely to have been due to forces simultaneously exerted to a point of overstretching the major sources of vaginal and uterine suspension, nor to have injured the levator ani itself, since it is situated lateral to the rectum (Fig. 13.1). Although the injury disrupted the anal sphincter, many of these patients will, by vigorously exercising the pubococcygei over a long period of time, produce an actual hypertrophy that results in a side-to-side sphincterlike action that helps hold the sides of the rectum in apposition and accomplishes a semblance of anal continence. Although this mechanism will not regain control of flatus, continence of the stool may be regained, particularly if the patient is careful to maintain a helpful degree of constipation.

RECTAL CONTINENCE

A network of neuromuscular receptors within the levator ani can detect rectal fullness and also can discriminate between gas, liquid, and solid content of the bowel. Stimulation of these receptors by increasing rectal content is followed by an increase in the tone of these muscles, which are never entirely at rest. The levator ani muscles are innervated by branches of the pudendal nerve, which similarly innervate the external anal sphincter. These muscles contract simultaneously and synergistically. They differ from the other voluntary muscles of the body in that they maintain, via this network of neuromuscular receptors, a constant state of tone proportional to the quantity of the rectal contents. Their unique capacity for discrimination can permit the slow escape of rectal gas even during sleep while retaining solid content. Because intestinal peristalsis continues even during sleep, it is this reflex contraction of these voluntary muscles that maintains continence. The ability of these muscles to contract effectively depends, therefore, on both their intrinsic integrity and the integrity of their nerve supply, primarily the pudendal or the accessory pudendal nerves.

A backup system of continence occurs through the internal anal sphincter, which is an involuntary smooth muscle continuation of the wall of the large intestine. By a complex interaction, the internal sphincter reflexively relaxes preceding and during the act of defecation to permit the unimpeded transit of stool. When the levator ani, the external anal sphincter, or their nerve supply have been effectively compromised, the internal anal sphincter may remain as the sole barrier to rectal incontinence.

315

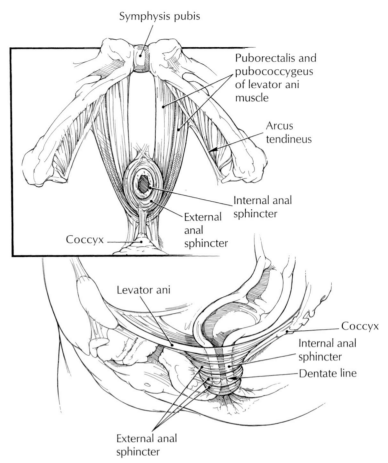

Symphysis pubis

Puborectalis and pubococcygeus of levator ani muscle

Arcus tendineus

Internal anal sphincter

External anal sphincter

Coccyx

Levator ani

Coccyx

Internal anal sphincter

Dentate line

External anal sphincter

Figure 13.1. Phantom drawings showing the anatomy of the puborectalis, pubococcygeus, and anal sphincter muscles. The relationships of the muscles to the rectum are shown in both frontal and sagittal views. When midline fourth-degree perineal laceration occurs, only the anal sphincters are torn apart and at the 12 o'clock position. The levatores ani, being lateral to the rectum, are undamaged. Notice the size and extent of the divisions of the striated external anal sphincter muscle. The internal sphincter is a caudal continuation of the smooth muscle of the rectum.

In addition to the previous mechanism, reflex contraction of the intact pubococcygei creates an anorectal valve that can be described by the angulation of the anorectal junction, whereby the anterior wall of the rectum covers the central lumen when the pubococcygei are contracted. Relaxation of this angulated valve promotes transit of stool.

ANAL INCONTINENCE

Anal incontinence is socially devastating to the afflicted patient, because it includes the inability to control and retain rectal gas as well as stool, both of which may be lost involuntarily under most inappropriate circumstances. The patient probably will have already undergone one or more external anal sphincter plication procedures with or without a coincident perineorrhaphy, which did not restore continence. In such patients, the surgeon must make a distinction between frequent bowel movements, as might be seen with an irritable colon or diverticulosis, and anorectal incontinence, the latter characterized by the addition of involuntary rectal soiling (10). Persistent rectal incontinence may also be demonstrated in a patient in whom the external anal sphincter is intact but suffers a faulty innervation. The pelvic diaphragm and levator ani are supplied primarily by the paired pudendal and accessory pudendal nerves, which also supply the muscular fibers of the external anal sphincter. These muscles function in concert with one another.

Partial or total denervation of the external anal sphincter and of the levator ani can result from a combination of many factors (15–17). Occult damage can be measured even after uncomplicated vaginal delivery, although it generally heals rapidly. Straining at stool may contribute to further damage, as may damage to the motor nerve roots of S3 and S4 from coincidental disc disease or spinal canal stenosis from osteoarthritis. Manning and Pratt (7) described their surgical results as best following the first repair; they noted difficulty in finding the frayed ends of the external anal sphincter when they were buried in scar tissue.

Classic descriptions of the transected external anal sphincter characterize it as a narrow bundle to be sought just beneath the perianal skin and distinctly caudal to the internal sphincter (3, 14). More recent studies using magnetic resonance imaging (MRI) come to quite a different conclusion. Aronson and colleagues (1) have observed from their MRI studies that the external sphincter normally is a strong ellipsoidal cylinder complex that surrounds the distal portion of the internal anal sphincter in the adult for a distance of 3 to 4 cm and is thicker anteriorly and posteriorly than laterally. They submit that surgical reapproximation of this entire muscular cylinder should more effectively restore sphincter function than reapproximation of just the superficial subcutaneous portion of the external anal sphincter. We agree, and no longer make a decisive effort to dissect the external anal sphincter away from its surrounding tissues, or to separate it from the internal anal sphincter at this level. The free but scarred ends of the lacerated external sphincter should be sought and grasped so that they may be sewn together as a part of the perineal reconstruction, but combining this with full perineal reconstruction will produce the best anatomic and functional result. Fecal continence is the result of effective interaction and support between not only the external and internal anal sphincters, but with the whole of the pelvic diaphragm, including its puborectalis portion (6).

Fecal incontinence after childbirth may be due to either obstetric rupture or muscular denervation of the external anal sphincter system. These may coexist. Delayed sphincter repair gives excellent results provided that denervation is not present. Denervation can be identified by electromyography, but postoperative improvement may follow reinnervation within a year, and improvement in continence can be demonstrated by electromyography (4).

Incontinence tends to get worse with the advancement of years, possibly related to some damage of the nerve supply which has been progressive over a long period of time. This may not become evident until some 25 years or so following the parturient correction of a fourth-degree laceration. By this time the patient's health care provider may well be a different person than the one who repaired the original laceration. Therefore, the mediolateral episiotomy can be recommended (2) for the following reasons:

1. Extension to fourth-degree perineal laceration is uncommon.
2. There are a reduced number of rectovaginal fistulas.
3. The above does not guarantee that there will not be any future incontinence because occasional but coincident pudendal nerve damage develops slowly and may not make itself known for many years.

To demonstrate anal incontinence, an enema may be given in the office to see if the patient can retain it. An alternate procedure would be to compose a mixture of mashed potato mix, water, and barium, place this into a caulking gun, and inject it into the rectum. This will permit x-ray studies of the rectum and its continence.

Rectal soiling may be preceded by loss of sensory discrimination between liquid, solid, and gaseous rectal content. When there is no evident mechanical disruption of the anal sphincter, such a patient must be considered at risk for future rectal prolapse.

A patient will present herself for repair of a complete perineal laceration at any time, even years after the original injury. Miller and Brown (9) have emphasized three fundamental principles essential to successful repair: (a) evidence of a good blood supply, (b) absence of infection in the tissues to be involved, and (c) closure of the repair without tension on the sutures as the tissues are reapproximated. It is equally important to excise all scar tissue to ensure tissue characteristics similar to those of a fresh fourth-degree laceration. Layer-by-layer reconstruction of rectal wall, submucosa, muscularis, perirectal connective tissue, anal sphincter, and rectovaginal septum before closure of the overlying vaginal floor should be accomplished by terraced rows of fine absorbable suture, but there is a tendency for such a repair to break down with formation of rectovaginal fistula. Such a discouraging result is particularly likely in the postmenopausal patient whose tissues are atrophic and have a reduced blood supply.

Intestinal peristalsis is reduced by age, particularly in the postmenopausal years. It also may be reduced indirectly by nicotine withdrawal of someone who has suddenly stopped smoking. The best anatomic and functional results are obtained when an obstetric laceration is properly repaired immediately after delivery, when the vascularity of the perineum and perivaginal tissues favors rapid healing. On the occasion of a later secondary repair, scar tissue is appreciable, wound healing is poorer, and recurrence of the fistula from a breakdown of the repair is more likely (10, 11).

A technique of repair providing an optimal chance of a good result with the first repair is obviously a procedure of choice. The Noble-Mengert-Fish (8, 12) anterior rectal flap operation has often been recommended. Primary healing with restoration of function also usually follows the Warren-Miller-Brown (9, 18) vaginal flap operation.

The choice between the Noble-Mengert-Fish (8, 12) rectal flap operation and the Warren-Miller-Brown (9, 18) operation can often be made on the basis of the size of the vagina. The vaginal flap operation makes the vagina measurably smaller and therefore would be used when this is a desired goal, whereas the rectal flap operation can be used in a patient with a smaller vagina, since it does not remove vaginal membrane. The rectal flap operation is particularly useful if an old fourth-degree laceration extends no more than 3 or 4 cm into the anal canal. Freeing up and pulling down the anterior rectal wall permits placement of anchoring sutures near the edge of the mobilized segment of the anterior rectal wall to the undersurface of the anal sphincter. The cut edge of the anterior rectal wall after resection is sewn to the perineal skin outside of the former anal canal and will cover the area where postoperative disruption of sutures not protected by such a flap might occur. In principle and usefulness this procedure is not unlike the mucosal flap operations for rectovaginal fistula, as described in Chapter 12, but it is indicated preferentially when external anal sphincter integrity has been disturbed.

TECHNIQUE OF THE RECTAL FLAP OPERATION

After a preoperative bowel preparation, the rectal flap (Noble-Mengert-Fish [8, 12]) procedure may be accomplished as follows: The scarred edge of the anterior rectal wall is grasped with several Allis clamps along the inverted U-shaped defect in which the anal membrane has by scarring become fused to the posterior vaginal wall. A transverse semilunar incision is made across the posterior wall of the vagina immediately above this scar tissue, and the rectovaginal space is entered (Fig. 13.2). Once this space has been identified, the separation of the rectum from the vagina is accomplished by blunt dissection into the rectovaginal space. With a guiding finger in the rectum and Allis clamps supported in the palm of the same hand, separation of vagina from rectum can extend all the way to the vault of the vagina and then is carried laterally the full width of the rectovaginal space. The Allis clamps attached to the anterior rectal will provide gentle trac-

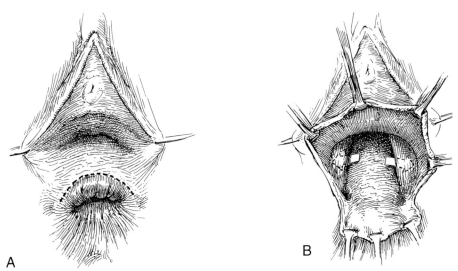

Figure 13.2. The rectal flap operation (Noble-Mengert-Fish). **A.** The mucocutaneous incision needed to restore the anal sphincter is identified by the *dashed line*. **B.** The edges of the incision are grasped by Allis clamps and dissection is carried upward to the rectovaginal space. Pararectal connective tissue is separated from the anterolateral surface of the rectum as shown by the *arrows*.

tion and permit some sliding and gentle stretching of the now mobilized anterior rectal wall until it may readily reach the site where it is to be anchored to the anal sphincter and perineal skin. The retracted ends of the anal sphincter are then sought at the site of the identifying dimples and freed if possible. The use of a "Bovie" electrosurgical needle electrode will aid hemostasis. Its brief electrical stimulation or that of a nerve or muscle stimulation also will help identify the striated muscle of the external anal sphincter. The partially mobilized ends of the sphincter are grasped by Allis clamps and the ends of the sphincter pierced by two mattress sutures of 2-0 delayed absorbable synthetic suture such as polydioxanone (PDS), to be tied after the sutures restoring the perineal body have been placed and tied. If the retracted ends of the sphincter cannot be isolated because they have become deeply buried in the scar tissue and have lost recognizable identity, there need be no concern as long as the operator brings the two sides of anal sphincter scar tissue (which can be demonstrated by traction to contain the sphincter ends) together in the midline before completing the associated perineorrhaphy.

The suitably denuded and mobilized lateral soft tissues necessary to form a reconstructed perineal body are then united in the midline by a series of interrupted 0 polyglycolic acid-type absorbable sutures in the fashion of an extensive perineorrhaphy, over the intact portion of the mobilized anterior rectal wall (Fig. 13.3). Ridges and shelving of tissues are to be avoided by careful suture placement. These sutures are then tied without strangulation of the tissue, and excess skin and mucosa are appropriately trimmed. The lower edge of the flap of the anterior rectal wall is fixed to the skin of the perineum by several interrupted 2-0 absorbable polyglycolic acid-type sutures placed not more than 1 to 2 cm apart. An occasional stitch should include a superficial bite of the anal sphincter.

The reconstructed anal canal should admit one finger breadth comfortably; if not (due to retraction and shortening of the anal sphincter fibers), the paradoxical sphincter incision described by Miller and Brown (9) can be performed. Such an incision should be made between the 4 and 5 o'clock positions, cleanly through the perineal skin and anal sphincter and perpendicular to the muscle fibers of the sphincter (see Fig. 13.4). The sphincter remains relaxed, and ultimate continence is reduced until healing in effect

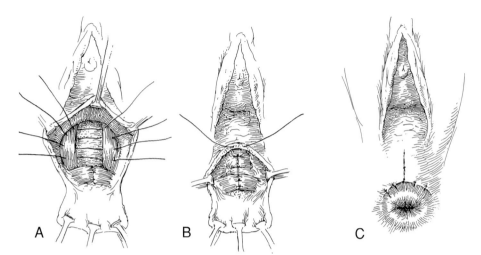

Figure 13.3. Reunification of the ends of the external anal sphincter. **A.** The ends of the external anal sphincter have been united and stitches placed in the pararectal tissues. **B.** They are tied, and the posterior vaginal wall will be closed from side to side. A perineal body is reconstructed with interrupted sutures. **C.** The vaginal and perineal skin is closed, and the excess flap is trimmed.

reunites the sphincter ends with scar tissue, restoring a degree of functional competence. It requires between 8 and 12 postoperative weeks for this to take place, and the patient should be so informed.

Incompetence of the anal sphincter is almost invariably the result of obstetric laceration, the integrity of the sphincter generally having been interrupted in the midline near the 12 o'clock position. The anterior wall of the rectum may or may not have been torn as well. When total healing has not taken place after repair of the fresh injury, various combinations of healing may occur: (*a*) The rectal tear may have healed but not the sphincter or perineal body. Sphincter incontinence results. (*b*) The perineal body and skin may have healed but not the rectal laceration. (*c*) The sphincter repair or some part thereof may or may not have healed. (*d*) A rectovaginal fistula is present, with or without sphincter incontinence.

When the healing process has been stabilized after injury or previous repair, and any raw areas have become epithelialized, planned reconstruction should take place provided the patient is symptomatic and desires a restoration.

TECHNIQUE OF THE VAGINAL FLAP OPERATION

After preoperative cleansing of the bowel by means of an electrolyte purge (GoLYTELY, NuLYTELY, or CoLYTE) the day before surgery and enemas until clear the morning of surgery, an inverted V-shaped incision is made in the posterior vaginal wall of such a width that when the sides of the vagina are subsequently united, the introital width will be of the desired caliber (Fig. 13.4). The base of this vaginal flap is continuous with the margin of the anterior rectal wall (9, 11, 18).

By sharp dissection through any scar tissue, the avascular space between the rectum and vagina is developed for several inches, mobilizing the anterior rectal wall. Stretching it by traction may bring it and the V-shaped vaginal flap to beneath the site of the external anal sphincter.

The buried ends of the external anal sphincter are grasped, and appropriate mattress sutures of 2-0 long-lasting but absorbable suture (PDS) are placed without tying.

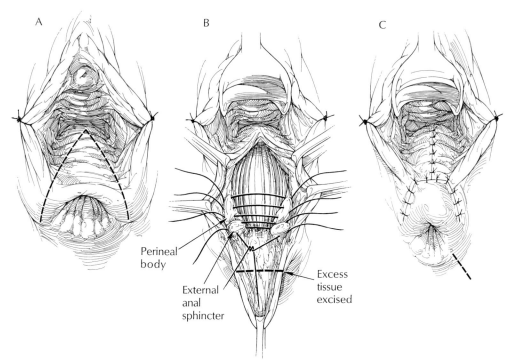

Figure 13.4. The vaginal flap operation (Warren-Miller-Brown). **A.** An inverted V-shaped incision is made through the full thickness of the vagina and skin of the perineum, opening into the rectovaginal space. **B.** Traction is applied to the vaginal skin overlying the rectum at the apex of the flap. This flap is freed laterally from the surrounding scar tissue, exposing the site of the perineal body and the ends of the anal sphincter. These are united from side to side with a series of interrupted stitches of long-lasting absorbable polyglycolic acid-type sutures. **C.** When the perineal body has been restored and the sphincter ends approximated, the flap is trimmed as shown and turned up to cover the sphincter repair. The posterior vaginal wall and skin of the perineum are closed by a series of interrupted sutures. If the reconstructed anal canal does not generously admit one finger breadth, the paradoxical sphincter incision of Miller and Brown can be performed (see text) at the site shown by the *dashed line.*

The perineal body is reconstituted by several side-to-side sutures that are tied. Then the anal sphincter stitches are tied and the perineal skin closed from side to side.

The undersurface of the vaginal flap is sewn to the reunited external anal sphincter and perineal skin. The excess vaginal flap is trimmed and removed, and the cut edge is sewn to the perineal skin.

RESTORATION OF CONTINENCE BY REPAIR OF A LACERATED ANAL SPHINCTER

This operation (as described by Novak [13]) is designed to restore sphincter integrity and anal continence to a patient in whom this has been lost by laceration, most commonly after a fourth-degree obstetric laceration, and often one in which the rectal component may have healed after its repair at delivery but there was postoperative breakdown of the anal sphincter repair and occasionally of the perineum. The operation provides good exposure to the critical areas, particularly the ends of the lacerated anal sphincter as well as the tissue from which the perineum will be reconstructed. As an essential step, stitches are placed to reinforce or restore the integrity of the perineal body and take much of the tension from the ends of the recently approximated external anal sphincter, splinting or bracing this repair and aiding in the integrity of its healing. If this tissue has been adequately identified and mobilized, it is *not* necessary to bring the medial borders of the pubococcygei together in front of the rectum, thus lessening the chance for painful ridges in the newly approximated tissue with production of subsequent dyspareunia. Polyglycolic acid-type suture is used, size 0 or 00. When the perineum has "disappeared," it must be mobilized and reconstructed as an integral part of the repair, which will effectively take much of the strain from the sphincter repair during its healing phase.

Symptoms of anal sphincter insufficiency are those of rectal incontinence, that is, inability to control rectal gas and/or feces, especially when liquid. At times, soiling may precipitate a troublesome vaginitis.

The gynecologist must also be mindful of the anorectal incontinence produced by nerve damage, often the pudendal nerve, which may be sufficient to essentially denervate the pelvic diaphragm and the external anal sphincter (16). This can be suspected during the preoperative pelvic examination when the patient cannot voluntarily contract her pubococcygei and her external anal sphincter. The diagnosis can be confirmed by electromyography. This nerve damage, when acquired, is probably the consequence of straining at stool or from difficult or prolonged labor. Myoplasty will tighten a loose external sphincter system; but if the muscles have been denervated, the prognosis for functional improvement is guarded. Residual postsurgical function will be improved in the patient with unilateral or partial residual innervation remaining. Rectal continence will be aided by a good internal (involuntary) sphincter system.

Other less common causes of anal incontinence include peripheral neuropathy as in some diabetics, diseases of the central nervous system or spinal cord or cauda equina, and postsurgical trauma as after laminectomy. It may be associated with the perineal descent syndrome (see Chapter 14). Some persons complaining of chronic diarrhea may really harbor an underlying undiagnosed sphincter incompetence secondary not only to sphincter laceration but also to sphincter denervation. Rectal sphincter weakness is usually not effectively treated by a sphincter plication in a patient who has not sustained a previous sphincter laceration. Long-term medical treatment including loperamide hydrochloride (Imodium) may be helpful.

TECHNIQUE FOR RESTORATION
OF ANAL SPHINCTER COMPETENCE

The bowel should be cleansed preoperatively by electrolyte wash (drinking 4 liters of chilled polyethylene glycol [PEG] 3350 electrolyte solution [NuLYTELY, GoLYTELY, CoLYTE]) the morning of the day before surgery followed by enemas until clear the morning of surgery. Three traction stitches are placed as shown in Figure 13.5*A* (13). The damaged tissues must be dissected and mobilized carefully and scar tissue freed by sharp dissection. None of the tissue need be discarded. The torn ends of the sphincter will be buried in scar tissue and are identified by the subcutaneous dimples as shown. An incision resembling the letter W is made with the knife through the skin margin between the vagina and rectum and extended upwn incision resembling the letter W is made with the knife through the skin margin between the vagina and rectum and extended upward *laterally* to the cut ends of the sphincter. The rectovaginal space is entered and the vagina carefully separated from the anterior wall of the rectum up to the site of the previously placed traction suture, as shown in Figure 13.5*B*.

Allis forceps grasp the cut edge of the vagina. Scar tissue is freed by both sharp and blunt dissection with wide mobilization of vagina from rectum. The caudal portion of the rectovaginal space and site of the perineum are clearly exposed. A traction stitch is placed in the muscularis of the anterior rectal wall, as shown in Figure 13.5*C*. When up-

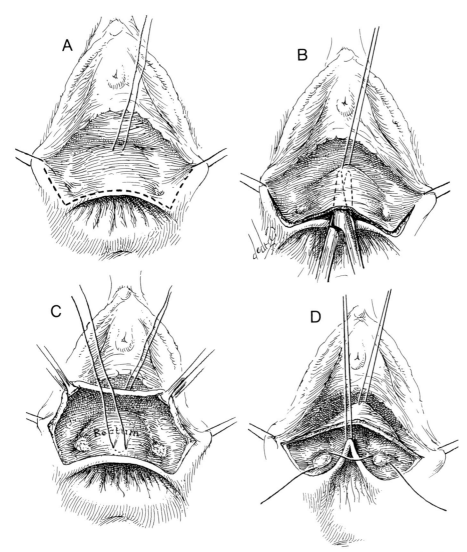

Figure 13.5. Sphincterplasty (Novak). **A.** The perineal defect has been displayed by the three traction sutures as shown. An initial incision along the mucocutaneous border is followed by incisions lateral to the dimples identifying the ends of the torn anal sphincter. The configuration is not unlike the letter W. **B.** The rectovaginal space is identified and entered and the vagina carefully separated from the rectum by sharp dissection that extends lateral to the divided ends of the anal sphincter. **C.** A traction suture is placed in the anterior wall of the rectum. **D.** When upward traction is applied to the rectal traction stitch, the torn ends of the sphincter stand out even more clearly. They are grasped with Allis clamps and freed from the surrounding tissue by sharp dissection, and a stitch of long-lasting polyglycolic acid-type suture is placed in each end of the torn sphincter. Any previous laceration of the anterior rectal wall is approximated from side to side with two layers of interrupted stitches if the mucosa is intact; otherwise the traction suture on the rectal wall has to be placed higher up, the laceration totally excised, and the freshened rectal wound approximated with two layers. **E.** The ends of the torn anal sphincter are approximated by tying the previously placed stitch, and an additional reinforcing mattress stitch or two is placed in the sphincter muscle and tied. **F.** The perineal body is reconstructed by a series of interrupted stitches approximating it from side to side. **G.** The skin of the vagina and perineum is closed vertically. (*Continues on following page.*) (Modified from Abram C. In: Novak F. Surgical gynecologic techniques. New York: Wiley, 1978:164–170. Used with permission.)

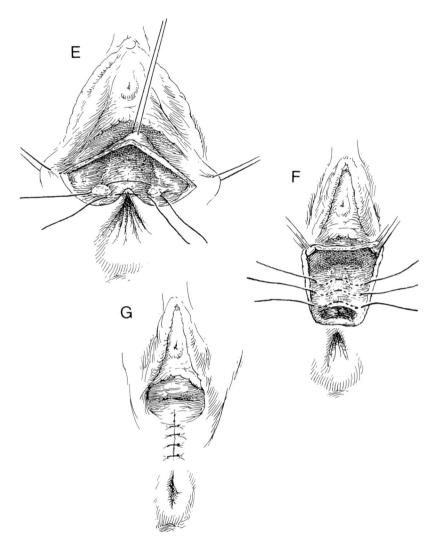

Figure 13.5, E to G.

ward tension is applied to this latter suture, the dimpling identifying the scar of the torn edges of the external anal sphincter will be more noticeable, and the edges may be grasped with Allis clamps or Kocher forceps. The scarred ends of the sphincter may be excised from the surrounding scar tissue by sharp dissection and a PDS or polyglycolic acid-type suture placed in the retracted scarred ends of the sphincter, as shown in Figure 13.5D. If the freed sphincter is long enough, the ends can be overlapped. For recurrent cases a suture of a permanent monofilament—Prolene, Surgilene, or Novafil—can be used provided it can be buried effectively.

If there is a V-shaped defect in the anterior anal wall, it is approximated by interrupted submucosal polyglycolic acid-type sutures (Fig. 13.5E), and a second reinforcing layer is placed to take the tension off the first layer.

The perineal body is reinforced or reconstructed by a series of horizontally placed interrupted sutures (Fig. 13.5F), the stitch in the anal sphincter is tied, a second and perhaps third reinforcing mattress suture is placed in the muscle itself and tied, and the perineal skin is closed vertically (Fig. 13.5G).

POSTOPERATIVE CARE

Postoperative care for all of these procedures is much like that after repair of any type of rectovaginal fistula. A clear liquid and low-residue diet should be employed for 5 days, during which period constipation is to be encouraged. A rectal tube, however, may be used for short intervals to overcome any difficulty in expelling flatus. Stool softeners are started the third postoperative day and a gentle laxative the fourth, and after 3 weeks a gradual return to house diet is initiated. Stool softeners are given for a month postoperatively. An initial bowel movement is usually desirable by the seventh postoperative day, after which softening of the stool should be maintained for the following 3 weeks.

References

1. Aronson MP, Lee RA, Berquist TH. Anatomy of anal sphincters and related structures in continent women: studies with magnetic resonance imaging. Obstet Gynecol 1990;76:846.
2. Crawford LA, Quint EH, Pearl ML, DeLancey JOL. Incontinence following rupture of the anal sphincter during delivery. Obstet Gynecol 1993;82:527–531.
3. Hirschman LJ. Synopsis of ano-rectal disease. 2nd ed. St. Louis: Mosby–Year Book, 1942:18–19.
4. Jacobs PPM, Scheuer M, Kuijpers JHC, Vingerhoets MH. Obstetric fecal incontinence: role of pelvic floor denervation and results of delayed sphincter repair. Dis Colon Rectum 1990;33:494–497.
5. Kelly HA. Operative gynecology. New York: D Appleton, 1898;l:211.
6. Madoff RD, Williams JG, Caushaj PF. Fecal incontinence. N Engl J Med 1992;326:1102–1107.
7. Manning PC, Pratt JH. Fecal incontinence caused by lacerations of the perineum. Arch Surg 1964;88:569–576.
8. Mengert WF, Fish SA. Anterior rectal wall advancement. Obstet Gynecol 1955;5:262–267.
9. Miller NF, Brown W. The surgical treatment of complete perineal tears in the female. Am J Obstet Gynecol 1937;34:196–209.
10. Nichols DH. Recurrent anal incontinence. In: Nichols DH, ed. Reoperative gynecologic surgery. St. Louis: Mosby–Year Book, 1991:219–225.
11. Nichols DH. Repair of rectal fistula and of old complete perineal laceration. In: Nichols DH, ed. Gynecologic and obstetric surgery. St. Louis: Mosby–Year Book, 1993:472–496.
12. Noble GH. A new operation for complete laceration of the perineum designed for the purpose of eliminating danger of infection from the rectum. Trans Am Gynecol Soc 1902;27:357.
13. Novak F. Surgical gynecologic techniques. New York: Wiley, 1978:164–170.
14. Oh C, Kark AE. Anatomy of the external anal sphincter. Br J Surg 1972;59:717–723.
15. Snooks SJ, Henry MM. Fecal incontinence due to external anal sphincter division in childbirth is associated with damage to the innervation of the pelvic floor musculature: a double pathology. Br J Obstet Gynecol 1985;92:824–828.
16. Swash M. New concepts in incontinence. Br Med J 1985;290:4–5.
17. Swash M, Henry MM. Unifying concept of pelvic floor disorders and incontinence. J Roy Soc Med 1985;78:906–911.
18. Warren JC. A new method of operation for the relief of rupture of the perineum through the sphincter and rectum. Trans Am Gynecol Soc 1882;7:322.

Retrorectal Levatorplasty

There is an uncommon major disorder of the integrity of the levator ani in which the pelvic diaphragm and the levator plate sag to such a degree that the patient actually sits upon her anus (Fig. 14.1). At times, this is accompanied by an unusual bearing-down sensation and difficulty with evacuation. The harder the patient strains attempting evacuation, the more difficult a movement becomes, as levator funneling in this condition becomes greater with straining, with a decrease in anal and stool diameter.

The condition is demonstrated while examining the patient when she is sitting on the examination table and the examiner's hand is introduced beneath the anus. As the patient strains the anus descends still further. This descent or prolapse of both anus and perineum must be clearly differentiated from rectal prolapse, which is an actual intussusception of the bowel through the anal sphincter (14). Variations in the angular relationship between the rectal inclination and the pelvic floor can be measured radiographically with a high degree of accuracy (3). Examination of the pelvis with the patient in the lithotomy position reveals a pathologic and almost vertical vaginal and rectal axis, and a short and tipped levator plate posterior to the rectum. In the perineal descent syndrome, the anus is the most dependent portion of the perineum.

This dependent location of the anus contrasts with its usual position in the intergluteal fold, and may be associated with chronic constipation or even obstipation requiring digital manipulation to achieve evacuation, or the deliberate abuse of laxatives to achieve an almost chronic state of diarrhea. This combination of anatomic displacement of the anus and chronic constipation or obstipation in the absence of rectal intussusception or prolapse is called the perineal descent syndrome. Some patients may evacuate by sitting on a board with a 3-inch hole, the edges of which extend counterpressure around the sides of the anus (DM Gallagher, personal communication). At times the condition produces the characteristic but uncommon symptom complex described, along with a feeling of pelvic and rectal pressure of falling out when standing. On occasion it becomes very difficult for the patient to sit comfortably. Prolapse of the anus and perineum appears to result from a variety of causes, including trauma, obstetric damage, defective innervation (11, 12, 23–25), aging, and chronically increased intra-abdominal pressure.

There appear to be two kinds of perineal prolapse. One is the result of traumatic multiparous stretching of the pelvic diaphragm, associated with constipation or obstipation; and the other is neuropathically induced, probably from stretching of the pudendal nerve consequent to obstetric labor or to long-standing constipation and straining at stool (12, 25). It is more common in the parous patient. This neuropathy probably leads to histologically demonstrable and more or less irreversible degeneration of the muscular cells of the levator ani. There may be an increased association with urinary stress incontinence (12). Although neuromuscular activity can be measured electromyographically (10, 12, 25, 28, 30), it can to some measure be predicted by the apparent inability of the patient

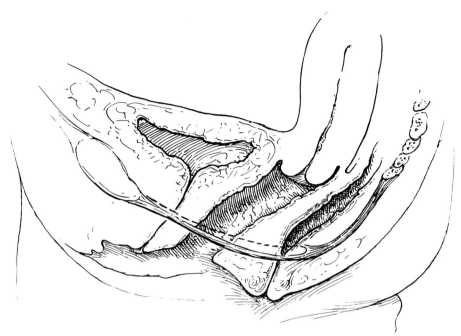

Figure 14.1. Sagittal section of the pelvis showing elongation and sagging of the levator plate. The usual angle between the anal canal and the rectum has been lost, as well as the horizontal axis of the rectum and the upper vagina.

to voluntarily contract her pubococcygei and external anal sphincter. The muscle and fascia stretching type may be effectively treated by timely retrorectal levatorplasty with colporrhaphy; the nerve stretching type may be augmented by the Parks postanal repair.

Perineal prolapse can be prevented by the proper conduct of labor, as well as subsequent lifelong establishment of good bowel habits and even the use of a mild laxative or suppository, if necessary, with increased bulk in the diet. Increased water intake (remembering that some degree of systemic dehydration is more common coincident with the diminution of thirst that grows greater with aging) and regular pubococcygeal isometric resistive exercises are helpful.

With perineal descent, constipation may appear as an early symptom due to loss of the integrity of an intact pelvic diaphragm during bearing-down efforts. As the phenomenon of strong voluntary bearing down effort becomes more regular and intense, the pudendal nerve may be damaged by stretching (11, 12, 23, 25), disturbing the innervation of both the pelvic diaphragm and the external anal sphincter, with resultant partial paralysis and atrophy of these muscles.

This may sometimes produce perineal prolapse with first obstipation and later rectal incontinence if the protective internal sphincter mechanism becomes overburdened. When perineal prolapse also correlates with a decreased perception of subjective feelings of rectal fullness, there may be degeneration of some of the neuromuscular receptors within the levator ani. This, in turn, may correlate with a less favorable prognosis after anatomic surgical reconstruction.

Bowel function is to a large extent a phenomenon of habit, and the esophogoanal and gastrocolic reflexes regularly assist. Providing there is content in the sigmoid colon, defecation is achieved by voluntarily first relaxing the pelvic diaphragm and external anal sphincter and then unlocking the colic valve, letting normal intestinal peristalsis take over with relaxation of the involuntary internal anal sphincter. Movement is then aided by modest increases in intra-abdominal pressure as by voluntary bearing down. A disorder of any of these steps may predispose to constipation.

It is possible that reconstruction of a damaged levator muscle with an intact nerve supply may produce a functionally more favorable result than when the nerve supply has been significantly defective, whatever the cause.

The levator plate, formed by fusion of the bellies of the pubococcygeus muscles, for the most part posterior to the rectum, extends to the insertion of these muscles upon the coccyx and lower portion of the sacrum (2, 9, 24). When the plate is intact, it is more or less horizontal in position; but when markedly attenuated, it becomes a loose hammock (Fig. 14.2). As the plate sags it tips, and with increases in intra-abdominal pressure may permit those structures that lie upon it to literally slide downhill (9). The latter structures, principally the vagina and rectum, in addition to descending, on occasion

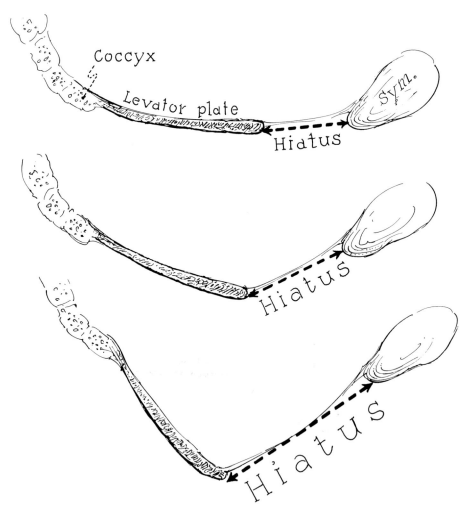

Figure 14.2. Drawings depicting sagging of the levator plate. As the levator plate sags, the genital hiatus becomes larger. In addition, the pull of gravity and the forces of intra-abdominal pressure accentuate the strain upon the pelvic suspensory system. *Sym.*, symphysis pubis. (After Berglas BB, Rubin IC. Study of the supportive structures of the uterus by levator myography. Surg Gynecol Obstet 1953;97;672–692. Used with permission of Surgery, Gynecology & Obstetrics, now known as the Journal of the American College of Surgeons.)

may exhibit telescoping when their respective axes are in the direction of increases in intra-abdominal pressure.

Uniting the medial portions of the pubococcygei beneath the vagina and anterior to the rectum does thicken the tissues of the perineum by interposing a muscular layer not initially well developed here (see Chapter 11). However, this neither shortens the muscles, nor restores the defective axis of the plate, nor corrects the pathologic descent of the anus and rectum (Fig. 14.3). The literature has not recorded much surgical technique or experience in achieving these goals, although lengthening of the levator plate has been described by the transperineal approach of Lange (17) and by the transabdominal surgery approach using various modifications of the operation of Roscoe Graham (6, 7, 8).

Although a surgeon can plicate the pubococcygeal muscles posterior to the rectum using a transabdominal approach, the exposure is difficult and deep within the pelvis, and pathologic vaginal displacements with associated cystocele and rectocele cannot be approached satisfactorily through the same operative exposure. Barrett (1) suggested a transperineal approach by incision and dissection between the anus and vagina, "posteriorly to the rectum in properly selected cases and the separated levator reunited with attachment of the rectal wall to this muscle," but apparently did not document pursuit of his idea.

Clinical interest in the Kraske or sacral transperineal approach to some surgical lesions of the rectum has reaffirmed the safety of this route (3, 4, 8, 13, 15, 16, 18, 19, 22, 31), and we have described a procedure using this approach to correct the levator deficiencies described above (20, 21). This transperineal retrorectal approach shortens the pubococcygei and puborectalis as necessary, and unites the medial bellies of these muscles in the midline posterior to the rectum, thus lengthening the levator plate and advancing the genital hiatus anteriorly. The posterior rectal wall is attached to the internal periosteum of the lower sacrum by a series of interrupted sutures, reestablishing or con-

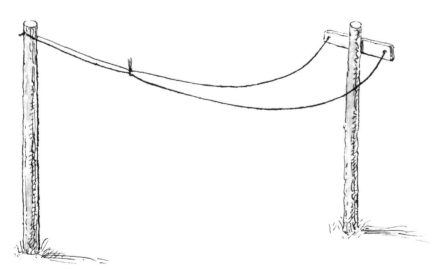

Figure 14.3. Representation of pathologically elongated pubococcygei. When elongated, the pubococcygei may be likened to a sagging clothesline suspended between two fixed poles. Tying one side to the other, as shown, will bring each side closer to the other but will not shorten the lines or reduce the sagging. For this reason, perineorrhaphy, per se, is ineffective in the treatment of the anal and perineal prolapse that is secondary to pathologic elongation of the pubococcygeal portion of the pelvic diaphragm. The clotheslines (as well as the pubococcygei) can effectively be shortened only by decreasing their length.

structing a relatively horizontal axis to the rectum and to the vagina overlying it. This procedure permits suspension of the elongated rectum (5, 15, 27) and, by the addition of appropriate supplemental anterior and posterior colporrhaphy (26, 29), the correction of any coexistent cystocele and rectocele. Any enterocele should be excised (32).

Significant individual variation in the strength and length of the anococcygeal raphe and the rectococcygeus muscle or ligament has been noteworthy.

The essential steps of the operation are as follows: The patient is positioned in the Kraske jackknife position (Fig. 14.4), although the standard lithotomy position may be used in those patients with plenty of pelvic room and on whom coincident colporrhaphy will be performed. A midline incision is made from the sacrum to the site of the external anal sphincter. The anococcygeal raphe is identified and separated from the coccyx; the latter is grasped in a towel clip but is not removed. Fat is displaced to identify the undersurfaces of the pubococcygei and the levator plate, which is usually incised in the midline, separating the right muscle belly from the left. The rectum is identified and separated from the levator muscles and plate. The rectococcygeal muscle or ligament is identified, if present, and transected, the retrorectal (or presacral) space thoroughly explored (Fig. 14.5), and the undersurface of the sacrum cleansed of fat and loose connective tissue, exposing the periosteum.

At least three plication stitches are placed in the posterior rectal wall 1 cm apart and are tied but not cut (Fig. 14.6). Using an overglove, a rectal examination is done to determine any suture penetration of the rectal mucosa, which if found would require replacement of the suture. These sutures are then sewn to the presacral fascia (Fig. 14.7). Polyglycolic acid-type sutures (Dexon, Vicryl, PDS or Maxon) are used throughout the operation. A large dental mirror and fiberoptic headlight are most helpful for visualizing the placement of these stitches. After all stitches have been placed, they are tied, beginning with the most cranial suture.

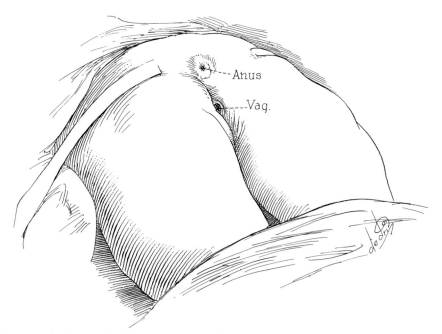

Figure 14.4. The "jackknife" or Kraske position. A sandbag has been placed beneath the hips, and the gluteal muscles are pulled apart by wide strips of adhesive tape fastened to the edges of the operating table.

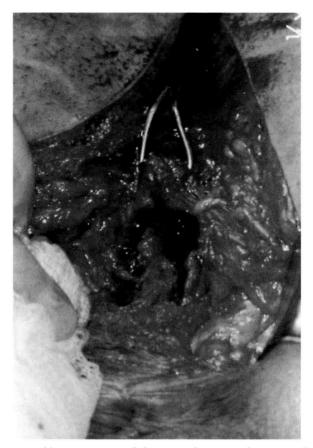

Figure 14.5. Retraction of the coccyx. A towel clip retracts the coccyx, the retrorectal space is entered, and the attenuated levator plate is cut in the midline to expose the posterior surface of the rectum.

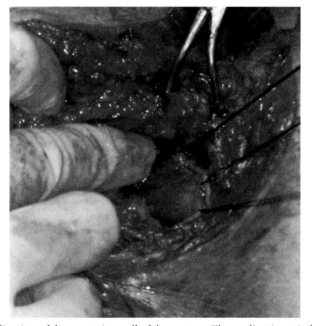

Figure 14.6. Plication of the *posterior* wall of the rectum. Three plication stitches have been introduced into the posterior wall of the rectum and tied.

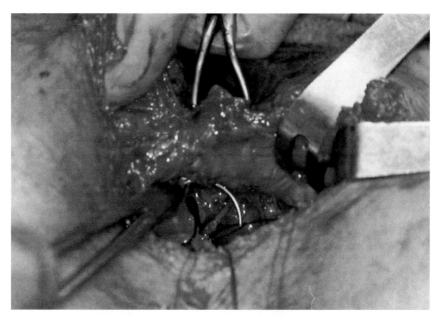

Figure 14.7. Sewing the tied plication stitches to the sacral periosteum. These are sewn to the presacral periosteum and, when tied, will bring the rectum back into the hollow of the sacrum.

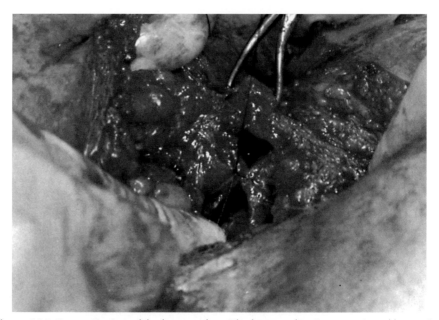

Figure 14.8. Reconstitution of the levator plate. The levator plate is reconstituted by sewing the borders of the pubococcygei muscles together posterior to the rectum. The first of several of these stitches has been placed and tied.

The coccyx usually is not removed, and the middle sacral artery is ligated only if essential to improve the anterior sacral exposure in a particular case or if the artery has been traumatized during dissection.

Using a series of interrupted sutures (Fig. 14.8), the medial borders of the levators (pubococcygei and puborectalis) are sewn together in the midline posterior to the rectum, restoring the levator plate (Fig. 14.9) and displacing the rectum forward.

The undersurface of both right and left limb of each pubococcygeus muscle (part of the anterior portion of the pelvic diaphragm) is shortened with Z-type sutures (see Fig. 14.9). The lower rectum is reattached to the medial surfaces of the pubococcygei, suspending the rectum higher within the pelvis than was seen preoperatively. The anococc-

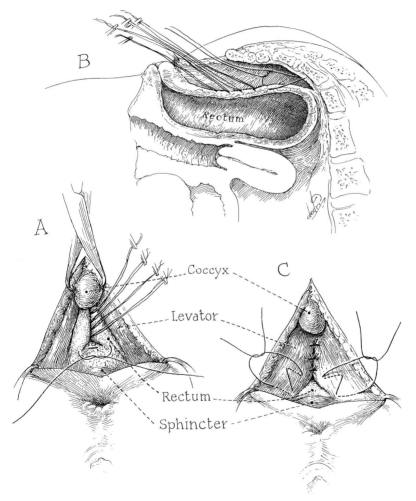

Figure 14.9. Summary of the three essential parts of the operation. **A.** A series of plication stitches are placed 1 cm apart in the posterior wall of the rectum, tied, and left long. **B.** The stitches are then anchored individually to the anterior periosteum of the sacrum. **C.** The levator plate is restored and lengthened by bringing the pubococcygei of each side together in the midline between the coccyx and rectum. The bellies of the pubococcygei may be shortened by a "Z" stitch placed as shown. (From Nichols DH. Retrorectal levatorplasty for anal and perineal prolapse. Surg Gynecol Obstet 1982;154:251–254. Used with permission of Surgery, Gynecology & Obstetrics, now known as the Journal of the American College of Surgeons.)

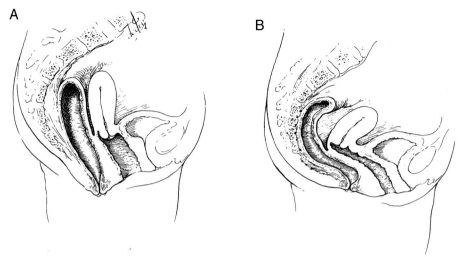

Figure 14.10. Comparison of preoperative with postoperative findings. **A.** Preoperative prolapse of the anus and perineum with tipping of the levator plate and elongation of the attachment of the rectum to the anterior surface of the sacrum. **B.** The result of surgery. The rectum has been approximated to the anterior periosteum of the sacrum, and the levator plate has been lengthened posterior to the rectum and shortened as necessary. The axes of the lower rectum and upper vagina now are more or less horizontal. An anorectal angulation is present, and the anus is no longer the most dependent portion of the perineum. (From Nichols DH. Retrorectal levatorplasty for anal and perineal prolapse. Surg Gynecol Obstet 1982;154:251–254. Used with permission of Surgery, Gynecology & Obstetrics, now known as the Journal of the American College of Surgeons.)

cygeal raphe is shortened as necessary and reattached to either the coccygeal periosteum or to the gluteal fascia. The subcutaneous tissue and the skin are closed with interrupted sutures.

Coincident anterior and posterior colporrhaphy, if indicated, and excision of any enterocele are performed with the patient repositioned to the conventional lithotomy position. If the perineal body has been separated from the connective tissue of the external anal sphincter, it may be reattached by a figure-of-eight stitch, thus further stabilizing both the perineum and anus. Sagittals section of the preoperative findings are shown in Figure 14.10*A*, and the postoperative result in Figure 14.10*B*.

This perineal prolapse is an uncommon type of genital prolapse and is characterized by descent of the anus and rectum and sagging of the normally horizontal levator plate. When the pathology is the consequence of damage to the anatomic integrity of the pelvic diaphragm, retrorectal levatorplasty with colporrhaphy may be curative of the coincident obstipation.

Rectal incontinence coincident with perineal prolapse suggests severe neuropathology and a less favorable postsurgical prognosis, although retrorectal levatorplasty with colporrhaphy or the Parks postanal repair (23) may recreate a useful anal valve that may be of help to the patient.

References

1. Barrett CW. Hernias through the pelvic floor. Am J Obstet Dis Wom 1909;59:553–569.
2. Berglas B, Rubin IC. Study of the supportive structures of the uterus by levator myography. Surg Gynecol Obstet 1953;97:672–692.
3. Boccasanta P, Segalin A, Bonavina L, Zennaro F, Salamina G, Velio P, Hofer C. L'inclinazione rettale posteriore nella diagnosi radiologica delle alterazioni della statica pelvi-rettale. Chirurgia 1995;8:38–42.
4. Crowley RT, Davis DA. A procedure for total biopsy of doubtful polypoid growths of the lowest bowel segment. Surg Gynecol Obstet 1951;93:23–26.

5. Davidian UA, Thomas CG. Transsacral repair of rectal prolapse. Am J Surg 1972;123:231.
6. Efron G. A simple method of posterior rectopexy for rectal procidentia. Surg Gynecol Obstet 1977; 145:75–76.
7. Goligher JC. The treatment of complete prolapse of the rectum by the Roscoe Graham operation. Br J Surg 1958;46:323–333.
8. Graham R. Operative repair of massive rectal prolapse. Ann Surg 1942;115: 1007.
9. Halban J, Tandler J. Anatomie und Ätiologie der Genitalprolapse beim Weibe. Wien: Braumüller, 1907, pp 52–3.
10. Haskell B, Rovner H. Electromyography in the management of the incompetent anal sphincter. Proceedings of American Proctologic Society, Cleveland, OH, June 1966.
11. Henry MM, Swash M. Assessment of pelvic floor disorders and incontinence by electrophysiological recording of the anal reflex. Lancet 1978;17:1290–1291.
12. Henry MM, Swash M, eds. Coloproctology and the pelvic floor. 2nd ed. Oxford: Butterworth-Heinemann, 1992.
13. Jenkins SG, Thomas CG. An operation for the repair of rectal prolapse. Surg Gvnecol Obstet 1962; 114:381–383.
14. Keighley M. Clinical features and pathophysiology of rectal prolapse. In: Henry MM, Swash M, eds. Coloproctology and the pelvic floor. 2nd ed. Oxford: Butterworth-Heinemann, 1992:316–321.
15. Klingensmith W, Dickinson WE, Hays RS. Posterior resection of selected rectal tumors. Arch Surg 1975;110:647–651.
16. Kraske P. Zur Extirpation Hochsitzender Mastdarmkrebse. Vehr Dtsch Ges Chir 1885;14:464–474.
17. Lange F. Intestinal and anal surgery. Quoted in Hadra BE, ed. Lesions of the vagina and pelvic floor. Philadelphia: McMullin,1888.
18. Lockhart-Mummery JP. Rectal prolapse. Br Med J 1939;1:345–348.
19. Mason AY. Trans-sphincteric surgery of the rectum. Prog Surg 1974;13:66–97.
20. Nichols DH. Retrorectal levatorplasty for anal and perineal prolapse. Surg Gynecol Obstet 1982;154: 251–254.
21. Nichols DH. Retrorectal levatorplasty with colporrhaphy. Clin Obstet Gynecol 1982;25:939–947.
22. O'Brien PH. Kraske's posterior approach to the rectum. Surg Gynecol Obstet 1976;142:412–414.
23. Parks AG. Anorectal incontinence. Proc Roy Soc Med 1975;68:681–690.
24. Parks AG. Modern concepts of the anatomy of the anorectal region. Postgrad Med J 1958;34:360–366.
25. Parks AG, Swash M, Urich H. Sphincter denervation in anorectal incontinence and rectal prolapse. J Br Soc Gastroenterol 1977;18:656–665.
26. Redding MD. The relaxed perineum and anorectal disease. Dis Colon Rectum 1965;8:279–282.
27. Romer-Torres R. Sacrofixation with marlex mesh in massive prolapse of the rectum. Surg Gynecol Obstet 1979;149:709–711.
28. Sharf B, Zilberman A, Shaft M, et al. Electromyogram of pelvic floor muscles in genital prolapse. Int J Gynaecol Obstet 1976;14:2–4.
29. Sullivan ES, Leaverton GH, Gary H, et al. Transrectal perineal repair: an adjunct to improved function after anorectal surgery. Proceedings of American Proctologic Society, New Orleans, LA, April 1967.
30. Taverner D, Smiddy. An electromyographic study of the normal function of the external anal sphincter and pelvic diaphragm. Dis Colon Rectum 1959;2:153–160.
31. Turner GG. Ideals and the art of surgery. Surg Gynecol Obstet 1931;52:273–311.
32. Wiersema JS. Treatment of complete prolapse of the rectum by the vaginal approach. Arch Chir Neerl 1976;28:25–31.

CHAPTER 15

Enterocele

Although by definition an enterocele is a peritoneum-lined sac between the vagina and the rectum, in most instances its symptoms are produced by traction upon its contents, which imply the presence of a long small bowel mesentery or omentum. Without the latter, the condition appears identical to that described as a "deep cul-de-sac," which is more frequently seen. The deep cul-de-sac will become an "enterocele" when small bowel mesentery and omentum have lengthened sufficiently to permit them to distend this deep cul-de-sac. Therefore, it should be obliterated coincidentally at surgery whenever it is found. The question may be asked, Does a long small bowel mesentery precede an enterocele sac or does it follow it?

It has been known for years (18, 19, 20, 32) that occasionally the posterior peritoneal cul-de-sac of Douglas will extend caudally between rectum and vagina to varying depths, even as far as the perineal body. When this space is filled with abdominal content, such as small bowel and omentum, the condition is known as enterocele. The length of the adult mesentery of the small intestine mesentery is usually about 15 cm (24), not long enough to permit a loop of small intestine to descend deeply into the pelvis. An abnormally long small intestinal mesentery is required to permit the bowel to descend this far. Because this content is not seen in all cases of deep cul-de-sac, one should distinguish those cases with bowel content and those without. The former are symptomatic with backache and a dragging sensation accentuated in the erect position and relieved by lying down, the discomfort probably the result of omental and mesenteric traction. The latter type, without bowel content, is generally asymptomatic. It is not known whether the two are etiologically different and whether the long intestinal mesentery is the cause or the result of the deep cul-de-sac when the two coexist. The weight of the bowel with a long mesentery may influence the possibility of recurrence of enterocele after treatment.

It is interesting that postoperative vaginal evisceration is so rare considering how often the vaginal vault is left open at the time of abdominal hysterectomy. Is this because the usual length of the small bowel mesentery is too short to permit routine pressure of the weight of the small bowel against the vault of the vagina?

In our experience, massive eversion of the vagina may occur with or without enterocele, though most commonly the former, and enterocele may occur with or without massive eversion (see Chapter 16). Enterocele and massive eversion often coexist, but are *separate* anatomic and clinical entities, each requiring separate, specific surgical treatment. It is essential that the gynecologist make these distinctions, since the treatment is quite different, as will be shown.

Strictly speaking, the term *enterocele* is a misnomer (10), since a hernia is named not according to its contents but according to its location. A better gynecologic term might be *hernia of the cul-de-sac*, but the present usage of the term *enterocele* has been accepted for so long that it would be hard to displace.

TYPES OF ENTEROCELE

An enterocele essentially consists of herniation of the lining of the peritoneal cavity, with or without portions of the abdominal viscera within the herniating sac, extending into areas of the pelvis where peritoneum is not usually found. Unrecognized and unrepaired, an enterocele tends to progress and causes increasing discomfort and, eventually, increasing disability.

Not infrequently, a competent gynecologic surgeon will repair a challenging enterocele with optimism and enthusiasm, only to find soon that as a result of the surgery a vagina with previously normal depth has become unexpectedly short and poorly supported. The surgeon may be unclear as to how an unacceptable vaginal shortening came about in one case but not in another. The surgeon may also be uncertain how to avoid repeating such an unsatisfactory result in the future.

It should be possible to recognize the possibility of such a problem ahead of time from the location of the enterocele. There seems to be a direct correlation between the location and the etiology. Using this information, a specific operative procedure can be selected that should prevent unexpected shortening of the vagina. Such consideration is the key to successful treatment, but it obligates the gynecologist to recognize etiologic factors in order to make a rational choice of the appropriate surgical procedure. The correct choice of operation will reduce the likelihood of a recurrence while avoiding an undesirable degree of vaginal shortening.

An enterocele may be identified as anterior, posterior, or lateral to the vagina (28), with or without secondary eversion of the vaginal vault. Efforts should always be made to distinguish an enterocele with accompanying vault eversion from one without such a complicating factor (27), because the etiology as well as the objectives and techniques of surgical reconstruction vary for each type of enterocele and are quite different when vaginal eversion is also present.

Figure 15.1 illustrates the significant relationships in the anatomy of enterocele that should suggest important differences in etiology. Figure 15.1A illustrates an enterocele posterior to the vault of the vagina, often associated with a *congenitally* deep pouch of Douglas and usually not associated with eversion of the vaginal vault. An unusually deep peritoneal pouch usually results from failure of normal fusion of the anterior with the posterior peritoneum of the cul-de-sac during late fetal development. If the soft tissue supports of the pelvis are otherwise intact, this type of posterior enterocele may exist quite independently of other lesions.

An enterocele associated with procidentia results from massive anterior segment damage as a result of both pulsion from above (20) and traction from below. As the cervix descends, it takes with it the anterior margin of the cul-de-sac, although the posterior peritoneal wall remains in situ and attached to the anterior wall of the rectum. The enterocele in Figure 15.1B is coexistent with eversion of the vault of the vagina and represents the result of *pulsion* from chronically increased intra-abdominal pressure; it is usually associated with the uterovaginal or sliding type of genital prolapse. This is a most massive form of damage, and descent of the entire upper vaginal suspensory apparatus is secondary to this descent. Reconstruction of this type involves not only excision of the enterocele sac but, more importantly, fixation or suspension of the vault of the vagina to some adequate structure capable of supporting it; if this is not done, permanent pathologic shortening of the vagina will be the inevitable result. Figure 15.1C illustrates another type of enterocele, also with eversion of the vagina but with associated cystocele and rectocele. This type of enterocele has developed as a result of *traction* to a poorly supported vaginal vault by the other pelvic structures that are already prolapsed. Enterocele with eversion of the entire vagina including the tissues caudal to the urogenital diaphragm, and thus the vesicourethral junction, is shown in Figure 15.1D. Note the change in the urethral axis when compared to Figure 15.1, A to C.

Iatrogenic alterations in pelvic anatomy may also play a role, as, for example, when development of an anterior enterocele (Fig. 15.2) is favored because of an unresected excess of anterior peritoneum that was not removed at the time of hysterectomy, or when the development of a posterior enterocele is favored because a surgical procedure

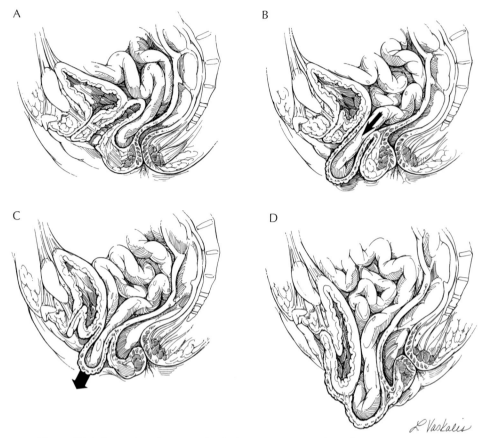

L. Vaskalis

Figure 15.1. Examples of enterocele. **A.** Posterior enterocele without eversion of the vagina. **B.** Pulsion enterocele; the upper vagina is everted and the enterocele sac follows the everted vault. Cystocele and rectocele are minimal. **C.** Traction enterocele; there is eversion of the upper two-thirds of the vagina with enterocele, cystocele, and rectocele. **D.** Eversion of the entire vagina, including the tissues distal to the urogenital diaphragm. Notice the change in the urethral axis.

changed the normally horizontal vaginal axis to a vertical inclination. Failure to recognize and correct an unusually deep cul-de-sac at the time of hysterectomy may favor the development of a posterior enterocele.

It would appear from the report of Burch (2) that enterocele may follow the vesicourethral "pin-up" operation in 11 to 15 percent of instances, probably because this operation induces a change in the vaginal axis that may leave the cul-de-sac unprotected and therefore subject to unusual stress from periodic increases in intra-abdominal pressure. For this reason, it appears desirable that specific intraperitoneal operative steps be taken to obliterate the cul-de-sac at the time of a vesicourethral "pin-up" operation, sparing the patient the risk of the secondary difficulty of subsequent enterocele. This may be accomplished by Moschcowitz (15) or Halban (5) sutures or even by the peritonealization following coincident hysterectomy. It is perhaps for these reasons that the incidence of subsequent enterocele should be less when surgery that changes the vaginal axis is performed by a thoughtful gynecologic surgeon who will open the peritoneal cavity and deliberately obliterate the cul-de-sac, particularly when there is pathologic widening of the posterior vaginal fornix, than it is when a thoughtless surgeon regularly performs a only a "pin-up" operation.

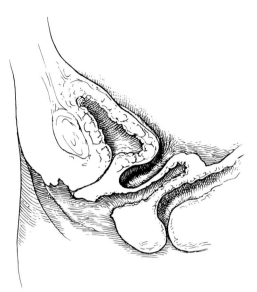

Figure 15.2. Posthysterectomy anterior enterocele between the bladder and the vagina. (From Nichols DH. Types of enterocele and principles underlying the choice of operation for repair. Obstet Gynecol 1972;40:257–263. Used with permission of Lippincott-Raven.)

With the congenital type of enterocele related to a pathologically deep cul-de-sac of Douglas, the anterior wall of the sac is attached to the undersurface of the posterior vaginal wall. This attachment is usually not present when acquired descent of the vaginal vault is coincident with general postmenopausal prolapse.

The incidence of enterocele *subsequent* to vaginal hysterectomy can only be determined by a long-term follow-up. A postoperative examination at 6 weeks gives no indication of this problem, for it is usually more than 6 months after operation before an enterocele occurs, and often it is not until after 1 or more years.

In Hawksworth and Roux's series (6), a 6-week follow-up was carried out on 944 patients after vaginal reconstruction. Only 3 were noted to have enteroceles causing symptoms that required subsequent operation. More than 1 year after surgery, 416 such patients were examined, among whom were 26 with enterocele symptoms requiring repair.

A noticeable defect in the attachments of the rectum may give rise to true rectal prolapse, which may coexist with or without an accompanying genital prolapse (see Fig. 5.5). As mentioned above, there is direct correlation between the principal locations of enterocele and the principal causes; when the etiologic factors have been identified, an appropriate selection of surgical repair may be made on a rational basis in order to lessen the chances of recurrence.

Whereas a cystocele and rectocele may precede a traction enterocele, they may follow a pulsion enterocele.

Coexistent enterocele may be either of the pulsion or the traction type, being either pushed down from above by pathologically increased intra-abdominal pressure or pulled down with a prolapsing cervix as a result of upper vaginal eversion. In a few instances, development of an enterocele will have been favored by a congenitally deep pouch of Douglas.

The four basic causes of enterocele—congenital, pulsion, traction, iatrogenic— should be recognized, and these may occur either singly or in combination. They are also the four different types of enterocele most frequently encountered, and each represents one of the basic etiologic factors. Because both pulsion and traction enteroceles are invariably progressive, they tend ultimately to pull with them the organs attached to the sides of the herniating peritoneal sac. As a result, there may be complete eversion of the vaginal vault, which usually, combined with a degree of lower vaginal eversion, requires repair. Subjective "bearing-down" symptoms are often related to mesenteric traction from the presence of bowel, omentum, or ovary within an enterocele sac. The pressure of a vaginal mass may also be noted, especially when standing. Identification of the enterocele as congenital, pulsion, traction, or iatrogenic becomes a matter of significance when surgical treatment is planned.

The argument as to whether anterior and posterior colporrhaphy is indicated whenever a vaginal hysterectomy is done should be settled in each instance on the basis of whether a significant degree of uterine prolapse is present, as determined by examination of the unanesthetized patient both while she is supine and while she is standing. Many surgeons elect the vaginal route when hysterectomy is indicated, when, for instance, there is dysfunctional uterine bleeding, with or without coincident small fibroids. Surgery by this route can often proceed quickly and with a minimum of postoperative discomfort and morbidity. However, an accompanying vaginal prolapse, if demonstrable but untreated, will be likely to progress in the postoperative years to a point requiring secondary operative reconstruction. A so-called pseudoprolapse may, however, warrant no other attention than recognition as such at the time of vaginal hysterectomy.

Progression of each of these types of true prolapse may finally result in massive eversion of the vagina. The correlation between etiology, location, and treatment of various types of enterocele is summarized (17) in Table 15.1.

It is important to distinguish pseudoenterocele from enterocele. Figure 11.4 illustrates pseudoenterocele in a patient whose midvaginal rectocele was not treated, although a simple perineorrhaphy had been performed. A precept in rectocele repair is that the repair should extend from a point cranial to the site of damage.

There are partial degrees of eversion that will generally progress if ignored at hysterectomy. See Figure 16.4A, which shows neither cystocele nor rectocele, but a vault that is coming down by pulsion. Figure 16.4B shows a traction eversion of the vault with cystocele and rectocele.

Table 15.1.
Correlation between Etiology, Location, and Treatment of Enterocele

Cause	Location	Treatment
Congenital	Sac between posterior vaginal wall and anterior rectal wall	Excision of the sac with high ligation of its neck; approximation of utero-sacral ligaments
Pulsion (pushed)	With eversion of vaginal vault	Restore vault depth by shortening cardinal-utero-sacral ligaments or culdeplasty if ligaments are strong. If ligaments are of poor quality, do sacrospinous fixation or sacrocolpopexy; coincident hysterectomy is often desirable
Traction (pulled)	Same as congenital, with lower eversion (cystocele and rectocele) pulling vault into eversion	Use same procedure as above plus anterior and posterior colporrhaphy
Iatrogenic	Anterior to vagina, or posterior from change in vaginal axis	Excise or obliterate sac and restore vaginal axis to normal if it is defective

From Nichols DH. Types of enterocele and principles underlying the choice of operation for repair. Obstet Gynecol 1972; 40:257–263.

Pudendal (1, 4) or lateral enterocele (Fig. 15.3) is most uncommon and may develop in sites of unusual weakness within or alongside the pelvic diaphragm or through the pelvic foramina. There may be a history of sudden traumatic increase in intra-abdominal pressure, either from the strain of exceedingly heavy lifting or from sudden massive abdominal compression, as from an explosion or blast. This traumatic increase has been reported when a patient has survived the trauma of having her abdomen run over by the wheel of a car. We have seen it in a patient on whose abdomen a horse had fallen. The enterocele may be brought to the patient's attention by the presence of a mass appearing alongside the vagina, but those that do not appear externally are likely to be diagnosed at the time of laparotomy for intestinal obstruction, in which the neck of the pudendal enterocele will be found to be the site of the mechanical obstruction.

RARE HERNIAS OF THE PELVIC FLOOR

Evacuation proctography may demonstrate rare hernias of the pelvic floor that are occasionally extraperitoneal. These are, in order of decreasing frequency: obturator, perineal, and sciatic.

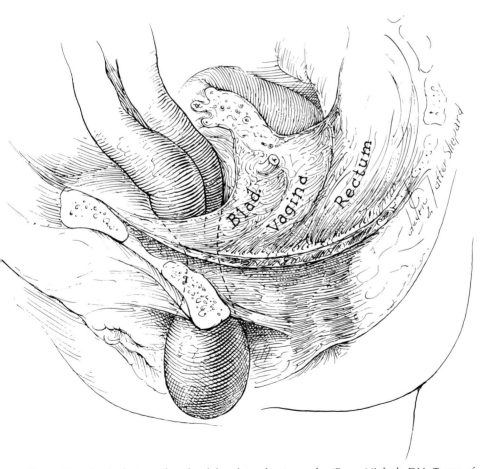

Figure 15.3. Sagittal view of pudendal or lateral enterocele. (From Nichols DH. Types of enterocele and principles underlying the choice of operation for repair. Obstet Gynecol 1972;40:257–263, with permission of Lippincott-Raven.)

Obturator Hernia

This is a rare type of pelvic hernia seen most commonly in elderly women and associated with a loss of weight. It occurs when the fatty plug that fills the obturator canal becomes atrophied and leaves a potential defect. Any condition that increases intra-abdominal pressure will increase the risk of a herniation (23, 26, 29). The surgeon must remember the relationship of the branches of the obturator artery lest it be cut during the repair of the hernia, resulting in severe hemorrhage. Because the sac is medial to the neurovascular bundle, the incision, if the sac cannot be reduced, should be made posteriorly and medially. The opposite side should be examined because there is a 6 percent incidence of bilaterality (21). Pressure on the obturator nerve by the hernia may elicit the so-called Howship-Romberg sign, which is characterized by intermittent pain referred to the medial thigh and knee and associated with abdominal pain. It may be of the Richter type (partial herniation only), although if bowel is trapped within the hernia the condition may produce an intestinal obstruction (29).

Perineal Hernia

This rare pelvic hernia is more common in females than males, possibly because of attenuation of the pelvic floor during pregnancy. It may be primary (congenitally acquired) or secondary (after exenteration or abdominoperineal resection), and either anterior or posterior to the transverse perineal muscle. It may be seen as a labial mass or a swelling between the anus and the ischial tuberosity (3), and may be associated with difficulty in defecation, although some are asymptomatic, presenting as a soft, reducible perineal mass. Intestinal incarceration and obstruction are uncommon because of the wide neck of the sac. The treatment is always surgical, involving closure of the neck of the sac and occasionally reinforcement of tissue defect by fascia transplant or permanent synthetic fabric.

Sciatic Hernia

This hernia is either congenital, due to maldevelopment of the piriform muscle, or acquired. Although exceedingly uncommon, it may be one of three types, depending upon location: through the greater sciatic foramen, cranial to the piriform muscle, or caudal to the muscle and through the lesser sciatic foramen beneath the sacrospinous ligament. Symptoms, when present, usually are those of intestinal obstruction, which is treated by appropriate laparotomy. Sciatic nerve compression may cause pain that radiates down the posterior thigh. When found, but asymptomatic, these hernias should be treated by obliteration or excision of the sac and tight closure of its neck, most likely transabdominally.

Other Hernias of the Pelvis

Hernias of the broad ligament either above or below the suspensory ligament of the ovary have been described, and may be the cause of intra-abdominal pain when intestine or omentum has become trapped in the pouch (7).

Rarely, a rectal hernia may protrude through a defect in the muscles of the pelvic floor, and when extraperitoneal, there will be no peritoneal sac. Cali et al. (3) have provided an excellent review of the rare hernias of the pelvic floor.

SYMPTOMS

Enterocele and vault prolapse are often associated with a feeling of pelvic heaviness and a bearing-down sensation, especially when standing, the result of the pull of gravity stretching the mesentery of the contents of the sac. If the cardinal and uterosacral ligaments are involved in the prolapse, downward traction on the uterosacral ligaments will often give rise to a backache that may worsen as the day goes on and is quickly relieved by lying down. There may be vaginal discomfort from the presence of a protruding vulvar mass; and coincident dyspareunia is common, accentuated by dryness of the exteriorized vagina. If the vaginal skin is ulcerated, there may be troublesome discharge and bleeding. When rectocele coexists, the patient may experience difficulty emptying the bowel, incomplete movements, and postevacuation discomfort. Urinary complaints are uncommon unless displacement cystocele coexists, which causes inability to empty the bladder, resulting in stagnation of urine with overflow incontinence. One should anticipate relief from the discomfort and distress of all of these symptoms by thoughtful and appropriate reconstructive genital surgery.

DIAGNOSIS

Descent of the cul-de-sac without enterocele is primarily related to a major defect in the pelvic diaphragm. It is usually, although not always, seen in a postmenopausal woman in whom the pelvic diaphragm sags, the levator plate tips, and the horizontal axis of the upper vagina is lost. It differs from enterocele, which is an actual herniation between rectum and vagina. The proper time to make this distinction is before the operation, because by that time the patient is recumbent, and damage that is obvious when the patient is awake and straining is now less evident. One must not forget the findings noted previously in the examining room.

An effective way of distinguishing between enterocele, prolapse of the vaginal vault, rectocele, and combinations of these weaknesses is by examination of the standing and unanesthetized patient as part of the initial physical examination. With an index finger in the rectum, the thumb is inserted into the vagina. The presence or absence of vault prolapse can be established when one replaces the vault of the vagina to its highest level within the pelvis and notes what happens when the patient is asked to bear down as by a Valsalva maneuver. If a peritoneal sac, containing omentum or a palpable loop of bowel, comes down between the thumb and index finger, the woman unquestionably has an enterocele (Fig. 15.4). Because an enterocele splits the fascia of Denonvilliers, it weakens the upper posterior vaginal wall. One often sees high rectocele coincident with enterocele, so often, in fact, that the presence of one should always suggest the presence of the other. The treatment of both should be coincident and will often require a transvaginal, rather than transabdominal, surgical procedure for optimal success.

Coexistent rectocele as well as a defective perineum can also be diagnosed by a finger in the rectum.

We believe that the importance of such preoperative evaluation relates to the fact that many enteroceles thought to have developed after vaginal surgery are aggravations of an unrecognized and, therefore, untreated process already existing at the time of the original pelvic operation.

The first principle in the management of enterocele is recognition of the entity and its probable cause. The gynecologist must remember that an enterocele can coexist with other manifestations of genital prolapse, but it is likely to be unrecognized when the patient is examined only when relaxed and in the lithotomy position. Preoperative rectovaginal examination and evaluation of the unanesthetized patient is, therefore, indicated with the patient both at rest and while straining, in both the lithotomy and standing positions. Contrast radiography will occasionally prove helpful (8, 9).

TREATMENT

The objectives of treatment for enterocele are as follows:

1. Restoration of normal anatomy and function
2. Prevention of recurrence as a result of the recognition and consideration of etiologic factors

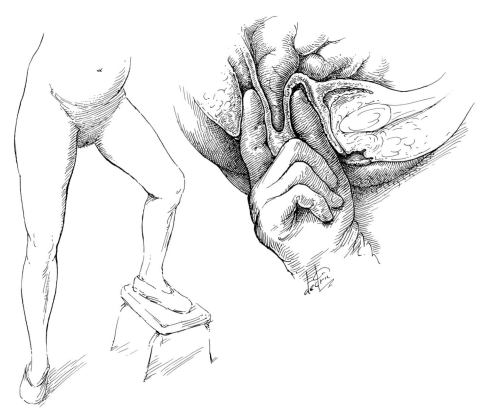

Figure 15.4. Examination for enterocele. Examination of the patient in a standing position permits the thumb in the vagina to note and replace any descent of the vaginal vault, while the index finger introduced into the rectum permits evaluation of any possible rectocele. When the patient strains, any enterocele present is evidenced by palpation of a bowel-filled sac prolapse dissecting the rectovaginal septum. (From Nichols DH. Repair of enterocele and prolapse of the vaginal vault. In: Barber H, ed. Goldsmith's practice of surgery. Woodbury, CT: Cine-Med Inc., 1981. Used with permission.)

   3. Appropriate surgical treatment of coexistent pelvic disease when indicated
   4. Recognition and treatment of any contributing medical disease.

Prophylaxis

Prophylaxis is important, and increased intra-abdominal pressure may be reduced by reducing weight appropriately, avoiding tight girdles and corsets, and refraining from cigarettes to decrease smoker's cough.

Pessaries are occasionally of temporary help in patients with coincident genital prolapse who are not candidates for surgery or whose personal schedule will not yet permit surgery, such as those with small children at home or with an aging relative who requires constant care. If a pessary can be retained, it will often be of the ring type, occasionally a rubber doughnut, or sometimes a Gellhorn. Isometric pubococcygeal contraction exercises are helpful in restoring muscle tone, but they are not curative.

At the time of initial vaginal hysterectomy and repair, one can do much to prevent postoperative enterocele (11). Enterocele may be present, but not obvious, in the patient who is anesthetized and in the Trendelenburg position, in which the pull of gravity is toward the head of the table. After the uterus has been removed and before the peritoneum has been closed, one should hook a finger in the cul-de-sac to see if there is extra cul-de-sac peritoneum; if present, this should be excised. If strong uterosacral ligaments are found, they should be shortened and used in an appropriate fashion to help support the vaginal vault. This may include the culdeplasty (14) that involves penetration of these now shortened uterosacral ligaments (see Chapter 8). This will draw the vault of the vagina back into the hollow of the sacrum, cranial and posterior to the point at which the peritoneum has been closed. The same stitches may be applied immediately after abdominal hysterectomy, along with transabdominal excision and side-to-side approximation of an appropriate wedge from the posterior vaginal vault if it is excessively wide. After vaginal hysterectomy, a high pursestring closure of the peritoneal cavity is often helpful, taking both uterosacral and round ligaments with good bites but being careful to avoid the ureter. This approximates the connective tissues to which the peritoneum is attached. If a large enterocele has been resected, one might wish to first close the peritoneum by a running front-to-back suture, followed by placement of two pursestring sutures, one caudal to the other, using a long-lasting polyglycolic acid-type suture (Vicryl, Dexon, PDS, Maxon).

Principles of Repair

The following are general principles for the repair of enterocele:

1. Expose, dissect, mobilize, and then excise or obliterate the entire sac.
2. Occlude the orifice of the sac by ligating as high as possible.
3. In performing all indicated repair, provide adequate support from below for the occluded orifice of the sac, and reconstitute a normal upper vaginal axis, if defective, so that the area of previous herniation will be held in place over a horizontal levator plate.

Choice of Operation

Our choice of surgical procedures is based on the following considerations:

Transvaginal procedures include recognition and excision of the sac with high ligation of the peritoneum (Fig. 15.5).

The transvaginal double-pursestring closure of the neck of the enterocele sac is essentially a low transvaginal Moschcowitz closure. Each pursestring takes some of the strain off the other. Bringing together two areas of peritoneum lining the neck of the sac instead of one produces a stronger scar (Fig. 15.6). It is useful if there is a coincident vault prolapse that is to be treated separately.

Our objection to the transabdominal Moschcowitz procedure for enterocele is that the original operation had been intended for a prolapsed or sliding rectum, which was then attached by concentric pursestring sutures to a fairly strong vagina and cervix. Gynecologists, however, appropriated this operation and reversed the principle by attaching a sliding vagina to the anterior wall of the rectum. The latter has rather poor structural support.

The Halban or Moschcowitz obliteration of the cul-de-sac is only useful in helping to prevent an enterocele; it will not treat a vault prolapse effectively. Neither the Halban nor the Moschcowitz stitch is able, in itself, to provide support for the vaginal vault; both obliterate the cul-de-sac, and neither requires removal of excess peritoneum. There are several other problems with the Moschcowitz or pursestring approach. Tying the top stitch at the pelvic brim may be difficult and, if any central opening remains, the little hole can provide access to a loop of small bowel, resulting in intestinal obstruction. The top stitch, because it is placed near the ureter, may be so close as to pull or displace the tissue to which the ureter is attached, and in this way it may kink the ureter on either side, with resultant obstruction.

Figure 15.5. Transvaginal repair of medium-sized enterocele. The enterocele sac has been resected and the peritoneal cavity will be closed by a pursestring suture of long-lasting synthetic material that incorporates the uterosacral and the round ligaments as shown. After this has been tied, a second pursestring stitch placed 1 cm distal to the first reinforces the closure.

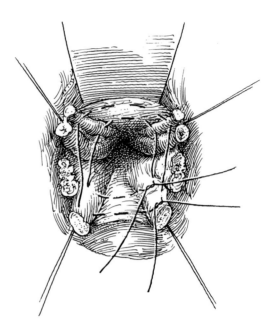

Sagittally placed Halban-type stitches are actually a *vertical* Moschcowitz type of suture placement but do not disturb the course of the ureter. They are especially useful when there is no coincident vault prolapse. They can be placed after either transabdominal or transvaginal operations (Fig. 15.7), but it must be remembered that neither type of enterocele repair alone will effectively support a poorly or unsupported vaginal vault.

The incidence of recurrent enterocele may be reduced by strengthening the scar following repair through the use of nonabsorbable suture material in its repair, and by closing the peritoneal sac with more than one layer of suture. An effective, fast, and safe method of repair for the large enterocele that does not involve much peritoneal resection is to obliterate a wide pouch of Douglas by sewing, from the front peritoneal surface to

Figure 15.6. Transvaginal double-pursestring closure. The first pursestring suture has been tied, closing the peritoneal cavity. A second pursestring has been placed 1 cm distal to the first, to be tied as well.

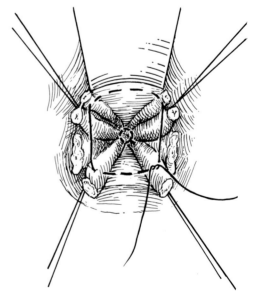

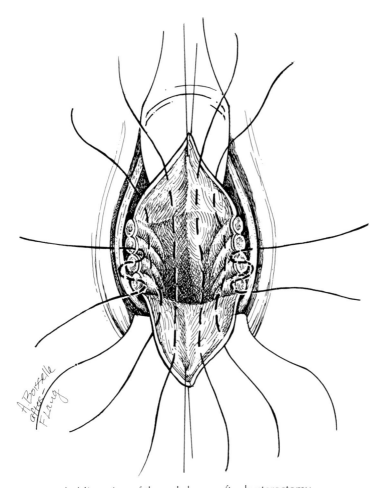

Figure 15.7. Sagittal obliteration of the cul-de-sac after hysterectomy.

the back surface, a transversely placed continuous synthetic monofilament suture that begins at the brim of the cavity. By alternate bites 1 cm apart between the anterior and the posterior cul-de-sac surfaces, the suture through both peritoneum and subperitoneal retinaculum is continued back and forth from one side of the pelvis to the other using a running locked stitch from the 3 o'clock to the 9 o'clock position. The knot is tied and the suture returned by a separate layer 0.5 cm distal to the first using a running stitch to the 3 o'clock position, where it is tied again. It is then followed by a pursestring suture a few millimeters distal to the transverse closure. This effectively creates a strong three-layered scar. The reverse of this may be applied to the large-neck enterocele that is occasionally encountered during transabdominal surgery: one places additional transverse rows each 1 cm or so cranial to its predecessor until the brim of the pelvis is reached, at which point the suture is tied. A final row of interrupted sutures 1 cm apart is placed at the pelvic brim (16).

Enterocele with prolapse of the vault posterior to the cervix in the patient whose uterus has been fixed by a Gilliam suspension or ventral fixation and there is no indication for hysterectomy is treated transvaginally by high ligation of the neck of the sac. This includes a deep bite or two into the lower posterior part of the cervix or lower uterine segment, then excision of the sac.

Midline approximation and shortening of the uterosacral ligaments is performed if they are strong; also indicated is repair of any coexistent cystocele and rectocele, the latter including the high full-length posterior colporrhaphy. If eversion of the upper vagina coexists and the strength of the cardinal and uterosacral ligaments is insufficient to support the vaginal vault securely, the vault may be sewn to the sacrospinous ligament(s) (see Chapter 16).

Transabdominal procedures include excision of redundant cul-de-sac peritoneum with approximation of uterosacral ligaments, longitudinal obliterative sutures of the Halban type (5) (Figs. 15.8 and 15.9), or circumferential obliterative sutures of the Marion-Moschcowitz type (12, 15). If there is a wide voluminous posterior vagina, this should be narrowed by wedging as suggested by both Waters (25) and Torpin (22). This can be done either transabdominally or transvaginally and will tend to approximate the uterosacral ligament attachments closer to the midline. The McCall transvaginal culde-

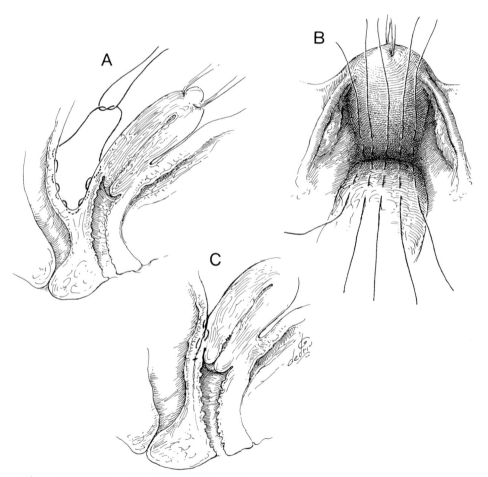

Figure 15.8. Obliteration of the cul-de-sac by a series of interrupted stitches placed from front to back. **A.** Sagittal section showing placement of the stitches. **B.** Stitches as viewed from the abdomen. **C.** Stitches after tying. If the uterus is no longer present, similar stitches are placed in the posterior wall of the vagina. (From Nichols DH. Repair of enterocele and prolapse of the vaginal vault. In: Barber H, ed. Goldsmith's practice of surgery. Woodbury, CT: Cine-Med Inc., 1981. Used with permission.)

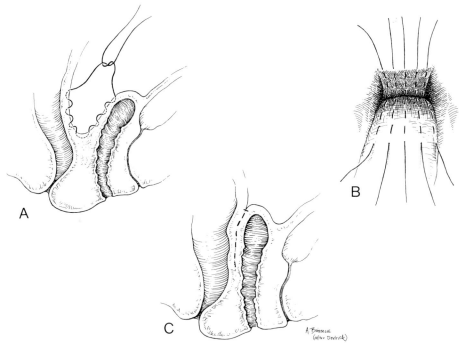

Figure 15.9. Obliteration of the cul-de-sac after transabdominal hysterectomy.

plasty may be useful if there are palpably strong uterosacral ligaments, as with the uterovaginal or "sliding" type of prolapse.

When coexistent eversion of the vagina is present and the abdomen is open, transabdominal colposacropexy might be considered to preserve vaginal length, although it must be remembered that any coincident cystocele and rectocele must be repaired by a separate procedure at a later date. When any transabdominal procedure is performed that changes the vaginal axis to a more vertical direction, such as the Marshall-Marchetti-Krantz (13) or the Burch (2) procedure, or ventral suspension or fixation (see Chapter 16), the cul-de-sac of Douglas should be adequately protected by surgical obliteration of the peritoneum-lined cul-de-sac anterior to the rectum. The increased exposure, vulnerability, and risk of enterocele if a deep anterior or posterior cul-de-sac is not obliterated should be more widely recognized. An anterior enterocele that develops after hysterectomy probably is best treated by transvaginal resection of the sac and redundant peritoneum, with restoration of the normal upper vaginal axis and correction of any defect in the levator plate.

Pudendal or lateral enterocele may be approached transvaginally if the margins of the neck of the sac are distinguishable and can be readily identified. If they are vague and ill defined, either a combined vaginal-abdominal or an abdominal approach should be considered.

SUMMARY

It is essential that the gynecologist recognize enterocele and any potential likely to result in an enterocele and correlate this with cause, symptoms, progression, and other coexistent pelvic damage. An enterocele may be any one of the following types: congenital, pulsion, or traction, and, occasionally, iatrogenic, spontaneous, or acquired. A pulsion enterocele may be followed by a cystocele and rectocele, whereas a traction enterocele is preceded by a cystocele and rectocele. An enterocele may occur with or without eversion of the vagina and with or without prolapse of the rectum. The location of the hernia will be determined by its cause. The etiology, symptoms, and principles of surgical treatment are considerably different for each of the various sites.

There is no one standard corrective operation for enterocele. A choice of the possible operative procedures should be made on a rational, correlative basis in accordance with the principles that have been suggested (Table 15.1).

References

1. Anderson WR. Pudendal hernia. Obstet Gynecol, 1968;32:802–804.
2. Burch JC. Urethrovaginal fixation to Cooper's ligament for correction of stress incontinence, cystocele, and prolapse. Am Obstet Gynecol 1961;81:281–290.
3. Cali RL, Pitsch RM, Blatchford GJ, Thorson A, Christensen MA. Rare pelvic floor hernias: report of a case and review of the literature. Dis Colon Rectum 1992;35:604–612.
4. Chase HC. Levator hernia (pudendal hernia). Surg Gynecol Obstet 1992;35:717.
5. Halban J. Gynäkologische Operationslehre. Berlin: Urban & Schwarzenberg, 1932.
6. Hawksworth W, Roux JP. Vaginal hysterectomy. J Obstet Gynaecol Br Commonw 1958;63:214–228.
7. Hunt AB. Fenestrae and pouches in the broad ligament as an actual and potential cause of strangulated intraabdominal hernia. Surg Gynecol Obstet 1934;58:906.
8. Lash AF, Levin B. Roentgenographic diagnosis of vaginal vault hernia. Obstet Gynecol 1962;20:427–433.
9. Lenzi E. L'Ernia Vaginale del Douglas O Elitrocele. Pisa: Edizioni Omnia Medica, 1959:65–69.
10. Lenzi E, Dino N, Liguori F, Paganelli A. Per una migliore nosografia dell'ernia del Douglas: elitrocele o enterocele? Riv Ost Gin Perin 1990;3:273–276.
11. Litschgi M, Käser O. The problem of enterocele. Geburtshilfe Frauenheilkd 1978;38:915–920.
12. Marion J. Quoted by Read CD. Enterocele. Am J Obstet Gynecol 1951;62:743–753.
13. Marshall VF, Marchetti AA, Krantz KE. The correction of stress incontinence by simple vesicourethral suspension. Surg Gynecol Obstet 1949;88:509–518.
14. McCall ML. Posterior culdeplasty: surgical correction of enterocele during vaginal hysterectomy, a preliminary report. Obstet Gynecol 1957;10:595–602.
15. Moschcowitz AV. The pathogenesis, anatomy and cure of prolapse of the rectum. Surg Gynecol Obstet 1912;15:7–21.
16. Nichols DH, (ed.) Gynecologic and obstetric surgery. St. Louis: Mosby–Year Book, 1993, p 428.
17. Nichols DH. Types of enterocele and principles underlying the choice of operation for repair. Obstet Gynecol 1972;40:257–263.
18. Nichols DH, Genadry RR. Pelvic relaxation of the posterior compartment. Curr Opin Obstet Gynecol 1993;5:458–464.
19. Pirogoff. Fig. 4, Plate XXI. In: Hart DB. Atlas of female pelvic anatomy. Edinburgh: W & AK Johnston, 1884.
20. Read CD. Enterocele. Am J Obstet Gynecol 1951;62:743–757.
21. Rogers FA. Strangulated obturator hernia. Surgery 1960;48:394–402.
22. Torpin R. Excision of the cul-de-sac of Douglas for the surgical sure of Hernias through the female caudal wall: including prolapse of the uterus. J Med Assoc Ga 1947;36:396–406.
23. Wakeley CPG. Obturator hernia: its aetiology, incidence and treatment, with 2 personal operative cases. Br J Surg 1939;26:515.
24. Warwick R, Williams PL. Gray's anatomy. 35th Br ed. Philadelphia: WB Saunders, 1973:1279.
25. Waters EG. Vaginal prolapse. Gynecology 1956;8:432–436.
26. Watson LF. Hernia. 2nd ed. St. Louis: CV Mosby, 1938.
27. Weed JC, Tyrone C. Enterocele. Am J Obstet Gynecol 1950;60:324–332.
28. Wilensky AV, Kaufman PA. Vaginal hernia. Am J Surg 1940;49:31–41.
29. Wilson JM. Pelvic relaxations and herniations. Springfield, IL: Charles C Thomas, 1954:58–62.
30. Zacharin RF. Pelvic floor anatomy and the surgery of pulsion enterocele. New York: Springer-Verlag, 1985.

CHAPTER 16

Massive Eversion of the Vagina

"The best defense (against vault prolapse) is a good surgical offense." Michael R. Smith, M.D.

SCOPE OF THE PROBLEM

There are few maladies in feminine life more disturbing to its quality than that of massive eversion of the vagina. It is specific, dramatic, obvious, frustrating, embarrassing, and progressive. It may occur with or without the presence of the uterus, since prolapse of the latter is the result and not the cause of the eversion. The malady is surgically curable with relief of symptoms and restoration of normal anatomic relationships.

The multiplicity of possible anatomic supportive defects that give rise to the combinations of clinically significant damage that may be encountered in examination of the patient with posthysterectomy vaginal eversion were studied and evaluated in 94 cadavers of various ages (11). The conclusions were that the upper third of the vagina is supported by vertical fibers of the paracolpium (i.e., cardinal ligament continuations that arise from a broad area on the pelvic sidewalls). Support of the paracolpium in the midvagina arises from attachment to the arcus tendineus, and in the lower vagina by fusion to the perineal body and its muscular and fibrous attachments. This study provides further support of the concept that damage to these support levels may occur singly or in any combination, and the gynecologic surgeon should identify each site of damage preoperatively and incorporate suitable remedial steps in the surgery of reconstruction. Symptomatic patients who are unidentified and untreated may require future reoperation with its attendant risks, suffering, and expense.

Massive eversion of the vagina is a complex disorder. Cystocele, rectocele, and enterocele may or may not coexist (Fig. 16.1), and the distinction is surgically important because each, when present, should be repaired. Comfort and normal vaginal function can be restored by carefully selected surgery.

More women are living longer, and there is much interest in maintaining a self-image of femininity and the capacity for sexual intercourse beyond the menopause.

Although some cases of massive eversion of the vaginal vault occur in the nullipara, probably related to congenital pelvic tissue weakness, defective innervation, or unusual trauma, the majority are seen in parous women. Among these women, the incidence might be reduced by obstetrically skillful management of labor and delivery. In various childbirth settings, there is less frequent use of timely and anatomically repaired episiotomy, and babies may be delivered by persons other than skilled obstetricians. With some resurgence of interest in home delivery, we should expect to see an increase in the incidence of genital prolapse as well as other gynecologic consequences of unattended childbirth.

That a "dropped uterus" is the result and not the cause of genital prolapse has not always been appreciated. "Routine" abdominal hysterectomy has been performed for

351

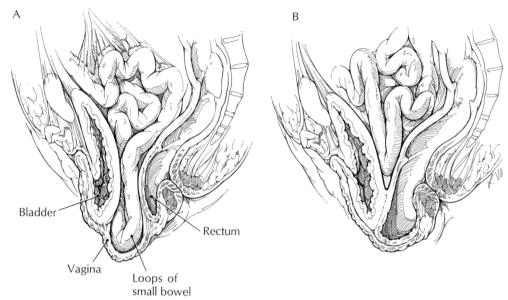

Figure 16.1. Massive eversion of the vagina. **A.** Massive posthysterectomy eversion of the vagina with enterocele. **B.** The less frequent massive eversion without enterocele. In this case, the connective tissue capsule of the bladder is fused with that of the anterior rectal wall.

uterine prolapse in the mistaken belief that if there is no uterus, there is no dropping. The vaginal vault prolapse persists whether or not the uterus is present, and these patients are seen in consultation some time after their primary surgery, frequently referred by the initial surgeon.

In taking the patient's history, one should carefully note whether there was a previous urinary stress incontinence when the patient was younger and which symptoms were relieved as the vaginal vault descended, suggesting a kinking of the urethra coincident with the prolapse. Such a patient is very likely to develop a recurrent urinary stress incontinence, when the vagina has been repositioned within the pelvis unless special appropriate steps are accomplished with the anterior colporrhaphy to lessen the likelihood of this possibility (27).

Urinary incontinence coexists more commonly in the postmenopausal patient with total eversion of the vagina. Although it is not frequent, it may be of several types and can be best demonstrated by examination of the awake patient with a partly filled bladder and with the vaginal vault digitally replaced and held in an intrapelvic position. The types of incontinence may include urinary stress incontinence, overflow incontinence from a bladder never completely empty, incontinence from significant detrusor or urethral instability, or incontinence resulting from low urethral pressure (a urethral closing pressure less than 20 cm H_2O). The causes of the latter, which are related to decreased urethral tone, are hard to pinpoint but may include contributions from decreased estrogen, decreased elasticity of the urethral wall, decreased vascularity, decreased muscle contractility, and a decrease in the effective support of the paraurethral tissues. The consequences, however, are usually obvious (i.e., troublesome postoperative urinary incontinence, in spite of coincident anterior colporrhaphy, resulting from unrecognized preoperative urethral kinking).

Because effective repair of the coincident low-pressure urethra (vesicourethral sling, periurethral injections, bulbocavernosus fat pad transplant, urethral plication) greatly improves patient satisfaction with surgery, it is vital that its presence be determined ahead of time. Low urethral pressure or compliance should be suspected in every instance of total vaginal eversion seen in a postmenopausal patient, especially among women who have not been participating in estrogen replacement therapy (ERT). In our experience, a low-pressure urethra will be found in 5 to 10 percent of such patients. Its prevalence in postmenopausal patients is a reason for prescribing biweekly vaginal instillations of 1 to 2 g of estrogen cream for 1 or 2 months preoperatively and weekly installations during at least the first year postoperatively.

If sophisticated urodynamic laboratory testing is not available to a patient, there is a simple method of demonstrating low urethral compliance. Preoperatively, in the examining room and with the patient's bladder partly full, the vaginal vault is manually replaced, and the patient, previously incontinence or not, is asked to cough and strain, and one observes whether urine is involuntarily lost. This examination is performed with the patient first in the lithotomy position and then standing.

If incontinence is demonstrated while straining, a condition of low-pressure urethra is strongly suspected. An inexpensive preliminary test is passing a no. 8 or 10 pediatric Foley catheter into the bladder, partially inflating the Foley bulb with 1 ml of saline, and gently making traction on the catheter to draw the bulb easily through the urethra. If this can be done, the diagnosis of low-pressure urethra is likely, and an appropriate surgical remedy should be incorporated in the primary reconstructive repair. If the bulb cannot be pulled through with gentle traction, 0.5 ml of saline is removed from the bulb and again traction is made to the catheter, whose bulb is partially inflated with the residual 0.5 ml of saline. If it can be drawn through the urethra with minimal resistance, the diagnosis of low-pressure urethra can be seriously entertained. This suspicion can, of course, be more fully "proven" by more sophisticated laboratory assessment if such a facility is available and is affordable.

In the operating room, near the end of the "corrective" surgery, the catheter pull-through "test" using the pediatric Foley catheter with the partly inflated bulb can be performed. The results can be expected to conform with the patient's future clinical behavior (i.e., correction of pathologically low pressure of the urethra and the prevention or correction of the often associated urinary incontinence).

The symptoms of vaginal vault eversion include backache, a feeling of vaginal fullness, and presence of a protruding vaginal mass when the patient is standing, because the pull of gravity aggravates the descent of the parts.

Vaginal vault eversion can occur as a consequence of an isolated deficiency in genital support, the vault coming down according to the attenuation of the vaginal portion of the uterosacral-cardinal ligament complex. Vaginal vault eversion is seen far more frequently as the consequence, usually progressive, of damage to the several levels of genital support (1, 6, 11).

There are three goals of reconstructive surgery:

1. Relieve the symptoms
2. Restore the anatomic relationships between the pelvic organs
3. Restore the function of each component organ system

To achieve a perfect surgical reconstruction, the surgeon must determine preoperatively the specific sites of damage (6, 11) and, in the operating room, must reaffirm the presence and extent of the damage by a careful examination under anesthesia immediately preceding the operation. Consideration of these observations determines the extend and details of the reconstruction.

There are essential differences between partial eversion of the vaginal vault (often diagnosed by examination of the patient while she is standing and bearing down or straining), subtotal eversion (protrusion of the vagina and organs to which it is attached above or cranial to the urogenital diaphragm), and total eversion of the vagina, which includes the above plus eversion of the vaginal tissues below or caudal to the urogenital diaphragm.

Simultaneous prolapse of the rectum and of the vagina is occasionally encountered (36). Surgical treatment of one element will not provide benefit to the other (24), but it is possible to treat both simultaneously. One method is transvaginal-transperineal, with colpopexy resection and repair of the prolapsed rectum, but, if there is need for transabdominal exploration, surgical treatment of both prolapses can be offered by laparotomy. In this instance, the rectal prolapse should be treated first, often by rectopexy with or without intestinal resection according to the amount of redundant bowel present. The site of sacrocolpopexy will be anterior to the rectal suspension and should be performed as the second procedure. The cul-de-sac should be obliterated before the abdomen is closed. Any necessary transvaginal repair of cystocele or rectocele should be accomplished separately.

When it is necessary to postpone surgery for a symptomatic prolapse, symptoms may be temporarily relieved by the use of an intravaginal pessary such as the Gellhorn (Fig. 16.2) or an inflatable pessary.

The chronically increased intra-abdominal pressure that was so often the cause of massive eversion of the vagina may also promote the coincident development of a hiatal hernia. Such a patient may give a history of heartburn when lying down, and bowel sounds may be heard during auscultation of the chest, especially in the lower left anterior portion of the thorax.

The patient should be examined when she is fully awake and when she is standing (see Chapter 15). One should replace the vault and reobserve any possible cystocele, rectocele, and enterocele. A notation should be made of all positive findings on examination, so that appropriate repair may be scheduled and remembered as part of the definitive surgery. When a decision has been made for repair of genital prolapse, a skilled surgeon should have several surgical techniques from which to choose. One should make the operation fit the patient, not make the patient fit the operation. Although a surgeon tends to concentrate on operations that he or she performs best, various combinations of damage necessitate thoroughly learning various techniques so that one may meet the need of the individual patient.

Generally, if weaknesses in these areas are present, even of minor degree, all should be repaired simultaneously. This will improve the overall surgical success of a reconstructive procedure and decrease the necessity for a separate future secondary operation.

Posthysterectomy vaginal vault eversion is related to the adequacy of support of the vaginal vault. Prevention of eversion is directly related to recognizing the strength and length of the patient's uterosacral ligaments at the time of surgery. If they are strong and long, they should be shortened before they are attached to the vaginal vault. A wide vaginal vault should be surgically narrowed, and the cul-de-sac obliterated or any enterocele excised. Sewing the uterosacral ligaments together at the time of posthysterectomy peritonealization is useful, and the New Orleans or McCall culdeplasty (see Chapter 8) can be used. When cardinal-uterosacral strength is lacking, the surgeon must use an alternate method of colpopexy.

The surgeon should attempt to restore normal vaginal depth and axis (see Chapter 1), particularly after any vesicourethral pin-up operation such as the Marshall-Marchetti-

Figure 16.2. Insertion of a Gellhorn pessary. **A.** The perineum is depressed, and the disc portion of the pessary is inserted. **B.** The pessary should rest comfortably and be retained above the pelvic diaphragm. **C.** Sagittal section showing that the properly fitted pessary elevates the vaginal vault and uterus to a position once again within the pelvis and, at the same time, relieves some of the distention of the cystocele and rectocele. (From Nichols DH, (ed.) Gynecologic and obstetric surgery. St. Louis: Mosby-Year Book, 1993. Used with permission.)

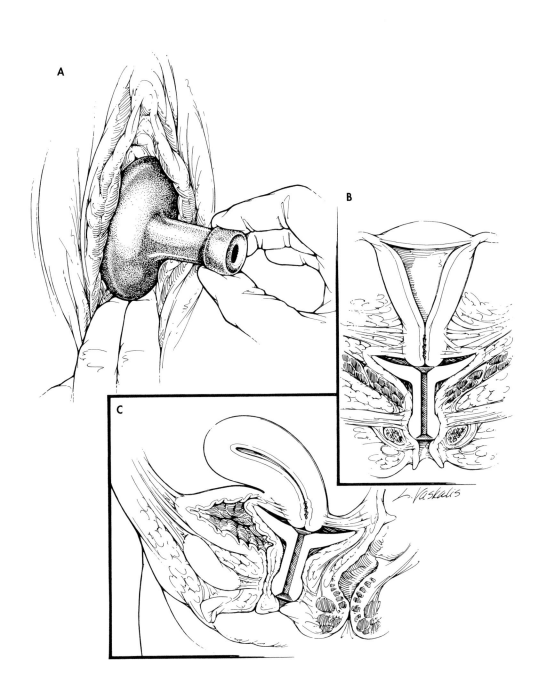

A

B

C

L. Vaskalis

Krantz (15) or the Burch modification (8), which pulls the vagina anteriorly. Many times this restoration can be aided by a perineorrhaphy and posterior colporrhaphy.

Although massive eversion of the vagina is more common in the postmenopausal patient, it also can occur in the young in whom the uterus may or may not be present. It is more common in the white patient than in the black, for reasons not totally understood. Progressive unrepaired uterine prolapse will often progress to procidentia, in which there is displacement of the entire uterus outside of the pelvic cavity. Surgically usable cardinal-uterosacral ligament strength may be absent in the patient with total genital procidentia, and colpopexy to a posteriorly located nongynecologic structure such as the sacrospinous ligament or the sacrum may be required to restore vaginal depth.

Because there are various etiologic factors, different surgical procedures are required for correction. Figure 5.7 shows an obvious protrusion of cervix beyond the vulva. Notice the rectocele and cystocele, but no enterocele. This condition represents general prolapse, usually postmenopausal, and includes weakness of the pelvic supporting tissues with consequent descent of the cul-de-sac. All the internal genitalia have dropped, but the relationship between the anterior rectal wall and the back of the uterus is unchanged. This relationship is the same as when the uterus and rectum were higher in the pelvis. Although the cul-de-sac is displaced, it does not dissect between the rectum and vagina as would be true of enterocele (5). One must make this distinction because both etiology and surgical therapy of prolapse with enterocele, shown in Figure 5.6, are entirely different. The cervix is outside the pelvis, and there is cystocele and enterocele but no rectocele. The relationship between the cervix and the anterior wall of the rectum is changed because the cul-de-sac and its peritoneum have dissected between the rectum and vagina, and the latter actually slides along the anterior wall of the rectum, the vaginal counterpart of rectal prolapse.

It is usually possible to predict with reasonable accuracy the patient with uterine procidentia who will require coincident sacrospinous colpopexy. This can be achieved, as suggested by Victor Bonney, by identifying the primary site of weakness as either in the upper or the lower vaginal supports with the patient in the lithotomy position on the examining table (7). The gynecologist should replace the prolapse within the pelvis, have the patient bear down, and observe which organs appear first. If the cervix and uterus or vaginal vault appear first followed by the cystocele and rectocele, the patient has a massive damage to the upper suspensory supports of the vagina, particularly the cardinal and uterosacral ligaments, and will probably require hysterectomy, colporrhaphy, and primary colpopexy as part of the initial procedure.

If, however, the cystocele and rectocele appear first and are followed by the cervix, the primary site of damage in all likelihood is concentrated on the supports of the lower pelvis, particularly the pelvic and urogenital diaphragms. This patient will probably be best treated by a skillful vaginal hysterectomy with colporrhaphy and will not require planning for a probable coincident sacrospinous or a transabdominal colpopexy.

Amreich (2) indicated the importance of preserving vaginal depth after hysterectomy. If, after removal of the uterus, the vagina is otherwise well supported and sits upon an intact levator plate, intra-abdominal pressure applied to the vagina will be countered by pressure in the opposite direction from the pelvic diaphragm. The vagina will be compressed between these two pressures and remain in place. But if the vagina is short after hysterectomy, and ends anterior to the levator plate (Fig. 16.3), it may telescope upon itself, becoming even shorter as intra-abdominal pressure is directed in the axis of such a vagina. An exception is the patient who has had a Wertheim or Schauta radical hysterectomy, in which the scarring in this area is so great that very little will disturb it. Preserving vaginal depth and axis are important prophylactic features of all genital surgery.

After total hysterectomy, the cardinal-uterosacral ligament complex is detached from the uterus and, if not deliberately reattached to the vaginal vault, undergoes atrophy. After a few months or years it may no longer be sufficiently strong to be of use in the surgical reconstruction of any future vault eversion.

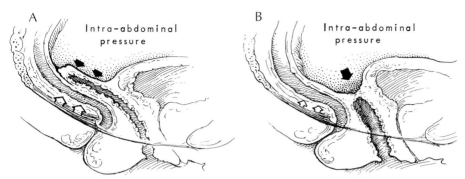

Figure 16.3. The importance of preserving vaginal depth. **A.** A deep vagina after hysterectomy tends to be squeezed or "sandwiched" in place between the forces of intra-abdominal pressure from above (*black arrows*) and the resistance of the levator place below (*white arrows*). **B.** When the vagina is so short as to end anterior to the levator plate, intra-abdominal pressure will be exerted in the axis of the vagina, tending to telescope it and make it even shorter. (From Amreich J. Äetiologie und Operation des Scheidenstumpf prolapses. Wien Klin Wochenschr 1951;63:74–77. Used with permission.)

There are also partial degrees of eversion which, if ignored at the time of hysterectomy or otherwise left unattended, will generally progress (Fig. 16.4).

METHODS OF SURGICAL TREATMENT

There are several methods of surgical treatment:

1. Vaginal hysterectomy and repair
2. LeFort colpocleisis or colpectomy
3. Other transvaginal reconstructive procedures, such as sacrospinous colpopexy with treatment of cystocele and rectocele through the same operative exposure
4. Transabdominal procedures, such as (*a*) ventral suspension or (*b*) sacrocolpopexy

Because there is no single operation that will correct all of the pathology that might be present in various types of prolapse, there is often a need for a combination of surgical procedures.

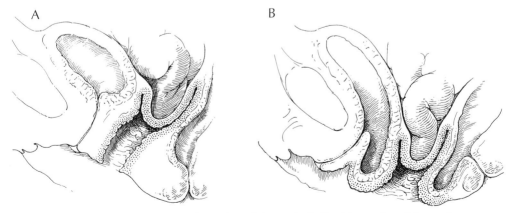

Figure 16.4. Posthysterectomy partial eversion of the vault. **A.** Partial eversion of the vagina after hysterectomy without cystocele and rectocele. **B.** Partial eversion of the vaginal vault after hysterectomy with obvious cystocele and rectocele.

Because pathologic descent of the uterus is the result of genital prolapse and is not its cause, hysterectomy, although often desirable, is not as important as the repair, nor should it be the prime objective of the operation. Hysterectomy may be useful as the means of mobilizing parametrial tissues for use in reconstructive surgery, but it serves as an adjunct to repair. For the patient who wishes to retain her uterus, colpopexy without hysterectomy can be elected.

Vaginal hysterectomy and repair constitute the procedure most often selected. If there are strong cardinal-uterosacral ligaments, they can be shortened and attached to the vault of the vagina, providing a satisfactory result (see Chapter 8). When enterocele coexists, the New Orleans or McCall-type culdeplasty is helpful (see Chapters 8 and 15). If the patient wishes to retain the uterine fundus, a Manchester-Fothergill operation may be considered (see Chapter 9), but the potential for subsequent pregnancy or for abnormal uterine bleeding must be understood. For the same reasons, the Watkins-Wertheim transposition operation is not recommended.

Partial colpocleisis (LeFort) or colpectomy have, at times, been popular in the aged patient. However, there are four problems specific to this type of operation: (*a*) It limits or destroys vaginal coital function. (*b*) Because the operation is extraperitoneal, colpocleisis or colpectomy will not remove any enterocele. (*c*) There is some increased potential for postoperative urinary stress incontinence caused by deliberate fusion of the anterior rectal wall to the base of the bladder, which flattens the posterior urethrovesical angle. (*d*) If the uterus is retained, the patient can bleed from it in the future from a number of causes, including carcinoma. Because the uterus and cervix are hidden behind the new vaginal septum, investigation is difficult. We do not often advocate colpocleisis.

Partial colpocleisis (Fig. 16.5) or total colpectomy can be effective and satisfactory in certain older patients of less favorable surgical risk for whom preservation of coital potential may be neither essential nor desirable. This is especially true when there is little

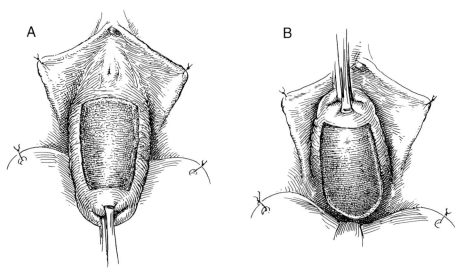

Figure 16.5. Partial colpocleisis (LeFort operation) for a massive eversion of the vagina and cervix. A preliminary D&C is performed and the vaginal tissues thoroughly infiltrated by 0.5% lidocaine in 1:200,000 epinephrine solution. **A.** The labia minora, if large, are temporarily stitched to the vulvar skin and a large rectangle of skin removed from the anterior vaginal wall. **B.** A matching-sized rectangle is removed from the posterior wall of the vagina. (*Continues on following page.*)

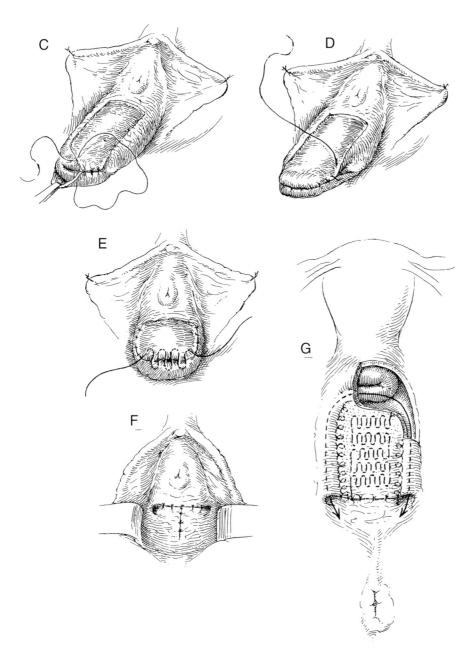

Figure 16.5 continued. C. The cut edge at the anterior vaginal wall is sewn to its counterpart, with each interrupted suture placed so that as it is tied the knot is turned into and remains in the epithelium-lined tunnel being established. **D.** This approximation is continued down each side of the vagina. **E.** The most dependent portion of the mass is inverted progressively and held in place by a front-to-back running fine suture with short bites in consecutively placed rows that will avoid side-to-side contractions and ensure smoother approximation of surfaces. **F.** This is continued until all the raw area has been approximated and the proximal transverse portion of the anterior vaginal wall is sewn to its counterpart. An appropriate perineorrhaphy may be performed as indicated by the vertical incision beneath the area of colpocleisis. **G.** Diagrammatic depiction of the end result with *arrows* showing the permanent transverse and lateral drainage canals.

tissue strength available for reconstruction (9, 22, 37). Colpectomy (Fig. 16.6) should be considered a destructive rather than a reconstructive operative approach. Furthermore, coexistent enterocele must be recognized and excised. Coincident colporrhaphy is preferred to lessen the potential for postoperative urinary stress incontinence. Because there is no route for subsequent uterine drainage, there is no place for colpectomy when the uterus has been retained. Symptomatic and troublesome vulvar hernias may be seen in patients who have experienced total colpectomy as a treatment for prolapse of the vaginal vault. In most instances, these represent enteroceles, either recurrent or unrecognized and untreated at the time of the original surgery.

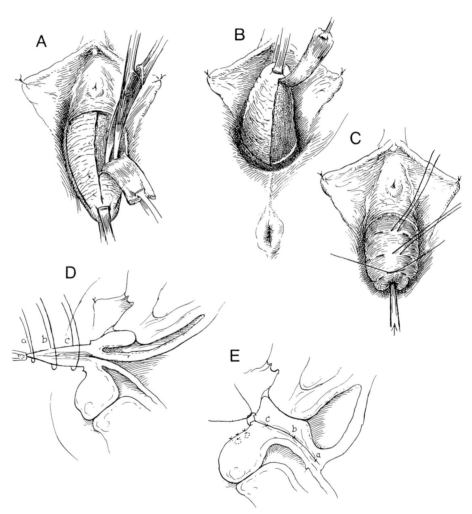

Figure 16.6. Colpectomy. **A** and **B.** After subcutaneous infiltration by lidocaine 0.5% in 1:200,000 epinephrine solution, the vagina is circumscribed by an incision at the site of the hymen and marked into quadrants. Each quadrant is removed by sharp dissection. **C.** A series of pursestring sutures using polyglycolic acid-type sutures is placed as shown. The vault of the soft tissue is inverted by the tip of a forceps as indicated by the *arrow*. **D.** The pursestring sutures are tied, *a* before *b* before *c*, with progressive inversion of the soft tissue before the tying of each suture. **E.** Sagittal section showing the final result. An appropriate perineorrhaphy may complete the operation.

OTHER TRANSVAGINAL RECONSTRUCTIVE PROCEDURES

A frequent problem encountered is that of an aging but sexually active patient with vaginal eversion, cystocele, and rectocele who cannot retain a vaginal pessary. There may have been progression of the genital prolapse associated with postmenopausal atrophic changes. The prolapsed uterus can be removed without difficulty, and, if there are strong cardinal and uterosacral ligaments, these should be shortened and used to support the vaginal vault, producing a satisfactory result (35).

Sometimes there is nothing of strength to use for support of the everted vagina. Descent of the vault without a true enterocele (19) occurs in about 20 percent of these cases. This condition usually represents a major problem in the integrity of all of the patient's endopelvic soft tissues, particularly of the pelvic diaphragm.

Although enterocele and massive eversion of the vagina often coexist, they are *separate* anatomic and clinical entities, each requiring definitive, specific surgical treatment. When eversion of the vagina follows hysterectomy, enterocele coexists two-thirds of the time. This disabling and uncomfortable consequence suggests that insufficient attention had been paid during surgery to a need for reinforcement and correction of weakened genital supports. If strong cardinal-uterosacral ligaments can be found at the sides of the everted vaginal vault, they can be shortened and the vagina attached to them for support (35), followed by excision of any enterocele and by high ligation of the peritoneum. However, after total hysterectomy, the remaining uterosacral ligament complex usually undergoes atrophy and, after a few months or years, is no longer sufficiently strong to be of much use in surgical reconstruction.

In the patient with total procidentia and severe laxity of the cardinal-uterosacral ligament complex, the surgeon should be prepared for vaginal hysterectomy with possible primary or coincident colpopexy and colporrhaphy, since the combined procedure may save the patient the trauma, expense, and suffering of reoperation to correct a posthysterectomy recurrent prolapse (10). In our experience this combination of massive prolapse with atrophic or poor uterosacral ligament support occurs in about 5 percent of patients with significant uterine prolapse. It can be identified in the examining room by making traction to a tenaculum applied to the posterior lip of the cervix and estimating the length and strength of the uterosacral ligaments. Their strength, or lack thereof, can easily be demonstrated by putting them on tension, and the appropriate surgical plan can then be formulated.

Primary sacrospinous colpopexy immediately after vaginal hysterectomy in a patient with uterine prolapse *without* surgically useful strong uterosacral-cardinal ligament support (general prolapse, see Chapter 5) is not common but is surprisingly easy to accomplish. This is because there has been no previous surgery to alter tissue planes and spaces. It can be added to the primary procedure by an experienced vaginal surgeon within an additional 15 minutes of operating time between the steps of peritoneal closure and the posterior repair.

If the symptomatic prolapse patient requires that the uterus be spared, possibly for future pregnancy, there are several options from which to choose. One is to wear an intravaginal pessary until after childbearing has been completed, followed by subsequent vaginal hysterectomy and repair. If the cervix is elongated, a transvaginal Manchester repair may be elected, provided there is adequate palpable strength of the cardinal-uterosacral ligament complex (see Chapter 9). If the complex is weak, however, transvaginal sacrospinous cervicopexy may be chosen, probably bilateral for maximum suspensory support. Alternately, the cervix may be attached transabdominally to the sacrum by construction of a retroperitoneal sacrocervical ligament.

An adequate reconstruction should incorporate steps designed to restore the normal depth and axis of the vagina. Chapter 1 called attention to the almost horizontal position of the upper half of the vagina. Normal position and relationships are maintained by connective tissue supports fused with the levator ani below (Fig. 16.7) and continuing with

Figure 16.7. The normal vaginal axis of the living. An almost horizontal upper vagina and rectum lie upon and parallel to the levator plate, which is formed by fusion of the pubococcygei muscles posterior to the rectum. The anterior limit of point of fusion is the margin of the genital hiatus. (From Nichols DH, Milley PS, Randall CL. Significance of restoration of normal vaginal depth and axis. Obstet Gynecol 1970;36:251–256. Used with permission of Lippincott-Raven.)

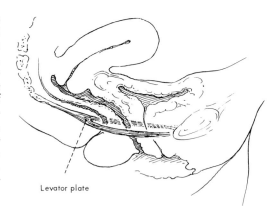

Levator plate

the supporting tissue also extending beneath the rectum (20). The fusion of levator muscle and fascia behind the rectum constitutes the levator plate, making direct surgical accessibility difficult. If the horizontal position of the levator plate is altered, the force of gravity and the stresses of day-to-day activities may pull upon the supports of the upper vagina to such a degree that they elongate and permit the upper vaginal axis to descend (Fig. 16.8). If the vault of the vagina moves anterior to the margin of the hiatus, it may literally slip over the edge of the levator plate, accentuating eversion of the upper vagina as it tends to turn itself inside out. When the plate is tipped forward, alternate methods of support and recreation of the normal vaginal depth and axis should be sought. Although obstetric trauma is the most significant and frequent factor in initiating vaginal eversion, the endocrine and nutritional changes during and after the menopause seem to accelerate progression of vaginal eversion by causing atrophic weakening of connective tissues. With minimal or negligible uterosacral strength, alternative methods of restoring vaginal depth and axis must be employed.

A number of techniques have been described in the relevant literature. Inmon (14) and later Symmonds and associates (35) then Shull and colleagues (31), and Peters and Christenson (23) stitched the vagina to the fascia of the pelvic diaphragm. Zweifel (41), in 1892, wrote that he had attached a weakly supported vagina to the sacrotuberous ligament. Transvaginal suture of the vagina to each arcus tendineus was described by White (40) in 1909. In 1951, Amreich (2) reported his experience using both a transgluteal (Amreich I) and transvaginal (Amreich II) approach to attach an everted vagina to the sacrotuberous ligament. Sederl (28) sewed the vagina to the sacrospinous ligament (Fig. 16.9). More recently, this approach has been reported by Richter (24, 25, 26) with enthusiastic accounts of his success, and it was Richter's early reports that stimulated our interest in this operation.

There are certain specific advantages to a transvaginal operation. First, it permits restoration of a functional vagina with a normal horizontally inclined upper vaginal axis atop the levator plate, thereby decreasing the chances of recurrence of vault eversion. Second, in contrast to abdominal sacropexy, it offers a convenient opportunity to correct cystocele, rectocele, or enterocele simultaneously through the same operative exposure. Third, it is a shorter procedure than the abdominal operation, and requires less duration and depth of anesthesia. Finally, because it is principally extraperitoneal, postoperative ileus, intestinal obstruction, incisional pain, and other hazards of transabdominal surgery are diminished.

As previously mentioned, primary sacrospinous colpopexy may be performed immediately after vaginal hysterectomy in the patient with extensive prolapse without a strong uterosacral-cardinal ligament complex (10). Although this is not a common problem, the operation is surprisingly easy to do if there are no adhesions from previous surgery to alter the tissue planes and spaces. If unilateral sacrospinous colpopexy is to be performed, it is necessary to narrow the vault to make the vagina much like a cylin-

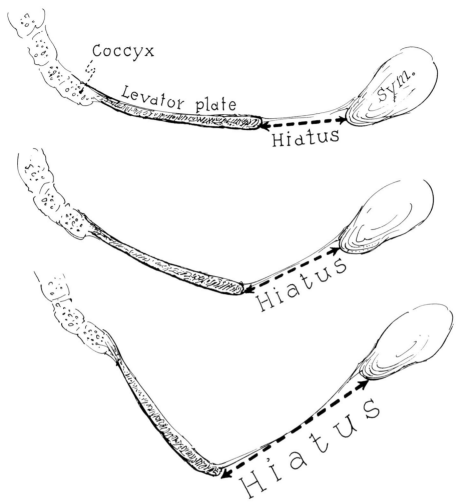

Figure 16.8. The effect of tipping of the levator plate. As the levator plate sags, the genital hiatus becomes larger. In addition, the pull of gravity and the forces of intra-abdominal pressure accentuate the strain upon the pelvic suspensory system. *Sym.*, symphysis pubis. (After Berglas B, Rubin IC. Study of the supportive structures of the uterus by levator myography. Surg Gynecol Obstet 1953;97:677–692, by permission of Surgery, Gynecology & Obstetrics, now known as The Journal of The American College of Surgeons.)

der (Fig. 16.10). If bilateral sacrospinous colpopexy is to be performed, the vaginal vault should be of sufficient width to be brought to each of the ischial spines simultaneously. The addition of sacrospinous colpopexy to vaginal hysterectomy with anterior and posterior colporrhaphy extends the operating time of the experienced surgeon by about 15 to 20 minutes. This is the time required for penetrating the rectal pillar and identifying and placing the vagina to one or both sacrospinous ligaments. A satisfactory increase in length of a now well-supported vagina has been achieved with restoration of independent bladder and rectal function and preservation of normal coital ability.

ANATOMY

The sacrospinous ligament is an aponeurosis located within the substance of each coccygeus muscle, which extends from each ischial spine to the lower portion of the sacrum. The ligament is identified by palpation, as the examining finger seeks first the

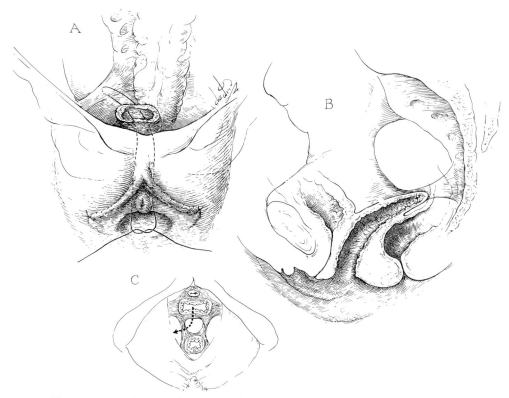

Figure 16.9. Technique of transvaginal sacrospinous fixation. **A.** After the posterior vaginal wall has been incised and the rectovaginal space has been opened, the operator perforates the right rectal pillar, proceeding from the rectovaginal space into the pararectal space. A Deschamps ligature carrier has perforated the right sacrospinous ligament, two finger breadths medial to the ischial spine. This suture, when passed through the vaginal wall and tied, fixes the vagina to the right sacrospinous ligament. **B.** Sagittal postoperative section showing the attachment of the vagina to the right sacrospinous ligament. **C.** The *dotted line and arrow* trace the path of incision from the vagina into the rectovaginal space, from the rectovaginal space through the right pillar to the right pararectal space, and then to the ischial spine and the sacrospinous ligament. (From Randall CL, Nichols DH. Surgical treatment of vaginal inversion. Obstet Gynecol 1971;38:330. Used with permission of Lippincott-Raven.)

ischial spine on either side and traces the fingerlike thickening of the ligament that runs posteriorly from this point to the hollow of the sacrum. To find it safely, one must understand the nature and boundaries of the connective tissue spaces (see Chapter 1). The sacrospinous ligament is located within the coccygeus muscle (16, 17, 23) in the lateral wall of the pararectal space, and in the surgical anatomy one notes the location of the pudendal nerve and vessels directly posterior to the ischial spine and the nearby sciatic nerve (Fig. 16.11). To avoid trauma to these structures, the surgeon should place the fixation stitches *through* the substance of the sacrospinous ligament one and one-half to two finger breadths *medial* to the ischial spine. It is easier for the operator who is right-handed to use the patient's right sacrospinous ligament, although the left can be used if desired. There may be some advantage to using both ligaments, if the upper portion of the vagina is sufficiently wide. When a unilateral sacrospinous colpopexy is being performed, the surgeon should deliberately narrow a wide vaginal vault by excising excess vagina. The width of posterior vaginal wall to be removed should be determined by the

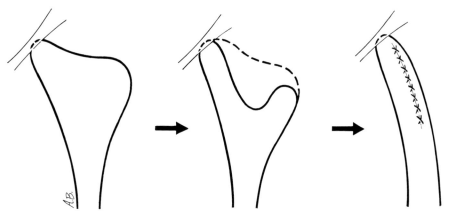

Figure 16.10. Narrowing a wide vaginal vault. Although bilateral sacrospinous colpopexy may be performed if the vaginal vault is wide, equally satisfactory results are usually obtained if unilateral colpopexy is performed, provided that a wide vault is surgically narrowed by excision of a proper width of tissue from the anterior and posterior vaginal walls preceding the colporrhaphy. This will convert the shape of the vagina to that of a cylinder of uniform diameter—since it is now an instrument of coitus and not parturition.

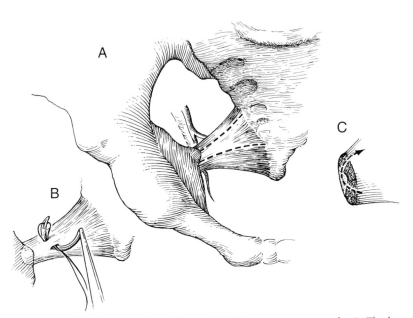

Figure 16.11. Location of sacrospinous ligament within coccygeus muscle. **A.** The location of the sacrospinous ligament deep within the substance of the coccygeus muscle is shown by the *dotted line*. The pudendal nerve and pudendal artery are shown behind the ischial spine. **B.** To avoid them, penetration of the coccygeus muscle and sacrospinous ligament is made one and one-half finger breadths medial to the ischial spine. Note that the ligature carrier has been placed through the muscle and ligament and not around them. **C.** The path of the ligature is shown by the *dotted line*; a cross section of the sacrospinous ligament is represented by the *stippled area* within the coccygeus muscle.

desired width and length of the vagina. A modestly shortened length may be found after the tissue excisions of previous operations. Excision of a narrower strip may permit an elastic vagina to be stretched to the region of the ischial spine.

In most instances, this distance from vulva to the ligament, and hence the length of the restored vagina, is greater than 4 inches, although rarely the distance may be but 3 or 3½ inches. When this distance is short, the fixation stitches should be placed closer to the sacrum and a greater effort made to build up the thickness and depth of the perineal body at reconstruction; at times, a Williams vulvovaginoplasty (Chapter 20) will be a useful supplement.

TECHNIQUE OF TRANSVAGINAL SACROSPINOUS FIXATION

Surgery for transvaginal sacrospinous colpopexy requires that the operator's fingers be of average length to be able to reach the hollow of the sacrum. An operator with short fingers has a distinct handicap.

With the patient in the dorsal lithotomy position, and after completion of any necessary hysterectomy, a V-shaped incision is made in the perineum, and its skin and the posterior vaginal wall are reflected from the perineal body until the avascular rectovaginal space has been entered. Development of this space is continued to the vaginal apex. The posterior vaginal wall is incised longitudinally as necessary, or if it is to be narrowed by planned colporrhaphy, excess vaginal wall is excised. Any enterocele sac is identified and opened. Alternatively, the most dependent portion of the dependent sac may be opened first (16, 17).

When massive eversion of the vagina follows total abdominal hysterectomy, the location of the vesical peritoneum may be different from that found when the eversion follows vaginal hysterectomy. This is because the peritonealization after total abdominal hysterectomy often brings the bladder peritoneum across the vault of the vagina, be it left open or closed, for attachment to the peritoneum of the anterior surface of the rectum. Peritonealization after vaginal hysterectomy, however, more often involves one or more pursestring applications, and the center of the pursestring more likely overlies the cut edge of the vaginal vault. Therefore, when one opens the sac of an enterocele coincident with massive eversion of the vagina after previous total abdominal hysterectomy, there is a slightly greater danger of unplanned cystotomy than when the opening and dissection of the enterocele follows total vaginal hysterectomy.

Once opened, the sac is mobilized, and after it has been determined by palpation that there is no surgically useful cardinal-uterosacral ligament support, it is closed by high, pursestring peritonealization, and the sac resected.

The right rectal pillar separates the rectovaginal space from the right pararectal space. It has two layers that may or may not be fused, consists primarily of a condensation of areolar tissue, and contains a few smooth muscle fibers and small blood vessels. It also includes a projection representing a posterior prolongation of the uterosacral ligament.

The ease of exposure of the coccygeus muscle–sacrospinous ligament complex depends upon the thickness of the rectal pillar, and whether it exists as one fused layer or two separate and distinct layers (see Chapter 1). It is necessary to penetrate *both* layers as the dissection proceeds from the rectovaginal space to the perirectal space.

The length and strength of the descending rectal septum seems to vary inversely with the diameter of the rectum; the septum is easier to penetrate in the patient with a large rectocele.

The connective tissue spaces are in reality but potential spaces, separated from one another throughout the pelvis by anatomically constant connective tissue septa; in this case, the descending rectal septum separates the rectovaginal space from the pararectal space. The operator's right index finger, introduced into the rectovaginal space, palpates the right ischial spine, usually at the 9 or 3 o'clock position, and notes the position and size of each sacrospinous ligament. During the progress of the surgeon's path from the rectovaginal space into the pararectal space, the descending rectal septum should be penetrated by either sharp or blunt dissection *closer to the undersurface of the vagina* than to the rectum, aiming directly at the site at which the ischial spine has been palpated.

The operator perforates the rectal pillar at a spot overlying the ischial spine and proceeds from the rectovaginal space into the pararectal space (Fig. 16.12). This penetration can be made bluntly with the fingertip if the pillar is thin or weak, or with scissor tips or a long hemostatic forceps, such as a tonsil forceps. A forceps tip may be inserted through this window in the right pillar, and the forceps or the tips of the Mayo scissors opened and spread, enlarging the penetration and exposing the superior surface of the pelvic diaphragm. A long and preferably straight retractor of suitable size (see Figs. 3.10, 3.16, and 3.17) is inserted deeply into the wound, displacing the rectum to the opposite side; another displaces the cardinal ligament and ureter anteriorly. (Similar exposure, although with less facility, can be obtained by three narrow Deaver retractors, but the curve of the Deaver offers no advantage and one must be especially careful not to let the tip of the retractor be pushed across the anterior surface of the sacrum, lest it risk dangerous damage to the sacral veins (33, 34).)

Direct adequate illumination of this deep area is essential and can be provided by a spotlight just over the operator's shoulder or by a suitable bright fiberoptic forehead lamp.

Loose areolar tissue is pushed to one side, exposing the superior surface of the pelvic diaphragm, and the blunt dissection easily proceeds to the ischial spine. The superior sur-

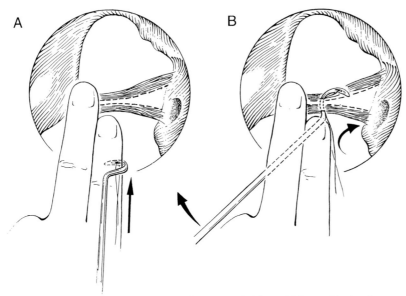

Figure 16.12. Palpating the sacrospinous ligament. **A.** The middle and index fingers of the operator's left hand have been inserted through a "window" in the rectal pillar into the right pararectal space. The lateral side of the tip of the middle finger touches the medial surface of the ischial spine. The Deschamps ligature carrier is positioned as shown and advanced down the index finger until its tip touches the right coccygeus muscle–sacrospinous ligament complex at a point one and one-half finger breadths medial to the ischial spine, safely away from the pudendal nerves and vessels. **B.** As it penetrates the muscle-ligament complex (the ligament within the muscle is shown by the *broken line*) by rotation of the handle, the latter is simultaneously swung to the operator's left *beneath* his or her palm so that the tip of the ligature carrier penetrates the ligament from below upward at right angles to the axis of the ligament.

face of the coccygeus muscle is clearly identified, running posteromedially from the ischial spine. Areolar tissue may be pushed from the surface of the right coccygeus muscle containing the sacrospinous ligament, if desired, using a "rosebud" or wisp sponge. Bleeding within the pararectal space exposure is uncommon, and is usually of anomalous venous origin, and can be controlled readily by medium-sized vascular clips.

If one is to use the right sacrospinous ligament, the middle finger of the left hand should be placed on the medial surface of the ischial spine, and under direct vision the tip of the long-handled Deschamps ligature carrier (Fig. 16.13) penetrates the coccygeus muscle–sacrospinous ligament at a point one and one-half to two finger breadths medial to the ischial spine. The carrier tip is pushed through (not around or under) the ligament. Considerable resistance is usually encountered, and this must be overcome by persistent forcefulness in the process of rotating the handle of the ligature carrier. Gentle traction to the handle will actually move the patient on the table, confirming proper placement. If no resistance is encountered, the ligature carrier could be either in front of the ligament or around the ligament rather than through it, exposing the structures behind the ligament to potential injury. Therefore, if no resistance is encountered as the ligature carrier is passed through the structure, the operator should remove the ligature carrier and reinsert it through the substance of the ligament. Obvious resistance should be encountered as the tip of the ligature carrier is being passed *through* the ligamentous tissue.

Early in his or her experience, the surgeon will wish to expose the area of fixation for suture placement to his or her direct vision, which requires appropriate anatomic dissection. Suture loop or needle retrieval must always be under direct visualization, however. The muscle and the ligament within it should often be grasped in the tip of a long Allis or Babcock clamp to help concentrate the tissue to be sutured and isolate it from any underlying vessels or nerves. The sutures in the Deschamps ligature carrier or needle should be inserted directly into the ligament one and one-half to two finger breadths medial to the ischial spine (Fig. 16.14). With increased experience and through a smaller incision into the septum, the tactile sense can be developed without compromising the

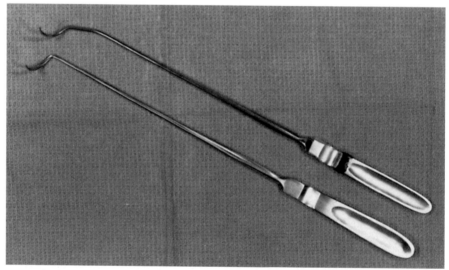

Figure 16.13. Long Deschamps ligature carriers. The angled Deschamps ligature carrier at the *top* (modeled after one modified by Rosenshein) is useful when the sacrospinous ligament is unusually deep. The handle must be swung through a wide arc. These instruments are available on special order from BEI Medical Systems, Zinnanti Surgical Instruments, Chatsworth, CA 91311; Codman & Shurtleff, Custom Device Dept., New Bedford, MA 02745; or Mr. William Merz, American V. Mueller, Chicago, IL 60648.

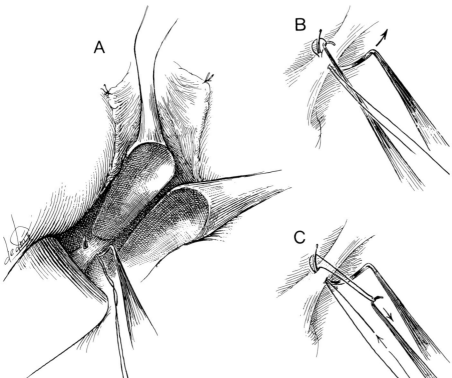

Figure 16.14. Retrieving the sutures from the ligature carrier. **A.** An upper retractor holds the transverse cervical ligament out of the way, and a similar retractor on the right displaces the rectum. The right sacrospinous ligament has been exposed and penetrated by the ligature carrier. **B.** The loop of suture within the ligature carrier is caught by the hook. **C.** Traction upon the hook brings the free end of the suture through the ligament, and the ligature carrier can be withdrawn.

accuracy of suture placement at a point one and one-half to two finger breadths medial to the ischial spine.

If the window made through the descending rectal septum is smaller than 3 cm in diameter, if difficulty is encountered in exposing the surface of the muscle, and if the operator is certain that the rectum has been displaced medially, it is possible to pursue an alternative approach to penetration of the ligament. The tip of the operator's middle finger is inserted through the window and along the inner surface of the pelvic diaphragm until the tip of the ischial spine and the sacrospinous ligament are identified. Keeping the lateral surface of the tip of the middle finger adjacent to the tip of the spine, the operator directs the tip of the long-handled Deschamps or the modified Deschamps ligature carrier (see Figs. 16.12 and 16.13) holding the suture along the undersurface of the operator's index finger until it reaches the sacrospinous ligament–coccygeus muscle complex. At a point clearly one and one-half to two finger breadths medial to the spine, and well away from the underlying pudendal nerve and vessels, the tip of the ligature carrier is rotated and made to penetrate the sacrospinous ligament. The fingers are withdrawn, the retractors suitably repositioned, and the tip of the ligature carrier visualized at this point. The suture is grasped by a hook, the suture carrier and Allis clamp removed, and the operation proceeds in the usual fashion. (Rarely, the nearby sacrotuberous ligament will be found to be stronger and more convenient than the sacrospinous, in which case suture to the sacrotuberous ligament may be substituted.)

The authors have not found the alternative of penetrating the sacrospinous ligament from above downward as by the Miya hook (16) to be of particular advantage, because retrieval of the suture from the Miya hook ligature carrier is sometimes cumbersome. We believe that penetration from beneath upward is generally more effective, and this can be accomplished by the use of the Deschamps ligature carrier or, more recently, by the use of the Shutt arthroscopic suture punch (30) (Fig. 16.15). The latter is of particular advantage to the operator with short fingers. The ligament is identified and grasped by the jaws of a long-handled Allis clamp and is penetrated by the hollow needle in the tip of the punch at a point one and one-half to two finger breadths medial to the ischial spine. The punch is closed, the suture is advanced through the hollow needle and retrieved, and the punch removed (Fig. 16.16). This may be repeated to bring additional sutures through the ligament if desired. A bilateral sacrospinous colpopexy may be considered if the vault of the vagina is wide enough to be stretched between the two ischial spines (Fig. 16.17).

When one follows the above steps, location of and entry into the pararectal space is consistent. When, however, the patient has a history of previous surgery in this area, the anatomic relationships may be distorted by fibrosis and adhesions secondary to the previous surgery, complicating the ease with which the surgeon can find the lateral wall of the pararectal space. A 2- or 3-cm fenestration through the rectal pillar overlying the ischial spine is all that is necessary to identify and expose a portion of the underlying coccygeus muscle and ligament sufficient to hold the necessary sutures.

The suture material is grasped at the tip of the ligature carrier (see Fig. 16.14*B*) and held with the hook, the loop is pulled through 2 or 3 inches, and the Deschamps carrier

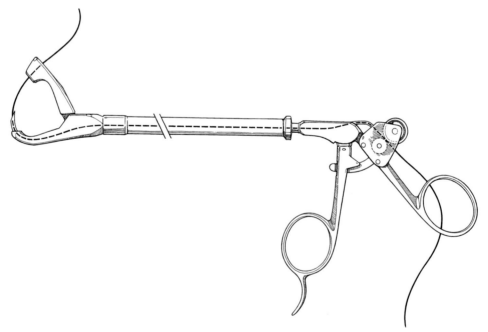

Figure 16.15. The Shutt suture punch. It consists of a long, hollow tunnel within the body of the forceps that terminates in a hollow needle. Monofilament suture is threaded through the tunnel; the suture passes beneath a friction wheel until it reaches the tip of the hollow needle. Then the direction of movement of the friction wheel is reversed so that the tip of the suture is withdrawn until it is barely within the substance of the hollow needle and no longer projects beyond it. The instrument is available from Linvatec, Largo, FL 34643.

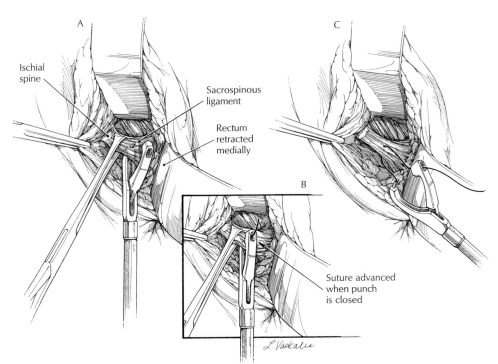

Figure 16.16. Penetration of sacrospinous ligament using Shutt punch. **A.** The right para-rectal space has been entered and the ischial spine identified. The coccygeus muscle–sacrospinous ligament complex running posteromedially from the ischial spine to the sacrococcygeal area is exposed and grasped by a long-handled Allis or Babcock clamp as shown. The tip of the Shutt punch is pushed under and through the ligament-muscle complex, the cardinal ligament being held out of harm's way by an anterior retractor as shown, and the rectum held medially by a second retractor. **B.** The jaws of the punch are closed, and the friction wheel rotated to propel the suture through the hollow needle and the fenestration in the upper jaw of the punch. **C.** The free end is grasped with a hemostat, the punch opened and removed, and the suture disengaged from the ligature carrier. Additional stitches may be placed as necessary. The long-handled Allis or Babcock clamp is removed.

is removed slowly and carefully in a counterclockwise fashion. The blunt point of the ligature carrier is less apt to lacerate nearby blood vessels than is the sharp point of the conventional swaged needle. The latter, being brittle because it is made of extruded wire, might break, and the broken tip may be hard to find and possibly lost. A second suture is similarly placed 1 cm medial to the first, and held. Alternatively, after pulling the first suture through as shown in Figure 16.14C, and while retaining both free ends, one cuts the loop in its center and pairs each end of the cut loop with its respective free suture end, thereby obtaining two sutures through the ligament but with only one penetration by the Deschamps carrier (Fig. 16.18).

A gentle tug to the ligature carrier or by the suture that has been grasped by the hook should actually move the patient a small degree on the table, indicating proper place-ment of the suture through the substance of the sacrospinous ligament. The ligature car-rier and Allis clamp are removed. Direct palpation of the suture and ischial spine con-firms the required distance between the two. If the suture seems too close to the ischial spine, traction is made upon it and a new suture is placed medial to the "offending" suture, which is then removed.

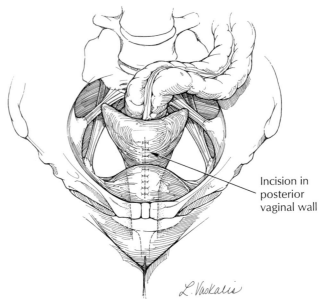

L. Vaskalis

Figure 16.17. Bilateral sacrospinous fixation, used when the vaginal vault is wide enough to reach from one side to the other. A phantom drawing shows the effect of bilateral sacrospinous colpopexy. This very effectively maintains a widened vaginal vault. The site of the posterior colporrhaphy closure is shown in the midline of the posterior vaginal wall.

Incision in
posterior
vaginal wall

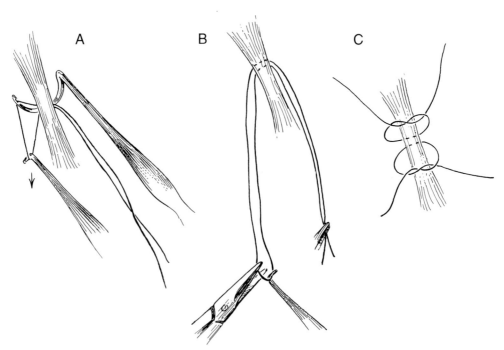

Figure 16.18. Cutting the suture loop. **A.** After the suture, doubled, has been passed through the ligament and caught by the hook, the ligature carrier is removed. **B.** The loop may be cut in the center and each end paired with its respective free suture. **C.** This results in two sutures through the ligament but with only one penetration by the Deschamps ligature carrier.

Postoperatively, in the patient with unilateral sacrospinous colpopexy the vault of the vagina deviates to the side of the patient to which the attachment was made, but this produces neither dyspareunia nor dysfunction.

The depth of the vagina to be realized after sacrospinous colpopexy is dependent upon the distance from the vulva to the point at which the vagina is fixed to the sacrospinous ligament(s). The sacrospinous colpopexy may be bilateral if the vault is wide enough to reach between the two ischial spines, if the prolapse is recurrent, if the patient has chronic obstructive pulmonary disease, or if the patient is prone to a lifestyle that requires lifting heavy objects.

The vagina normally is much wider at the vault. This is particularly evident when the vagina has turned inside out, as from massive posthysterectomy prolapse. Whether a colpopexy should be unilateral or bilateral depends upon the width of the vaginal vault. If it is wide and the operator intends to keep it that way, the colpopexy should be bilateral. If the vault is narrow or if the operator has deliberately made it narrow, then the colpopexy should be unilateral. If a wide vault is attached unilaterally, the unattached side, unless it is surgically narrowed, will gradually descend.

Satisfactory results are obtained if a unilateral colpopexy is performed provided that a wide vault is resected to convert the shape of a vagina from one resembling a light bulb to that of a cylinder of uniform diameter–since it is now an instrument of coitus, not parturition (see Fig. 16.10).

The free end of the sutures through the ligament is sewn to the underside of the vagina but not yet tied. If an anterior colporrhaphy has not yet been performed, a full-length repair of the anterior vaginal wall is usually done now. If the patient has been shown to have "stress" urinary incontinence coincident with a low urethral closure pressure, a vesicourethral sling procedure at this point in the operation will be performed to reduce the risk of postoperative urinary stress incontinence. If the patient with a low urethral closure pressure is not incontinent, even upon replacement of the prolapse within the pelvis, a series of "Kelly" stitches (see Chapter 10) will be placed and added to a full-length urethral plication. Then the upper part of the posterior colporrhaphy is begun, and when the upper 2 inches of posterior vaginal wall have been approximated, traction is made to the free end of the pulley stitch, all slack is taken up, and the pulley stitch and each of the other colpopexy stitches are tied, fixing the vaginal vault in the hollow of the sacrum, after which the remainder of the posterior colporrhaphy and perineorrhaphy is completed.

If a narrow vault is attached bilaterally, the undersurface of the vagina cannot reach the surface of the coccygeus muscle–sacrospinous ligament complex without suture bridges. If these are absorbable sutures, the ultimate scar will be weak and recurrence of the prolapse likely, but if they are of nonabsorbable Novafil, Prolene, or Surgilene, the vault probably will stay in place.

The vagina ideally should be sewn to the muscle-ligament as a firm tissue-to-tissue approximation. One method of bringing the soft movable vagina to the surface of the coccygeus muscle and ligament might be described as a "pulley." After the stitch has been placed in the ligament, one end of the suture is rethreaded on a free needle and sewn and tied by a single half-hitch to the full thickness of the fibromuscular layer of the undersurface of the vaginal apex, while the free end of the suture is held long. Traction to the free end of the suture at the proper time will pull the vagina directly onto the muscle and ligament (Fig. 16.19) (20, 21), where a square knot will fix it in place. When the vagina is thin or if greater vaginal length is desired, each end of the a long-lasting colpopexy stitch such as polydioxonone (PDS) may be inserted *through* the vagina, as shown in Figures 16.20 and 16.21. This should be done after an appropriate segment of posterior vaginal wall has been excised as part of the posterior colporrhaphy, and the sides of the upper half of the vagina have been united by side-to-side approximation with a running subcuticular stitch of polyglycolic acid suture. Tying the fixation stitch before this latter step reduces visibility for exposure of the vaginal vault, making suture of the colporrhaphy more difficult. It is essential that the pulley stitch be tied snugly so there

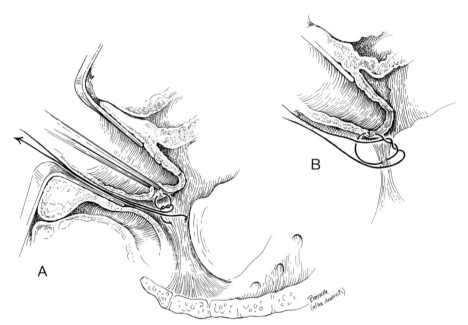

Figure 16.19. The "pulley" stitch. **A.** One end of the suture through the sacrospinous ligament has been sewn to the undersurface of the cut edge of the vaginal vault. Traction to the other end of the suture draws the vagina up and laterally to the surface of the ligament, and the ends are tied together, fixing the vagina to the ligament at this point. **B.** A second "safety" stitch similarly placed through the ligament is sewn to the subepithelial tissues of the vaginal wall and tied.

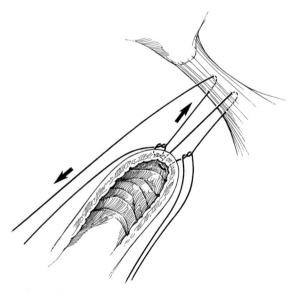

Figure 16.20. Tying the calpopexy sutures, knots buried. When the vaginal wall is thin and scarred but there is not much room in which to work or excessive exposure, the nonabsorbable monofilament suture may be placed as a pulley stitch as shown. The monofilament absorbable suture may be placed through the full thickness of the posterior vaginal wall with penetrations about 1 cm apart for tying after the pulley stitch has been tied.

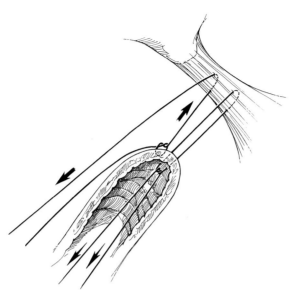

Figure 16.21. Tying the copopexy sutures—one knot exposed. In fixing the colpopexy stitches to the vagina, whether the colpopexy has been unilateral or bilateral, both permanent and long-lasting absorbable sutures are used. Permanent sutures should be placed through the fibromuscular wall of the vagina to which the stitch is tied, fixing it in position on the vagina as shown. The long-lasting but absorbable stitch may be placed through a very thin posterior vaginal wall with a double penetration in which the intervening wall serves as a bolster to improve the purchase of the sutures. Since this stitch is introduced from outside in and then inside out, the knot will be tied and buried beneath the posterior vaginal wall.

is no void or gap between the vagina and the ligament (Fig. 16.22). Such a gap would be called a *suture bridge* and should be avoided because once an absorbable suture has been absorbed, there would be less in the way of strong scar tissue to hold the vagina to the ligament, and if the vagina pulls away, the prolapse may recur. We now use size 1 polydioxanone (PDS) monofilament delayed absorbable or size 1 or 2 polyglycolic acid-type suture (Dexon or Vicryl) for this suture, since too fine a suture in this ligament might act somewhat like a saw and actually cut through the ligament while being tied. The no. 2 size thickness has good knot-tying strength and, being of controlled slow absorbency, will last for several weeks. This is in contrast to catgut, which retains its maximal strength and continuity for only 7 to 10 days. A monofilament synthetic nonabsorbable suture such as size 1 Novafil, Prolene, or Surgilene is usually added, particularly in the patient with significant chronic respiratory disease or with recurrent prolapse, though care should be taken any nonabsorbable suture and its knot are buried beneath the vagina.

Permanent sutures such as monofilament synthetic nonabsorbable suture (Novafil, Prolene, or Surgilene) size 0 or 1 can be recommended as the principal colpopexy stitches in the following circumstances:

1. Recurrent vaginal vault eversion
2. A patient with chronic respiratory disease
3. A patient with a short vagina of insufficient length to reach the ischial spine; in this circumstance, one may create a deliberate suture bridge between the top of the vault of the short vagina and the surface of the coccygeus muscle–sacrospinous ligament
4. A patient who will be required to perform heavy lifting after her convalescence

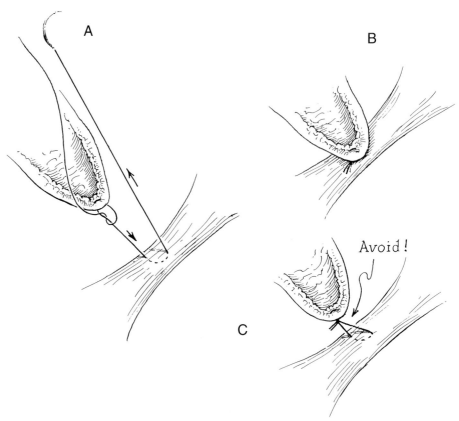

Figure 16.22. Avoiding a suture bridge. **A.** A suture has been passed through the sacrospinous ligament and a firm bite taken into the tissues of the vaginal wall, to which it is fixed at this point by a single half-hitch. **B.** Traction to the opposite free end of the suture will use the point of passage through the firm tissue as a pulley, bringing the movable tissue to this point where the two tissues are now in direct contact with one another; a conventional knot is tied, fixing the new relationship. **C.** A suture bridge should be avoided.

Figure 16.23 shows the effect on the vesicourethral junction of bringing an everted vault of the vagina back into the hollow of the sacrum.

The pulley stitch need be done with only one of the suture pairs. The second or "safety" stitch can be inserted *through* the wall of the vagina. The suture penetrations should be 1 to 2 cm apart, so the often thinned vaginal wall may be used as a bolster but not tied until the pulley stitch has brought and tied the vagina securely to the sacrospinous ligament. The second or safety stitch is later readily tied with a simple square knot either beneath or within the vagina (see Fig. 16.19*B*). Any needed anterior colporrhaphy is now accomplished.

It is now time to tie the sacrospinous fixation stitches. By traction to the free end of the stitch(es) (opposite to that which had been fixed to the undersurface of the vagina), the vaginal wall is drawn to rest squarely upon the surface of the sacrospinous ligament–coccygeus muscle complex, and the knots are tied. The posterior colporrhaphy and perineorrhaphy are then completed. The whole operation is shown in Figure 16.24 (color insert). The vault of the vagina will be found to lie in its normal horizontal axis; however, if the colpopexy was unilateral, it will be deviated slightly to the side. The vagina can be packed lightly with iodoform gauze for 24 hours. Because the right rectal pillar is now compressed between the vagina and the sacrospinous ligament, immediate post-

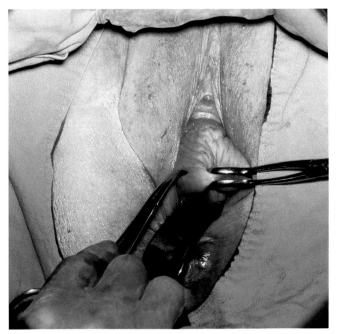

Color Figure 16.24 A. The scar at the apex of the vagina is grasped by a sponge forceps. The hemostat marks a small dimple; this is the site at which the right uterosacral ligament was attached to the vagina at hysterectomy almost 30 years earlier.

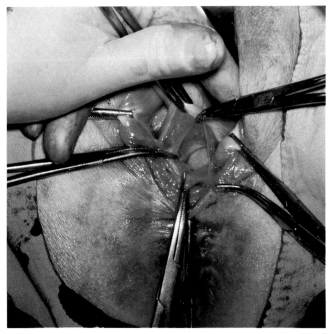

Color Figure 16.24 B. An enterocele is identified, opened, and mobilized before resection.

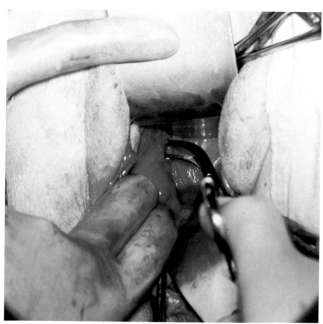

Color Figure 16.24 C. The right rectal pillar is penetrated at a spot overlying the right ischial spine. The penetration is here being enlarged by opening the tips of a long, pointed forceps.

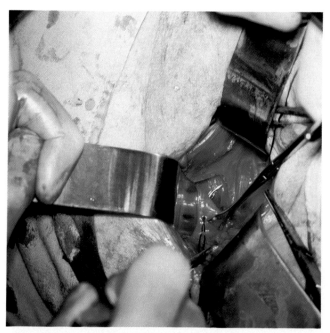

Color Figure 16.24 D. The sacrospinous ligament within the coccygeus muscle is grasped in a long Babcock clamp, about 4 cm medial to the ischial spine. At a point about 3 cm medial to the spine, the sacrospinous ligament and coccygeus muscle are penetrated by the tip of a Deschamps ligature carrier into which has been inserted a suture of no. 1 Novafil or Prolene.

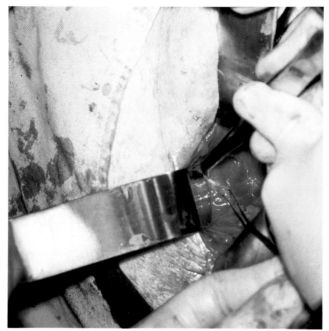

Color Figure 16.24 E. The Deschamps ligature carrier has been removed. This shows placement of the Novafil suture through the sacrospinous ligament and coccygeus muscle. Traction to the suture will move the patient on the table. The location of the ischial spine is indicated by the tip of the forceps in the upper part of the picture. One can readily see that the ligament has been penetrated 2.5 to 3 cm medial to the spine.

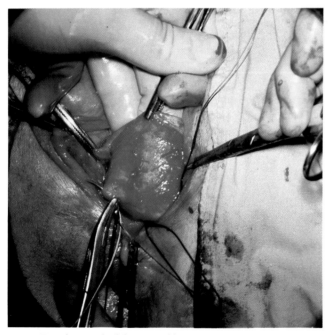

Color Figure 16.24 F. A free end of the Novafil suture is sewn through the undersurface of the full thickness of the fibromuscular wall.

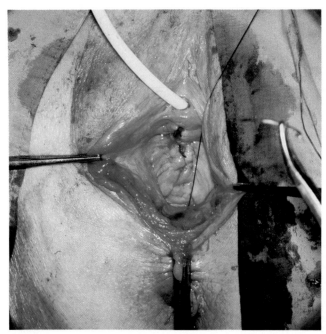

Color Figure 16.24 G. The remainder of the posterior vaginal wall is closed from side to side with a running subcuticular stitch, and the perineal body reconstructed.

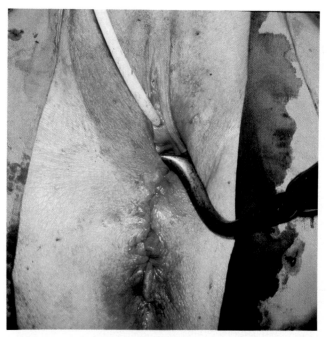

Color Figure 16.24 H. The vagina now has a relatively normal depth and axis, as shown by insertion of the Breisky-Navratil retractor. Digital examination confirms the integrity of the rectum. (Photographs by Lester V Bergman, courtesy of LTI Medica and The Upjohn Company. Copyright 1982 by Learning Technology Incorporated. Used with permission.)

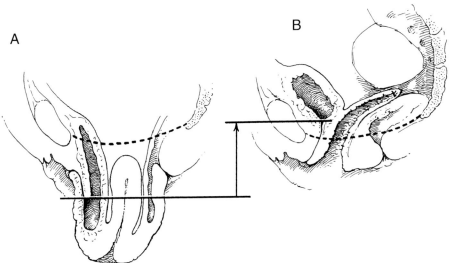

Figure 16.23. Sagittal section showing the relationship of the vesicourethral junction to the pubis and pelvis. The usual location of the pelvic diaphragm is indicated by the *dotted line*; the vesicourethral junction is indicated by the *solid line*. **A.** Advanced genital prolapse, showing that eversion of the vagina may pull on tissues supporting the vesicourethral junction, exteriorizing the latter. **B.** The effects of restoring vaginal depth and axis. Repositioning of the vagina has provided upward traction to tissues of the vesicourethral junction, helping to restore them once again to a position within the pelvis. (From Nichols DH. Effects of pelvic relaxation on gynecologic urologic problems. Clin Obstet Gynecol 1978;21:1766. Used with permission of Lippincott-Raven.)

operative examination will show the rectum to be pulled to the patient's side. Within a few weeks the pillar must elongate, for by then the rectum can again be found to be in the midline. Postoperatively, many patients observe a transient mild discomfort or pulling sensation deep in the buttock, without transmission of discomfort to the thigh, but as the edema subsides, this regresses within a few days or weeks. Examination usually shows excellent vaginal depth and axis (see Figs. 16.7, 16.9), and increased intra-abdominal pressure serves to press the vagina against the levator plate and accentuates the restored horizontal axis of the vagina. To date, no patient of ours has complained of dyspareunia after this type of vaginal fixation.

OPERATIVE COMPLICATIONS

If a needle tip penetrates the lumen of any adjacent viscus (the rectum would be most likely), the needle should be withdrawn and no additional treatment should be necessary. If a laceration is encountered, it should be repaired by a standard two-layered closure. If at any time during the procedure it has been determined by a rectal examination that a suture has transgressed the wall of the rectum, the suture should be promptly removed or cut and replaced by a stitch in a proper position outside the rectal lumen.

Pudendal or sciatic trauma, a rare complication of sacrospinous colpopexy, is recognized by immediate severe postoperative gluteal pain running down the posterior surface of the affected leg. It should be treated promptly by deligation and medial reposition of the fixation sutures.

In spite of the *full-length* anterior colporrhaphy usually done, a mild but usually transient urinary stress incontinence has been noted in an occasional patient, probably the result of temporarily straightening the posterior urethrovesical angle. It tends to disappear after several months as a new posterior urethrovesical angle becomes established. Estrogen replacement therapy and a long course of Kegel perineal resistive exercises are helpful. Rarely, suprapubic vesicourethral suspension may be recommended.

Recurrent but asymptomatic cystocele without stress incontinence is the most frequent complication of colpopexy (4, 13, 23, 32) and will usually become evident within the first 3 months postoperatively. It rarely requires treatment. Some cystoceles are probably the result of progression after under-repair at the time of surgery, some are the result of natural progression of the aging process, and some the result of unrecognized and unrepaired lateral (paravaginal) attenuation or avulsion. The presence and degree of the latter, when recognized preoperatively or intraoperatively, can be repaired as part of the reconstructive surgery (see Chapter 10).

Bleeding deep within the pelvis and along the pelvic sidewall (usually of venous origin) is easily controlled by the application of medium-sized hemaclips. Far more ominous is the rare instance of venous bleeding from trauma to the large vein within one of the sacral foramina (possibly caused by an assistant's inappropriate movement of the tip of a deeply placed retractor toward the opposite side of the pelvis). This may be controlled by occluding the foramen with a firmly pressed sterile thumbtack (33, 34, 39) or lag screw.

PELVIC SHELF RECONSTRUCTION

A transvaginal posterior "pelvic shelf" reconstruction with colporrhaphy was described by Seigworth (29) in which after ureteral catheters have been placed a midline suspension of the vagina is accomplished with a series of posterior pelvic pursestring polyglycolic sutures. The sutures are placed transperitoneally from one uterosacral ligament, the pelvic diaphragm medial and caudal to the ischial spine, and reef the peritoneum covering the anterior surface of the rectum. The stitch continues, incorporating the same structures on the opposite side, and when tied to the apex of the vaginal vault becomes, in effect, a vaginal Moschcowitz type (18) of closure that permits simultaneous colporrhaphy through the same operative exposure. The surgical use of the perirectal fascia for support of the vaginal vault (which may be the same tissue as the coccygeus muscle and its aponeurosis) (23, 38) emphasizes its potential usefulness. The vaginal axis is not unlike those following bilateral sacrospinous colpopexy with colporrhaphy, but the midline vaginal vault is wider and a little deeper with the latter procedure, which does not require ureteral catheters. The accompanying pursestring peritoneal closure of any enterocele also brings the uterosacral ligaments closer to the midline.

TRANSABDOMINAL SURGERY

There are some abdominal approaches to the solution of this difficult problem, but the success of these procedures is variable. Ventral fixation of the uterine fundus to the anterior abdominal wall was once popular. Although the patient may be reasonably comfortable for a while, the cause of the prolapse has not been relieved and, given enough time, continued progression of the prolapse will become evident. Although the uterine fundus may remain fixed to the abdominal wall, the uterus and cervix often will elongate until, ultimately, the vagina and those organs to which it is attached will come down again. The patient, meanwhile, has often forgotten the nature of her surgery many years before, and her operative records may have been lost and the surgeon may no longer be in practice. One may begin what appears to be a usual vaginal hysterectomy and repair only to find upon opening the peritoneal cavity that the fundus of the uterus extends all the way to the anterior abdominal wall (Fig. 16.25). A confirmatory tug on the cervix at that point will produce visible dimpling in the anterior abdominal wall. This adhesion between uterine fundus and anterior abdominal wall must be released in order for the

A   B

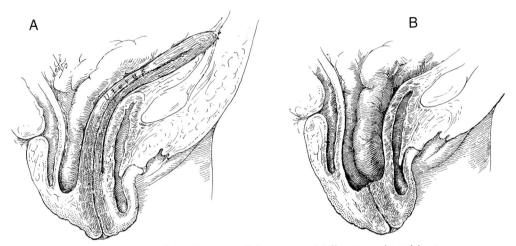

Figure 16.25. Vault prolapse following ventral fixation and following subtotal hysterectomy. **A.** Drawing showing the failure of ventral fixation of the uterus to retard progression of genital prolapse. An enterocele is developing from the now unprotected cul-de-sac. **B.** Eversion of the vagina after subtotal hysterectomy. Although on superficial external examination the two conditions resemble one another, the technical details of subsequent surgical treatment are vastly different.

hysterectomy and repair to proceed. This can usually be accomplished by sharp dissection at a quick transabdominal "minilap" without disturbing the vaginal surgical drapes.

A drawback of the procedure of ventral fixation of either uterine fundus or posthysterectomy vaginal vault is the now exposed cul-de-sac. By having changed the axis of the vagina, one has made the cul-de-sac even more vulnerable to increases in intra-abdominal pressure (Fig. 16.26). When Burch (8) presented his excellent results in treating incontinence by fixating the vagina to the Cooper ligament, it was pointed out that the incidence of subsequent enterocele was between 11 and 15 percent. The probable explanation is that the change in vaginal axis caused the now unprotected cul-de-sac to become more directly vulnerable to increases in intra-abdominal pressure. The cul-de-sac should be clearly obliterated as a separate step with any abdominal surgery that changes the normal horizontal axis of the vagina.

Sacrospinous colpopexy in a patient who has sustained a previous Burch, Marshall-Marchetti-Krantz (MMK), or needle suspension of the anterior vaginal wall requires that the vault be pulled in the opposite direction, which over a period of time may increase the risk of recurrence. Therefore, a transabdominal colpopexy should be considered as an alternate in those post-Burch or post-MMK patients who do not wish to accept this increased risk, estimated at 25 percent. A vesicourethral sling procedure, however, does not pull the vagina as significantly in an anterior direction, since the pull is concentrated on the urethrovesical tissues rather than the vaginal walls, and the recurrence rate of vault prolapse does not seem to be significantly increased.

Sacropexy

Arthur and Savage (3) and Falk (12) attached the fundus of the uterus to the periosteum of the sacrum. Better still, one can remove the uterus and attach the vagina to the sacrum by a retroperitoneal bridge of Mersilene mesh or fascia lata (21). This reestablishes a more or less horizontal vaginal axis, especially following any restorative transvaginal colporrhaphy.

The transabdominal method of retroperitoneal sacropexy is a satisfactory but complex procedure. This method is particularly attractive when the abdomen must be opened

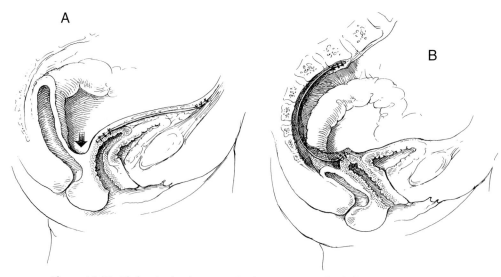

Figure 16.26. Abdominal colpopexy. **A.** The unprotected cul-de-sac left after ventral fixation of the vagina is noted by the *arrow*. **B.** The vagina has been fixed to the promontory of the sacrum by a retroperitoneal bridge of Mersilene mesh or of fascia. The cul-de-sac is no longer vulnerable. (From Nichols DH. Repair of enterocele and prolapse of the vaginal vault. In: Barber H, ed. Goldsmith's practice of surgery, 1981. Used with permission of Cine-Med Inc.)

for an unrelated reason, such as for removal of an ovarian tumor or when the vagina is too short to be brought to the ischial spine. Coexistent intestinal diverticulosis risks future perforation of a diverticulum at the site of the mesh, and is a relative contraindication to the abdominal approach. If the mesh bridge becomes infected, it must be removed. A risk with this approach occurs when cystocele and rectocele are present. To attempt a vaginal repair and simultaneous transabdominal sacral fixation of the vagina appreciably increases the risk of infection at the site of the nonabsorbable sutures and Mersilene mesh, and it is not recommended. The repair of the cystocele and rectocele should be done at another time. Transabdominal sacropexy will correct eversion of the vaginal vault but not eversion of the lower vagina.

If massive vaginal eversion is secondary to a ventral fixation of the vagina or uterus, it is difficult to return this type of vaginal axis to normal without freeing the vagina or uterus from its attachment to the anterior abdominal wall. Massive eversion of the vagina is by no means uncommon after even a single pregnancy in a patient with a history of exstrophy of the bladder, even if the patient had been delivered by Cesarean section. The obvious anatomic weakness of the anterior vaginal wall is no comfort at all to the surgeon in providing an anatomic basis for suitable surgical support, because so many of these patients previously have had a cystectomy. One possibility should there be an enormous appearance of a "cystocele" (namely, a massive relaxation of the anterior wall of the vagina with bulging and a feeling out and fullness), but the patient has no uterine descent, is an operation involving modification of the Watkins-Wertheim transposition in which the fundus of the uterus is sewn to the periosteum of the pubic rami. To this may be added the modification in which the cervix is amputated and the uterus is opened before the transposition. The entire endometrial cavity is excised. The limits of the endometrial cavity to be removed may be defined by the intrauterine installation of an ampoule of indigocarmine, which will stain all the tissue a deep violet color. The uterine wall is then reunited and the transposition finished.

The patient born with bladder exstrophy has a special potential problem following pregnancy. When procidentia accompanies a prolapse in this sort of situation, there often is no cardinal or uterosacral ligament strength to which to attach the vault of the vagina with confidence that it will stay there. An operation of Howard Jones (personal communication, 1990) has been employed successfully in which by a transabdominal approach the cul-de-sac of Douglas is obliterated and the vagina attached by an intermediate Mersilene strip to the periosteum of the pubis. Because there is no bladder to get in the way in this circumstance, this permits minimal displacement of the ureteral sigmoidostomy that may have been accomplished at the time of the preceding cystectomy, often in the patient's youth.

TECHNIQUE

Anticipating some possible contamination of the operative field from the vagina, a single dose of an appropriate "prophylactic" antibiotic should be given preoperatively. An obturator is inserted into the vagina or the vagina is carefully packed with iodoform gauze and a Foley catheter is inserted into the bladder. The lower abdomen is opened through a midline lower incision and the abdomen is explored. The vaginal vault filled with an obturator or packing is easily identified. A transverse incision is made in the peritoneum over the uppermost portion of the vagina, and the peritoneum is reflected both anteriorly and posteriorly for a distance of 2 to 3 cm. This line of cleavage should denude the musculoconnective tissue wall of the vagina. The bladder will be identified with its attachment to the anterior peritoneal reflection. Any appreciable enterocele sac should be identified and obliterated or excised. A Dexon or Vicryl 2-0 guide suture is placed on each side of the vaginal apex, and three pairs of 2-0 coated *nonabsorbable* braided synthetic sutures, such as Ethibond, are placed transversely 1 cm apart in the central portion of the vaginal vault through the full subepithelial fibromuscular thickness of the vaginal wall but not into the vaginal lumen. Any vaginal packing is then removed so that the surgeon may be certain that no stitches have fixed it to the vagina.

A longitudinal incision is made through the peritoneum over the sacral promontory and extended caudally for 5 to 6 cm. The peritoneal flaps on either side are caught in retraction sutures left long enough to permit an adequate exposure of the bifurcation of the aorta and the vena cava. The midsacral artery and any nearby vein may need to be coagulated or ligated to provide access to a 6- to 8-cm area of clean periosteum over the promontory of the sacrum between the common iliac veins. The exposed area of periosteum must be freed of all connective tissue, and hemostasis must ensure a dry field where a segment of fascia lata or plastic gauze is to be sutured to the periosteum.

A subperitoneal tunnel may be established by blunt dissection with a long, curved intestinal clamp or kidney stone forceps. The dissection should extend from the inferior edge of the incision over the sacral promontory beneath the peritoneum across the posterolateral aspect of the right side of the cul-de-sac to the cut edge of the peritoneum overlying the vaginal apex. Alternatively, the peritoneum of the cul-de-sac may be incised longitudinally and reflected.

Small blood vessels may be electrocoagulated to ensure a dry operative field. Three pairs of 2-0 braided nonabsorbable sutures (Ethibond) are placed in the sacral periosteum, using a strong but small half-circle needle with a trocar point. The midpoint of a 2- to 8-inch piece of Mersilene mesh folded longitudinally (alternatively, a large strip of fascia) is brought to the vaginal apex. The braided plastic sutures are threaded through it and tied securely. The curved intestinal clamp running through the tunnel grasps the free end of the mesh or fascia now attached to the apex of the vagina and draws it to the promontory of the sacrum as the clamp is withdrawn. A little slack is left in the strip; it is not pulled so tightly as to elevate the cul-de-sac of the peritoneum appreciably. The nonabsorbable sutures previously placed in the periosteum over the sacral promontory are now passed through the appropriate points of the intermediate bridge; when all have been satisfactorily placed, they are tied, fixing the bridge to the sacral periosteum. Excess ends of the bridge are excised and the peritoneum closed with fine absorbable suture. The cul-de-sac is obliterated and the parietal peritoneum closed. Unless one is planning an anterior colporrhaphy, a suprapubic pin-up of the vesicourethral junction will lessen the chance of an unwanted postoperative urinary stress incontinence. The vagina is redistended overnight with a splinting iodoform or gauze pack. The patient is permitted out of bed on the first postoperative day, and the urinary catheter is removed. It is our view that treatment of coincident rectocele and cystocele are best managed previously or at another time by a transvaginal approach directed at the sites of damage.

CONCLUSION

Vaginal hysterectomy and repair, although usually successful, will not serve all patients with massive eversion of the vagina equally well. There are various causes, tissue strengths, and damages that should be identified and correlated with a choice of different surgical procedures. For those patients with vaginal vault prolapse but without usable cardinal-uterosacral ligament support, supplemental techniques for support of the vault must be added. The ultimate goal is to relieve symptoms and restore the natural depth and position of the vagina, while at the same time effectively treating any coexistent pelvic disease, including cystocele, enterocele, and rectocele. This can be accomplished using techniques that will restore or preserve coital function.

It is usually unnecessary and often a distinct disservice to an active patient with prolapse to leave her with a short vagina or to perform partial or total colpectomy.

When colpectomy is performed, however, the results are better when any coexistent enterocele has been identified and the sac excised. Accurate perception, correct diagnosis, and an adequate procedure that will correct all the sites of weakness cannot help but improve the long-term result of the surgery employed.

References

1. Addison WA, Timmons MC, Wall LL, Livengood CH, et al. Failed abdominal sacral colpopexy: observations and recommendations. Obstet Gynecol 1989;74:480.
2. Amreich J. Äetiologie und Operation des Scheidenstumpf prolapses. Wien Klin Wochenschr 1951;63: 74–77.
3. Arthur HGE, Savage D. Uterine prolapse and prolapse of the vaginal vault treated by sacral hysteropexy. J Obstet Gynaecol Br Emp 1957;64:355.
4. Backen MH, Jr. Success with sacrospinous suspension of the prolapsed vaginal vault. Surg Gynecol Obstet 1992;175:419–420.
5. Baden WF, Walker TA. Physical diagnosis in the evaluation of vaginal relaxation. Clin Obstet Gynecol 1972;15:1060.
6. Baden WF, Walker TA. Surgical repair of vaginal defects. Philadelphia: JB Lippincott, 1992.
7. Bonney V. The sustentacular of the female genital canal, the displacements that result from the yielding of its several components, and then appropriate treatment. J Obstet Gynaecol Br Emp 1914;45:328–344.
8. Burch JC. Urethrovaginal fixation to Cooper's ligament for stress incontinence. Am J Obstet Gynecol 1961;81:2.
9. Cox OC. Hystero-culpectomy. Sibley Mem Hosp Alumni Assoc Bull 1958;1:9–16.
10. Cruikshank SH. Sacrospinous fixation: should this be performed at the time of vaginal hysterectomy? Am J Obstet Gynecol 1991;164:1072–1076.
11. DeLancey JOL. Anatomic aspects of vaginal eversion after hysterectomy. Am J Obstet Gynecol 1992; 166:1717.
12. Falk HC. Uterine prolapse and prolapse of the vaginal vault treated by sacropexy. Obstet Gynecol 1961; 18:113–115.
13. Heinonen PK. Transvaginal sacrospinous colpopexy for vaginal vault and complete genital prolapse in aged women. Acta Obstet Gynecol Scand 1992;71:377–381.
14. Inmon WB. Pelvic relaxation and repair including prolapse of vagina following hysterectomy. South Med J 1963;56:577–582.
15. Marshall VF, Marchetti AA, Krantz KE. The correction of stress incontinence by simple vesicourethral suspension. Surg Gynecol Obstet 1949;88:509.
16. Miyazaki FS. Miya hook ligature carrier for sacrospinous ligament fixation. Obstet Gynecol 1987;70: 286.
17. Morley GW, DeLancey JOL. Sacrospinous ligament fixation for eversion of the vagina. Am J Obstet Gynecol 1988;158:872.

18. Moschcowitz AV. The pathogenesis, anatomy, and care of prolapse of the rectum. Surg Gynecol Obstet 1912;15:18.
19. Nichols DH. Sacrospinous fixation for massive eversion of the vagina. Am J Obstet Gynecol 1982; 142:901.
20. Nichols DH, Milley PS, Randall CL. Significance of restoration of normal vaginal depth and axis. Obstet Gynecol 1978;36:241–246.
21. Parsons L, Ulfelder H. An atlas of pelvic operations. 2nd ed. Philadelphia: WB Saunders, 1968:280–283.
22. Percy NM, Pert JI. Total colpectomy. Surg Gynecol Obstet 1961;113:174–184.
23. Peters WA, Christenson ML: Fixation of the vaginal apex to the coccygeus fascia during repair of vaginal vault eversion with enterocele. Am J Obstet Gynec 1995;172:1894–902.
24. Richter K. Massive eversion of the vagina: pathogenesis, diagnosis, and therapy of the "true" prolapse of the vaginal stump. Clin Obstet Gynecol 1982;25:897–912.
25. Richter K. Die operative Behandlung des prolabierten Scheidengrundes nach Uterusextirpation Beitrag zur Vaginaefixatio Sacrotuberalis nach Amreich. Geburtshilfe Frauenheilkd 1967;27:941–954.
26. Richter K, Albrich W. Long term results following fixation of the vagina on the sacrospinal ligament by the vaginal route (vaginaefixatio sacrospinalis vaginalis). Am J Obstet Gynecol 1981;141:811.
27. Rosenzweig BA, Pushkin S, Blumenfeld D, Bhatia NN. Prevalence of abnormal urodynamic test results in continent women with severe genitourinary prolapse. Obstet Gynecol 1992;79:539–542.
28. Sederl J. Zur Operation des Prolapses der blind endigenden Scheide. Geburtshilfe Frauenheilkd 1958;18:824–828.
29. Seigworth GR. Vaginal vault prolapse with eversion. Obstet Gynecol 1979;54:255–260.
30. Sharp TR. Sacrospinous suspension made easy. Obstet Gynecol 1993;82:873–875.
31. Shull BL, Capen CV, Riggs MW, Kuchl TJ. Bilateral attachment of the vaginal cuff to iliococcygeus fascia: an effective method of cuff suspension. Am J Obstet Gynecol 1993;168:1669.
32. Shull BL, Capen CV, Riggs MW, Kuchl TJ. Preoperative and postoperative analysis of site-specific pelvic support defects in 81 women treated with sacrospinous ligament suspension and pelvic reconstruction. Am J Obstet Gynecol 1992;166:1764.
33. Sutton GP. Thumbtacks (letter to the editors). Am J Obstet Gynecol 1991;164:931.
34. Sutton GP, et al. Life-threatening hemorrhage complicating sacral colpopexy. Am J Obstet Gynecol 1981;140:836.
35. Symmonds R, Williams TJ, Lee RA, et al. Posthysterectomy enterocele and vaginal vault prolapse. Am J Obstet Gynecol 1981;140:852.
36. Tancer ML, Fleischer M, Berkowitz BJ. Simultaneous colpo-recto-sacropexy. Obstet Gynecol 1987; 70:951.
37. Thompson HG, Murphy CJ, Picot H. Hystero-colpectomy for treatment of uterine procidentia. Am J Obstet Gynecol 1961;82:743–753.
38. Thornton NW, Peters WA. Repair of vaginal prolapse after hysterectomy. Am J Obstet Gynecol 1983; 147:140–145.
39. Timmons MC, Kohler MF, Addison WA. Thumbtack use for control of presacral bleeding, with description of an instrument for thumbtack application. Obstet Gynecol 1991;78:313.
40. White R. An anatomical operation for the cure of cystocele. JAMA 1909;53:1707–1710.
41. Zweifel P. Vorlesungen über klinische gynakologie. Berlin: Hirschwald, 1892:407.

CHAPTER 17

Choice of Operation for Urinary Stress Incontinence

There is no doubt that instrumentation has advanced beyond our knowledge to comprehend the information obtained . . . be wary of simple solutions to what appears to be a very complex hydrodynamic problem. Douglas Marchant (57), 1981 p. 373.

There are a greater number of older women, and the essence of enjoying their longevity is their quality of life. When this is compromised by disorders in the uro-gynecologic system, it becomes the responsibility of the gynecologic surgeon to evaluate and offer appropriate therapy. This therapy must be affordable, however, and in these days of required cost containment and diminished length of hospitalization, the surgeon must not only choose to do the right thing correctly the first time, but must also correct all of the pathology at the initial operation so that it should not be necessary for the patient to be readmitted in the future for additional corrective surgery. A predictable necessity for reoperation is unbearably expensive.

The rules of the past no longer apply. The time when a surgeon *always* performs the same favorite operation for the same indication has passed. The surgeon of today must be experienced in a variety of procedures, some surgical and some not, with which to treat the same condition. The new rules are these:

1. These decisions must be based on accurate interpretation of contributing anatomic changes.
2. The surgeon must look for and measure alterations in physiology, including relevant neuropathy (81).
3. Treatment must be cost-effective.
4. The surgeon must realize that, for many patients, the best solution and first line of attack may not be surgical at all.

It is appropriate to not only consider realigning our own perspectives in urogynecology and reconstructive surgery but also to develop international perspectives, since the problems of women are much the same the world over. Our new theme is not how to do an operation, but whether or not to do it, and if not, what then, and why? One should determine, if possible, how long the incontinence has been present and, to exclude a transient incontinence, whether or not the condition is getting better by itself (which may require neither work-up nor treatment) or worsening (requiring analysis and intervention).

The International Continence Society (ICS) defines urinary stress incontinence (USI) as the involuntary loss of urine caused by an increase in intra-abdominal pressure, not mediated by a bladder contraction, in a quantity the patient considers unacceptable (1).

Because urinary incontinence is a symptom complex that includes etiologic components of varied relationships, it constitutes a mixture of symptoms that compete and combine to account for varying degrees of disability. Some components are inflammatory; some are the result of neurologic disturbances affecting the voiding mechanism; others are the result of congenital deficiency or of iatrogenic disease. Specific anatomic deficiencies may have so altered normal bladder physiology as to make it difficult for the patient to retain her urine at times of increased intra-abdominal pressure. When dominant, this component is referred to as urinary stress incontinence and may vary between such wide extremes as an occasional, almost incidental occurrence to a major and very real social disability.

The different anatomic and physiologic factors involved in the development of urinary incontinence should be separately identified, because they play a most important role in the selection of appropriate, individualized therapy for the woman. The hydrodynamics of micturition and stress incontinence have been summarized by Crisp (24) as follows:

1. The intracystic pressure is equal to, or slightly greater than, an intra-abdominal pressure under normal conditions, regardless of the degree of filling. It measures approximately 2 mmHg.
2. Intracystic pressure rises immediately and directly as the intra-abdominal pressure increases. This occurs whether the bladder is in normal position or in marked prolapse, since the law of hydrostatics (Pascal's law) states that when an external pressure is applied to the wall of a container of fluid, this pressure is transmitted equally in all directions.
3. Under conditions of rest, the pressure within the urethra is greater (2 to 6 mmHg) than the intracystic pressure. The pressure within the urethral segment rises proportionately to the increase in intracystic pressure. These observations, confirmed by Beck, Hsu, and Maughan [11], show that stress incontinence cannot occur without some incompetence of the urethral segment. Urethral pressure depends not only on the involuntary resistance, which includes the urethral mucosa, periurethral tissues, and vasculature, but also on the voluntary resistance of the midportion of the urethra and the pubourethral ligaments. The patient will not be incontinent as long as the voluntary muscular segment functions normally, maintaining the pressure of the urethra greater than the intravesical pressure with or without the additional intra-abdominal pressure that is associated with stress of coughing, etc.

Some observers have stated that the problem of stress incontinence is centered around the loss of the posterior urethrovesical angle. These authors give the impression that in order to be continent, the female must have an angle of obstruction that prevents incontinence but that she may lower to void. The loss of the posterior vesical angle is only a sign of, not the cause of, stress incontinence. Resistance of flow in any tubular structure is inversely proportional to the diameter of the pipe, and directly proportional to its length. Angulation of the pipe does not significantly change this principle. There is, of course, a degree of back-thrust of the urinary stream at the point of angulation, but it is probably insignificant. Some patients will have urinary incontinence from bladder or urethral instability, still others from overflow, and many from a mixture of causes.

To reiterate, intraurethral pressure is dependent upon good support of both segments of the urethra. Involuntary loss of urine occurs when intravesical pressure is greater than intraurethral pressure.

In the presence of a large cystocele, increases in intra-abdominal intravesical pressure will be transmitted largely to the most dependent portion of the cystocele (at the vaginal introitus), rather than against the attenuated urethrovesical junction. In addition, progressive development of prolapse of the bladder tends to angulate or to kink the urethra to some extent. Sometimes this action will "cure" the patient's incontinence or even overcompensate for the leakage, in that the bladder must be manually elevated before the patient is able to void. Careful search of the history of many patients who have maximal prolapse (who are continent, as a rule) will disclose a past history of stress incontinence, now relieved.

Cystoceles may cause voiding dysfunction, and lack of symptoms of stress incontinence is unreliable in patients with cystocele. They may be associated with other symptoms, most of which actually resolve after operative repair. Operative repair will resolve stress incontinence in the majority of patients with coincident cystocele (36).

Women with severe genitourinary prolapse may also be at risk for uninhibited detrusor contractions but not demonstrate incontinence. Urine loss may be masked in the presence of a prolapse, most likely because of urethral kinking (76).

As part of the preliminary physical examination, the patient with a genital prolapse should be examined in the office while standing, her bladder *unemptied*. The gynecologist should replace the prolapse within the pelvis, and while holding it there ask the patient to cough or strain. If, at this time, an otherwise continent patient leaks urine, this patient will require some coexistent surgical support of the vesicourethral junction during reconstructive surgery, or a postoperative urinary stress incontinence can be predicted and almost assured. Operative correction of the uterine prolapse and repair of the cystocele not only correct the urethral angulation but also direct any increases in intravesical pressure upon the atonic funneled neck of the bladder and urethra.

When a patient has this condition, the same attention should be given to the urethra as in a patient with severe stress incontinence, lest she be very wet and unhappy after repair of the cystocele and correction of the prolapse have been accomplished. At least 3 to 6 months should lapse before reoperative surgical correction. Mere repetition of a vaginal procedure or simple vaginal operation may not help. As a rule, a suprapubic or combined approach will be required. Primary operation is not indicated per se for an asymptomatic cystocele.

NEED FOR COMPARATIVE DATA

Much interest has been evidenced in comparing the reported success rates with the varied operative procedures for the relief of USI. For purposes of comparative study, the symptom complex of USI might well be divided into at least two major groups: (*a*) severe and socially disabling USI and (*b*) minor degrees of incontinence often coexistent with other more significant pelvic pathology for which surgery is indicated. In the latter group, treatment of the USI may be of relatively secondary importance, but failure to include indicated repair may be followed by a result that will be unsatisfactory from the patient's standpoint.

To compile and report, in terms of a single percentage figure, the "cure rate" of patients with varying causes and degrees of urinary incontinence, as has so frequently been done in the past, only contributes to the confusion. Different reported series containing widely divergent percentages of each of the possible types and degrees of incontinence must be supported by data reflecting success rates with each of the clinical and anatomic problems recognized. Otherwise, a meaningful comparison between the relative successes with the different surgical procedures becomes difficult if not impossible.

Obviously the criteria of "cure" and the duration of that cure are important, but the period of observation after surgery is of major importance. It would appear that the long-term successes of surgical procedures have been somewhat inversely proportional to the postoperative period of observation. A follow-up period of not less than 2 years seems adequate and reliable if one is to report conclusive and meaningful results. Follow-up reevaluations after more than 2 years can be misleading, however, since some of those being followed will begin to be affected by normal aging processes. Postmenopausal atrophic changes alone will confuse the evaluation of the operative procedures themselves by adding still another variable. A comparison of the results of various operations shows that the effects of the aging process upon USI are quite different among patients of different age groups. Therefore, for statistics to be meaningful, patients of the same age must be compared.

To a considerable degree, the symptoms of USI are subjective and of somewhat variable intensity, depending on the individual's social and physical activities, the degree of social acceptability, and the extent to which the patient will tolerate the situation. Because these factors are not necessarily interdependent, one must employ diagnostic methods of measuring the improvement that has resulted from surgery, in addition to subjective description.

DIAGNOSIS

History

The preoperative investigation of urinary incontinence need not be formidable and certainly should be individualized for each patient. There is no substitute for a careful, thoughtful, and detailed history. Questions should be meaningful, and close attention should be given to the patient's responses. One seeks to establish both the nature and the severity of the disability, as well as its duration. One wishes early on to identify various contributing components to the symptoms of incontinence, including urgency, detrusor instability, frequency, and stress. Because so many drugs have as side effects sympathetic, parasympathetic, or detrusor response (67), a detailed recitation of what medications the patient is taking is relevant, including a description of the effect on the patient's urinary symptoms.

Although the patient may be asked to fill out a questionnaire, reciting the questions verbally provides a broader opportunity for patient response and elaboration than a simple yes or no answer.

Suitable leading questions may be found among the following:

1. Do you lose your urine when you laugh, cough, or sneeze?
2. Is the loss immediate, or is it 30 to 45 seconds after you laugh, cough, or sneeze?
3. Do you lose urine when you are lying down?
4. Do you have to get up at night to pass your urine? Can you make it to the bathroom?
5. Have you a history of any bladder or kidney infections? Were they accompanied by chills, fever, or backache?
6. Does the sound of running water make you want to pass your urine?
7. When you put your foot in the bath to see if the water is too hot before you get in, does it give you a sudden urge to pass your urine? Do you pass it?
8. Have you had any change in bowel habits coincident with your change in bladder habits?
9. How often do you pass your urine during the day? During the night?
10. How much tea, coffee, cola drinks, or chocolate do you consume?
11. Did you have trouble with bedwetting as a child?
12. Did other members of your family have problems in holding their urine?
13. Did you have any trouble holding your urine during pregnancy?
14. Did you have any trouble passing or holding your urine after delivery?
15. What medications are you taking regularly?
16. Do you have any burning when you pass your urine?
17. After you have passed your urine and stand up, does it sometimes feel as though you have to go a second time? If you try to go a second time, do you find there was really no need? Is there any urinary dribbling after voiding?
18. Have you had any operations on the vagina, uterus, or bladder, and did they affect bladder function at all?

19. How long have you been having your problem?
20. Was the onset gradual or sudden?
21. Are you beyond the menopause?
22. Was your problem worse at the time of menopause?
23. Are you taking any hormone supplements? Have the hormone supplements helped your bladder function?
24. Do you ever lose urine during intercourse?
25. How many times can you stop and start the stream?
26. When the urine involuntarily begins to leak, can you stop the stream?
27. How much sanitary protection do you wear? Only when you have a cold or respiratory infection, or must you wear something all the time?

Walters (88) has listed some of the types of medication that can affect lower urinary tract function (Table 17.1).

Prazosin (Minipres) and phenoxybenzamine (Dibenzyline) are antihypertensive alpha-adrenergic blockers, but in some women they may lower urethral pressure because there are many alpha receptors in the urethra. This may mimic USI (26). A careful history should be taken to determine if this may be the case, and if so, the medication eliminated and the patient reevaluated before any surgical therapy is contemplated.

Differential Diagnosis of Bladder Control Disorders

Green (39) has characterized the disorders responsible for the *symptom* of USI as follows:

"1. True anatomic USI (75 to 85 percent of cases): There is abnormal configuration and location of the urethrovesical junction, with the proximal urethra displaced outside the intra-abdominal field of force. Urethra, bladder, detrusor function, and neuropharmocologic control are normal.
  2. Detrusor dyssynergia (15 to 20 percent of cases): A hyperirritable detrusor reflex is involuntarily triggered by a sudden increase in intra-abdominal pressure or by a critical volume of bladder urine. Incontinence is of an "involuntary voiding" type and occurs despite a normal urethrovesical support and anatomic configuration.
  3. Combination of true anatomic USI and detrusor dyssynergia (5 to 10 percent of cases).

(con't)

Table 17.1.

Types of Medication That Can Affect Lower Urinary Tract Infection

Type of Medication	Lower Urinary Tract Effects
Diuretics	Polyuria, frequency, urgency
Anticholinergic agents	Urinary retention, overflow incontinence
Alcohol	Sedation, impaired mobility, diuresis
Psychotropic agents	
antidepressants	Anticholinergic actions, sedation
antipsychotics	Anticholinergic actions, sedation
sedatives/hypnotics	Sedation, muscle relaxation, confusion
Alpha-Adrenergic blockers	Stress incontinence
Alpha-Adrenergic agonists	Urinary retention
Beta-Adrenergic agonists	Urinary retention
Calcium-channel blockers	Urinary retention, overflow incontinence

Adapted from Walters (89).

4. Miscellaneous disorders (5 to 10 percent of cases):
   a. Rigid, frozen, "pipe-stem" urethra: There is low resting intraurethral pressure, and any sudden increase in intra-abdominal pressure is not transmitted to the proximal urethral lumen sufficient to equal and offset the pressure increase. This occurs despite normal urethrovesical anatomy and support. The disorder is seen most often in patients who have had multiple surgical procedures in the region of the bladder neck.
   b. Urethral diverticulum: The diverticulum may fill during voiding and then be emptied by a sudden cough or change in position.
   c. Short urethra syndrome (or total urinary incontinence): The urethra is too short (0.5 to 1.5 cm) to maintain adequate intraurethral pressure, either at rest or with sudden increases in intra-abdominal pressure. Although the patient experiences a stress-type leakage, actually she has total urinary incontinence and leaks constantly."

Green (39) has listed the symptoms of true anatomic USI:

"1. Urgency, frequency, and urgency incontinence are usually absent. (Minimal urgency and frequency are occasionally seen in patients with marked funneling of the vesical neck.)
2. Leakage of urine occurs at the instant of physical stress.
3. A variable but limited volume of urine is lost instantaneously and simultaneously with the physical stress.
4. Leakage will occur with stress even though the bladder has recently emptied and contains only a small volume of urine.
5. Leakage occurs only in the upright position (usually only in the standing position). Usually simple changes in position are not accompanied by leakage. Incontinence never occurs at night in bed.
6. Most often, leakage is caused by coughing, sneezing, laughing, vigorous athletic activity, and similar stresses that produce sudden large increases in intra-abdominal pressure. Ordinarily, the sound of running water or normal walking or running activity do not cause loss of urine.
7. Patients usually can stop their stream while in the act of normal voiding.
8. There is no associated psychosomatic disorder.
9. There are no spontaneous remissions or exacerbations, although there may be progressive increase in the frequency and severity of USI with the passage of time.
10. Usually, there is no past history of functional disorders of bladder control. There may be a history of transient stress incontinence during and for a short time after one or more earlier pregnancies. Then the symptom fails to clear up after a subsequent pregnancy and persists and often worsens over the years."

Green (39) has also identified contrasting symptoms of uninhibited involuntary detrusor contraction:

"1. Urgency, frequency (nocturnal as well), and painless incontinence are usually prominent.
2. Usually there is a considerable latent period or lag of several seconds between the physical stress and the onset of leakage.
3. A large volume of urine is lost, often in gushes, a steady stream, or prolonged dribbling, and the leakage occurs over a protracted interval of several seconds. (Actual uninhibited involuntary voiding is occurring.)
4. Leakage is more likely to occur when the bladder is moderately full; each patient seems to have her own critical volume at which frequency, urgency, and stress-induced incontinence are most likely to be experienced.
5. Leakage may occur in any position and often is triggered by a change in position. Leakage may occur even in bed.
6. Walking or running or the sound of running water often trigger incontinence, whereas coughing, sneezing, or laughing do so less consistently.
7. Patients usually find it difficult to halt the stream during normal voiding.
8. An underlying, generalized anxiety or depressive state is often discernible.
9. Often there are spontaneous remissions and exacerbations in relation to changes in the total life situation. Usually, fluctuations involve weeks, months, or even several years, but in some patients there may be daily variations, with symptoms tending to disappear at night.
10. There is often a history of voiding and bladder difficulties, including enuresis, dating back to early childhood."

Urinary stress incontinence is sometimes coexistent with that from detrusor instability. The conditions, though usually of separate etiology, are synergisti, and the mere presence of one tends to make the other worse. Generally speaking, the detrusor instability is more difficult to cure than the stress incontinence, so it should be approached first. If urodynamic testing equipment is unavailable, it may be possible to judge the extent of the patient's urinary instability by placing her on a few days of therapy with an anticholinergic and asking her to call and report in a few days. Occasionally, one will observe that when the detrusor disability has been controlled, the stress component will no longer be severe and surgery will be unnecessary. Bladder reeducation and drills can be implemented as a long-term program of treatment for the instability. To treat the stress component first, as by surgery, may make the urinary urgency and precipitancy worse, and the patient more uncomfortable and harder to treat effectively.

Diagnostic Procedures

The Marshall- or Bonney-type test is an important and simple diagnostic procedure for the demonstration of stress incontinence. It is readily performed in the office and can easily be combined with a simplified cystometric evaluation (74).

MARSHALL STRESS TEST

The patient is asked to void before examination and then is catheterized to measure residual urine volume. The urine sample is put aside for analysis, and the glass or plastic funnel of a sterile 60-ml Asepto syringe is attached to the catheter. The bottom of the syringe is held about the level of the patient's pubis, and sterile saline in increments of 50 ml is poured into the syringe (Fig. 17.1). The patient is asked to identify the first urge to void. The volume of saline instilled is recorded, after which increments are added until

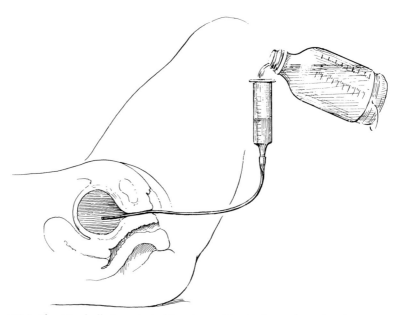

Figure 17.1. The Marshall stress test. After the residual urine volume has been measured, sterile saline is instilled in increments of 50 ml, and the bladder capacity is measured. The fluid level in the syringe is watched closely. If it rises, a detrusor contraction is occurring. The catheter and all but 250 to 300 ml are removed, and a Marshall or Bonney test is done with the patient first in the recumbent, then in the standing position.

maximal patient discomfort is approached, at which time the total volume used is again noted. All but 250 to 300 ml of saline is permitted to run out, and the catheter is removed. The saline volumes and subjective feelings give a fairly valid estimation of bladder tone, helping to identify either hypertonia or hypotonia, and spontaneous uninhibited bladder contractions also can be identified by a rise in the column of saline in the glass syringe. (An observation of abnormality suggests the need for a more sophisticated urodynamic.) The patient is then asked to cough (53); if no urine is lost, the perineum should be depressed and the cough repeated (44). If urine is lost, the vesicourethral junction should be elevated by the examiner, care being taken not to occlude the urethra by pressure, and the patient is asked to cough again. If no urine is lost with coughing when the patient is in the lithotomy position, she should be asked to stand and to cough again. The test is considered positive if no additional urine is expelled by coughing when the vesico-urethral junction is so elevated.

If the Marshall test in the supine position is negative, one should determine whether, by depressing the perineum and asking the patient to laugh, cough, or sneeze, it becomes positive (44). It should also be determined whether the patient can voluntarily contract her pubococcygeal muscles and external anal sphincter. Failure to be able to do so may correlate with anal incontinence and possibly a pudendal neuropathy (82, 83).

In evaluating a presumably positive Marshall test, one should note carefully the time interval between the cough and the loss of urine. If the condition is truly one of urinary stress incontinence, the loss will be immediate and usually can be stopped by the patient's voluntary pubococcygeal contraction. If there is a delay of several seconds between the cough and the loss of urine, the patient is probably experiencing a provoked detrusor contraction, which is a form of bladder instability and not stress incontinence. The patient may be unable to stop the stream. In this instance, the investigation should be centered around a probable diagnosis of detrusor instability, for which the treatment is generally nonsurgical (30, 33, 49). A surgeon should be most cautious about recommending surgery to correct USI in the presence of a negative Marshall test without first obtaining a confirmatory urethrocystometrogram. If there has been a history of pyelonephritis or previous chronically recurrent cystitis, urine cultures and an intravenous pyelogram are indicated. The results should be considered carefully and appropriate treatment given.

SIMPLIFIED CYSTOMETRIC EVALUATION

Necessary equipment includes a graduated commode insert, a stopwatch, an indwelling catheter, sterile water, and a 50-ml irrigation syringe.

When the patient feels her normal urge to void, she is asked to void in private using the commode insert to collect the urine. She should start the stopwatch at the onset of flow and stop it when flow stops. The mean flow rate (volume/time) should exceed 10 ml/sec; a low flow rate may not be valid if the voided volume is less than 200 ml. A catheter is inserted and the residual volume is measured and the specimen sent for urinalysis. The residual urine volume should be less than 100 ml. (Low flow rates and high residuals are indications for a more complex urodynamic evaluation.) Increments of 50 ml of saline at room temperature are added while watching the level of the fluid on the syringe. A rise would indicate a detrusor contraction (see Fig. 17.1).

Standing, simple incremental cystometry appears to be superior in detecting detrusor instability than does that performed on the recumbent patient (20, 35, 79). It may offer an alternative for the presumptive diagnosis of detrusor instability when multichannel urodynamics are not available (78).

With the catheter still in place, the bladder is emptied and the patient is allowed to stand with the 50-ml Asepto-type syringe (without piston or bulb) attached to the catheter and held above the level of the bladder in preparation for "eyeball cystometry." The bladder is slowly filled by gravity by pouring 50-ml aliquots of sterile room-temperature saline into the syringe. The patient should note her first sensation of fullness (usually 150 to 200 ml) and her maximum capacity (usually 400 to 600 ml). If a detrusor contraction occurs, the level of the water in the syringe will rise. At maximum cystometric capacity, the patient should be asked to cough, bounce on her heels, and listen to running water in an effort to provoke contractions. If contractions occur, the patient should attempt to suppress them. Sustained increases in bladder pressure or an unusual degree of urgency at inappropriately low volumes during cystometry is an indication for further testing.

The catheter is removed and the patient is asked to cough forcefully. Leakage of urine from the urethra at the apex of the cough should be observed. An inability to demonstrate this sign is a contraindication to continence surgery without further testing.

URETHROCYSTOMETRY

Interpretations of the Marshall stress test may be correlated with pre- and postoperative endoscopy and with direct simultaneous intraurethral intravesical pressure measurements. Simultaneous measurement of intraurethral and intravesical pressures (4, 8, 11, 41, 42, 66) (urethrocystometry) should be strongly considered when the stress incontinence is recurrent or when there is a history of enuresis, spontaneous voiding, inability to stop the stream, suspected neuropathy involving bladder function (disc, spina bifida, multiple sclerosis, diabetic neuropathy, central nervous system lues, etc.), or the finding of a high postvoiding urinary residual volume without evident outlet or urethral obstruction. A comprehensive urodynamic testing system is illustrated in Figure 17.2.

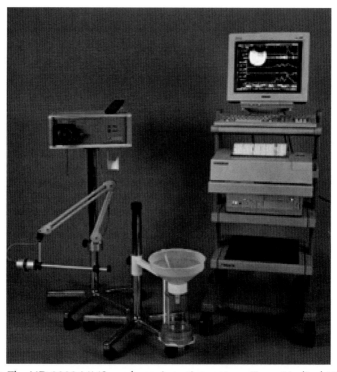

Figure 17.2. The UD-2000 MMS urodynamic testing system. (From Medical Measurement Systems USA, Inc., Wheaton, Illinois. Used with permission).

Mattox and Bhatia (59) have suggested that the indications for referral of incontinent patients for a multichannel urodynamics, high-risk profile should be the following:

1. Failed prior anti-incontinence surgery
2. Age over 60
3. Prior radical pelvic surgery
4. Continuous incontinence
5. History and physical examination suggestive of neurologic disorder
6. Uterine procidentia, complete vaginal vault inversion, grade III cystocele
7. Significant abnormalities on basic work-up:
   a. Low or high bladder capacity
   b. Negative Q-tip test (fixed urethra)
   c. No urine loss demonstrable
   d. No sensation of filling
   e. High postvoid residual

We would recommend multichannel urodynamic testing as part of the preoperative work-up of any genital prolapse patient with a history of previous spinal fusion on laminectomy.

Urethrocystometric testing should be performed with the patient both supine and standing (79). Urethral instability is not uncommon and should be diagnosed and treated (89). Gleason et al. (38) suggested that the results obtained from a water-filled system for urethrocystometry have fewer false-positive results than those using gas or air, despite the obvious convenience of the latter. However, direct urethroscopy using a gas medium is of help in evaluating the urethra and the competency of the vesical neck (75).

Bergman, Koonings, and Ballard (15) have called attention to the importance of urodynamic testing in even the continent patient with significant genitourinary prolapse to identify those women at risk of developing postoperative urinary incontinence (19) so that appropriate prophylactic measures can be undertaken at the time of surgery.

Since women with stress incontinence *and* low urethral closure pressure are significantly older (85), it is important to make an accurate diagnosis to help determine the treatment of choice. A low urethra closure pressure is generally one of less than 20 cm of water. Perhaps a measurement of the "leak point pressure" should also be studied. This is a measurement of the pressure necessary to *open* the urethra, not to close it, and it should be above 60 cm of water.

The invasion of the bladder necessitated by urodynamic evaluation produces post-instrumentation bacteriuria in about 15 percent of women. Coliforms are isolated most frequently. Most of these infestations appear to be self-limited. If the posttest culture is positive, the patient probably should be treated by appropriate antibiotics or antibacterials (70).

BEAD-CHAIN URETHROCYSTOGRAMS

Comparison of pre- and postoperative bead-chain urethrocystograms of urethrocystocolpograms, when now used, is primarily as part of the investigation of certain individuals with recurrent incontinence, or when the patient is part of a special study group. A urethral chain, radiopaque to show the axis of the urethra, may be introduced inside a split rubber catheter. A modification of urethrocystography in which the urethra is opacified without a chain has been described by Morgan (personal communication). The advantage of his modified technique is that there is no chain or catheter to splint or, by its weight, depress the urethra artificially, altering the view of the relationship with the bladder. The technique is as follows:

1. A 5% solution of sodium iodide and 30 ml of Lipiodol are instilled into the bladder.
2. Barium paste (5 ml) is instilled into the urethra.
3. If coincident colpography is desired, 5 ml of barium paste may be instilled into the vagina.

Without the splinting of the catheter, this technique demonstrates the S-shaped curve of the urethra and any funneling or changes in luminal size at different levels within the urethra, and may provide visualization of any urethral diverticulum or an occasional urethrovaginal fistula.

PERINEAL ULTRASOUND

Perineal ultrasound, which does not distort or displace the vesical neck from an intravaginal probe, may be of advantage because there is no radiation given and no catheter, and only a thin "slice" of pelvic tissue is visualized, permitting more accurate measurement (80).

Adequate preoperative incontinence study requires suspicion, evaluation, definition, and elimination of the dissimilar but occasionally coexistent etiologies of urinary incontinence (46) and the incontinence resulting from poor voiding habits. These individuals, if pre- and postoperative comparison are not carried out will confuse the degrees of surgical success attributed to a specific technique for the relief of stress incontinence. Coexistent urgency incontinence is so often present that when unrecognized and untreated it, too, will affect the rate of surgical cure. The patient does not know why she is losing her urine, but she wants relief. The burden of investigation is upon the doctor who must recognize and treat correctly each of the various factors accounting for the patient's symptoms.

TREATMENT

The surgeon responsible for treatment must not only recognize the need for and interpret adequate preoperative studies, but also must be skilled and experienced in the full range of operative procedures that can be employed and choose the one best suited for a particular patient. No competent gynecologist will restrict all choice to a single procedure or recommend only the procedure that he or she may be best able to perform.

The choice of an inappropriate operation usually compounds the patient's problem. One can hope to achieve a 2-year cure rate of urinary incontinence approaching 95 percent only by a well-considered appraisal of a patient's problem and selection of the proper operation for that problem. Without making such effort and exercising such judgment, both patient and surgeon needlessly settle for a failure rate as high as 20 percent.

Nonsurgical Treatment

Nonsurgical treatment of urinary stress incontinence, which also is useful often as both a preoperative and postoperative supplement, includes (*a*) planned courses of perineal resistive exercises; (*b*) estrogen supplementation to the postmenopausal patient; (*c*) avoidance of tight abdominal garments that unnecessarily increase intra-abdominal pressure; and (*d*) correction of chronic respiratory illness, stopping smoking, and so forth.

A long program of voluntary Kegel perineal resistive exercises (47) should be started preoperatively and continued postoperatively (31). The patient should start on a period of daily perineal resistive exercises employing isometric contractions, 15 to 20 in a row, 3 seconds per contraction. This should be repeated as a sequence six times a day, starting when first arising, then at midmorning, lunchtime, midafternoon, suppertime, and bedtime. Some estimate of the effectiveness of the patient's pubococcygei in controlling urinary incontinence may be obtained by determining how many times the patient can stop and start the stream during the process of voiding. If the muscles are effective and strong, a patient should be able to stop and start the stream six to eight times when voiding from a full bladder. When the muscle is weak and ineffective, the patient may be unable to stop the stream at all or, at most, once or twice; this gives some evidence of the value that might be obtained by a course of isometric contraction exercises. Developing strength from perineal resistive exercises requires about 3 months of daily effort to bring about a significant improvement, and the patient should be cautioned not to expect vast improvement overnight. The beneficial effect of adequate pelvic floor training continues for years (50).

If, however, the patient is unable to voluntarily contract her pubococcygei effectively, a program of regular galvanic stimulation of the pelvic muscles, supplemented by biofeedback, will in time produce increased muscular bulk to raise intraurethral pressure. Occasionally, the relief obtained will be enough to negate a recommendation for surgery. For patients with troublesome incontinence who are not candidates for surgical repair, electrical stimulation of the muscles of the pelvic floor by means of a single vaginal or anal electrode at relatively high intensity for 20 minutes a day has given considerable relief. There are no specific, simple pretreatment tests that will predict success, but urodynamic evaluation and endoscopy to rule out urethritis or interstitial cystitis are desirable. Fall and Lindstrom have given an excellent summary and analysis of this medium (29).

A pessarylike, plastic, bladder neck support prosthesis with prongs to support the vesicourethral junction has been found effective in relieving stress urinary incontinence among women not ready for surgery (25). This device, as well as a Smith-Hodge pessary, may be useful in predicting the outcome from surgery (16).

Estrogen supplementation for the postmenopausal patient is useful, both as a substance to be taken internally and as a vaginal cream to be applied locally on a weekly basis. This program should be of long duration, providing there is no contraindication, such as a history of previous adenocarcinoma of the endometrium or metastatic cancer of the breast.

Some patients can also learn how to avoid incontinence in some situations. If the Marshall test is positive, one should ask the patient to tighten her levator muscles and repeat the cough. If she is dry when coughing in the presence of voluntarily contracted pubococcygei, she can use this safeguard as an almost "automatic reflex" so that whenever it is necessary for her to laugh, cough, or sneeze, she contracts her pelvic muscles just *before* the stress rather than just after. In many cases, this may be all the treatment the patient requires (65).

Women with both detrusor instability and genuine stress incontinence may be cured by effective colporrhaphy or suprapubic surgery only about 30 percent of the time. Therefore, in such patients medical treatment of the bladder instability with training, anticholinergics, and coincident Kegel perineal resistive exercises should be initiated before a surgical procedure is performed (77).

Surgical Treatment

The prudent surgeon will not offer a surgical relief for someone's incontinence until certain of the etiology. One must consider the possibility of a small but undiagnosed fistula, especially in a patient with a history of previous pelvic surgery.

One must also be cautious of making sweeping recommendations and assurances of good postoperative prognostic results in a patient with a history of coincident rectal incontinence, because this suggests the problem of pudendal denervation, usually from childbirth. It may also suggest chronic straining that may not be surgically remedial and that may follow a long history of constipation and obstipation with stretching of the pudendal nerve, resulting in partial denervation of the structures thus innervated by it, that is, the levator ani and the external anal sphincter. Onset of constipation coincident with urinary incontinence, particularly after a fall, suggests the possibility of herniation of an intervertebral disc. This should be diagnosed from appropriate neurologic examination and study, but one must be mindful that if this occurs within the cauda equina it may not appear on a myelogram. There are halfway or partial degrees of success in surgical relief. A result that is less than 100 percent successful in a particular patient is not necessarily a failure if her disability has been reduced from a major and socially unacceptable degree of incontinence to a minor and acceptable problem.

Wall, Norton, and DeLancey (87) have suggested a classification of surgical procedures for genuine stress incontinence:

I. Anterior colporrhaphy with Kelly plication
II. Abdominal bladder neck suspension operations designed to correct anatomic hypermobility
   A. Retropubic bladder neck suspension
       1. Marshall-Marchetti-Krantz operation
       2. Burch colposuspension
   B. Paravaginal bladder neck suspension
       1. Paravaginal repair
       2. Vagino-obturator shelf procedure
   C. Needle suspension procedures
       1. Pereyra procedure
       2. Subsequent minor modifications
III. Operations for intrinsic sphincteric weakness or dysfunction
   A. Sling operations
       1. Organic materials
           a. Autologous materials, e.g., rectus fascia, fascia lata
           b. Heterologous materials, e.g., porcine dermis, ox dura
       2. Synthetic materials
   B. Periurethral injections
       1. Teflon paste
       2. GAX collagen
IV. Salvage operations
   A. Purposefully obstructive sling operations
   B. Periurethral injections
   C. Artificial urinary sphincter
   D. Urinary reconstruction and/or diversion

Some correlation with patient diathesis in type is important as well. Irrespective of her urethrovesical configuration, an obese woman may have different problems with intra-abdominal pressure than a thin patient, and these may affect the long-term success after surgical treatment for USI. Similarly, a chronic asthmatic or a patient with hay fever, bronchitis, or chronic cough is prone to have much less long-term success after certain procedures than an individual without a respiratory problem.

A statement that operation A is better than operation B will only be meaningful if it is qualified by a description of (a) what the condition was, (b) what coexistent related symptoms and findings were present, (c) what degree of disability the patient had experienced, (d) which specific surgical approach was used, and (e) for how long the result has been observed.

An operative procedure should so improve urethral tone and pressure that it may exceed intravesical pressure both at rest and when intra-abdominal pressure is increased. This will be favored by elevating the vesicourethral junction to a point once again above the bottom of the hydrostatic column of water. As a result, changes in intra-abdominal pressure will be transmitted to the proximal urethra as well as the bladder.

IS COINCIDENT HYSTERECTOMY OF VALUE?

Up to 30 percent of women may demonstrate unexpected urinary dysfunction following total hysterectomy. Although much of this resolves spontaneously within a year, its very existence should dampen the surgeon's enthusiasm for coincident hysterectomy at the time of surgical treatment for urinary stress incontinence, unless there is some clear-cut indication for removing the uterus (69).

Anterior colporrhaphy with correction of funneling of the vesicourethral junction by Kelly-type plication stitches and plication of the posterior pubourethrovaginal ligament portion of the urogenital diaphragm without skeletonizing the urethra has been very successful in our hands. It relieves the symptoms of urinary stress incontinence provided that a long-lasting suture material (such as polydiaxanone) has been used as described in Chapter 10.

For anterior colporrhaphy to be effective in the treatment of urinary stress incontinence, Beck (12) has noted that proper plication of the periurethral tissues of the urogenital diaphragm will elevate a hypermobile urethra only when these stitches effectively elevate the vesicourethral junction.

We presume that a measure of urethral funneling or low urethral closure pressure may be present in a patient if we have preoperatively been able to pull the partly inflated (0.5 ml) bulb of a no. 8 Foley catheter through the urethra. These patients, continent or not, will be given sufficient suburethral plication over a transurethral no. 16 Foley catheter to reduce the urethral diameter (34).

URETHRAL FUNNELING

Funneling or vesicalization of the urethra lowers the physiologic vesicourethral junction and also activates the detrusor contractibility reflex. This reflex then functions when the patient is not voiding, particularly when she is in a nonsupine position and gravity has pulled even small amounts of urine into the pathologically dilated urethra (9). For this reason, the presence of funneling, once diagnosed, should be corrected as a part of any surgical procedure designed for the treatment of a patient's urinary stress incontinence.

Urethral funneling may be diagnosed by several methods. (a) A lateral cystogram may be taken; one should also look for flattening of the posterior urethrovesical angle at rest. (b) The patient can be examined standing, with the examiner's finger placed lightly under the lower anterior vaginal wall, seeking the palpable transmission of a cough impulse into the proximal urethra. (c) Direct urethroscopy may be used; it is not necessarily diagnostic, but it may help diagnose urethral smooth muscle sphincter insufficiency. The latter and funneling appear to be two different entities, although they may coexist. (d) Urethral pressure profilometry may be used, which may demonstrate an unexpectedly low slope starting at the proximal urethra. (e) The surgeon may visualize the funneling at surgery. Urethral funneling is even more significant when coincident with rotational descent of the bladder neck.

When urethral funneling or vesicalization is present, Kelly-type mattress stitches will restore the urethral lumen to normal size and improve the effectiveness of local muscular tone in reestablishing a mechanism for closure of the vesical neck.

Urethral detachment, or rotational descent of the bladder neck, however, implies damage to the ligamentous or fibromuscular support of the urethra. When this is coincident with a drop in urethral tone so that intraurethral pressure no longer exceeds intravesical pressure, involuntary incontinence may take place (11). Treatment consists of surgically elevating the vesicourethral junction so that it is once again within the range of effective response to increases in intra-abdominal pressure. This may be accomplished by transvaginal techniques.

URGE INCONTINENCE

Before deciding upon the best operation for a specific patient's stress incontinence, the surgeon must decide first if it is stress incontinence that is to be treated, or whether the patient's complaint is really urgency or even simply the result of poor voiding habits. When urgency and stress incontinence coexist, it is generally best that the urgency component be treated first because it is well known that infection, when present, increases detrusor irritability. Once the urgency has been relieved, many patients will no longer be incontinent. Conversely, the swelling and trauma of surgery can make an untreated urgency component worse for several months; the patient will not be likely to make the subtle distinction between the two types, and she is likely simply to conclude that she is worse than before surgery.

From the number of cases of urge incontinence treated unsuccessfully by inappropriate surgery, it is apparent that the subtle distinction is not always being made between detrusor instability and USI. The operation will be recorded as a surgical failure when, in fact, it should not have been performed in the first place. An inappropriate operation compounds the patient's problem. A proper choice of the initial operation properly performed offers the best chance for cure and should be made by the surgeon who is to do the procedure. The surgeon who depends on someone else to tell him or her what to do should generally not be the one to do it.

COEXISTENT CONDITIONS

When USI is quite mild, often inconstant, and not of itself sufficiently disturbing to have motivated the patient to seek a repair, that degree of incontinence alone is not likely to warrant the disability and risks of surgery; but when a similarly mild degree of incontinence coexists with other indications for repair (e.g., rectocele, genital prolapse), adequate coincident transvaginal surgical reconstruction of the anterior vaginal wall should indeed be advised.

Pubourethrovaginal ligament plication as part of an anterior colporrhaphy is ideal when used with surgical treatment for a coexisting genital prolapse, and this plication may be used to prevent urinary incontinence resulting from the straightening out of a posterior urethrovesical angle during the course of an anterior colporrhaphy. The White (91) or Figurnov (32) transvaginal reattachment of paraurethral tissue to the pubic end of the arcus tendineus (5, 92) is useful when one finds either insufficient tissue strength for midline plication or evidence of lack of sulcus support. Pathologic damage to the levator plate may be measured indirectly by urethrocolpography, and appropriate surgical remedy should be instituted. If a reason is present for coincident primary laparotomy (ovarian tumor, large uterine leiomyoma, etc.), a primary suprapubic procedure may be elected, though any posterior cystocele should be corrected separately. Coincident transabdominal obliteration of a deep or wide cul-de-sac is desirable to prevent the future development of a postoperative enterocele, such as might result from a change in the vaginal axis from pulling the vagina anteriorly, which leaves a cul-de-sac (particularly a wide one) unprotected.

An intraoperative choice between a Marshall-Marchetti-Krantz operation, which sews periurethral tissue to the back of the pubis, and the Burch procedure, which sews perivaginal tissue to Cooper ligament, may be made according to whether the pubic periosteum can securely hold the sutures placed into it. Anterior plication of the urethra may be added if urethral funneling is evident (54). It has been reported that only 50 percent of patients were completely dry 5 years after the Burch procedure, even though permanent suture material had been used, and 30 percent needed further incontinence surgery (28).

NEEDLE SUSPENSIONS

We are emerging from a 35-year experience with needle suspension as a "simple" treatment for the symptomatic or potentially symptomatic patient with urethral hypermobility. Enthusiasm has waned in recent years as a consequence of objective failure of symptom relief and lack of long-term clinical success beyond the initial 2 to 5 years. In many instances reevaluation and reoperation have been required.

We were once fond of the Pereyra needle suspension procedures (71, 72) for a relatively simplified elevation of the vesicourethral junction in patients with socially unacceptable urinary stress incontinence and a pathologically hypermobile urethra. However, the fall in cure rate over several postoperative years has been discouraging, to the point where the late Pereyra (personal communication) no longer recommended the operation. This less than acceptable cure rate is probably the consequence of attaching a strain-bearing soft tissue to another soft tissue, rather than to a fixed structure.

One does see in consultation a number of the needle suspension patients of others who have developed a chronic retropubic infection involving the permanent sutures or any plastic bolster through which the sutures have been passed. A chronic draining sinus has formed with persistent bloody vaginal discharge and abundant granulation tissue. The latter recurs rapidly following local removal. The only treatment of value has been surgical removal of the infected suture material or bolus that has become an infected foreign body. This removal, usually suprapubic, is occasionally simple; one only needs to identify the sutures and their knots superficial to the surface of the rectus fascia, cut the sutures, and extract them. Removal of the infected bolus, however, is tedious and sometimes formidable. The surgeon should follow the uncut suture down to the bolus by sharp dissection and extract them together. The use of permanent sutures whenever a sling procedure is performed will improve the long-term results (51). Surprisingly many of the postoperative patients retain their newly restored urinary continence, probably as a result of the retropubic scar tissue and fibrosis that has developed coincident to the inflammatory process.

Because there are anatomic differences between the three principal types of needle suspensions in use, they are described here to hopefully aid the surgeon who must occasionally remove them. The Pereyra (71, 72) procedure to correct symptomatic hypermobility of the urethra is shown in Figure 17.3. Transvaginal incisions lateral to the vesicourethral junction are made, and a long-handled ligature carrier is inserted through an incision about two finger breadths cranial to the upper border of the pubis. The path of this ligature carrier will be extraperitoneal and extravesical. The safety of this passage may be monitored by pushing the tip of the ligature carrier to meet the operator's index finger inserted through the vaginal wound, as shown in Figure 17.3A. A second penetration is made on the opposite side of the urethra (Fig. 17.3B). A nonabsorbable suture that has been placed in a helical fashion in the periurethral supporting tissue is threaded through the eye of the needle and the ligature carrier withdrawn into the abdominal incision, as shown in Figure 17.3B. Just enough traction is made to the abdominal sutures to bring about closure of the vesical neck (Fig. 17.3C). The new vesicourethral angle is shown in contrast to the original flattening of this area (Fig. 17.3C, *dotted tissue*).

The Stamey variation (84) is shown in Figure 17.4. The long needle penetrates first the medial portion of the periurethral connective tissue, and a suture is withdrawn. The other end of the suture is passed through a Dacron bolster. The needle is passed from above a second time lateral to the first stitch, the suture threaded through the needle, and the needle withdrawn. The effect of this bolster is seen to the *right*. The cystoscope carefully monitors the integrity of the urethral and vesical mucosa and is used to judge the tension under which the stitches will be tied. The end point is the tension at which the vesical neck can be seen to be just closed. The wound in the anterior vaginal wall is closed, preferably by two layers. The bolster offers considerable resistance to postoperative traction of the suture through the tissues that it has penetrated to help hold the vesicourethral junction in place.

The Raz modification of the needle colpopexy (23) is shown in Figure 17.5. An inverted U-shaped incision is made in the anterior vaginal wall, which is dissected from

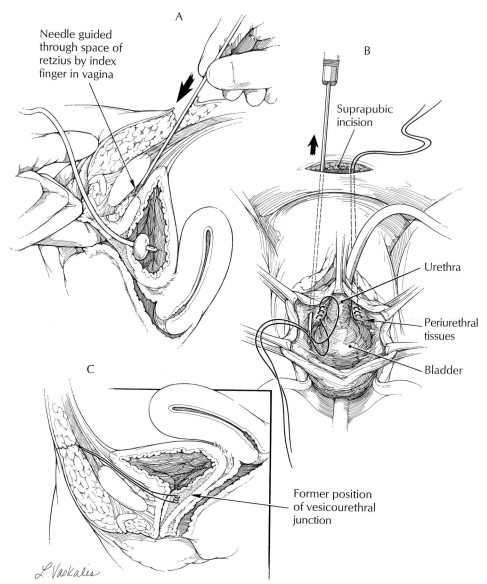

Figure 17.3. A Pereyra II needle urethropexy. **A.** A Foley catheter has been placed in the bladder, and an incision has been made in the anterior vaginal wall and deepened through the tissues of the urogenital diaphragm. Through a small, suprapubic incision a long Pereyra-type needle holder is inserted and advanced hugging the back of the pubis until the tip meets the operator's index finger. **B.** A helix of a nonabsorbable suture has been placed through the urogenital diaphragm lateral to the vesicourethral junction. The ends of the suture are attached to the suprapubic needle as shown. Traction to the needle will withdraw it along the path of its course to bring the suture with it. This has already been accomplished on the opposite side of the urethra on the *right.* **C.** Traction is made to the abdominal ends of the sutures, which are then tied in front of the rectus aponeurosis. This should be sufficient to elevate the vesicourethral junction to a point marking the junction of the lower third and the upper two-thirds of the back of the pubis and permitting the proximal urethral orifice to close as shown.

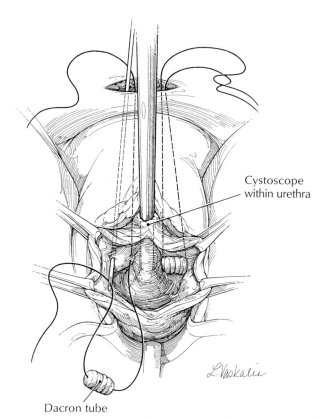

Cystoscope
within urethra

Dacron tube

Figure 17.4. The Stamey modification of the Pereyra needle suspension. A Dacron bolster is placed beneath each of the suture loops as shown. A cystoscope has been placed in the bladder to provide direct observation of the vesicourethral junction, and traction is made to the abdominal ends of the suspension sutures until the operator has noted that the internal urethral orifice has closed, having previously observed that there was no suture penetration of the bladder mucosa. At this point the sutures are fixed to one another anterior to the rectus aponeurosis.

the underlying tissue and the dissection advanced posteriorly. The nonabsorbable suture is sewn in a helical fashion to the periurethral connective tissue and vaginal wall by a long needle passed from above as shown, and the suture is threaded onto the long needle, which is then withdrawn through an abdominal incision. The wound in the anterior vaginal wall is closed with interrupted sutures.

The differences between three types of needle suspension are shown in coronal section in Figure 17.6. In the modified Pereyra (Fig. 17.6*A*), the ends of the sutures are tied to one another over the fascia of the rectus aponeurosis. The wound in the vagina has been closed using side-to-side approximation. The Gittes and Loughlin modification (37) is shown in Figure 17.6*B*. No incision has been made in the vagina, but the pointed needle has been passed through the vaginal membrane and the suture made to loop through one further penetration of the vaginal membrane and returned to the surface of the rectus aponeurosis. The same thing is repeated on the opposite side and the sutures tied to each side of the rectus aponeurosis. In Figure 17.3*C*, the Stamey bolsters are shown as they have been buried beneath the vaginal epithelium. The wound in the anterior vaginal wall has been closed with interrupted stitches.

There may be some enthusiasm for the "no-incision urethropexy" of Gittes and Loughlin (52). However, the falloff rate of cure compared to other types of needle sus-

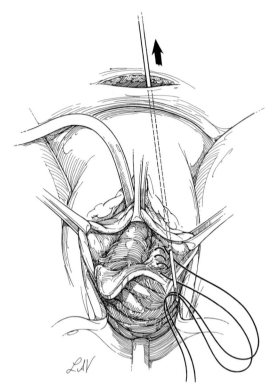

Figure 17.5. The Raz modification of needle colpopexy. The attachment to the periurethral connective tissues is made beneath an inverted U-shaped incision in the anterior vaginal wall as shown. When the suture has been withdrawn through the tunnel on each side, it is sewn to the periurethral connective tissue and the subepithelial anterior vaginal wall. It is then tied over the rectus fascia, and the anterior vaginal wall incision is closed by a series of interrupted sutures.

pension may increase after 2 years, particularly in postmenopausal patients in whom the integrity of vaginal connective tissue strength is compromised.

Following needle suspension, some residual stress incontinence has been reported in 49 percent of patients, most of whom still were still wearing protective padding. The incidence of recurrent stress incontinence rose 23 percent beyond the 2-year postoperative period (48). A good review of the needle suspension procedures for urinary stress incontinence has been provided by Cornella and Ostergard (23).

RECURRENT URINARY STRESS INCONTINENCE

Sling Procedures

A high percentage of success should be expected from fascial sling procedures in patients with complicated stress incontinence. However, an occasional patient will demonstrate persistent stress incontinence, and some will have troublesome urge incontinence. In the occasional patient with a neurogenic bladder, postoperative urinary retention can be expected and should be treated with intermittent self-catheterization (17). The operation is especially useful in reconstructive pelvic surgery, when there is insufficient periurethral tissue for more conventional anti-incontinence procedures.

A   B   C

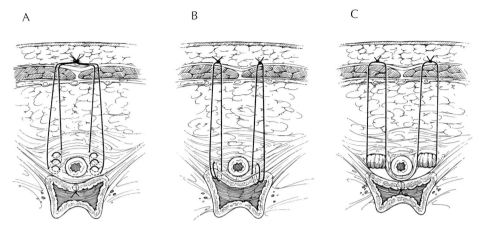

Figure 17.6. Different types of needle urethropexies. **A.** In the Pereyra II procedure, the helical stitch is used, and one side is tied to the other anterior to the rectus muscles. **B.** The Gittes-Loughlin modification. The sutures have been passed through the unincised vagina and unthreaded from the needle, which then penetrates closely parallel to the original path. When it enters the vagina a second time, the suture is rethreaded to the eye of the needle, and the ligature carrier and suture are withdrawn. When this has been accomplished from the opposite side, each suture is tied anterior to the rectus fascia. **C.** In the Stamey modification, each suture has been passed through a short piece of Dacron tubing to form a bolster. Each suture is then tied anterior to the rectus fascia.

Hawksworth and Roux (40) long ago wrote that most successful surgical means of supporting the vesicourethral junction are "sling" procedures of one type or another, whether the lateral walls of the vagina or urethra are plicated to tissues normally found in that area, whether the vagina is attached to the back of the pubis as in the pin-up operation, or whether a material is used as a transplantable sling to actually elevate the vesicourethral junction. The sling can be abdominal fascia that has been relocated, a graft such as fascia lata, or a foreign material such as Mersilene mesh. The effect is similar in all cases because the vesicourethral junction is elevated to a point within the pelvis where the proximal urethra and bladder are simultaneously subject to increases in intra-abdominal pressure. A comparison is shown in Figure 17.7, and the mechanical effect of a sling is shown in Figure 17.8.

The sling procedure as we know it, using a transplantable material, has been one of several methods used to treat severe and socially disabling urinary stress incontinence.

Choice of Material. When we have decided to use a suprapubic vesicourethral sling procedure for the treatment of severe or recurrent socially disabling urinary stress incontinence (42, 43, 68, 73), our choice of material from which the sling is made (7, 92) has often been between Mersilene mesh (never the narrower Mersilene tape) or fascia lata (61, 63, 64, 90). Mersilene mesh, by its thinness and flexibility, seems to be superior to other plastics as a choice of synthetic sling material. It also saves the patient the uncomfortable leg that follows from obtaining a strip of fascia lata.

Tissue reaction to expanded polytetrafluoroethylene (Gore-Tex) suburethral slings for urinary incontinence has been studied. There was a 23 percent reaction or removal rate for these procedures postoperatively, and infection was not prevented by prophylactic antibiotic coverage (14). We have noted a similar experience and no longer use this material (Gore-Tex soft tissue patch).

Surprisingly, about half the patients from whom the Gore-Tex sling has been removed will remain continent, presumably the consequence of fibrosis in this area induced by the infection within the sling material. The reaction site is most commonly the vagina, although occasionally it might be seen at the abdominal end of the sling. Amaz-

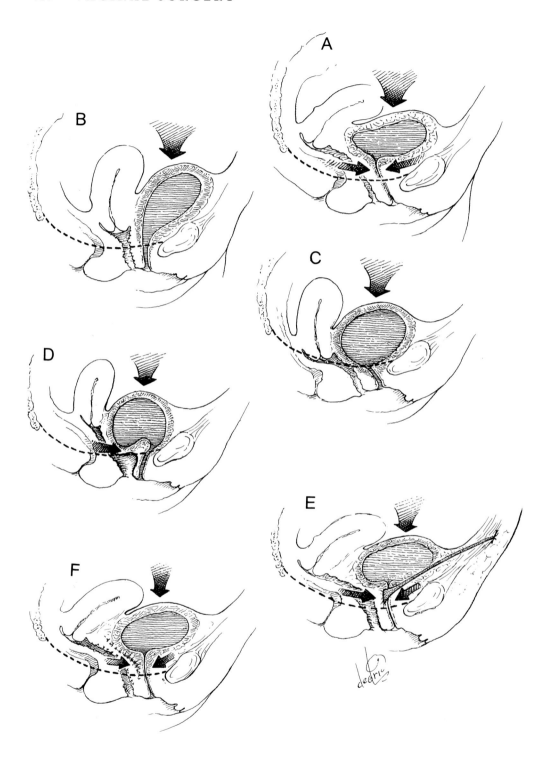

ingly, this reaction may develop at an advanced postoperative time, even 1 to 2 years postoperatively, suggesting that bacteria may have been dormant within the sling material from the time of the original surgery and ultimately the bacterial growth proliferated.

When one is using the single-layered, porous Mersilene mesh, the length and width of the sling or hammock can be predetermined and the material cut to size. Macrophotography of the unstretched weave Mersilene mesh (Fig. 17.9) shows by the configuration of the spaces between the threads why it will stretch in one direction more than the other. The Mersilene mesh hammock (available from Ethicon, Inc., Sommerville, NJ, catalog no. RM 43 or RM 54) measures no more than 2.5 cm maximum width at the center of its belly and tapers to 1.5 cm at each end of the hammock; it measures 32 cm in length. It is important that the maximum width of the plastic hammock be no greater than 2.5 to 3 cm to aid in optimum positioning beneath the vesicourethral junction. Any wider diameter would bring the posterior margin of the synthetic hammock too far onto the posteroinferior surface of the bladder, and one much narrower might strangulate the urethra. Moir (61) has stressed the importance of cutting the sheet of gauze in the direction of least stretch.

Particularly in situations where there is risk of postoperative vaginal necrosis, such as atrophic vagina, previous radiation, or extensive scarring from previous repair, the surgeon might wish to select a sling made of fascia lata, as championed by Ridley (74, 75), as a modification of the Goebell-Frankenheim-Stoeckel procedure. This material is a homograft and not likely to be rejected or to harbor prolonged infection even if delib-

---

Figure 17.7. Illustration of the relationship between increases in intra-abdominal pressure and intravesical and intraurethral pressures. **A.** The continent state of the anatomically normal patient. An increase in intra-abdominal pressure is noted by the *large arrow* being applied directly to the bladder. Increases applied to the proximal urethra are indicated by the *smaller arrows.* The lower limit of the physiologic "body cavity," or usual position of the pelvic diaphragm, is indicated by the *dotted line.* **B.** There is loss or straightening of the urethrovesical angle, and increases in intra-abdominal pressure are being applied to the bladder but not to the urethra. In this situation, intravesical pressure will exceed intraurethral pressure, and incontinence will result. **C.** There is loss or lengthening of urethral support with rotational descent of the urethrovesical junction at rest, and the urethra is effectively displaced to a point below the physiologic "abdominal cavity." Increases in intra-abdominal pressure are transmitted primarily to the bladder and not to the urethra; at these moments, intravesical pressure will exceed intraurethral pressure, and incontinence will result. **D.** The effect of a Marshall-Marchetti-Krantz procedure or any of its modifications. In this instance, the tissues lateral to the urethra have been fixed to the posterior surface of the pubis and the urethrovesical junction restored to a point within the body cavity. Increases in intra-abdominal pressure are applied to the bladder (as noted by the *large arrow* above) and to the posterior surface of the proximal urethra (*smaller arrow*). **E.** The effect of a sling procedure. The urethrovesical junction has been elevated with prompt restoration of this junction to a point within the body cavity. Integrity of the bladder base plate has been restored. Increases in intra-abdominal pressure are applied to both the bladder (as noted by the *large arrow*) and the anterior and posterior surfaces of the urethra (*smaller arrows*). **F.** The effects of appropriate anterior colporrhaphy, which has included plication and elevation of the urethrovesical junction. The *large arrow* indicates the transmission of intra-abdominal pressure to the bladder, and the *smaller arrows* indicate similar transmission of the increase in pressure to the proximal urethra. Thus transmission of intra-abdominal pressure to the proximal urethra as well as the bladder is shown in A, D, E, and F. A positive ratio is preserved between intraurethral and intravesical pressure when the bladder is at rest, restoring urinary incontinence. (From Nichols DH. Anatomic considerations in stress urinary incontinence. In: Slate WB, ed. Disorders of the female urethra and urinary incontinence. 2nd ed. Baltimore, Williams & Wilkins, 1982. Used with permission.)

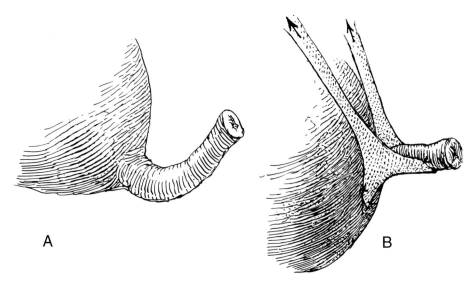

A

B

Figure 17.8. The mechanical effect of a sling. **A.** Preoperative deficiency in support of the vesicourethral junction at rest, which permits flattening of the vesicourethral angle, often resulting in urinary stress incontinence. **B.** Diagrammatic representation of the effect of the suburethral sling after it has been sewn in place. The vesicourethral junction is elevated over a wide area, reducing any tendency toward strangulation and pressure necrosis. (From Nichols DH. The Mersilene mesh gauze hammock for severe urinary stress incontinence. Obstet Gynecol 1973;41:88–93. Used with permission.)

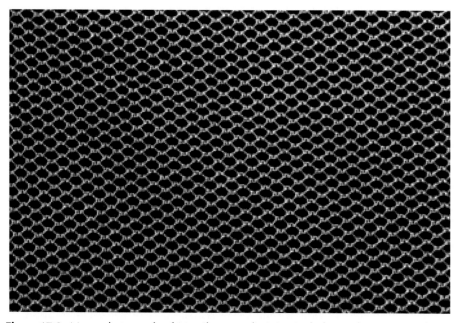

Figure 17.9. Macrophotograph of Mersilene mesh. It is single-layered, porous, and very flexible.

erately exteriorized in the vagina, as might be planned when the vaginal wall is particularly thin (74, 75, 90) (Fig. 17.10).

Rectus fascia obtained through the conventional midline or Pfannenstiel incision is less than optimal, because the direction of fibers in the strip so obtained is oblique and, therefore, not of maximal strength. To obtain a suitable long strip from an abdominal incision would require a crescent-shaped incision that would be cosmetically unattractive. Furthermore, cutting strips from the midline rectus fascia is associated with an increased risk of postoperative wound hernia.

A strip of fascia lata is obtained by the technique suggested by Ridley (74) and shown in Figure 17.11. Its overall width may be increased somewhat by increasing the distance between the parallel incisions shown in Figure 17.11B and curving the strip inside the Masson stripper. When the strip is too narrow, the suburethral pressure of the strap may be concentrated in too small an area, increasing the risk of pressure necrosis of the urethra. If the central belly of the sling is still too narrow, it may widened by central incisions. If there is evidence of funneling within the proximal urethra, or a low urethral closure pressure has been demonstrated preoperatively, the tissues surrounding the urethral wall at the vesicourethral junction may be strengthened and supported by imbrication with one or more Kelly-type plication stitches, using fine polyglycolic-type suture. (Moir once commented that the addition of such suburethral plication to a sling procedure was analogous to a man's lack of confidence by wearing both a belt and suspenders. However, we see no harm in using these funnel-plication sutures.)

The position of the urethrovesical junction is carefully reconfirmed by palpating the site of the inflated Foley catheter bulb. The tissues of the urogenital diaphragm on each *paraurethral* side of the vesicourethral junction are perforated bluntly with the tips of

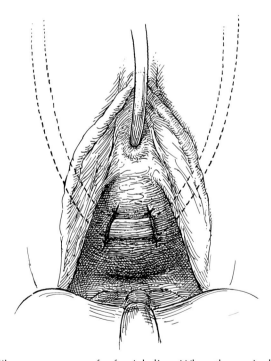

Figure 17.10. Deliberate exposure of a fascial sling. When the vaginal wall is unusually thin, the belly of a fascial sling may remain exteriorized and exposed in the vagina. The *dotted lines* indicate the retropubic path of the tails of the sling. Epithelialization is complete in about 6 weeks.

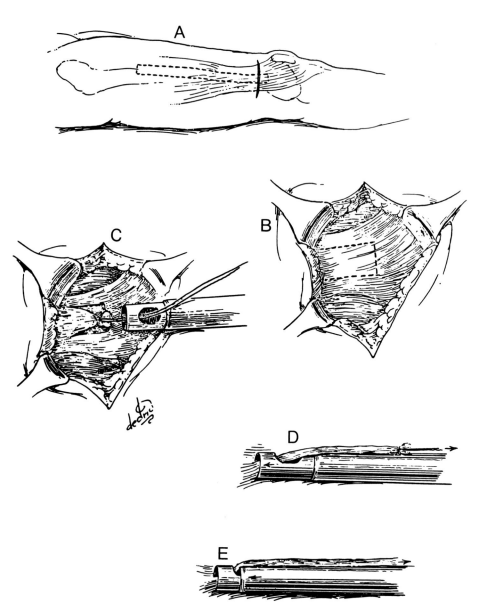

Figure 17.11. The location and technique for obtaining a fascia lata homograft. **A.** A skin incision is made in the right thigh above the patella; the piece of fascia to be excised is indicated by the *dotted line*. **B.** The incision in the distal portion of the fascia lata is identified. **C.** This portion is threaded into the distal end of a Masson fascia stripper. The stripper is passed subcutaneously as far as it will go while countertraction is made at the distal end of the fascial strip, which is held by a Kocher hemostat. **D and E.** When the stripper can proceed no further, the outer sleeve is unscrewed and slid distally as a guillotine over the central barrel, transecting the fascia at its proximal end. The fascia and fascia stripper are removed, the visible remaining fascia lata defect can be closed with a few interrupted polyglycolic acid-type sutures, and the skin incision is closed. (From Nichols DH. The sling operations. In: Cantor EB, ed. Female urinary stress incontinence. Springfield: Chas. C. Thomas, 1979.)

the curved Mayo scissors, which are directed upward and laterally away from the bladder toward the previously established retropubic inguinal tunnel, into the space of Retzius. The scissors are opened 1 to 2 cm and withdrawn, enlarging the opening. It is important to stay close to the pubic rami but to avoid the periosteum. Some venous bleeding is occasionally seen and responds readily to gauze-sponge tamponade. The sterile packs are removed from the abdominal incisions and an abdominal approach is resumed. The surgeon inserts the tip of the left index finger through the abdominal incision on the patient's right and introduces the tip of a uterine dressing forceps, convex side toward the operator, into the transvaginal tunnel through the urogenital diaphragm on the patient's right, until it meets the left index fingertip posterior to the obturator foramen.

The synthetic plastic hammock is not a cure-all, but it appears more advantageous than the Marshall-Marchetti-Krantz because it permits variation in intraurethral pressure, as the sling is tightened coincident with rectus muscle contraction associated with coughing and other such actions. This is in contrast to the fixed, relatively inflexible rigidity resulting from the Marshall-Marchetti-Krantz procedure. Both operations tend to restore or elevate a dropped urethrovesical junction to within the pelvis where it can respond again to changes in intra-abdominal pressure, thereby equally affecting both intraurethral and intravesical pressures. Even in the presence of sudden changes in intra-abdominal pressure, as with coughing or sneezing, continence will be maintained if the resting or nonvoiding intraurethral pressure remains greater than the intravesical pressure.

When the sling is too short, there is risk that the strap may be sewn to the rectus aponeurosis too tightly, which will prevent the patient from voiding or completely emptying her bladder. The tension under which a sling of inelastic fascia lata must be placed is more critical than that of the more flexible and slightly elastic Mersilene mesh. Although the length may be increased by splicing two strips of fascia together, an alternate method of lengthening the strip is shown in Figure 17.12, which does not require joining two separate strips together beneath the urethra at their most vulnerable point. In

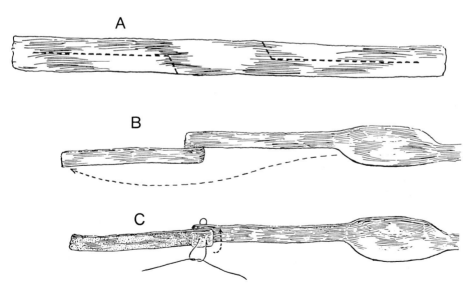

Figure 17.12. A means of increasing the length of the fascia strip. **A.** Incisions are made along the path of the *dotted lines*. **B.** The strips are folded back; drawing shows only the left incision. **C.** The strips are folded over, and a single stitch made to fix the folded fascia in place. The same procedure is accomplished on the opposite end of the fascial strip in place. (From Nichols DH. The sling operations. In: Cantor EB, ed. Female urinary stress incontinence. Springfield, Chas. C Thomas, 1979.)

this modification, a longitudinal incision is made from the lateral edge of the central belly of each end of the strap to within 1 to 2 cm of its lateral end. It is then folded back upon itself and overlapped, and a stitch is required to hold the folded strip until scarring fuses it. The sling is more likely than the "pin-up" operation to restore a broken bladder "base plate," which possibly accounts for its 5 percent better long-term result.

Technique of the Sling Operation. The anesthetized patient is placed in modified lithotomy position (Fig. 17.13), and the abdomen, vulva, and vagina are scrubbed, painted with antiseptic solution, and draped. The operation is commenced suprapubically with a 5-cm incision through the skin overlying each groin, parallel to the inguinal ligament. The incision is medial to the pubic tubercle and extends laterally toward the anterior iliac spine. For the patient with a previous Marshall-Marchetti-Krantz procedure (58), these incisions are lateral to the site of retropubic scarring, which need not be disturbed. If the patient has previously experienced a Burch-type (21) suspension of the vagina to the Cooper ligament, a conventional Pfannenstiel incision is made through the skin and fascia, the stitches of the Burch procedure are identified and cut, and the vesicourethral junction is freed by sharp dissection from the back of the pubis. (Any cystotomy here should be closed in two layers, if possible.) Each incision is deepened to the rectus sheath, which is opened by a 3-cm incision parallel to the skin incision. Each rectus muscle is penetrated by the tips of the curved Mayo scissors, with the curve directed toward the pubis, and the operator's index finger or the closed scissor tips are advanced

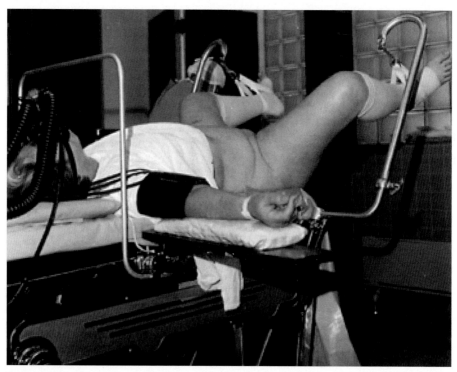

Figure 17.13. Placement of patient for sling operation. Elastic stockings have been applied to each leg. After abdomen, vagina, and perineum have been prepared and draped, further redraping and repings have been applied to each leg. After abdomen, vagina, and perineum have been prepared and draped, further redraping and repositioning of the patient on the operating table later in the procedure become unnecessary. Even in the markedly obese patients, the inguinal incision can be made below the panniculus. The arrangement of operating table, patient, and stirrups is not unlike that used for laparoscopy.

extraperitoneally through the transversalis fascia into the space of Retzius. If scissors are used, the tips are opened somewhat and withdrawn, enlarging the deeper incision. Blunt finger dissection continues to the posterior surface of the obturator foramen. A sterile pack is placed in each wound, the operator and assistants reposition themselves, and the vaginal portion of the operation commences. If the stirrups are in the position chosen for laparoscopy, it is not necessary or desirable to reprepare and redrape the patient between the different phases of the operation. A transurethral no. 16 silicone-coated Foley catheter is inserted into the bladder, and 50 ml of sterile evaporated milk or commercial infant formula is instilled to better identify any unrecognized penetration of the bladder during the course of the procedure. Prompt appearance of the milk will be obvious, but it does not stain the surrounding tissue for the duration of the case, as would be true were methylene blue or indigo carmine used. The bulb on the Foley catheter is identified, and the vaginal wall is picked up between two Allis clamps placed at the 3 and 9 o'clock positions, proximal to the position of the Foley bulb.

A longitudinal full-thickness vaginal incision is made between the clamps into the vesicovaginal space and carried anteriorly by sharp dissection, separating the vagina from the urethra to within 1.5 cm of the urethral meatus. The separation of bladder from vagina is carried posteriorly well beyond the bulb on the catheter—the full distance to the vault of the vagina if a cystocele is to be repaired—and the dissection is carried laterally as far as the pubic rami. Lateral dissection of the vaginal wall from the vesicourethral junction in previously operated patients may release troublesome scar tissue that may have been holding the internal urethral orifice open. The uterine dressing forceps is advanced, keeping contact with the surgeon's left index finger so as to avoid unwanted penetration of bladder or peritoneum, until the tip appears at the skin surface of the incision in the right groin. Here, the tip of the clamp grasps one end of a long heavy silk pilot suture, which is withdrawn through the retropubic tunnel. A similar procedure is accomplished on the patient's left (Fig. 17.14).

The fascia lata strap or a precut Mersilene mesh hammock is held in place transversely beneath the posterior urethra, and the ends are temporarily clamped to the drapes by two hemostats at the 3 and 9 o'clock positions. The anterior margin of the wide hammock belly is tacked and fixed to the undersurface of the lateral paraurethral connective tissue by two interrupted 00 nonabsorbable synthetic sutures, and the posterior edge of the belly is sewn to the posterolateral surface of the bladder capsule. An additional interrupted tacking suture or two is placed in the posterior midline of the gauze hammock belly, fixing it to the bladder capsule. This stretches the hammock anteroposteriorly, without tension but with sufficient pull to remove most of the wrinkles from the belly of the strap. Each silk pilot suture is tied to the respective tail end of the plastic mesh or fascial strap and drawn through its tunnel (see Fig. 17.14B).

If an anterior colporrhaphy is to be accomplished, it is completed now. Thin or defective vaginal walls require that the plastic Mersilene gauze be covered by a Martius bulbocavernosus transplant, or if the vagina is sufficiently wide, the vaginal lapping operation may be used to advantage. Any cystocele repair is completed, and the edges of the anterior vaginal wall, trimmed only if necessary, are approximated in two layers: a deep or buried layer of interrupted 00 polyglycolic sutures, followed by a superficial layer of interrupted mattress sutures (also of 00 polyglycolic) (Fig. 17.15). Any tension on the vaginal suture line should be relieved by lateral vaginal relaxing incisions (see Chapter 20).

Any necessary posterior colporrhaphy or perineorrhaphy is next accomplished, and the vagina is packed overnight with iodoform gauze. The packing itself acts as a bolster in supporting and elevating the vesicourethral junction. When it is in place, the operator's attention is redirected to the abdomen and the sling is sewn to the point where it penetrates the rectus aponeurosis, only tightly enough to take up any slack that may be present. It may be presumed that, when the patient is subsequently standing, the vesi-

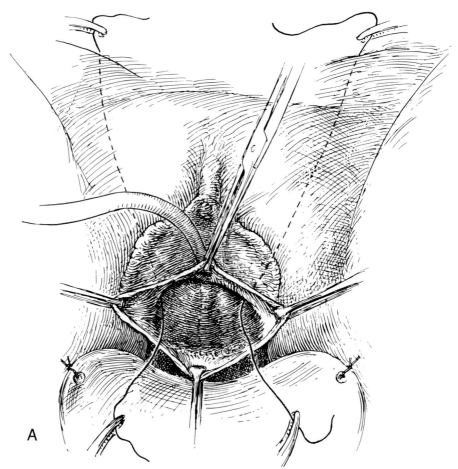

Figure 17.14. The sling operation. **A.** A short abdominal extraperitoneal incision has been made through each rectus aponeurosis into the space of Retzius. The anterior vaginal wall has been opened and the urogenital diaphragm penetrated. A silk pilot suture has been placed through this tunnel on each side. (*Continues on following page.*)

courethral junction, supported by the properly placed sling, will be at the same position that it occupied when the packing was in place, having restored the proximal urethral to an intra-abdominal position. Vesical neck closure can be confirmed by urethroscopy.

After the free ends of the hammock have been securely anchored to the rectus fascia using nonabsorbable synthetic sutures, the excess tails are trimmed and removed from the operative field, and any remaining rectus fascia incision is closed with interrupted sutures. The skin is closed with skin clips or interrupted silk mattress sutures. The wide belly of this sling distributes suburethral pressure over a wide area, and the sling neither constricts the urethra nor decreases its lumen, although it does appear to increase both urethral tone and intraurethral pressure by providing a firm support upon which the urethral may rest. In the rare event of unexpected bladder penetration during placement of the sling, any externally visible opening can be repaired. If good exposure is not available, the sling may be repositioned so as to be away from the penetration, the edges of the penetration permitted to fall together, and the catheter decompression of the bladder maintained a full 14 days, permitting the bladder to heal.

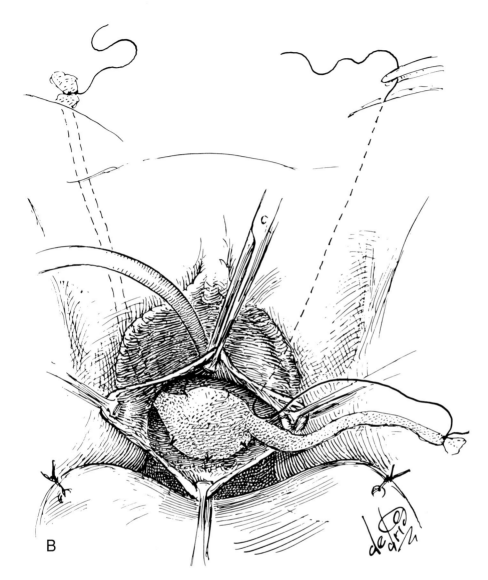

B

Figure 17.14 continued. The sling operation. **B.** The belly of the strap or hammock has been tacked by interrupted synthetic nonabsorbable 000 sutures to the undersurface of the periurethral connective tissue anteriorly, and to the bladder capsule posteriorly. The ends of the hammock have been tied to the vaginal pilot sutures, and traction upon the pilot suture on the patient's right has drawn the strap through the preformed tunnel. The end of the strap to which the pilot suture was tied appears in the wound in the patient's right groin. A similar maneuver will be performed on the patient's left, and the vaginal wall closed with two layers of interrupted 00 polyglycolic acid-type sutures, a deeper buried layer and a superficial layer of interrupted mattress sutures. An iodoform-impregnated gauze vaginal pack is inserted. Without repositioning the patient, the ends of the hammock are sewn without extra tension to the rectus aponeurosis, and the incision in each groin is closed. (From Nichols DH. The Mersilene mesh gauze hammock for severe urinary stress incontinence. Obstet Gynecol 1973;41:88–93. Used with permission.)

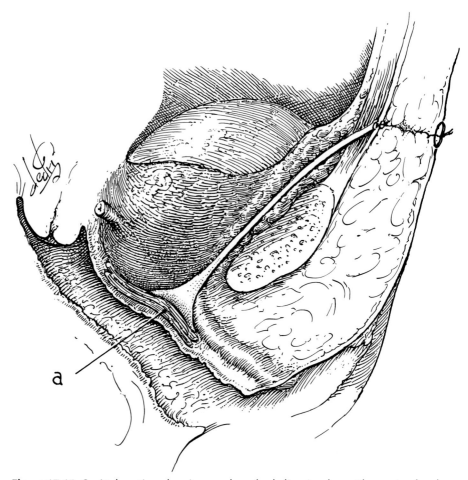

Figure 17.15. Sagittal section showing a suburethral sling in place. The vagina has been closed in two layers (*a*) to insulate the belly of the sling from the vagina. (From Nichols DH. The sling operations. In: Cantor EB, ed. Female urinary stress incontinence, Springfield: Chas. C. Thomas, 1979. Used with permission.)

A challenging situation may arise with the development of stress incontinence in a patient previously subjected to colpectomy or colpocleisis. Because exposure of the vesicourethral junction is difficult in these instances, one can consider a divided sling technique (73), wherein, through a transabdominal incision, each urethral end of a half-sling may be attached to the paraurethral fibromuscular tissue on each respective side and fixed to the rectus aponeurosis. Blind tunneling beneath the urethrovesical junction, as is necessary with the Millin-Reed sling procedure (60), is not recommended because of the increased risk of urethral or vesical penetration.

Postoperative Adjustments in Sling Tension. If the sling, of whatever material has been used, has been placed too loosely to achieve an increase in intraurethral pressure sufficient to restore continence, this will become evident shortly after the Foley catheter has been removed in the immediate postoperative period. Similarly, if it has been placed too tightly, the patient may not be able to empty her bladder. To lessen the chance of traumatic necrosis of the overlying flap of vagina, the approach of choice to tighten the sling is by a transabdominal approach through one of the groin incisions. This is easiest within the first 7 to 14 days after surgery when there is as yet minimal fibrosis and scarring around the sling. Simply releasing one end of the sling from its attachment to the abdominal aponeurosis is sufficient to relieve the tension of a sling applied too tightly. (Weeks or months later it is more difficult to find the abdominal end of the sling, by this time buried in scar tissue, but the end will be found adherent to the underside of the lower edge of the incision through the rectus aponeurosis. Alternatively, it may be severed through a transvaginal incision.) Alterations in tension need be applied to but one end of the sling; thus only one of the groin incisions needs to be reopened.

The degree to which the sling should be tightened or loosened can be judged by simultaneous direct urethroscopy in the operating room. After the abdominal end of the sling has been mobilized, the sling is fixed at such a point under direct visualization that the internal urethral orifice has just closed. This requires a two-team approach: an abdominal operating team and a urethroscopist. Lacking a urethroscope, a cystoscope, hysteroscope, arthroscope, or laparoscope can be used transurethrally. In the absence of urethroscopy, a less precise method of determining sling tension can be elected. One can choose the point at which sudden manual abdominal compression against the full bladder will not produce leaking, or, if the patient is under spinal anesthesia, she can be asked to cough, and the sling tension chosen at at the point when there is no transurethral leakage.

Combined Procedures

When the patient's primary symptom is recurrent, severe, and socially disabling USI, the surgeon may consider a combined procedure. A combined approach may be of special interest if urethral vesicalization or funneling is present that will permit plication of both anterior and posterior urethrovesical angles (6) followed by a Marshall-Marchetti-Krantz (58) procedure, a Burch (21), or a sling type of repair. In the absence of demonstrable funneling, plication of the vesicourethral junction or bladder neck may be omitted to lessen the chance of a subsequent stricture.

Using the pubourethrovaginal ligament plication stitch (see Chapter 10) with a complementary perineorrhaphy (44, 56, 62), we have approached rotational descent of the bladder neck (urethral detachment) by a primary vaginal procedure that elevates the vesicourethral junction. If midline defect of urethral support is lacking, the alternative of paravaginal attachment (3, 32, 91)(BH Word Jr, HA Montgomery, personal communication) is available (see Chapter 10); depending upon the extent of damage, both may be employed. Because this operation relocates the vesicourethral junction at a higher level within the pelvis and is supported by an appropriate perineorrhaphy, it accomplishes more than simple urethral plication. When there is flattening of the posterior urethrovesical angle without rotational descent of the bladder neck, one may choose a vaginal, suprapubic, or combined approach, depending on the severity of the patient's symptoms, the presence of coexistent medical disease such as asthma or hay fever, or coexistent vaginal or intra-abdominal pathology, which requires simultaneous correction. If the vaginal operation is chosen for the correction of urinary stress incontinence, the operator's attention is directed to the requirement that the repair emphasize plication and support of the vesical neck and the proximal urethra with its supporting tissues, with less emphasis on cystocele repair posterior to the vesicourethral junction.

When the cystocele and lateral sulci but not the vault of the vagina come down when a patient strains but the lateral sulci do not go back when the patient contracts her pubococcygei, this is good evidence of a lateral vaginal attachment defect that might be made a part of the patient's surgical repair (5). Very little if any vaginal membrane should be resected in this circumstance, but complementary perineorrhaphy is usually indicated with each anterior colporrhaphy and will aid in the support of the urethra.

There are specific but uncommon circumstances in which the operator might wish to combine a vaginal hysterectomy and appropriate colporrhaphy with a retropubic suburethral sling procedure, such as for symptomatic and progressive genital prolapse in a patient with recurrent severe and socially disabling USI, often accompanied by a chronic respiratory disease or a coincident low urethral closure pressure. The technique of the combined operation should begin with an incision in each groin through the rectus aponeurosis, bluntly through the rectus muscle and the transversalis fascia, and extraperitoneally to the obturator foramen in the space of Retzius on each side. Then the vaginal hysterectomy and excision of any enterocele are accomplished and the anterior colporrhaphy begun. The suburethral sling is tacked beneath the vesicourethral junction and pulled through the tunnel on each side into the space of Retzius to appear at the wound in the groin, and the anterior colporrhaphy is finished. Any necessary posterior colporrhaphy is done, the vagina is packed, elevating the vesicourethral junction, and the operator's attention is redirected to the abdominal groin incision where the ends of the sling are fixed on each side to the rectus aponeurosis.

A suprapubic operative procedure for the relief of severe and socially disabling USI might be considered when either or both of the following criteria are present: (*a*) The incontinence is secondary to failure of a previous repair. (*b*) There is coexistent contributing medical disease: emphysema, asthma, hay fever, heavy smoking, chronic bronchitis, obesity, and so forth.

Although adequate performance of the Marshall-Marchetti-Krantz procedure does relieve a rotational descent of the bladder neck, it does not treat a distention cystocele. In the sling procedure, the vaginal wall is opened at the time the sling is to be fixed, and this exposure permits the operator to treat surgically any coexistent cystocele while fixing the sling in place.

When pubourethrovaginal ligament support is poor, there is coincident low urethral closure pressure (less than 20 cm of water), or the tissues are excessively thin or scarred, a suprapubic procedure is especially attractive. Although the Marshall-Marchetti-Krantz pin-up procedure (21, 58), or any one of its various modifications, "pulls" the urethrovesical junction back into the pelvis, it does not necessarily restore the integrity of a damaged bladder base plate (45, 86), nor does it treat coincident distention-type cystocele. The vesicourethral junction is now permanently fixed in a retropubic position from which it will no longer descend physiologically during voiding.

A suprapubic sling procedure "pushes" the vesicourethral junction back into the pelvis and tends to restore the competence of a damaged base plate. As the rectus muscles and the levator ani relax during voiding, the vesicourethral unction will descend to some extent.

It is evident that when one has chosen to use a suburethral sling procedure for the surgical treatment of severe or recurrent USI, there are various materials and techniques that may be selected to remedy the patient's disability. Several of these have been described, along with the circumstances whereby one might favor one over another. We emphasize that the surgeon should be familiar with and experienced in several techniques in order to be able to select those materials and technical steps that will best serve the needs of each individual patient.

Periurethral Bulking Agents

Cross-linked collagen preparations (GAX) can be used to increase urethral closure pressure in patients following previous failed incontinence operations, particularly when the urethrovesical junction is otherwise well supported (27). When an incontinent patient with a low urethral closure pressure (but without urethral hypermobility) has been identified, and particularly when a previous surgical procedure has failed to cure the incontinence, a submucosal injection of bovine collagen may be made on each side of the urethra as shown in Figure 17.16. The point of the needle tip (bevel toward urethral lumen) is visualized beneath the surface by a cystoscope held by the same person doing the injection. A similar procedure is repeated on the opposite side. The cystoscope is periodically withdrawn a bit so that one may observe the end point at which the two sides of the urethra make gentle contact with one another.

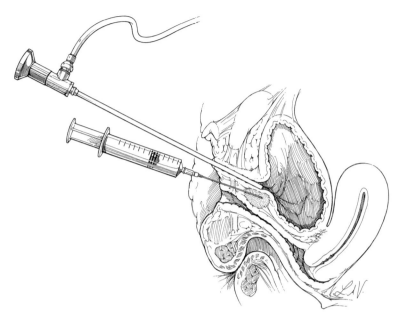

Figure 17.16. Injecting bovine collagen. The tip of a cystoscope has been placed at the vesi-courethral junction. The tip of a long needle attached to a syringe containing the collagen paste has been placed beneath the urethral mucosa, where its position can be verified by observation through the cystoscope. Several milliliters of the paste is slowly injected, and a similar penetration and injection are made on the opposite side sufficient to cause the internal mucosal surfaces to touch one another.

As an alternative treatment to surgery or for the patient in whom major surgery is neither safe nor suitable, a satisfactory additional method of treating decreased outflow resistance when this is required to remedy bladder outflow incompetence may be obtained in the patient without a hypermobile urethra by submucosal injections of polyte-trafluoroethylene (polytef, or Teflon) or GAX collagen (Contigen) (2). Concerns over particle migration have reduced the utility of polytef (which is *not* biodegradable), especially in younger patients. When periurethral injections of polytef (Teflon) were studied in female dogs and male monkeys, particles were found in the pelvic nodes and lungs and later the brain, kidneys, and spleen (55). Since these granulomas that were found signify chronic foreign body reaction, and since the long-term effects in humans are as yet unknown, we believe that polytef paste should not be used in children or young adults with normal life expectancy. Now that collagen is available as an alternate (GAX), it is probably a preferable medium to be injected, although its long-range results have not yet been studied for a large number of people.

Contigen is a sterile, nonpyrogenic material composed of highly purified bovine dermal collagen that is cross-linked with glutaraldehyde and dispersed in phosphate-buffered physiological saline. When it has been determined by preliminary intradermal inoculation 4 weeks before the planned treatment that the patient is not sensitive to the collagen, it may be injected transurethrally or periurethrally. The urethra is anesthetized by 1% plain lidocaine injected at the 3 to 9 o'clock position. Then a 22-gauge spinal needle with obturator is placed periurethrally at the 4 o'clock position with the bevel directed medially and is slowly advanced while its progress is followed through the 17F 0- or 30-degree cystoscope until the needle tip is subepithelial and at the vesi-courethral junction. The obturator is removed, and using one hand to stabilize the cystoscope, the 3-ml syringe is attached to the spinal needle and the Contigen is injected until the bulge produced reaches the midline. The needle is removed and the process is repeated at the 8 o'clock position on the opposite side. The injection is continued under direct cystoscopic visualization of the vesicourethral junction until the mucosal tissue of one side just touches that of the opposite side. Presumably, the collagen elicits an inflammatory response without granuloma formation that enables eventual replacement of bovine collagen with the patient's own collagen; this is in contrast to polytef, which remains and exerts its effect as a foreign body. Appell has described his considerable success and enthusiasm for this procedure (2).

The Wolf aspiration-injection system (Richard Wolf Medical Instruments Corp., Vernon Hills, Illinois) is most helpful in stabilizing the injection needles to allow accurate submucosal injection. The oblique tip design of its 21F urethroscope-cystoscope sheath allows visualization of the needle immediately as it emerges from the sheath, permitting accurate endourethral placement of the needle tip into the submucosal tissues. The cystoscope is *not* reintroduced, lest it compress the collagen and laterally distort the recent mucosal approximation. About 8 to 10 percent of patients will experience transient urinary retention, and their bladders can be emptied by intermittent self-catheterization. An indwelling Foley catheter should not be placed lest it press the collagen to the sides, disturbing the mucosal approximation.

Contigen, which is biodegradable, appears to be safe and efficacious, particularly in patients who do not manifest detrusor problems and have a urethrovesical junction that is fairly well stabilized in position. Contigen begins to degrade 12 weeks after injection. It stimulates and is replaced by the body's own collagen, retaining the effect of being a bulking agent. About a third of the patients will require a second injection of 15 ml of Contigen after 30 days if they are not dry, and patients have then reported that they have remained dry for at least 12 months (2). Follow-up, however, has been short.

For the 4 percent of patients shown by skin test to be sensitive to bovine collagen, autologous subcutaneous fat (22) obtained by liposuction can be substituted. This is less successful than GAX (18).

Although good results may be seen immediately following periurethral Teflon injection, these good results fall off rapidly in the following years, and many of these people will have to be retreated (13). Some have reported that only 25 percent of patients are relieved or continent after 5 years, even when polytef (Teflon paste) has been used.

CONCLUSION

Accurate diagnosis, confirmation, and individual assessment of each patient's complaint of urinary stress incontinence must precede treatment if optimal results are to be expected and attained. The gynecologist must clearly understand how the patient perceives her problem and the depth of her description of an acceptable solution. Only then can an effective recommendation for treatment be given with the expectation of relief. Simple confirmatory diagnostic procedures will suffice when the sole symptom is stress incontinence, and a clearly positive stress test may suffice before starting treatment, which may be nonsurgical, surgical, or both.

A course of electrical stimulation with biofeedback should precede specific surgery for the patient with poor voluntary pubococcygeal contractile ability. It may cure the symptom and obviate a surgical solution. Estrogen supplementation should be given to the postmenopausal patient and continued indefinitely if effective. For the patient with symptoms of incontinence of mixed etiology, or in whom there was prior failed surgery, the help of sophisticated urodynamic laboratory assessment should be required. Ultimately, however, the decisions about treatment must be made by the individual patient, and not the laboratory, as she weighs the options and recommendations available to her.

A urodynamic computer is a poor witness to the patient's symptoms. Dionysios K. Veronikis (personal communication, 1995).

References

1. Abrams P, Blaivas JG, Stanton SL, Anderson JT. The International Continence Society Committee on Standardization of Terminology. The standardization of terminology of lower urinary tract function. Scand J Urol Nephrol 1988;114S:5.
2. Appell RA. Injectables for urethral incompetence. World J Urol 1990;8:208–211.
3. Appell RA. New developments: injectables for urethral incompetence in women. Int Urogynecol J 1990;1:117–119.
4. Asmussen M, Ulmsten U. Simultaneous urethro-cystometry with a new technique. Scand J Urol Nephrol 1976;10:7–11.
5. Baden WF, Walker TA. Evaluation of the stress-incontinent patient. In: Cantor EB, ed. Female urinary stress incontinence. Springfield, IL: Charles C Thomas, 1979:157–158.
6. Ball TL. Gynecologic surgery and urology. 2nd ed. St. Louis: Mosby, 1963:165–209.
7. Barton DPJ, Armstrong MJ, O'Sullivan JF. A review of the gauze-hammock sling operation for patients with recurrent stress incontinence following surgery. J Obstet Gynecol 1989;9:226–228.
8. Bates CP, Loose H, Stanton SLR. The objective study of incontinence after repair operations. Surg Gynecol Obstet 1973;136:1722.
9. Beck RP, Arnusch D, King C. Results in treating 210 patients with detrusor overactivity incontinence of urine. Am J Obstet Gynecol 1976;125:593–596.
10. Beck RP, Hsu N. Relationship of urethral length and anterior wall relaxation to urinary stress incontinence. Am J Obstet Gynecol 1964;89:738–741.
11. Beck RP, Hsu N, Maughan GB. Simultaneous intraurethral and intravesical pressure studies in patients surgically treated for stress incontinence. Am J Obstet Gynecol 1965;91:314–319.
12. Beck RP, McCormick S, Nordstom L. A 25-year experience with 519 anterior colporrhaphy procedures. Obstet Gynecol 1991;78:1011–1018.
13. Beckingham IJ, Wemyss-Holden G, Lawrence WT. Long-term follow-up of women treated with peri-urethral teflon injections for stress incontinence. Br J Urol 1992;69:580–583.
14. Bent AE, Ostergard DR, Zwick-Zaffuto M. Tissue reaction to polytetrafluoroethylene suburethral sling for urinary incontinence: clinical and histological study. Am J Obstet Gynecol 1993;169:1198–1204.
15. Bergman A, Koonings PP, Ballard CA. Predicting postoperative urinary incontinence development in women undergoing operation for genitourinary prolapse. Am J Obstet Gynecol 1988;158:1171–1175.
16. Bhatia N, Bergman A. Pessary test in women with urinary incontinence. Obstet Gynecol 1985;65:220–226.
17. Blaivas JG, Jacobs BZ. Pubovaginal fascial sling for the treatment of complicated stress urinary incontinence. J Urol 1991;145:1214–1218.
18. Blaivas JG, Santarosa RP. Periurethral fat injection for sphincteric incontinence. Neurourol Urodynam 1992;11:403.
19. Borstad E, Rud T. The risk of developing urinary stress incontinence after vaginal repair in continent women: a clinical and urodynamic follow-up study. Acta Obstet Gynecol Scand 1989;68:545–549.
20. Bump RC. Urinary incontinence. In: Quilligan EJ, Zuspan FB, eds. Current therapy in obstetrics and gynecology. Philadelphia: Saunders, 1990:122–123.
21. Burch JD. Urethrovaginal fixation to Cooper's ligament for correction of stress incontinence, cystocele, and prolapse. Am J Obstet Gynecol 1961;81:281.
22. Chalchir A, Benzaquen I. Fat-grafting injection for soft-tissue augmentation. Plast Reconst Surg 1989;84:921–924.
23. Cornella JL, Ostergard DR. Needle suspension procedure for urinary stress incontinence: a review and historical perspective. Obstet Gynecol Surv 1990;45:805–816.
24. Crisp W. Urinary pressure incontinence in the female. Ariz Med 1966;23:513–516.
25. Davila GW, Osterman KV. The bladder neck support prosthesis: a nonsurgical approach to stress incontinence in adult women. Am J Obstet Gynecol 1994;171:206–211.
26. Dwyer PL, Teele JS. Prazosin: a neglected cause of genuine stress incontinence. Obstet Gynecol 1992;79:117–121.
27. Eckford SD, Abrams P. Para-urethral collagen implantation for female stress incontinence. Br J Urol 1991;68:586–589.
28. Eriksen BC, Hagen B, Eik-Nes SH, Molne K, Mjølnerød OK, Romslo I. Long-term effectiveness of the Burch colposuspension in female urinary stress incontinence. Acta Obstet Gynecol Scand 1990;69:45–50.
29. Fall M, Lindström S. Electrical stimulation: a physiologic approach to the treatment of urinary incontinence. Urol Clin North Am 1991;18:393–407.
30. Fantl JA, Hurt WG, Dunn LJ. Dysfunctional detrusor control. Am J Obstet Gynecol 1977;129:299–303.
31. Ferguson KL, McKey PL, Bishop KR. Stress urinary incontinence: effect of pelvic muscle exercise. Obstet Gynecol 1989;75:671–675.
32. Figurnov KM. Surgical treatment of urinary incontinence in women. Akush Ginekol 1949;6:7–13 (in Russian).
33. Fliegner JR, Glenning PP. Seven years experience in the evaluation and management of patients with urge incontinence of urine. Aust N Z J Obstet Gynaecol 1979;19:42–44.

34. Frewer WK. Foley catheter urethrography in stress incontinence. J Obstet Gynaecol Br Commw 1971; 78:660–663.
35. Frigerio L, Ferrari A, Candiani GB. The significance of the stop test in female urinary incontinence. Diagn Gynecol Obstet 1981;3:301–304.
36. Gardy M, Kozminski M, DeLancey JOL, Elkins T, McGuire EJ. Stress incontinence and cystoceles. J Urol 1991;145:1211–1213.
37. Gittes RF, Loughlin KR. No-incision pubovaginal suspension for stress incontinence. J Urol 1987; 138:568–570.
38. Gleason DM, Bottaccini MR, Reilly RJ. Comparison of cystometrograms and urethral profiles with gas and water media. Urology 1977;9:155–160.
39. Green TH. Urinary stress incontinence: differential diagnosis, pathophysiology, and management. Am J Obstet Gynecol 1975;122:368–400.
40. Hawksworth W, Roux JP. Vaginal hysterectomy. J Obstet Gynaecol Br Commonw 1958;63:214.
41. Henriksson L, Ulmsten U. A urodynamic evaluation of the effects of abdominal urethrocystopexy and vaginal sling urethroplasty in women with stress incontinence. Am J Obstet Gynecol 1978;131:77–82.
42. Hodgkinson CP. Stress urinary incontinence. Am J Obstet Gynecol 1970;108:1141.
43. Hodgkinson CP, Kelly WT. Urinary stress incontinence in the female III: Rounded-ligament technique for retropubic suspension of the urethra. Obstet Gynecol 1957;10:493–499.
44. Howkins J, Stallworthy J. Operations for Stress Incontinence In: Bonney's gynaecological surgery. 8th ed. London: Balliere Tindall, 1974:550–551.
45. Hutch JA. Anatomy and physiology of the bladder trigone and urethra. New York: Appleton-Century-Crofts, 1972:133–173.
46. Jeffcoate TNA, Francis W. Urgency incontinence in the female. Am J Obstet Gynecol 1966;94:604–618.
47. Kegel AH. Progressive resistance exercise in the functional restoration of the perineal muscles. Am J Obstet Gynecol 1948;56:238–248.
48. Kelly MJ, Roskamp D, Knielsen K, Leach GE, Bruskewitz R. Symptom analysis of patients undergoing modified Pereyra bladder neck suspension for stress urinary incontinence: pre- and postoperative findings. Urology 1991;27:213.
49. Khanna OP. Disorders of micturition. Urology 1976;8:316–328.
50. Klarskov P, Nielsen KK, Kromann-Anderson B, Maegaard E. Long-term results of pelvic floor training and surgery for female genuine-stress incontinence. Int Urogynecol J 1991;2:132–135.
51. Korn AP. Does use of permanent suture material affect outcome of the modified Pereyra procedure? Obstet Gynecol 1994;83:104–107.
52. Kursh ED. Factors influencing the outcome of a no-incision endoscopic urethropexy. Surg Gynecol Obstet 1992;175:254–258.
53. Langmade CF, Oliver JA. Simplifying the management of stress incontinence. Am J Obstet Gynecol 1984;149:24–27.
54. Lee RA. Correcting recurrent stress incontinence. Contemp Obstet Gynecol 1978;12:3341.
55. Malizia AA, Reiman HM, Myers RP, Sande JR, Barham SS, Benson Jr, RC, Dewanjee MK, Utz WJ. Migration and granulomatous reaction after periurethral injection of polytef (Teflon). JAMA 1984; 251:3277–3281.
56. Malpas P. The choice of operation for genital prolapse. Prog Gynecol 1957;3:663–673.
57. Marchant D. Urinary incontinence. Obstet Gynecol 1981;58:372–374.
58. Marshall VF, Marchetti AA, Krantz KE. The correction of stress incontinence by simple vesicourethral suspension. Surg Gynecol Obstet 1949;88:509.
59. Mattox TF, Bhatia NN. Anatomy, physiology, and pathology of pelvic support. In: Moore TR, Reiter RC, Rebar RW, Baker VV, eds. Gynecology and Obstetrics: a longitudinal approach. New York: Churchill-Livingstone, 1993:731–733.
60. Millin T, Reed CD. Stress incontinence of urine in the female. Postgrad Med J 1948;24:51.
61. Moir JC. The gauze-hammock operation. J Obstet Gynaecol Br Commonw 1968;75:1.
62. Nesbitt REL, Holmann JC. Management of urinary stress incontinence in the female. Surg Gynecol Obstet 1971;132:588–596.
63. Nichols DH. The Mersilene Mesh Gauze-Hammock in repair of severe on recurrent urinary stress incontinence. In: Taymor ME, Green TH, eds. Progress in gynecology. New York: Grune & Stratton, 1975;6:689–704.
64. Nichols DH. The sling operations. In: Cantor EB, ed. Female urinary stress incontinence. Springfield, IL: Charles C Thomas, 1979:235–260.
65. Novak F. Surgical gynecologic techniques. New York: Wiley, 1978.
66. Obrink A, Bunne G. Urethral pressure profile at pubococcygeal repair for stress incontinence. Acta Obstet Gynecol Scand 1980;59:433–437.
67. Ostergard DR. The effect of drugs on the lower urinary tract. Obstet Gynecol Surv 1979;34:424–431.
68. Parker RT, Addison WA, Wilson CJ. Fascia lata urethrovesical suspension for recurrent stress urinary incontinence. Am J Obstet Gynecol 1979;135:843.
69. Parys BT, Haylen BT, Hutton JL, Parsons KF. Urodynamic evaluation of lower urinary tract function in relation to total hysterectomy. Aust N Z J Obstet Gynecol 1990;30:161–165.

70. Payne SR, Timoney AG, McKenning ST, der Hollander D, Pead LJ, Maskell RM. Microbiological look at urodynamic studies. Lancet 1988;2:1123–1126.

71. Pereyra AJ. A simplified surgical procedure for the correction of stress incontinence in women. West J Surg 1959;67:223.

72. Pereyra AJ, Lebherz TB, Growdon WA, Poers JA. Pubourethral supports in perspective: modified Pereyra procedure for urinary incontinence. Obstet Gynecol 1981;59:643–648.

73. Ridley JH. Surgery for stress urinary incontinence. In: Ridley H, ed. Gynecologic surgery: errors, safeguards, salvage. 2nd ed. Baltimore: Williams & Wilkins, 1981.

74. Ridley JH. Urinary incontinence not curable by sphincter plication. In: TeLinde RW, Mattingly RF, eds. Operative gynecology. 4th ed. Philadelphia: JB Lippincott, 1970.

75. Robertson JL. Genitourinary problems in women. Springfield, IL: Charles C Thomas, 1977.

76. Rosenzweig BA, Pushkin S, Blumenfeld D, Bhatia NN. Prevalence of abnormal urodynamic test results in continent women with severe genitourinary prolapse. Obstet Gynecol 1992;79:539–542.

77. Sand PK, Bowen LW, Ostergard DR, Brubaker L, Panganibar R. The effect of retropubic urethropexy on detrusor stability. Obstet Gynecol 1988;71:818–822.

78. Sand PK, Brubaker LT, Novak T. Simple standing incremental cystometry as a screening method for detrusor instability. Obstet Gynecol 1991;77:453–457.

79. Sand PK, Hill RC, Ostergard DR. Supine urethroscopic and standing cystometry as screening methods for the detection of detrusor instability. Obstet Gynecol 1987;70:57–60.

80. Schaer GN, Koechli OR, Schuessler B, Haller U. Perineal ultrasound for evaluating the bladder neck in urinary stress incontinence. Obstet Gynecol 1995;85:220–224.

81. Smith ARB, Hosker GL, Warrell D. The role of pudendal nerve damage in the aetiology of genuine urinary stress incontinence in women. Br J Obstet Gynaecol 1989;96:29–32.

82. Snooks SJ, Badenoch DF, Tiptaft RC, Swash M. Perineal nerve damage in genuine stress urinary incontinence: an electrophysiological study. Br J Urol 1985;57:422–426.

83. Snooks SJ, Swash M, Henry MM, Setchell M. Risk factors in childbirth causing damage to the pelvic floor innervation. Int J Colorect Dis 1986;1:20–24.

84. Stamey TA. Endoscopic suspension of the vesical neck for urinary incontinence. Surg Gynecol Obstet 1973;136:547–554.

85. Summitt RL Jr, Bent AE, Ostergard DR, Harris TA. Stress incontinence and low urethral closure pressure. J Reprod Med 1990;35:877–880.

86. Uhlenhuth E, Hunter de WT. Problems in the anatomy of the pelvis. Philadelphia: JB Lippincott, 1953.

87. Wall LL, Norton PA, DeLancey JOL. Practical urogynecology. Baltimore: Williams & Wilkins, 1993:153–190.

88. Walters MD. Evaluation of incontinence: history, physical examination, and office tests. In: Walters MD, Karram MM. Clinical urogynecology. St. Louis: Mosby, 1993:49–61.

89. Weil A, Miege B, Rottenberg R, et al. Clinical significance of urethral instability. Obstet Gynecol 1986;68:106–110.

90. Wheeless CR, Wharton LR, Dorsey JH, et al. The Goebell-Stoeckel operation for universal cases of urinary incontinence. Am J Obstet Gynecol 1977;128:546–549.

91. White GR. Cystocele: a radical cure by suturing lateral sulci of vagina to white lines of pelvic fascia. JAMA 1909;53:1707–1709.

92. Zoedler D. Die operative Behandlung der Weiblichen Ahninkontinenz mit dem Kinststaff-Netz-Band. Actuelle Urol 1970;1:28.

CHAPTER 18

Urethral Diverticulum and Fistula

URETHRAL DIVERTICULUM

Suburethral diverticula are not as uncommon as is widely believed, and the number found will be proportional to the diligence of the gynecologist in searching for them.

There is no need to repair an asymptomatic urethral diverticulum. Dribbling, dysuria, or dyspareunia, however, are symptoms that suggest indications for surgery.

Those symptomatic diverticula found in the distal urethra are prone to be associated with postmicturition dribbling, as Asmussen and Miller (1) have indicated:

The leakage can lead to a suspicion of stress incontinence because of the effect of straining and movement. Leakage, however, occurs soon after micturition, while in stress incontinence this is the one time when a patient can be almost certain that she will not leak, simply because the bladder is empty. After leakage has occurred from the diverticulum there is a tendency for the patient to be dry until after the next micturition. In stress incontinence the reverse is the case–she leaks more when the bladder is full.*

Significant urinary leaking is less common in patients in whom there is a diverticulum of the proximal urethra, but dysuria and dyspareunia are of greater intensity, proportional to the degree of diverticular infection (1). Intradiverticular stones may be found in those present for a long period of time, and are secondary to chronic urinary stasis. The stones may precipitate hematuria and may contribute to the cause of urethral malignancy, which must be thoughtfully diagnosed.

Urethral diverticula are most frequently found arising from the middle third and less commonly from the posterior or posterolateral wall of the upper urethra, and about 15 percent from the distal urethra (7). An opening from the anterior wall of the urethra is uncommon. The walls of diverticula adhere to all nearby structures with which they are in contact, including the wall of the vagina. The sac of a diverticulum may occasionally extend ventrally alongside the urethra on one or both sides.

The origin of urethral diverticula is not clear, but when the wall includes only fibrous tissue and is without an epithelial lining, it is believed that the condition is one acquired from infection and obstruction of a paraurethral duct (8, 9). When muscle is present in the diverticular wall, as is true of bladder diverticula, a possibly congenital origin is suggested. It should be differentiated from a Gartner duct cyst, which contains mucus, has a distinct epithelial lining, and does not communicate with the urethral lumen.

The condition should be suspected when there is a history of dysuria, dribbling, and dyspareunia, but positive findings are not always obvious on physical examination, because the contents of some urethral diverticula may be easily discharged into the urethral

---

* From Asmussen M, Miller A. Clinical gynaecological urology. Oxford: Blackwell Scientific Publications, 1983:173. Used with permission.

lumen, producing temporary collapse of the sac. If infection of the sac or stones are present, tenderness will be elicited upon palpation of the suburethral tissues. Urine or exudate obtained from stripping the urethra is suspicious, and the diagnosis may be confirmed by radiography (in which the sac may be filled with contrast medium injected under pressure using a special double-ballooned catheter such as the Davis) or by direct urethroscopy.

There is some evidence that the urethral pressure profile of a woman with a urethral diverticulum will have a biphasic shape, the pressure decrease being found at the anatomic location of the diverticular orifice (2), but this is of low specificity (10). Direct visualization and documentation on radiographic studies, which can be brought to the operating room for orientation at surgery, are most useful.

Cystourethroscopy is likely to be accurate, and the size and number of diverticula can be best determined by lateral urethrography, in which the diverticula have been filled by radiopaque material instilled into the urethra under pressure. Since only 60 percent of diverticula are palpable, diagnosis by vaginal ultrasonography may be useful, especially in the patient with a history of chronic recurrent urinary tract infection (7).

The primary treatment of symptomatic urethral diverticula is surgical and requires adequate preoperative diagnosis and preparation for possibly extensive dissection involving mobilization of all tunnels and ramifications of the diverticulum. Because diverticula are often the site of chronic infection and not uncommonly of calculus formation, patience is required to identify, mobilize, and excise every bit of the tract of a diverticulum. When the urethral defect is large, one may use a portion of the mobilized wall of the diverticulum to bridge the gap (Fig. 18.1).

When a diverticulum is acutely infected, it may be impossible to separate its wall with the orifice from its fusion to the adjacent muscular wall of the urethra without risking unwanted resection of a major portion of the latter. In this case, after it has been separated from the vagina, the sac is entered and as much as can be safely dissected is removed,

the ostium visualized, and closed . . . without attempt to resect the sac at its neck. The remaining sac wall is then sutured side-to-side as a second layer over the ostial closure. The cavity is thus obliterated. A third layer of periurethral tissue which surrounded the sac is used, if available.*

Diverticulectomy should be accomplished *only* if the diverticulum can be palpated at the time of surgery. If a formerly palpable diverticulum is not demonstrable at surgery, it is desirable to fill the diverticulum at the start of the procedure. This is probably best accomplished by using a Davis double-balloon catheter.

Multiple diverticula can be present, and it is important to recognize each and treat of all the tracts present. Because of occasional instances of troublesome postoperative incontinence, we have not found marsupialization of urethral diverticula (8) to be especially useful.

Following are the possible complications of urethral diverticulectomy:

1. Hemorrhage and infection
2. Postoperative urinary incontinence consequent to disturbance the neuromuscular or muscular statics in the vesicourethral junction or the sphincter mechanism
3. Urethrovaginal fistula
4. Recurrence (were there two ostia present?)
5. Urethral stricture
6. Progression of coexistent undiagnosed urethral carcinoma

The incidence of these complications can be lessened by meticulous attention to detail and careful hemostasis, often achieved by frequent use of the electrocautery (6).

*From Tancer ML, Hyman R. Suburethral diverticulitis in the female. Am J Obstet Gynecol 1962;84; 1853–1858. Used with permission.

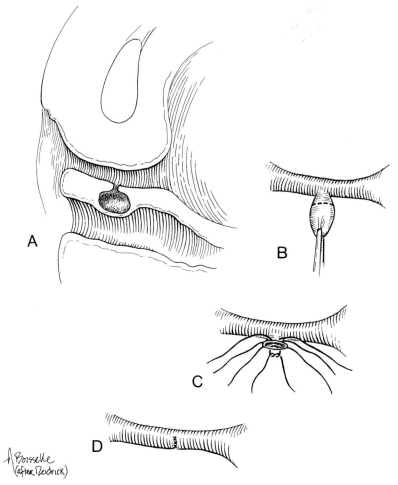

A Boisselle
(after Deidrick)

Figure 18.1. Excision of a urethral diverticulum. **A.** Sagittal drawing shows the diverticulum arising from the midportion of the urethra. An incision is made in the anterior vaginal wall, and the diverticulum is mobilized by sharp dissection. **B.** If the ostium is narrow, it may be tied and the diverticulum amputated, but if wide, the diverticulum may be cut across as shown. **C.** The remaining wall is united transversely by interrupted sutures placed transversely to the axis to reduce the chance for urethral stricture. **D.** The sutures are tied, the repair insulated from the vaginal incision by a bulbocavernosus fat pad transplant, and the vaginal incision closed using interrupted sutures. The vagina is packed overnight.

During a subsequent pregnancy a successful repair is no contraindication to future vaginal delivery.

The patient usually should have been placed in the lithotomy position, with a 10- to 20-degree Trendelenburg tip of the table. Adequate illumination of the operative field is essential; and if it cannot be provided by overhead lights or spotlight, a suitable fiberoptic headlamp for the operator should be used.

URETHRAL DIVERTICULECTOMY

Some effective techniques of repair are illustrated in Figures 18.1 and 18.2. The technique of Asmussen and Miller (1) is especially helpful, since closure of the U-shaped incision in the anterior vaginal wall lessens the chance of fistula formation by covering the

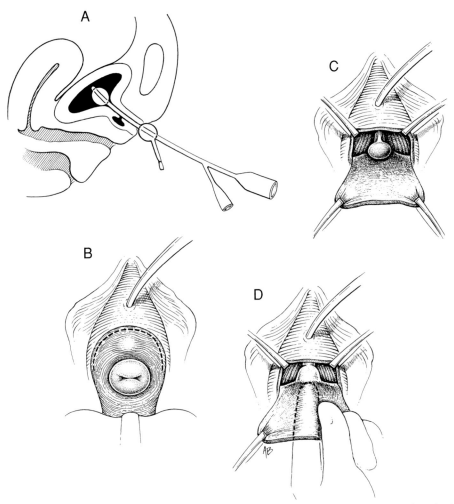

Figure 18.2. Excision of urethral diverticulum. **A.** Sagittal section shows a midurethral diverticulum. A double-ballooned catheter is in place, and the urethra and diverticulum are filled with a colored solution. **B.** The double-balloon catheter is then removed and replaced by a transurethral no. 12 silicone-coated Foley catheter and its bulb inflated. An inverted U-shaped incision is made in the anterior vaginal wall (*broken line*). **C.** Traction to some Allis clamps folds the flap during sharp dissection toward the surgeon, exposing the diverticulum. **D.** Stretching the vagina over the operator's finger aids in the usually difficult dissection. The diverticulum is removed and the ostium closed using 4-0 PGA suture. If the diverticulum is opened, the fenestration is enlarged sufficiently to admit the surgeon's finger, after any stones have been removed, and the remainder of the diverticular sac is carefully dissected from the surrounding scar tissue and excised. The anterior vaginal wall is replaced and the incision closed using interrupted stitches (I). The vagina is packed overnight. Catheter drainage will be maintained for 7 to 10 days.

repair with the full uninterrupted thickness of the vagina. Lee (6) emphasizes that similar security can be achieved by a vest-over-pants lapping closure to avoid superimposed suture lines (see Fig. 19.17). If upon dissecting the sac of the diverticulum upward and laterally it may be found that the diverticulum originates from the anterior surface of the urethra, the diverticulum is excised and the neck of the diverticulum transected and permitted to retract with no attempt to close the defect in the urethra, as suggested by Lee.

The desirability of a postoperative suprapubic cystotomy for diverting urine away from the recently repaired defect in the urethra can depend on the number of ostia that have been identified and repaired, as well as their proximity to the vesical neck.

URINARY FISTULAS: SUPRAPUBIC CYSTOSTOMY

There is only a small risk of unwanted penetration of nearby organs by the tip of the introducing forceps when the blind method of suprapubic cystostomy is employed. Although not required, we recommend that this method be performed at the beginning of the operation rather than at the end, so as not to chance disruption of the repair that has been completed. A Bozeman uterine dressing forceps is inserted through the urethra into the bladder (Fig. 18.3). The tip of the forceps is then directed anteriorly against the

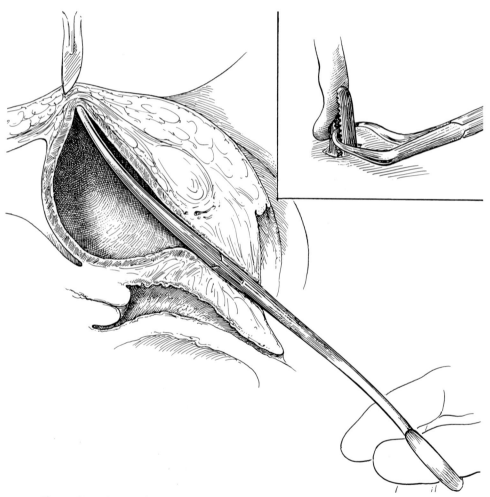

Figure 18.3. Suprapubic cystostomy. Before repair of the anterior vaginal wall, Bozeman uterine dressing forceps with the tips directed to the anterior abdominal wall can be inserted through the urethra into the bladder, which is distended with 300 ml of sterile saline. When the tip of the forceps can be palpated, a 1-cm skin incision is made over the tip. The forceps are advanced and opened slightly with a towel clip (*inset*) sufficiently to grasp the end of a Foley catheter. As the forceps are withdrawn the catheter is pulled into the bladder, where the Foley bulb is inflated; the uterine dressing forceps are removed. A temporary second transurethral splinting Foley catheter may be inserted later to help identify the vesical neck and urethra, but such a splinting catheter should be removed after the repair.

abdominal wall until it can be palpated suprapubically beneath the skin, at which point a small incision is made through the skin, underlying extraperitoneal tissues, and bladder wall to expose the tip of the forceps. The forceps are then pushed further through this incision until the tip appears outside the abdomen. The tip is spread slightly, sufficiently to grasp the tip of a Foley catheter. As the forceps are withdrawn, the Foley catheter is pulled into the bladder, after which the bulb is inflated. The dressing forceps are promptly removed so that the operation may proceed as originally planned.

Alternatively, a transabdominal suprapubic cystostomy can be performed if the bladder can be distended with 300 to 500 ml of saline, lessening the chance of an unwanted penetration into the peritoneal cavity (Fig. 18.4).

URETHROVAGINAL FISTULAS

Urethrovaginal fistulas present special problems in repair that Keettel et al. (4) have identified:

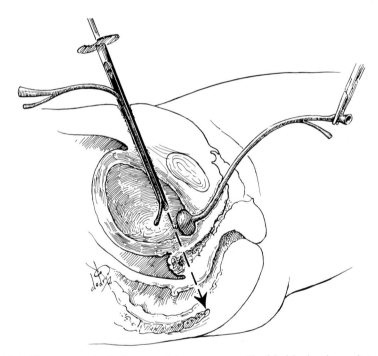

Figure 18.4. Alternate method of suprapubic cystostomy. The bladder has been distended by 400 ml of sterile saline solution instilled through a transurethral Foley catheter, shown in place and clamped. At a midline point two finger breadths above the superior border of the pubis, a no. 22 spinal needle is introduced through the anterior abdominal and bladder wall and pointed toward the coccyx. When a free flow of clear urine has been observed, the needle is immediately removed and a 1.5-cm transverse incision is made through only the skin using a no. 12 scalpel blade at the site of the needle puncture. The operator, having noted the approximate depth at which the spinal needle entered the bladder, bluntly introduces the Campbell-type trocar in the same direction until the characteristic "give" is noted. The sharply pointed obturator of the trocar is withdrawn about an inch, the blunt end of the sleeve is inserted an additional inch or two, and the obturator is removed. There is prompt escape of urine and saline, and immediately a no. 16 Foley catheter is inserted through the trocar into the bladder as shown. The 5-ml bulb is inflated, the trocar is removed, and a brief tug on the catheter until resistance is encountered brings the now inflated bulb to the undersurface of the fresh cystostomy. (From Nichols DH, Milley PS. A simplified technique for suprapubic cystostomy. Ob/Gyn Digest 1970;12:30–35. Used with permission.)

1. Extensive urethral damage
2. Involvement of the vesicourethral junction
3. Extensive scarring
4. Often insufficient tissue for a second-layer closure

A fistula involving the middle or lower third of the urethra may not produce incontinence, but the fistulous opening permits urine to be discharged into the vagina at the time of urination. There will likely be an unpleasant uriniferous odor in the vagina, and the postmicturition dribbling from the vagina is certain to have been noticed. Openings that develop in the upper third of the urethra, closer to the vesical neck, are likely to be associated with either intermittent or, at times, total urinary incontinence, mainly dependent upon the extent to which a functionally sphincterlike tone has or has not been maintained (5).

An asymptomatic urethrovaginal fistula may occasionally be found on routine pelvic examination, perhaps to the surprise of the examining physician as well as the patient. Such a fistula may have been accounting for no discernible or troublesome complaint, and it need not be repaired if unassociated with chronic urinary infection, not responsible for an unpredictable stream when voiding, and unaccompanied by evidence of neoplasia. When the history suggests, or there is record of a previous operation for excision or drainage of a urethral diverticulum or suburethral abscess, the site and origin of a urethral fistula are immediately suspect. When the fistula is associated with a chronic bloody vaginal discharge or hematuria, however, the possibility of malignant disease must be the first considered, and appropriate biopsy must be taken before surgical reconstruction is considered. Urethroscopy and cystoscopy should be included in the investigation, and, during surgery, areas of hard tissue found not to represent calculus formation should be promptly biopsied and submitted for immediate tissue diagnosis.

When biopsy of the urethra or adjacent tissue is reported to indicate invasive malignant disease, treatment should be that appropriate for the malignancy and will usually involve radiation and/or surgery, the details of which are beyond the scope of this discussion.

When a fistula indicates surgical reconstruction of the urethra, the choice of operative procedure should be determined by the need for restoration or improvement in function. Consideration of involuntary urinary incontinence, whether continual or intermittent, is of paramount importance.

When reconstruction of a major portion of the urethra is required, the technique described by Symmonds and Hill (11) is valuable and should be accomplished over a catheter stent (Fig. 18.5). A subsequent suprapubic vesicourethral sling may be necessary to establish continence after total urethral reconstruction (see Chapter 17).

If incontinence is not a consideration, the surgeon should first mobilize the urethra, undercutting the wall of the vagina to the extent necessary to permit excision of the fistulous track and closure of the defect without tension. Alternately, the fistulous opening may be inverted into the urethral lumen without excision of the track as long as the subepithelial connective tissues of the urethra can be approximated without tension, using interrupted fine absorbable sutures. Such a defect should usually be closed transversely to avoid or minimize the postoperative urethral stricture. Repair should be accomplished with a catheter in the urethra. The site of repair may be insulated from the vaginal incision by the vaginal flap technique (3), as described in Chapter 19.

The repair of a fistula at or near the vesical neck often requires a special technique. After preliminary infiltration with dilute lidocaine-epinephrine solution and insertion of a transurethral Foley catheter, an inverted U-shaped incision is made through the full thickness of the anterior vaginal wall. The vaginal wall is carefully reflected by sharp dissection to expose the full length of the fistulous tract, and the dissection is carried around and cranial to the fistula (Fig. 18.6A). The tract is excised from the wall of the urethra or

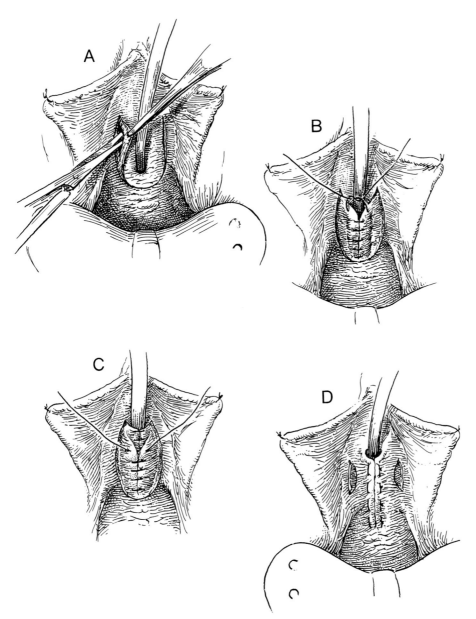

Figure 18.5. Construction of a neourethra. The labia minora have been stitched out of the way to improve the operative exposure, and a Foley catheter has been inserted into the bladder. The tissues to be mobilized may be infiltrated by epinephrine-lidocaine solution to reduce blood loss. **A.** A U-shaped incision is made. **B.** The flap is undermined medially so that the medial margins of the incision may be joined together in the midline, surrounding the catheter. **C.** A second layer approximates the subepithelial connective tissue. **D.** The lateral incisional margins are brought together by a series of interrupted mattress stitches. Any tension on the suture line is relieved by lateral relaxing incisions as shown. In a sense, this operation is a miniaturized counterpart of the Williams vulvovaginoplasty (see Chapters 20 and 21). Placement of a fascia lata vesicourethral sling as a future procedure may be required to establish continence (see Chapter 17).

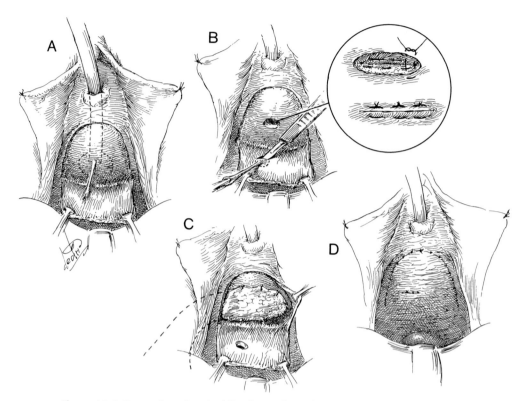

Figure 18.6. Correction of vaginal fistula involving the proximal urethra at the bladder neck. Bladder drainage may have been conveniently obtained by suprapubic cystostomy and a separate transurethral Foley catheter insertion. **A.** An inverted U-shaped incision is made in the anterior wall at the hymenal margin from the 8 o'clock position on the patient's right to the 4 o'clock position on the patient's left, and the cut edges of the vagina are grasped with Allis forceps. **B.** By sharp and blunt dissection, the full thickness of the anterior vaginal wall is separated from the underlying connective tissue and displaced posteriorly. This mobilization continues around the fistula until the neck has been mobilized 1.5 to 2 cm in all directions, after which only the tract is excised, as shown. If located at the vesical neck, the surroulized 1.5 to 2 cm in all directions, after which only the tract is excised, as shown. If located at the vesical neck, the surrounding bladder muscle will retract to some extent, and the vesicourethral opening of the fistula will appear even larger than the original vaginal opening. No sutures penetrate the bladder lining, and no knots are tied within the bladder. The submucosal connective tissue around the fistula is closed transversely with a running horizontal mattress stitch of 3-0 PGA absorbable suture material reinforced by a second layer of interrupted mattress stitches (*inset*). Transverse closure in this area reunites the vesical and urethral portions of the trigone and, by its direction, lessens the chance of postoperative stricture. **C.** It is often desirable to reinforce this repair with an additional layer of living tissue from either a pubococcygeus muscle transplant or a bulbocavernosus fat pad transplant, as described in Chapters 12 and 19. **D.** The inverted U-shaped incision in the anterior and lateral vaginal wall is closed with interrupted sutures, any episiotomy or Schuchardt incision is repaired, and the vagina is lightly packed for 24 hours. If the bladder is to be drained by suprapubic cystostomy, the transurethral catheter may be removed to avoid any subsequent contact between the catheter and the vesicourethral side of the fistula repair.

bladder neck, as well as from the vagina (Fig. 18.6B). The urinary defect is closed by a deep layer of running mattress suture of fine absorbable suture (3-0 polyglycolic [PGA]) and a superficial layer of interrupted mattress sutures of the same material (Fig. 18.6B, *inset*). A bulbocavernosus fat pad may be transplanted to insulate the bladder or urethral repair from the vagina (Fig. 18.6C). The incision in the anterior vaginal wall is closed by interrupted sutures and the vagina packed overnight with iodoform gauze. The transurethral Foley catheter is removed in favor of 7 to 10 days of postoperative suprapubic catheter drainage to keep the catheter away from the site of the repair.

MARTIUS BULBOCAVERNOSUS FAT PAD TRANSPLANT

This tissue has been employed as a means of bolstering the vesicourethral junction, but, because it contains a large amount of fat, the tissues are physiologically inert. We have elected to use this technique principally to reinforce a fistula repair (Fig. 18.7) by interposing a layer of living tissue and its new blood supply between the sites of repair in adjacent organs.

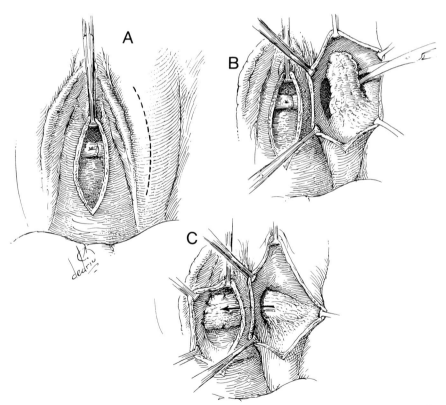

Figure 18.7. The bulbocavernosus fat pad transplant. **A.** A longitudinal incision is made to the central position of the left labia majora in the site shown by the *dashed line*. **B.** By sharp dissection, a thumb-thick pedicle of fat and bulbocavernosus muscle is freed from all but its inferior attachment. **C.** A tunnel is established beneath the vulvar and vaginal skin, and the freed margin of the pedicle is brought through the tunnel without constriction and sewn to the undersurface of the vaginal flap of the opposite side.

When incontinence due to vesical neck incompetence coincident with fistula repair is expected, some additional supplementation or reinforcement of the tissues beneath the vesicourethral unction should be considered, either simultaneous with the primary repair or as a future secondary procedure. The pubococcygeus muscle transplant (see Chapter 10) will provide the security of intermittent striated muscle contraction. This seems to offer an advantage over the Martius bulbocavernosus fat pad translocation in this situation because, although the latter brings additional blood supply into the area and bolsters the suburethral connective tissue, it does not provide for any eventual contribution to sphincteric contraction. Lateral vaginal relaxing incisions in a sagittal plane (see Fig. 20.5) may be necessary to avoid tension in a new suburethral suture line. Both local and systemic estrogen therapy, preferably started before surgery, may be helpful in the healing of the vaginal wound of a postmenopausal patient.

References

1. Asmussen M, Miller A. Clinical gynaecological urology. Oxford: Blackwell Scientific Publications, 1983:172–175.
2. Bhatia NN, McCarthy TA, Ostergard D. Urethral diverticula: urethral closure pressure profile. In: Zinner NR, Sterling AM, eds. Female incontinence. New York: Alan R Liss, 1981:239–242.
3. Judd GE, Marshall JR. Repair of urethral diverticulum or vesicovaginal fistula by vaginal flap technique. Obstet Gynecol 1976;47:627–629.
4. Keettel WC, Sehring FG, deProsse CA, et al. Surgical management of urethrovaginal and vesicovaginal fistulas. Am J Obstet Gynecol 1978;131:425–431.
5. Kunz J. Urological complications in gynecological surgery and radiotherapy. Basel: S Karger, 1984:73–74.
6. Lee RA. Atlas of gynecologic surgery. Philadelphia: WB Saunders, 1992:269–272.
7. Lee RA. The repair of urethral injuries, diverticula, and fistula. In: Nichols DH, ed. Gynecologic and obstetric surgery. St. Louis: Mosby-Yearbook, 1993.
8. Spence HM, Duckett JW Jr. Diverticulum of the female urethra: clinical aspects and presentation of a simple operative technique for cure. J Urol 1970;104:432–437.
9. Spraitz AF, Welch JS. Diverticulum of the urethra. In: 1964–1965 collected papers in surgery from the Mayo Clinic and the Mayo Foundation. Philadelphia: WB Saunders,1965;56:195–198.
10. Summitt RL Jr, Stovall TG. Urethral diverticula: evaluation by urethral pressure profilometry, cystourethroscopy, and the voiding cystourethrogram. Obstet Gynecol 1992;80:695–699.
11. Symmonds RE, Hill M. Loss of the urethra: a report on 50 patients. Am J Obstet Gynecol 1978; 130:130–138.
12. Tancer ML, Hyman R. Suburethral diverticulitis in the female. Am J Obstet Gynecol 1962; 84:1853–1858.

CHAPTER 19

Vesicovaginal and Other Urogenital Fistulas

The various sites of the urogenital fistulas are seen in Figure 19.1. Fistulas involving the female genitalia may be the result of trauma, necrosis secondary to invasion by neoplastic growth, or, rarely, the reaction to certain types of necrotizing inflammation. Genital tract trauma is by far the most common cause.

Unrecognized or unrepaired full-thickness trauma involving the urinary or the intestinal system will usually result in fistula formation, which explains the necessity of immediately recognizing unexpected penetration of a neighboring viscus at the time of any gynecologic operation or obstetric procedure. The presence of a *small* amount of urine in the bladder is desirable at the time of vaginal hysterectomy or anterior colporrhaphy, because its appearance in the operative field will usually alert the surgeon to the likelihood of a penetrating injury. When such an injury is even suspected, the question must be answered and an appropriate repair accomplished without delay. The incidence of accidental penetration is small and becomes smaller as the experience of the operator increases. Nevertheless, accidental injuries due to unexpected relationships will occur occasionally with every surgeon, whether he or she operates occasionally or frequently. The techniques of repairing fresh injury and the postoperative management of such repair are considered in detail in Chapter 22.

VESICOVAGINAL FISTULA

Lee (15) has correctly stated, "A vesicovaginal fistula with its constant odorous, scalding, unimpeded leakage of urine is one of the most devastating surgical complications that occur in women." This type of urinary fistula is likely to develop as a result of unrecognized or inadequately repaired sites of trauma. A history of previous low cervical cesarean section is a predisposing factor during hysterectomy because of the altered tissue relationships between the bladder and cervix. It is important to remember that a history of previous cesarean section will be present in about 20 percent of the present generation of parous patients requiring hysterectomy in the future. Preoperative intravesical instillation of 60 ml of indigo carmine or methylene blue solution is especially helpful when operating on the patient with a history of previous cesarean section. Not only can the violet-stained bladder mucosa be sometimes seen *before* it might be opened, but violet-stained urine in the operative field is evidence of unwanted penetration.

When vesicovaginal fistula follows hysterectomy, it is likely to be located at the very apex of the vagina if the vaginal cuff was not closed, or just anterior to the suture line if it was. Vesicovaginal fistula in the lower vagina is more likely to follow previous colporrhaphy or as a complication of labor and delivery.

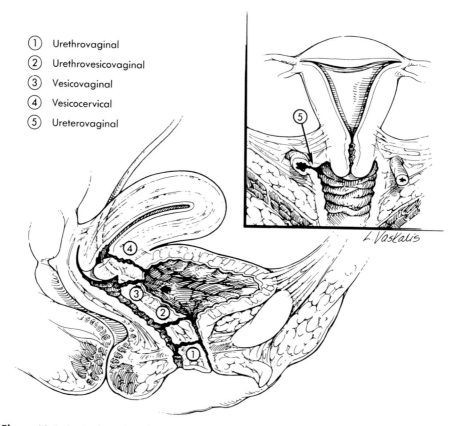

1. Urethrovaginal
2. Urethrovesicovaginal
3. Vesicovaginal
4. Vesicocervical
5. Ureterovaginal

L. Vaskalis

Figure 19.1. Sagittal section showing the various sites of the more frequently seen urogenital fistulas. A combination of fistulas is possible, and the tracts may course through several structures. One or more fistulas may exist at the same time. (From Nichols DH: Gynecologic and obstetric surgery St. Louis, Mosby-Year Book, 1993. Used with permission.)

Vesicovaginal fistula rarely may be seen from erosion through the anterior vaginal wall and bladder wall by a long-standing, forgotten, or neglected intravaginal pessary. Temporary pessary use is often desirable in elderly patients with genital prolapse. However, although generally used as a temporary medium of pelvic support for patients awaiting surgery, a pessary can be dangerous if it is forgotten for a long period of time (8). Such a fistula can be repaired promptly if examination shows that the fistula borders are neither macerated nor infected.

A fistula first recognized after hysterectomy is usually the result of an unrecognized penetration or laceration at the time of the primary operative procedure, the result of trauma recognized but inadequately repaired, or perhaps the result of postoperative necrosis of a small area of bladder epithelium secondary to an infected hematoma or to devascularization by a suture placed into or immediately adjacent to the lumen of the bladder. Carelessly placed hemostatic mattress sutures in the bladder wall near the cut edge of the vagina may devitalize the spot of tissue in which they have been placed. Incomplete surgical separation of the bladder from the vaginal cuff during hysterectomy will place it at risk.

The presence of unsuspected postoperative hematuria after the initial operative procedure should alert the operator to the possibility of a later fistula, particularly when bloody urine persists longer than the first 48 postoperative hours. Inspection by cystoscopy is then desirable, and catheter drainage should usually be prolonged for a number of days beyond the usual period. When a fistulous tract, even though small, is relatively short, incontinence is the rule. When the tract is longer, and particularly when tortuous, incontinence is likely to be intermittent because the flow of urine through the tract may be inversely proportional to the amount of urine within the bladder. This type of intermittent incontinence seems especially prone to infection and calculus formation along the tract.

The presence of an intermittent, spontaneous, bloody urethral or urinary discharge is particularly ominous, and when present, the coexistence of malignant disease relating to the fistulous tract must be evaluated by adequate study and biopsy, followed when indicated by treatment appropriate to the malignant disease.

The possibility of multiple fistulas must always be considered during the investigation of any patient with a recognized fistula. Should an additional tract escape recognition, an apparently successful surgical correction of the one recognized fistula will in no way eliminate a continued incontinence resulting from an unrepaired coexistent fistula, leading both operator and patient to suspect a treatment failure when, in fact, the failure may not have been due to the treatment but rather to the inadequacy of the preoperative study and appraisal. Careful review of the history and circumstances preceding recognition of a fistula is always indicated.

The differentiation between a vesicovaginal and a ureterovaginal fistula is of prime importance. In making this distinction, the tampon test (17, 24) is helpful and may be performed as follows. The operator injects 6 to 8 ounces of strongly colored methylene blue or indigo carmine solution into the bladder and then inserts a rather long menstrual tampon in the vagina. The patient is instructed to walk about for 10 or 15 minutes, after which the tampon is examined. If the lowest part alone is wet and blue, the patient presumably suffers from stress incontinence of urine or detrusor instability. If the upper thirds are wet and blue, the indication is a vesicovaginal fistula; if the upper third is wet but not blue, the diagnosis is of a damaged ureter.

There are several excellent techniques of repair, adaptable to a variety of clinical circumstances, but we will consider those that seem most applicable to the women seen in urban communities and in whom coexistent neoplastic disease of the pelvis has been excluded. In younger patients with a history of urinary loss, particularly when there is evidence of congenital malformation in the genitalia, thorough inspection of the urinary as well as the genital tract is indicated. Intravenous pyelography may be the only way an aberrant or third ureter opening into the vagina will be demonstrated. It is equally important to know whether the urinary fistula patient has bilateral ureteral patency with two normally placed ureters, or perhaps only a single kidney and ureter. This latter situation should certainly be known to the operator before the repair of a urinary fistula is planned or undertaken. The relationship of a fistula to the ureteral orifices, bladder neck, and trigone should be studied by preoperative cystoscopy. The operative preparation of the patient should therefore include a pyelogram as well as cystoscopic investigation.

Electrosurgical or chemical cautery of a very small fistulous opening has been recommended by others (6) from time to time on the basis and with the hope that coagulation will destroy the epithelial lining of the tract and may be effective in permitting spontaneous healing in a small percentage of cases of tiny fistula. It is followed by immediate decompression of the bladder by constant drainage for 2 to 3 weeks, and is most likely to succeed when the fistula is only 1 or 2 mm in diameter, follows an oblique course, and exists with a thick, healthy bladder around the fistulous tract, as may be seen after an inadvertent stitch through the bladder wall.

TIMING OF FISTULA REPAIR

If the injury follows an obstetric laceration, a repair should be accomplished within 24 hours of the injury. If a fistula develops some days after hysterectomy or failure of a previous fistula repair, a usual interval of between 3 and 6 months, preferably the latter, should pass to permit adequate lymphatic drainage to return to the tissue and the infection, swelling, and edema of surgery to subside.

The timing for surgical repair remains controversial. If the leakage from the vagina occurs in the immediate postoperative period from the primary surgical procedure, one can assume that there was an injury consisting of either an unrecognized puncture or tear of the bladder that occurred during the procedure. Because the injury is less likely to have produced an extending area of necrosis of the bladder wall, healing following prompt repair would be more likely to occur. An intravenous pyelogram and a cystoscopy are necessary, however, to exclude the possibility of multiple fistulas, or of a coincident uretero-vaginal fistula (18). Clean, uncomplicated vesicovaginal fistulas can often be repaired as soon as they are diagnosed, providing that good operative exposure can be achieved. The surgeon should anticipate a high, but not total, rate of success.

A fistula that occurs later in the postoperative course may be the consequence of ischemia and necrosis of the bladder wall following hysterectomy, and bladder distention and its resulting ischemia may be a potential contributing factor. In this circumstance, it is well to insert a catheter in the bladder for decompression for about 6 weeks, during which time the necrotic tissue will slough and fresh granulation tissue will develop, thus defining the margin of healthy tissue. When viewed cystoscopically, the area around the fistula will at first be of a dusky gray color, frequently with exudate surrounding it. As healing progresses, the fistula will either close, or the margins will stand out amid the neighboring bladder tissue, which will assume a healthy pink appearance. In this circumstance it is better to wait about 3 months from the time of fistula diagnosis until repair is undertaken. Preoperative urine culture is appropriate with antibiotic coverage as indicated. Local vaginal estrogen cream may be used preoperatively to improve the vaginal tissue. If there is a history of carcinoma in this area, the patient should be examined with particular care and a biopsy of any hard or suspicious areas obtained preoperatively.

If the fistula appears after necrosis from irradiation, the vagina should be given effective estrogen supplementation and the repair postponed at least a year to permit the causative endarteritis obliterans to have ceased progression (27). When active malignancy has been excluded by biopsy of any suspicious area in the margin of the fistula, successful repair generally requires not only delicate handling and approximation of tissue, but also introduction of a new layer of tissue, bringing with it a new blood supply between the repair of the organs involved. If the labia are fleshy, one may use for this new layer a bulbocavernosus fat pad transplant including a patch of attached skin to cover the defect (24). If the labial tissues are atrophic, a nonirradiated graft of omentum, blood supply intact, may be brought down and sutured in place to provide the new blood supply and the necessary insulation (15, 27).

While awaiting repair, some temporary but socially welcome relief can be obtained by wearing a contraceptive diaphragm modified for the collection of body fluids by cementing a Foley catheter to a fenestration in the diaphragm and attaching the catheter to a leg bag (3, 4, 29) (Fig. 19.2). The resulting improvement will relieve the physician of some of the burden so often imposed by the patient anxious for a quick repair at a time when the condition of the tissues may not be favorable or optimal for surgical repair. We have had no experience with cortisone treatment to accelerate tissue preparation for surgery and prefer to wait the necessary time required for inflammation and edema to subside.

PRINCIPLES OF REPAIR

It is desirable to examine both sides of the fistulous tract in choosing the appropriate surgical procedure for the repair of a genital fistula. This will reveal information about the size of each aperture and will afford better opportunity to appraise edema, inflammation, scarring, fibrosis, and the possibility of multiple openings.

It is important to remember that a fistula has both a high-pressure and a low-pressure side, since material flows from the high-pressure to the low-pressure area and not vice versa. Since the bladder is the high-pressure area when dealing with a vesicovagi-

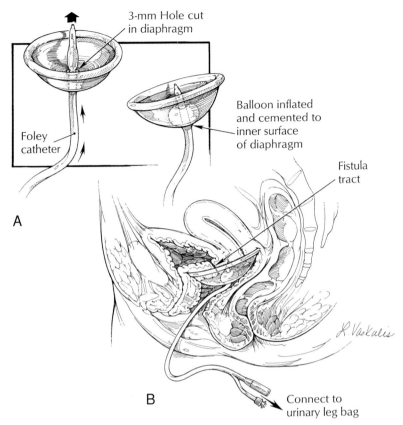

Figure 19.2. Modified diaphragm urine-collecting device. **A.** The tip of a Foley catheter has been placed through a 3-mm hole in the center of a contraceptive diaphragm as shown in the drawing to the upper left. **B.** The balloon has been inflated and cemented to the inner surface of the diaphragm. It is placed in the vagina, as shown in the sagittal section, and the Foley connected to a urinary leg bag.

nal fistula, it is essential for cure that the flow of urine be stopped at the high-pressure side. Closing the low-pressure or vaginal side, although very desirable, is of secondary importance.

Principles of urinary fistula repair include the following:

1. Postpone the repair until infection and inflammation have subsided and healthy granulation tissue is present.
2. Dissect, mobilize, and excise the epithelialized tract and adjacent scar tissue until healthy, normal tissue is reached, converting the lesion to a fresh wound. A fresh wound of bladder or rectum should heal promptly and primarily if initial repair is adequate and appropriate. The wound should be closed without tension.
3. Try to interrupt the continuity of the fistulous tract so that the orifice of repair in one viscus no longer overlies or underlies its counterpart.
4. Approximate anatomically strong layers or flaps and, when available, interpose between the previous fistulous orifices a strong layer of tissue with an independent blood supply.
5. When infection or abscess formation is likely, provide for adequate drainage of the low-pressure side of the previous tract.

6. Decompress the bladder postoperatively.
7. If the ureter is adjacent to or incorporated in the fistula, catheterize it at the time of the repair to avoid unintentional operative ureteral stricture; if it appears likely that it will be compromised by the repair, a coincident ureteroneocystostomy may be desirable.
8. Supplement or begin estrogen replacement pre- and postoperatively if the patient is postmenopausal.
9. Use lateral vaginal relaxing incisions if the repair has been closed under tension.

A few special instruments can be very helpful at the time of fistula repair, such as a pair of fine dissecting scissors, right-angled scissors, Sims hooks, and Sims or Breisky retractors. A small suction tip is desirable.

A variety of scalpel blades and handles should be available to the operator, particularly nos. 11 and 15 blades and the no. 7 scalpel handle. Knowledgeable, interested assistance at surgery can also be of great help, as will a flexible operative time schedule that permits the operator to employ as much surgical time as necessary for the particular reconstruction, because the length of an adequate operation is not always predictable.

Adequate exposure of the fistula is of paramount importance; and if for any reason this cannot be obtained with the exaggerated lithotomy position, an alternate choice would be the knee-chest position or even the jackknife or Kraske position, in which the patient is face down and the hips well flexed, the table being bent at this point with extra padding under the hips (Fig. 19.3). This will enable the operator to look directly down on the fistula (Fig. 19.4). Adequate, well-focused lighting is equally important, and at times the operator may find it advantageous to wear a forehead fiberoptic light to concentrate illumination and reduce annoying shadows.

Mobilization of a fistulous tract can be improved by insertion of a small or pediatric-sized Foley catheter (no. 8, 9, or 10) into the bladder through the fistula itself. When the bulb on the Foley is inflated, traction on the catheter serves as an identifying handle and

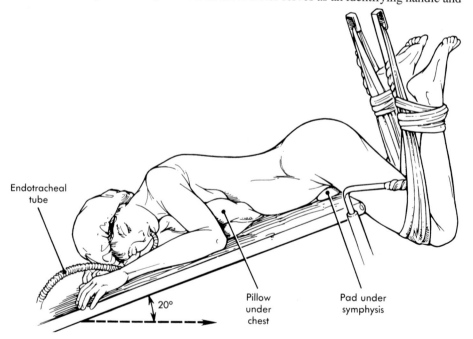

Endotracheal tube

20°

Pillow under chest

Pad under symphysis

Figure 19.3. The jackknife position. The prone position may improve the surgeon's view of the operative field when a vesicovaginal fistula is adherent to the pubic symphysis. (From Nichols DH: Gynecologic and Obstetric Surgery St. Louis, Mosby-Year Book, 1993.)

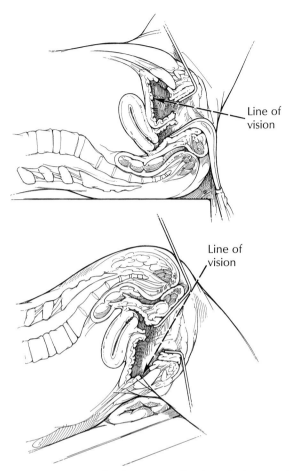

Figure 19.4. Visualization of a large fistula. **A.** Visualization of a large vesicovaginal fistula adherent to the pubic symphysis may be difficult when the patient is in the usual lithotomy position. **B.** It may be improved with the patient in the knee-chest position as shown in the drawing at the bottom.

permits traction to the fistula in all directions (11). If the fistulous opening is too small to permit the entry of a pediatric Foley catheter, the opening can be enlarged gently by spreading the tips of a small hemostat or inserting a small Hegar dilator. Infiltration of the area by dilute epinephrine-lidocaine solution offers hemostatic effect, and, by the local hemostatic effect, small sponges (wisps, pushers, or "peanuts") soaked in the solution of epinephrine often improve the surgeon's visibility, especially when the healthy mucosal tissue is being dissected and mobilized. There may be considerable oozing but few vessels are large enough to clamp and tie.

Most experienced gynecologic surgeons will repair vesicovaginal fistulas using a transvaginal approach, reserving the transabdominal route (18, 20, 25) for very unusual situations in which mobility is limited, the ureter is involved, there have been repeated previous failures, or sometimes when the fistula has developed in tissues previously irradiated. Moir (F.I.G.O. conference, 1978) was once asked why he preferred a transvaginal to a transabdominal exposure and replied, "If you were going to have your tonsils taken out, would you prefer they be removed through your mouth or through an incision in the side of your neck?" Käser, Iklé, and Hirsch have emphasized that no operation for fistula repair should be done routinely. The surgery should be adapted according to the conditions that prevail in a given case (13).

OPERATIVE TECHNIQUES

Latzko Technique

If the patient has a deep vagina and there is a posthysterectomy fistula located at the very apex of the vagina, the simplest and most effective operative repair will often involve the Latzko colpocleisis (14, 19, 22)(L Tancer, personal communication). This technique can be useful also for a small residual vault fistula remaining after previous closure of a larger fistula. The anatomy of a vesicovaginal fistula is seen in Figure 19.5. If any problem in exposure of the fistula is encountered, a preliminary episiotomy or Schuchardt-type incision (see Chapter 8) is strongly recommended to improve accessibility and ensure visibility of the fistula. Adequate exposure is an essential ingredient of a successful operative closure.

In this technique (Fig. 19.6), a 1.5 to 2 cm disk divided into quadrants and comprising the vaginal epithelium only is excised from around the fistulous opening. When approximated by suture, the collar will effectively close the area turned into the bladder lumen for vesical epithelialization. It is essential to have excised outward from the line of the initial incision a wide enough collar of vaginal membrane to ensure that the subepithelial connective tissue layer (vaginal wall denuded of epithelium by excision of the epithelial collar) can be brought together as a thickened supporting layer beneath the segment of vaginal membrane being invaginated into the bladder lumen (Fig. 19.6, A–C). The excised collar of vaginal epithelium should be ovoid rather than round, usually with the long axis of the ovoid transverse across the vault of the vagina to avoid constriction of vaginal caliber by the infolding of a portion of the former diameter of the vagina. When the depth of the vagina is likely to be more critical than the diameter, the long axis and repair of the denuded ovoid of connective tissue surrounding the invaginated segment of vaginal membrane can parallel the length rather than the width of the vagina. The sutures of the first layer should be so placed as to bring together the narrow layer of preserved vaginal wall surrounding the fistula in what should effectively serve as a subcuticular closure of the denuded segment of vaginal wall, precluding a postoperative bladder diverticulum (Fig. 19.6, D to F). To avoid tangling the sutures that have been placed but not yet tied, the free end pairs may be clamped in small hemostats, each handle of which is then placed over the free tip of a long hemostat whose handle has been clamped to the drape by two towel clips, as shown in Figures 19.7 and 19.8.

The watertightness of the repair may be observed by the instillation of sterile milk into the bladder, and any leakage must be promptly corrected. The best results will be achieved by observing the following: (*a*) Mobilization must be sufficient to permit

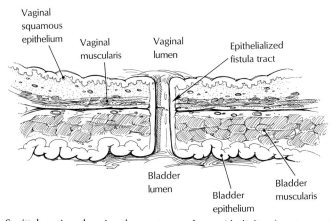

Figure 19.5. Sagittal section showing the anatomy of an epithelialized vesicovaginal fistula.

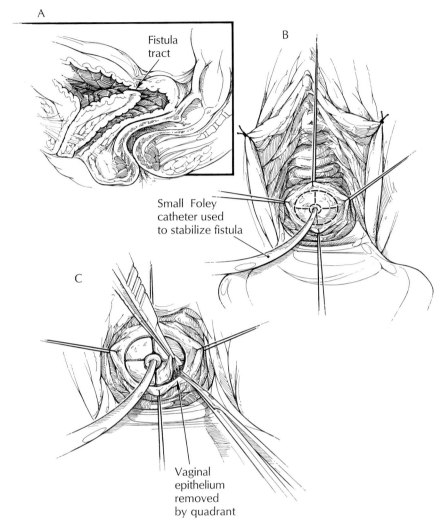

A

Fistula
tract

B

Small Foley
catheter used
to stabilize fistula

C

Vaginal
epithelium
removed
by quadrant

Figure 19.6. The Latzko procedure. **A.** Sagittal drawing of the pelvis shows a posthysterectomy vesicovaginal fistula at the vaginal vault. **B.** The fistula is exposed as shown. Note that the fistula is just anterior to the hysterectomy scar in the vault. Four guide sutures are placed, and a pediatric-sized Foley catheter is placed into the bladder through the fistula. One may enlarge the fistula to accommodate the catheter, if necessary, by spreading the tip of a fine-pointed hemostat in the fistula. The surrounding tissues may be infiltrated by a subepithelial liquid tourniquet. The vaginal epithelium to be excised surrounding the fistula is marked off in quadrants. **C.** Incisions are made through the vaginal wall. The separate removal of each quadrant is begun in the posterior half of the operative field. (*Continues on following page.*)

approximation of the supporting connective tissue layer with no tension and with no irregular buckling of the surfaces as they are brought together, obliterating the angle at each side of the vault. (*b*) No suture material should go into the lumen of the urinary tract or through both bladder and vaginal walls into the lumen of the vagina (Fig. 19.9).

Two or more additional layers of interrupted stitches are placed to coat the denuded vesical musculature, and the vaginal wall is closed with interrupted sutures. If it is desirable to not overlap the vaginal closure over the vesical suture line, as in repair of a

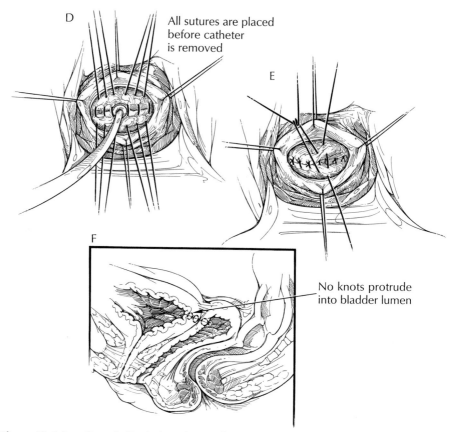

Figure 19.6 (continued). D. A deep layer of interrupted fine polyglycolic acid sutures is placed in a transverse axis. When all have been placed, the Foley catheter through the fistula is removed and the sutures tied. **E.** The watertightness of the suture line is tested and confirmed and a second layer of interrupted mattress sutures is placed. When all stitches have been inserted, each is tied, and a final layer of interrupted sutures is placed through the edges of the incision. **F.** The final result is shown in sagittal section in F. Note that no knots protrude into the bladder.

recurrent fistula, the modification of Hurd (10) (Figs. 19.10 and 19.11) is effective but requires some undermining of the vaginal wall through an area of dense scar tissue, shortening the vagina a bit more. If the bladder opening is too large to close from side to side without unusual tension, a flap of vaginal wall (28) may be transposed to cover the defect (Fig. 19.12).

Postoperatively, the bladder is usually decompressed by catheter drainage for 10 to 14 days, but generally the patient should be ambulated the day after surgery. The patient should take stool softeners for 2 to 3 weeks so that she can evacuate without straining.

The Latzko technique, when employed at the apex of the vagina, may shorten the vagina as much as an inch. Should the shortened vagina constitute a marital problem, a distal additional depth can be created using a Williams vulvovaginoplasty (Chapter 21). As with all postoperative care after any type of fistula repair, no coitus should be permitted for 2 postoperative months.

One might expect a 6 percent failure rate for the operation. If watertightness is not demonstrated at the conclusion of the operation, the stitches should be removed and the wound reapproximated as part of the same operation. If there is a failure, usually recognized promptly postoperatively, and the patient wishes re-repair, this can be done 2 or

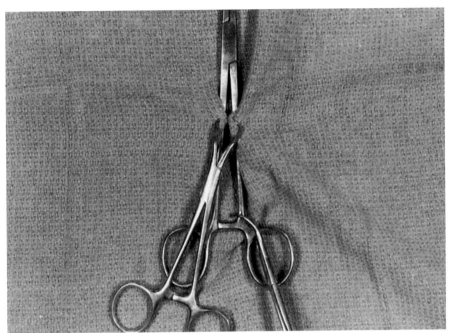

Figure 19.7. A method for keeping multiple sutures from becoming entangled before they have been tied. The handle of a straight hemostat is fixed by two pointed towel clips to the surgical drape as shown.

3 weeks later by taking down the repair and repeating the procedure, paying special attention to dissecting and repairing the lateral tissues of the wound.

Modern Sims Technique

Moir (17) reintroduced a modification of the standard Sims vaginal operation for repair of a vesicovaginal fistula, particularly for those distal to the vaginal apex. The operation does not shorten the vagina and has proved popular for many years.

A classic Sims repair is shown in Figure 19.13. Moir modified the classic Sims "saucerization" repair in two ways (17). In the first, he proposed an undercutting of the vaginal wall through the dense scar tissue that so often surrounds the fistula using a no. 11 scalpel blade or a right-angled scissors. This mobilizes just enough of the wall of the bladder to permit a deeper layer of interrupted mattress sutures which do not include the vesical mucosa. A layered closure is the second modification. The superficial or vaginal layer is of interrupted fine nylon mattress sutures that produce an eversion of the vaginal edge and that are left in place for a minimum of 21 days postoperatively. If there is any tendency toward tension in the closure of these suture layers, one or more vaginal relaxing incisions should be made. Moir has correctly emphasized that these sutures should be tied only tightly enough to approximate the tissue securely, but not so tight as to strangulate the tissue. The ends of any nonabsorbable sutures should be left long to facilitate their removal about the 21st postoperative day. At the time of removal, the patient is given a brief general anesthetic. Because vaginal vault exposure is difficult in most instances, a blunt hook is introduced under each suture (the tissue edema beneath having long since subsided), and the suture is cut with either the fine-pointed scalpel or the fine scissors just inside the knot so that the knot and deeper sutures can be removed

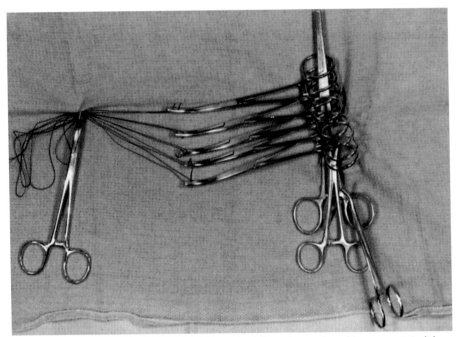

Figure 19.8. Pairs of the free ends of sutures (which have been placed but not yet tied) have been clipped to the ends of hemostats, the handles of which are threaded over the free end of the straight hemostat. The sutures do not become tangled before they have been tied. They are subsequently tied in the reverse order from which they had been placed.

easily. The surgeon carefully notes the number of stitches that are removed and compares them with the original operative report that describes that number that were placed so that none are left behind.

A Modern Sims Technique

After suitable exposure has been obtained, the margins of the fistulous tract, often quite vascular, may be injected or infiltrated by a few milliliters of 0.5 percent lidocaine in 1:200,000 epinephrine solution. A small Foley catheter is inserted through the fistula (enlarged if necessary by the tip of a small hemostat) into the bladder, and the bulb is inflated. Traction on the catheter will stabilize the position of the fistula and bring it closer to the operator (Fig. 19.14, *A* and *B*).

The circumference of the fistula is circumscribed by the point of the scalpel blade 1/2 to 1 cm from the edge of the fistula. A sagittal incision is made completely through the vaginal wall (but not into the bladder muscularis or cavity) for a distance of 1 cm superior and inferior to the fistula using a no. 11 taper-pointed Bard-Parker blade, and the vaginal wall is undercut about 1 cm along each side of the fistulous tract (Fig. 19.14, *C* to *E*). Undercutting is continued until the bladder adjacent to the fistulous tract is mobilized sufficiently to facilitate closure without tension.

A circular incision is made through the full thickness of the bladder wall, and the fistulous tract and Foley catheter are removed. Any remaining fibrous tissue is carefully excised to a point where normal tissue vascularity is apparent, because it is desirable to remove as much scar and fibrous tissue as possible in order to convert the edges of the defect to a state resembling a fresh operative wound. If necessary for hemostasis, the bladder mucosa is approximated with a layer of running 3-0 polyglycolic or chromic

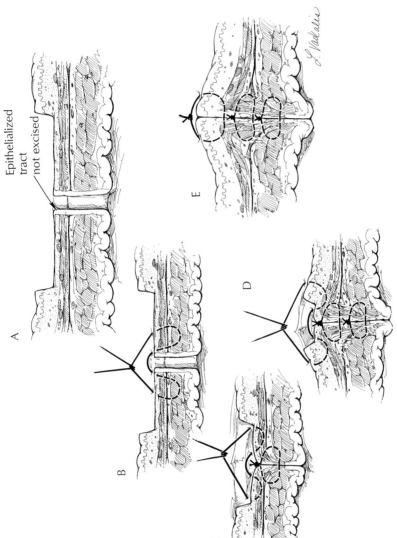

Figure 19.9. The Latzko repair as seen in cross-section. **A.** A small, deep layer of vaginal epithelium remains following excision of the four quadrants of vaginal epithelium surrounding the fistula site. **B.** The first layer of imbrication sutures is placed. **C** and **D.** After it has been tied, a second buried layer of sutures is placed and tied. **E.** The full-thickness of the covering wall is closed.

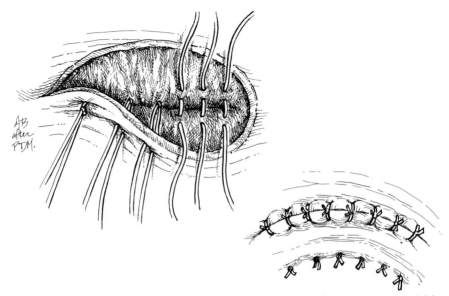

Figure 19.10. Hurd's alternate method of closing the vault (10). This method is useful for a recurrent fistula. The posterior vaginal wall margin has been undermined for 1.5 cm and the ends of the final reinforcing layer of stitches approximating the bladder wall are tied, reinserted through the full thickness of the vaginal wall as shown, and tied again to avoid overlapping of the closure of the bladder with that of the vagina. The edges of the vaginal incision are closed separately.

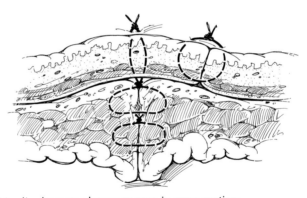

Figure 19.11. Hurd's alternate closure as seen in cross section.

suture, using a subcuticular stitch that inverts any exposed bladder mucosa into the lumen of the bladder (Fig. 19.14, *F* and *G*). The watertightness of the closure may be tested by instilling sterile milk or infant formula into the bladder, and additional sutures are inserted if necessary. If the cut edge of the vaginal incision appears ragged, torn, or suspiciously thin, it may be trimmed and the full thickness of the vaginal membrane closed from side to side with vertical mattress sutures of 2-0 monofilament nylon (Fig. 19.14, *H* and *I*). This second layer of closure takes much of the tension from the stitches of the first layer. All of these interrupted stitches are best placed and held before they are tied, and when tied, the operator should be certain to incorporate a double turn on the first cast of each knot followed by four additional casts of the suture to obviate postoperative slipping. The nonabsorbable sutures are removed on the 21st postoperative day.

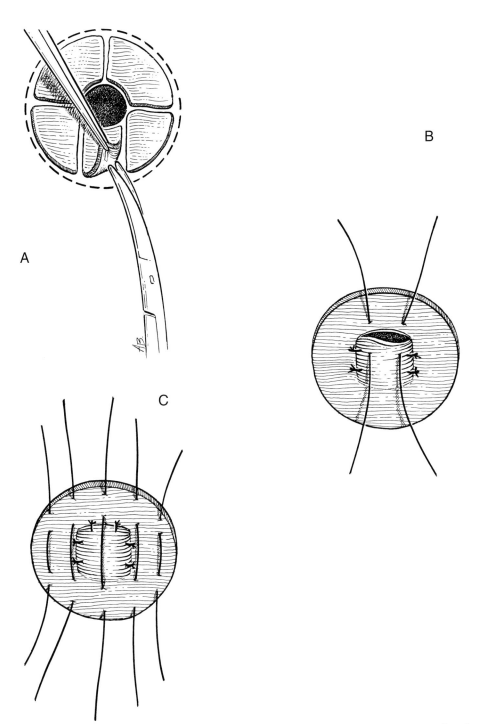

Figure 19.12. Ueda's (28) alternate method of closing a large fistula. **A.** The vaginal wall around the fistula is divided into five sections as shown. Four are removed, but the fifth, the width of the fistula, is developed as a flap. **B.** The vaginal flap is turned to cover the fistula and sewn in place by several interrupted sutures, sufficient to make the closure watertight. **C.** A second layer of sutures approximates the exposed tissues, and when these have been tied, the cut edges of the vagina are approximated by interrupted through-and-through sutures.

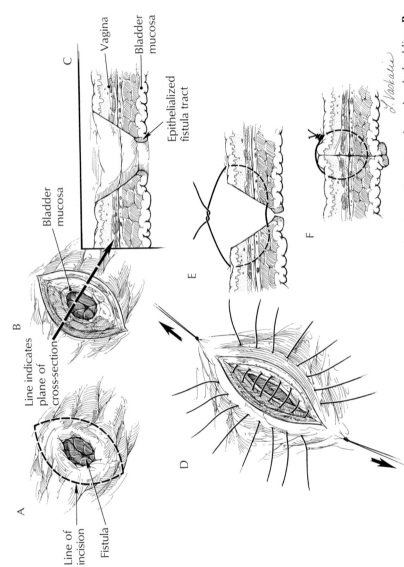

Figure 19.13. The Sims saucerization. **A.** The fistula is excised by sharp dissection along the *dashed line.* **B** and **C.** The dissection continues down to, but does not include, the bladder mucosa. **D** to **F.** The defect is closed by vertical nylon matress stitches.

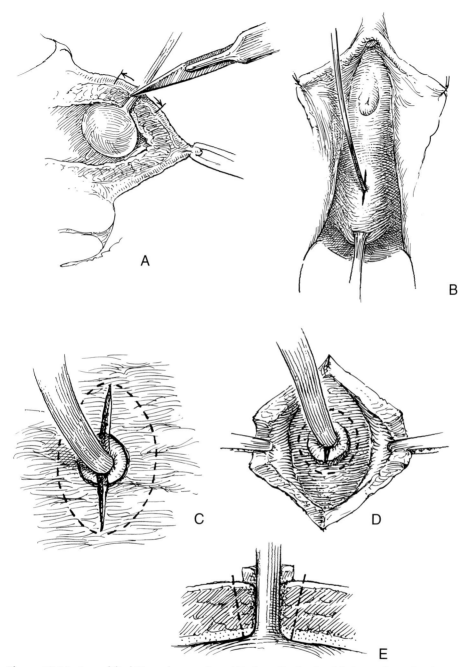

Figure 19.14. A modified Sims closure. **A** and **B.** A pediatric-sized Foley catheter has been inserted through the fistula and a linear incision made in the anterior vaginal wall. **C.** The fistulous tract is circumscribed by an incision (A) and the anterior vaginal wall undermined by sharp dissection to the limits indicated by the *broken line.* **D** and **E.** The flaps are mobilized (D) and the round segment containing the fistula and surrounding cicatrix excised along the pathway indicated by the *broken line* in D and E, leaving a circular defect in the bladder wall. (*Continues on following page.*)

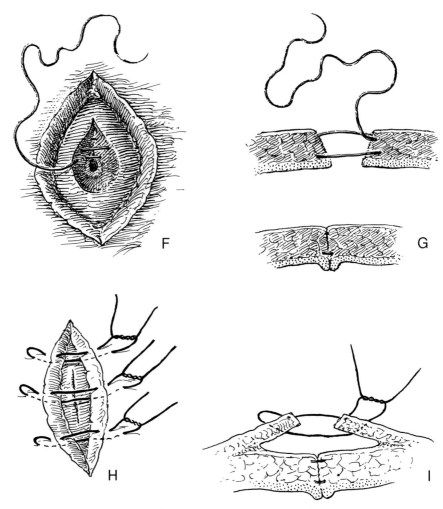

Figure 19.14 (continued). F and **G.** The muscularis of the bladder wall is reunited by a suture line of running or fine mattress sutures, with no knots protruding into the lumen of the bladder. If there has been sufficient mobilization and the bladder wall edges can be brought together without tension, the axis of bladder closure may be at right angles to that planned for the vagina. A second layer may be placed to insure watertightness. **H** and **I.** The vaginal wall is closed by interrupted vertical mattress sutures.

Full-thickness lateral vaginal relaxing incisions, as noted in Chapter 20, may be made to relieve any tension on the suture line, after which the vagina should be loosely packed with iodoform gauze for 48 hours. An indwelling catheter is inserted and constant drainage initiated to ensure bladder contraction for 10 days. If the patient is postmenopausal, both local and systemic estrogen should be administered through the postoperative period.

Futh Repair

The Futh repair is of particular value in the less common circumstance of a medium-sized vesicovaginal fistula in which the uterus is still present and the fistula is not too high in the vagina (Fig. 19.15*A*). It requires that the vaginal vault be mobile so that traction upon the cervix can bring the site of operative repair closer to the surgeon (13, 21).

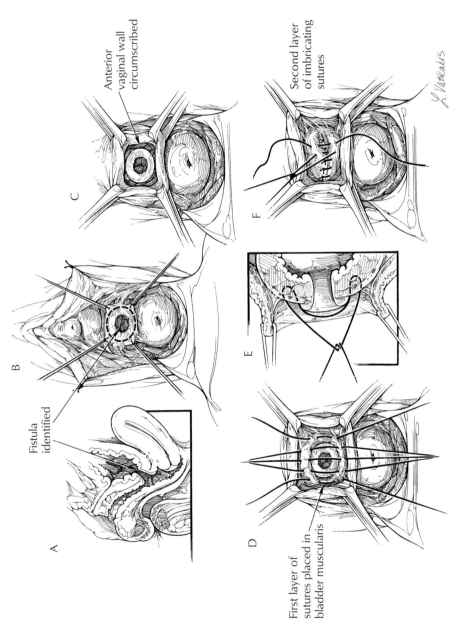

C

Anterior
vaginal wall
circumscribed

F

Second layer
of imbricating
sutures

B

Fistula
identified

E

D

First layer of
sutures placed in
bladder muscularis

Figure 19.15. The Futh repair of a vesicovaginal fistula. **A.** Sagittal section showing the location of the fistula in the anterior vaginal wall. **B.** The fistula is readily identified. **C.** A circular incision is made through the vaginal wall at least 1 cm lateral to the fistula, and the lateral vaginal wall is freed by undercutting its edges. **D** and **E.** A series of interrupted vertical mattress sutures is placed in the bladder muscularis. **F.** When these have been tied, a second layer is placed and tied. (*Continues on following page.*)

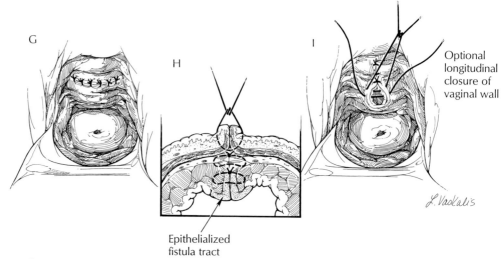

Figure 19.15 (continued). **G** and **H.** The vaginal wall may be closed transversely by a series of interrupted through-and-through sutures of polyglycolic acid sutures. Notice how the fistulous tract has become inverted into the vagina. **I.** If it would favor vaginal dimensions, the anterior wall may be closed longitudinally.

The labia minora are sewn out of the way to improve the operative exposure (Fig. 19.15*B*), and Allis clamps or four traction sutures are placed through the vaginal wall lateral to the site of fistula repair. The latter are not tied, but are held in hemostats. The tissues around the fistula are infiltrated by a liquid tourniquet (such as 1:200,000 epinephrine in 0.5 percent lidocaine), and using a no. 11 scalpel blade, the fistula is "circumcised" by an incision made 1 cm lateral to the margins of the fistula (Fig. 19.15*C*). The operator makes the incision in such a fashion that the vagina is undercut lateral to the button containing the fistula, being careful to avoid a buttonhole penetration of the bladder, which would complicate the repair considerably. Interrupted vertical mattress sutures of polyglycolic acid material are placed in the bladder muscularis about three-fourths ($\frac{3}{4}$) of a centimeter apart and tied after all have been placed (Fig. 19.15, *D* and *E*). A second layer of vertical mattress sutures is placed superficial to the first layer, imbricating it thoroughly (Fig. 19.15*F*). The vagina is then closed with a third layer of interrupted sutures placed either transversely or longitudinally, depending on the axis of the residual vagina (Fig. 19.15, *G* to *I*).

Bulbocavernosus Fat Pad Transplant

Reiffenstuhl (21) has suggested the option of interposing a Martius bulbocavernosus flap between the vagina and the most superficial layer of closure in the bladder muscularis (Fig. 19.16). This might be particularly applicable to the patient in whom the fistula is postmenopausal, has occurred in a field of pelvic radiation, or is recurrent.

Technique of Vaginal Lapping

For the larger vesicovaginal fistula, it is particularly important to adequately mobilize the vaginal wall from the bladder wall by a more extensive dissection so that one may interpose a significant layer of subcutaneous tissue between the sutures closing the bladder and those closing the defect in the vagina. When the vaginal wall is suitably redundant, a vaginal lapping technique emphasized by Aldridge (1) and Judd and

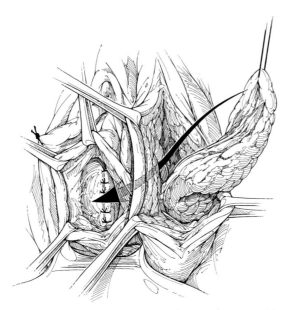

Figure 19.16. The bulbocavernosus fat pad transplant. A linear incision is made in the labium majora and a thick pedicle of bulbocavernosus muscle with its surrounding fat pad freed by sharp dissection. A wide attachment at its base is maintained to preserve its blood supply. A tunnel has been made beneath the skin, connecting with vesicovaginal space. The fat pad is gently led through this tunnel in the direction of the arrow and with no constriction to its blood supply. It will then be sewn to the underside of the vaginal wall of the opposite side, insulating the repair, and bringing a fresh blood supply into the area.

Marshall (12) may provide a useful means of insulation and reinforcement because it interposes an additional layer of supporting tissue between closure of the bladder wall and closure of the vaginal incision.

If a hysterectomy has been performed immediately preceding the operation to be described, the anterior vaginal vault has been already opened. The full thickness of the anterior vaginal wall may then be incised in the midline, creating an inverted T-shaped incision of the anterior half of the vaginal membrane. If no hysterectomy has been performed and none is to be performed, this incision (Fig. 19.17, *A* and *B*) is made through the full thickness of the anterior vaginal wall in the midline, entering the vesicovaginal space (see Chapter 10).

This incision should be deep enough to leave all vaginal fibromuscular connective tissue attached to the vaginal flap. Equivalent full-thickness vaginal flaps are developed by dissecting to the full lateral limit of the vesicovaginal space on each side. This mobilization is extended almost to the pubic ramus on each side.

The urogenital diaphragm containing the pubourethrovaginal ligaments is now identified and may be plicated beneath the vesicourethral junction (Chapter 10), but this plication suture should be tied and held long, rather than cut, to facilitate identification later in the procedure (Fig. 19.17, *C* and *D*). The connective tissue "capsule" of the bladder is then plicated to any degree that seems advisable, using 2-0 polyglycolic suture. Care must be taken to avoid tying these sutures too tightly to prevent tissue strangulation at the points of approximation. A satisfactory degree of plication should reduce the transverse diameter of the bladder wall that had been sagging into the vesicovaginal space and at the same time should thicken the bladder capsule and somewhat decrease future tension on the flap by limiting potential bladder expansion in this area.

The underlying fibromuscular layer of the right vaginal flap is then split from the vaginal epithelium (Fig. 19.17, *E* and *F*) to the lateral margins of the vesicovaginal space.

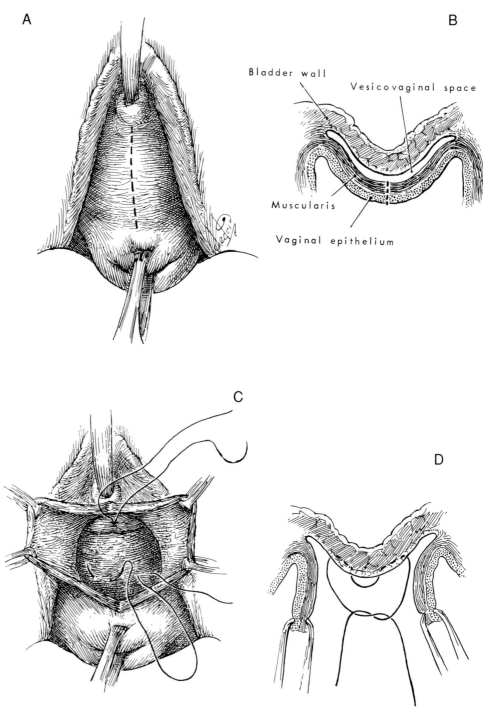

Figure 19.17. The vaginal lapping technique. **A** and **B.** An incision is made through the full length and full thickness of the anterior vaginal wall into the vesicovaginal space, as shown by the *dotted line.* **C** and **D.** The vaginal wall has been freed and retracted laterally, the pubourethrovaginal plication stitches have been placed and tied, and the bladder capsule is being plicated with interrupted sutures to reduce the transverse diameter of the vesicovaginal space and thus thicken the bladder capsule. (*Continues on pages 455–457.*)

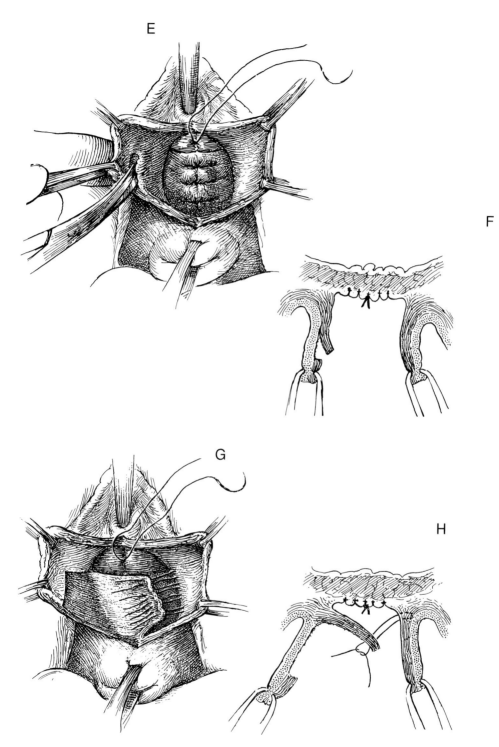

Figure 19.17 (continued). E and **F.** The fibromuscular layer of the right vaginal flap is dissected from the superficial vaginal skin as shown. **G** and **H.** The fibromuscular layer of the right vaginal flap is sewn to the undersurface of the unsplit left vaginal wall. (*Continues on following page.*)

Figure 19.17 (continued). I. The pubourethrovaginal "ligament" stitch is sewn to the undersurface of the vagina. **J** and **K.** The excess of the split right vaginal flap (*a*) is trimmed, as shown by the *broken line*. The fibromuscular layer of the right flap (*c*) is sewn to the undersurface of the unsplit left flap (*b*). (*Continues on following page.*)

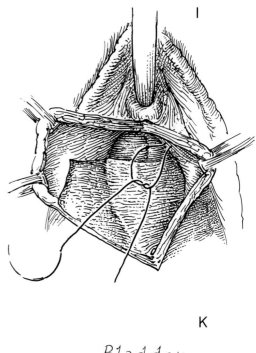

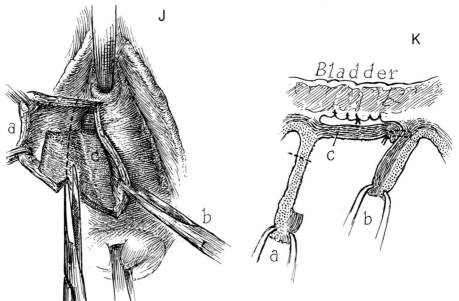

This line of cleavage should separate the musculoelastic layer of the vaginal wall from the overlying layer of vaginal epithelium. The vaginal flap of the left side is not similarly split, however, and all connective tissue should remain attached to the epithelial layer of the left flap of the vagina in order to preserve as much of its blood supply as possible.

The medial edge of the right inner vaginal or fibromuscular flap is sewn to the undersurface of the unsplit full-thickness flap of left vaginal wall, along the lateral extent of the vesicovaginal space, by a series of interrupted sutures of 2-0 polyglycolic suture (Fig. 19.17, *G* and *H*). Each untied suture is held loosely until all have been placed, and then all are tied.

The ends of the suture previously placed to shorten the pubourethrovaginal ligaments are sewn to the undersurface of the vaginal flap and again tied, but not too tightly, reestablishing fusion between the urogenital diaphragm and the vagina (Fig. 19.17*I*).

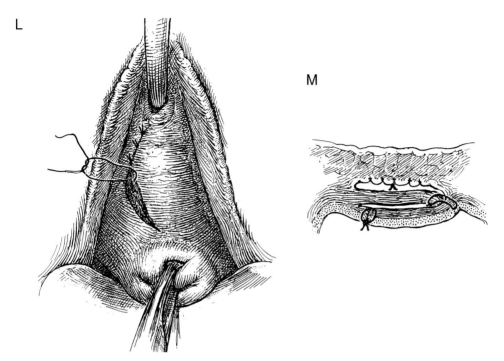

Figure 19.17. L and **M.** The full thickness of the left flap is sewn to the right.

An appropriate amount of the right epithelial covering layer of vaginal flap is then trimmed along the left lateral margin of the vesicovaginal space (Fig. 19.17, *J* and *K*), at which point the edges of the vaginal membrane again become adjacent and roughly parallel, overlying the now doubled fibromuscular tissue layers. Finally, the full thickness of the unsplit left vaginal flap should be attached along the cut edge of the right flap by a series of interrupted sutures of 2-0 polyglycolic suture (Fig. 19.17, *L* and *M*).

Leaving the vaginal muscularis attached to the epithelium on one side ensures preservation of its blood supply. The procedure, as described, effectively doubles the thickness of the subepithelial connective tissue layers of the anterior vaginal wall supporting the bladder.

Any significant damage or relaxation of the posterior vaginal wall and perineum should also be repaired. Postoperatively, it is advisable to place postmenopausal patients on estrogen with to improve the vascularity and wound healing in these estrogen-sensitive tissues.

An ingenious transvaginal repair has been described by Scott (23). The patient is upside down and in a jackknife position, the legs adducted. Using adequate retraction and many stay sutures, the fistula is exposed and the edges freshened (although the fistula is not excised) sufficiently to get rid of the epithelial surface of the fistula itself. The vagina is carefully separated from the bladder and undermined in all directions for about 1.5 to 2 cm from the fistula. Traction by sutures placed in the deeper layers of the fistula enables one to undermine the mucosa of the bladder until the mucosa is free. Bleeding is controlled by electrocautery when necessary. The tissues are closed in layers with either a pursestring technique using 000 polypropylene (Prolene) sutures or a running horizontal stitch. These sutures are placed as "pull-out" sutures that pierce the vagina and then run with a series of bites before they pierce the vagina again. The wound will close only as tension is applied to the suture. After the second or third layer of suture is in place, all are closed. The sutures are then threaded and tied over buttons and the vagina lightly packed. If drainage from the transurethral Foley catheter is without significant bloody component, transurethral drainage is used, but if the irrigation fluid return is grossly bloody, then a suprapubic drain may be placed. The sutures and buttons are removed on the 10th postoperative day and the indwelling catheter 1 day later. Scott believes that not closing the mucosa is important. His study with experimental animals has shown that stitches placed through the mucosa invite delayed healing and the likely recurrence of the fistula, whereas stitches placed beneath the mucosa are more likely to heal primarily.

The Ocejo Operation

Under rare circumstances, if unusual thinness of the anterior vaginal wall and preservation of full vaginal depth and width is strongly desired, the Ocejo modification of the Watkins-Wertheim interposition operation may be useful in patients in whom the uterus is still present. The modification championed by Gallo (7), in which the cervix is amputated and the endometrium is excised (Fig. 19.18) through a longitudinal incision in the anterior wall of the uterus, safely removes this future source of potential endometrial trouble or symptoms.

MASSIVE POSTOBSTETRIC VESICOVAGINAL FISTULA

Massive postobstetric vesicovaginal fistulas are rare in the Western world but not uncommon among the population of the rural areas of undeveloped countries like Africa (5, 9). Their repair requires most careful tissue dissection and approximation without tension, followed by appropriate postoperative bladder decompression during the healing phase. Postoperative vaginal strictures can sometimes be prevented by the use of a modified *myocutaneous* Martius bulbocavernosus graft, cut of a size to fill the vaginal defect, and sewn in place (Fig. 19.19) (16, 24).

VESICOUTERINE FISTULA

Vesicouterine or vesicocervical fistula with its accompanying incontinence is almost invariably the aftermath of a cesarean section at which the integrity of the bladder

Figure 19.18. Ocejo transposition operation. The uterine corpus may be transposed between the bladder and the vagina in certain cases of vesicovaginal fistula when the blood supply is poor. In Ocejo's (7) modification, the endometrium has been removed by sharp dissection and the cavity obliterated by sutures, as shown. An elongated cervix will have been amputated.

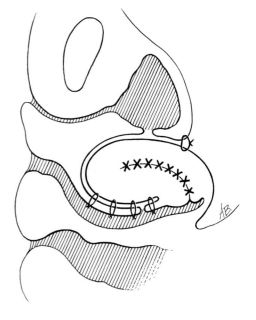

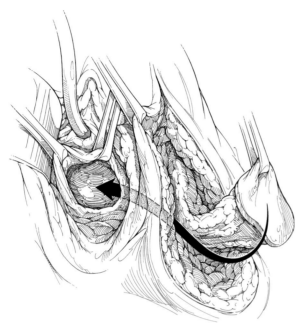

Figure 19.19. Myocutaneous bulbocavernosus transplant. When the defect in the vagina is of such size that its edges could not be approximated without tension and postoperative stenosis, a myocutaneous bulbocavernosus fat pad transplant can be accomplished as shown. A full-thickness labial skin incision has been made circumscribing a piece of labial skin of a size sufficient to fill the defect in the anterior vaginal wall. The underlying fat pad and bulbocavernosus are carefully mobilized, and a tunnel created by sharp and blunt dissection to unite the two incisions in the direction of the arrow and of a width sufficient to permit the myocutaneous flap to pass without compromising its blood supply. It has been sewn to the edges of the vaginal defect by a series of interrupted through-and-through sutures.

was compromised by a suture used in the repair of the uterine incision. It occasionally follows uterine rupture with precipitate labor (2). Surgery requires the anatomic dissection and separation of the bladder from the uterus at the site of the fistula, with freshening of the edges and separate repair of each organ using long-lasting absorbable suture. A period of not less than 10 days of postoperative catheter decompression of the bladder is desirable.

VESICOCERVICAL FISTULA

Urinary incontinence may not always be evident with vesicocervical fistula; and occasionally, the sole symptom will be menstrual hematuria, erroneously suggesting endometriosis of the bladder. In such instances, some valvelike arrangement due to a flap effect within a fistulous tract permits fluid to pass from the uterus to the bladder but not in the reverse direction.

POSTHOSPITALIZATION CARE FOLLOWING REPAIR OF VESICOVAGINAL FISTULA

The bladder is usually decompressed by catheter drainage for 2 weeks following discharge from the hospital. Attachment of the catheter to a leg bag will facilitate ambulation. Although the bladder that has been totally incontinent as a result of a vesicovaginal fistula for a number of years is usually capable of physiologic regeneration and restoration of function within a few weeks as the result of its long period of rest, after repair the patient should be expected at first to demonstrate a relatively small bladder capacity and should have been warned to expect a certain amount of urgency and need to empty her bladder frequently for the first few postoperative weeks following removal of the catheter, even during the night. It might be suggested that she set an alarm clock to arouse her for this purpose in order to avoid nocturnal bladder overdistention. Because primary healing is so very important, a fistula repair patient should be maintained on urinary antisepsis for several weeks from the time of surgery.

URETEROVAGINAL FISTULA

Although freshly damaged or transected ureters may be transvaginally reimplanted into the bladder at the time of the initial injury if the operator is familiar with the technique of repair (25, 26), the postoperative ureterovaginal fistula is most often approached through a transabdominal route, either for reconstruction or reimplantation. The related techniques cannot be included within the scope of this text.

References

1. Aldridge AH. Modern treatment for vesicovaginal fistula. J Obstet Gynaecol Br Emp 1953;60:1.
2. Al-Juburi A, Aloosi I, Khundra S. Unusual vesicocervical fistulas. J Obstet Gynaecol 1984;4:264.
3. Banfield PJ, Scott G, Roberts HR. A modified contraceptive diaphragm for relief of utero-vaginal fistula: a case report. Br J Obstet Gynaecol 1991;98:101.
4. Dotters DJ, Droegemueller W. Diaphragm catheters for vesicovaginal fistula management. Contemp Obstet-Gynecol Technology 1992 (special issue) 1992:45–46.
5. Elkins TE. Surgery for the obstetric vesicovaginal fistula: a review of 100 operations in 82 patients. Am J Obstet Gynecol 1994;170:1108–1120.
6. Falk HC, Orkin LA. Nonsurgical closure of vesicovaginal fistulas. Obstet Gynecol 1957;9:538–541.
7. Gallo D. Ocejo modification of interposition operation. In: Urologica Ginecologica. Guadalajara: Gallo, 1969.
8. Goldstein I, Wise GJ, Tancer ML. A vesicovaginal fistula and intravesical foreign body: a rare case of the forgotten pessary. Am J Obstet Gynecol 1990;163:589–591.
9. Hamlin R, Nicholson C, Zacharin R. Massive vesicovaginal fistula. In: Nichols DH, ed. Gynecologic and obstetric surgery. St. Louis: Mosby-Yearbook, 1993:869–880.
10. Hurd JK. Vaginal repair of vesicovaginal fistula. In: Libertino JA, Zinman L, eds. Reconstructire urologic surgery. Baltimore: Williams & Wilkins, 1977.
11. Janisch H, Palmrich AH, Pecherstorfer M. Selected urologic operations in gynecology. Berlin: Walter de Gruyter, 1979.
12. Judd GE, Marshall JR. Repair of urethral diverticulum or vesicovaginal fistula by vaginal flap technique. Am J Obstet Gynecol 1976;47:627–629.
13. Käser O, Iklé FA, Hirsch HA. Atlas of gynecologic surgery. 2nd ed. New York: Thieme-Stratton, 1985: 20.1–20.21, 1985.
14. Latzko W. Postoperative vesicovaginal fistulas. Am J Surg 1942;58:211–228.
15. Lee RA. Atlas of gynecologic surgery. Philadelphia: WB Saunders, 1992:280–291.
16. Margolis T, Elkins TE, Seffah J, Oparo-Addo HS, Fort D. Full thickness Martius grafts to preserve vaginal depth as an adjunct in the repair of large obstetric fistulas. Obstet Gynecol 1994;84:148–152.
17. Moir JC. The vesicovaginal fistula. London: Balliere, Tindall & Cassell, 1967.
18. Nanninga JB, O'Connor VJ Jr. Suprapubic repair of vesical vaginal fistula. In: Carlton SE Jr, ed. Controversies in urology. Chicago: Yearbook, 1989:176–180.
19. Nichols DH. Transvaginal repair of bladder injuries and of urogenital and vesicovaginal fistula. In: Nichols DH. Gynecologic and obstetric Surgery. St. Louis: Mosby-Yearbook, 1993:847–868.
20. O'Connor VJ Jr. Repair of vesicovaginal fistula with associated urethral loss. Surg Gynecol Obstet 1978;146:251–253.
21. Reiffenstuhl G, Platzer W. Atlas of vaginal surgery. Philadelphia: WB Saunders, 1975:668–681.
22. Robertson JR. Vesicovaginal fistulas. In: Slate WG, ed. Disorders of the female urethra and urinary incontinence. 2nd ed. Baltimore: Williams & Wilkins, 1982.
23. Scott FB. The case for vaginal repair of vesical vaginal fistula. In: Carlton CE Jr, ed. Controversies in urology. Chicago: Yearbook, 1989:180–189.
24. Symmonds RE. Incontinence: vesical and urethral fistulas. Clin Obstet Gynecol 1984;27:499–514.
25. Thompson JD. Transvaginal ureteral transection with vaginal hysterectomy and anterior colporrhaphy. In: Nichols DH, Delancey JOL, eds. Clinical problems, injuries and complications of gynecologic surgery. 3rd ed. Baltimore: Williams & Wilkins, 1995.

26. Thompson JD, Benigno BB. Vaginal repair of uteteral injuries. Am J Obstet Gynecol 1971;3:601.
27. Turner-Warwick R. The use of pedicle grafts in the repair of urinary tract fistulae. Br J Urol 1972;44:644.
28. Ueda T, Iwatsubo E, Osada Y, et al. Closure of a vesicovaginal fistula using a vaginal flap. J Urol 1978;119:742–743.
29. Wolff HD, Gililand NA. Vaginal diaphragm catheters. J Urol 1957;78:681.

CHAPTER 20

The Small Vagina

When the mature vagina cannot admit or contain one's sexual partner with comfort, there is a major threat to conjugal harmony. Disproportion in size is a frequent cause of pain and discomfort.

The etiology is varied, including such congenital deformities as absence of the vagina and uterus, absence of the lower half of the vagina, and obstructive transverse septa at any level, including an imperforate hymen. A longitudinal vaginal septum may exist with duplication of the birth canal, and the presence of a rudimentary uterine horn may produce dyspareunia as well as dysmenorrhea. Thick lateral bands connecting the external urethral meatus to the hymenal margin may be a source not only of dyspareunia but, by dragging upon the meatus during coitus, may invite recurrent postcoital cystitis (KG Cummings, RP Gibbons, RJ Correa, et al., scientific exhibit, American College of Obstetricians and Gynecologists, 1976).

Menopausal change may be a factor, especially when there has been pelvic irradiation or when the aging process has been accompanied by an unusual degree of progressive atrophy and shrinkage. The coital problem may be compounded by some relative flaccidity of the sexual organ of the marital partner, making vaginal penetration difficult.

Iatrogenic causes are significant and range from postepisiotomy scarring and discomfort to the posthysterectomy vagina that is too short, especially after radical surgery with partial vaginectomy. The vaginal diameter may be too narrow as a consequence of excessive subepithelial plication or excision of a more than adequate amount of vaginal membrane with colporrhaphy. Subepithelial ridges that have been produced become more tender as the fibrosis of postoperative scarring progresses.

Contributing psychosomatic factors must be added to the above, including fear of being hurt, the psychologic scarring after rape, the fear of becoming pregnant, fear based on lack of knowledge concerning sexual practices, and, to some, an unconscious or conscious desire to inflict punishment upon oneself or one's marital partner.

These factors may be etiologically grouped in any combination, and successful treatment requires identifying and paying proper attention to each contributing factor.

PRESERVING VAGINAL DEPTH

A hallmark of treatment is prevention. If the patient is postmenopausal, and particularly if there is sign of mucosal or vulvar atrophy, more or less permanent estrogen replacement will strengthen, restore, and preserve vaginal elasticity and blood supply in estrogen-sensitive pelvic tissues.

Proper techniques of either vaginal or abdominal hysterectomy, particularly when some degree of genital prolapse is present, require shortening of the elongated cardinal and uterosacral ligaments, which should be firmly attached to the vault of the vagina. When these ligaments are hypertrophic, the technique of culdeplasty (see Chapter 8) is useful in preserving or restoring vaginal length. In principle, this fixes the vaginal vault to the undersurface of strong uterosacral ligaments, which have been brought together behind the vagina, lessening any tendency toward enterocele formation. This technique can be used successfully with either vaginal or abdominal hysterectomy, but with the latter the surgeon must be especially careful not to produce ureteral obstruction.

Effort should be made to identify actual or potential enterocele, and any excess peritoneum should be excised coincident with high peritonealization. The vaginal vault can be strengthened by excising any excess width.

Preserving vaginal depth by fixing the vault above the levator plate will lessen any tendency for telescoping since increases in intra-abdominal pressure compress the vagina against the levator plate. If strong and surgically useful cardinal-uterosacral ligaments are lacking, alternative methods of colpopexy to support the vault must be used even at the time of hysterectomy (see Chapter 16). As Amreich (1) has pointed out, a short vagina ending anterior to the levator plate will tend with time to become even shorter, since intra-abdominal pressure may be transmitted in the axis of the vagina.

PRESERVING VAGINAL WIDTH

It is essential that the surgeon carefully calculate the amount of the vagina to be excised with colporrhaphy that will permit a coitally acceptable postoperative vaginal width. There should be suitable allowance for any anticipated shrinkage with aging and hormone withdrawal (i.e., all other things being equal, one would excise less vaginal membrane from a premenopausal patient in whom postoperative vaginal shrinkage has yet to occur). Allowance should be made for the age and genital size of the patient's marital consort. In the temporary absence of sexual activity, periodic insertion of a vaginal obturator will be of value if there is any tendency toward stricture or stenosis.

CONGENITAL ANOMALIES

With lower vaginal agenesis, a tunnel is dissected through the vestibular area toward the upper vagina. If a functional uterus is present, a hematocolpos will have been confirmed by rectal examination. The upper vaginal canal can be mobilized, opened, stretched, and sewn to the skin of the vestibule to cover the raw lower area. It should not be necessary to perform a graft. When a vaginal obturator has not been worn during a convalesence following construction of a neovagina, the vaginal cavity may shrink a great deal as a consequence of unrestrained scarring and fibrosis (11). Under this circumstance coitus may be impossible.

The uterus may be present in a patient with any level of a transverse vaginal septum. Interestingly, there is no associated urinary tract anomaly, suggesting a significant difference from the Rokitansky-Küster-Hauser syndrome. A vaginal septum or imperforate hymen is treated by appropriate excision.

THE SHORT VAGINA

When upper vaginectomy is required, sufficient depth may be retained by closing the vaginal vault from side to side (Fig. 20.1). When the vagina is short, as from previous radical pelvic surgery that has included partial vaginectomy, the distal vulvovaginoplasty of Williams (14) may add 1 to 2 inches to the length provided that the labia majora are fleshy (see Chapter 21). For those requiring still more depth, construction of a new upper vagina by a partial McIndoe procedure may be accomplished (Figs. 20.2 and 20.3). Additional depth may be created as well as maintained by the use of appropriate vaginal obturators (3, 5). Occasionally, the Vecchietti operation (12) may be offered. It is described in some detail in Chapter 21.

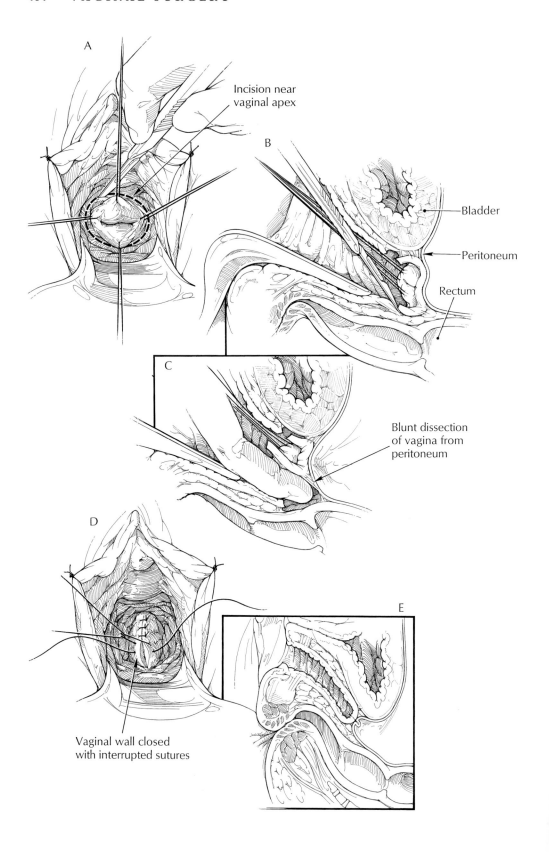

A

Incision near
vaginal apex

B

Bladder

Peritoneum

Rectum

C

Blunt dissection
of vagina from
peritoneum

D

E

Vaginal wall closed
with interrupted sutures

When the vagina is narrow or constricted at a specific point, additional width can be obtained by surgery at an appropriate level, the technique and procedure depending upon the site of the constriction.

Most commonly, this occurs at the perineum, often after overenthusiastic perineorrhaphy or hurried inadequate reapproximation of an episiotomy. This is particularly true when the pubococcygei have been approximated anterior to the rectum (see Chapter 11). A midline perineotomy with a suture of the wound in the direction at a right angle to the incision may be all that is required, although this will shorten the vagina a small bit. If atrophy is present, a bilateral episiotomy with sliding of the skin margins (13) (Fig. 20.4) will widen the introitus.

CORRECTION OF A MIDVAGINAL STRICTURE OR STENOSIS

Stricture of the midportion of the vagina may be overcome by the use of lateral relaxing incisions made through the full thickness of the vagina (Fig. 20.5). The margins of the incision are undercut, and the vaginal caliber is maintained by a suitable obturator during epithelialization and healing. If the freshly excised vaginal wall is still on the

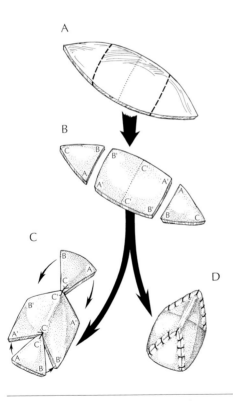

Figure 20.2. "Tent" full-thickness skin graft for vaginal foreshortening. **A.** A full-thickness piece of skin has been removed from the iliac crest using two elliptical incisions. **B.** All subcutaneous fat is scraped away, and triangles are cut from each end of the ellipse. **C.** The triangles are rotated so that site C is sewn to C'. **D.** The remainder of the cut edges are brought together by interrupted stitches. This tent will be placed with the rough edge external into the depths of the recipient site in the vaginal wall. The bottom edges may be tacked to the cut margin of the upper edge of the vaginal canal, fixing the graft in place. The cavity is thoroughly packed with sterile cotton balls soaked in saline to obliterate any dead space that may be present. These must be left in place for a minimum of 5 days.

Figure 20.1. Removal of the proximal vagina. **A.** View showing the area of the vaginal apex to be removed. Guide sutures are placed as shown, and an incision will follow the path of the *dashed line*. **B.** Sagittal section showing sharp dissection extending circumferentially up to the peritoneum. **C.** With traction to the guide sutures, the vagina is bluntly dissected from the peritoneum. **D.** Following removal of the vaginal apex, the vaginal incision is closed from side to side by interrupted stitches to help preserve vaginal depth. **E.** The end result as seen in sagittal section.

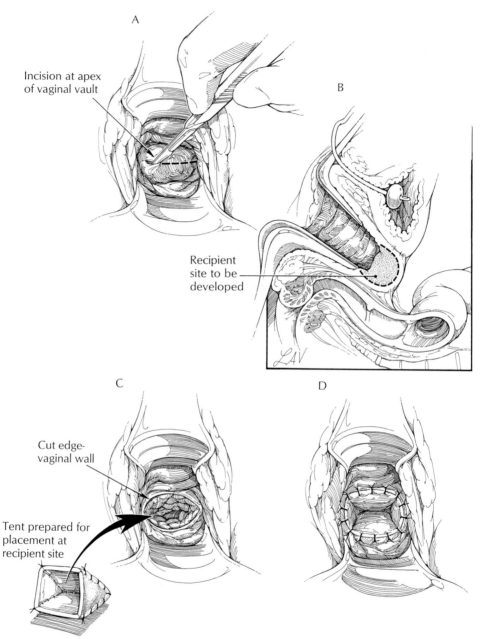

Figure 20.3. Site development and skin grafting of a new proximal vagina. A rather short vagina has been demonstrated following previous surgery and hysterectomy. There is somewhat dense scar tissue in this area, but it is possible to elongate the vagina by developing an extraperitoneal excavation at the vaginal vault using both sharp and blunt dissection. **A.** A transverse incision is made through the full thickness of the vaginal vault. **B.** Sagittal view of the site to be developed. **C.** After this cavity has been formed and hemostasis secured, the "tent" of full-thickness skin from the iliac crest is placed into the donor site. **D.** The tent is sewn to the cut edge of the vagina. The tissues are tightly packed with saline-soaked sponges and left to rest for 5 days. The sponges are then removed, the cavity irrigated, and the patient given an obturator to wear until healing is complete.

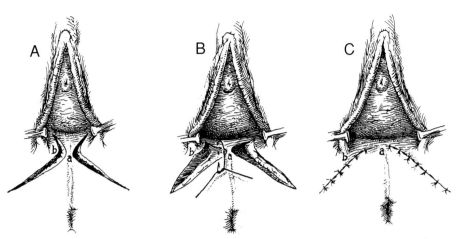

Figure 20.4. Bilateral episiotomy. **A.** The skin and perineal tissues are cut. **B.** Repair is begun at the medial edge in such a fashion that *b* is no longer adjacent to *a* but is in fact moved laterally on each side a distance sufficient to enlarge the introitus as much as is necessary. **C.** The now widened introitus.

scrub nurse's table, a patch may be cut of a size sufficient to fill the defect in the lateral vaginal wall and sewn in place as a full-thickness graft (Fig. 20.6).

Lateral vaginal relaxing incisions can be made in a constricted vagina at any time, even years later, although a brief rehospitalization and anesthetic is required. The technique and aftercare are precisely the same as when done in the fresh surgical patient. When a full-thickness graft of abdominal skin is used to fill the defects, healing and rehabilitation are significantly faster (8, 9) (Fig. 20.7).

With moderate constriction of the lower vagina, as seen for example in the patient with congenital adrenal hyperplasia, a fasciocutaneous flap from the labia may be developed and swung into place to bridge the defect created by a fresh episiotomy (10). This thick flap must include *all* of the attached fat and subcutaneous tissue, bringing with it the relevant blood supply. For this reason it may be made in almost any length regardless of the width, because the usual 1.5:1 length-width ratio of thinner flaps does not apply. This is illustrated in Figure 20.8.

According to McGregor (7), "The natural resistance of the perineum to its normal flora would appear to extend to skin grafts, and infection is seldom a problem given good contact between graft and recipient site and no dead space full of hematoma or tissue fluid to provide a culture medium" (p. 181). One can strengthen this contact between the graft and underlying vagina by covering it first with a coating of fibrin glue and then sewing the graft in place after adequate hemostasis has been achieved. The vagina can then be packed securely to hold the graft against its underlying raw areas.

Skin advancement techniques for filling small defects with flaps from adjacent tissue are discussed in Chapter 4. Large musculocutaneous grafts as from the thigh may be used when massive vaginal reconstruction is required (2).

CORRECTION OF LOWER VAGINAL STRICTURE

Extensive constriction of the lower half of the vagina from either congenital underdevelopment or postoperative stricture consequent to the surgical excision of too much tissue may be relieved by the use of full-thickness skin flaps (6) from the inner thigh, a

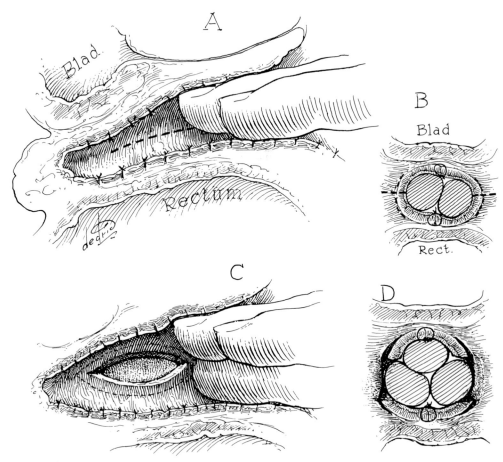

Figure 20.5. Lateral relaxing incisions of the vagina. **A.** Digital examination of the vagina immediately after colporrhaphy discloses an unexpected stenosis in the upper half that will admit but two finger breadths. **B.** The sites of the lateral relaxing incisions are indicated by the *dashed lines*. **C.** These incisions are made through the lateral wall of the vagina to a depth sufficient for the vagina to comfortably admit three finger breadths. **D.** The vaginal wall is undercut for a centimeter in each direction. Any obvious bleeding vessels are clamped and tied, and a firm vaginal packing is inserted. This may be replaced within a day or so by a large vaginal obturator or mold to keep the cut edges of the relaxing incisions apart until healing and epithelialization are well under way, usually by the fifth postoperative day, after which the obturator or dilator may be worn at night for an additional 2 or 3 months. Thus the integrity of the colporrhaphy incisions in the anterior and posterior vaginal walls is not compromised.

modification of the Graves operation (4) for construction of a neovagina. Convalescence requires several weeks of relative rest and several months' use of a vaginal obturator.

The Graves Procedure

The Graves procedure (4) was described as a method of treating congenital absence of the vagina in which a tunnel between the bladder and rectum was established and lined by four full-thickness flaps of skin. Two were raised from the medial surface of the thighs, and two were raised from the full thickness of the skin medial to the labia majora and including the labia minora, which were spatulated. The edges of these were all sewn

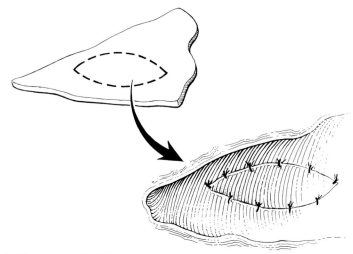

Figure 20.6. Placement of a full-thickness vaginal wall graft. A full-thickness graft may be cut from the vaginal membrane previously excised with the colporrhaphy. The proper size of the graft is that which will fit the defect in the lateral vaginal wall created by the relaxing incisions. It is held in place by a few interrupted stitches, as shown.

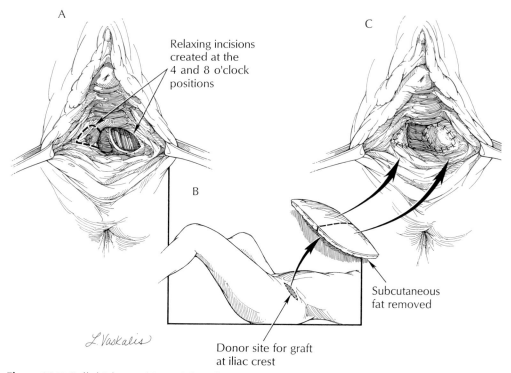

Figure 20.7. Full-thickness skin graft for relieving midvaginal stenosis. **A.** Large relaxing incisions have been made through the full thickness of the lateral vaginal wall at the 3 and 8 o'clock positions, exposing the underlying muscle of the pelvic sidewall. The opening of this tissue can be seen on the *right*. The size to be expected from a similar relaxing incision on the *left* is indicated by the *dashed line*. **B.** These raw areas can be effectively covered by a full-thickness graft of skin taken from the iliac crest. **C.** All subcutaneous fat is removed, the donor graft bisected along the path of the *dashed line*, and the free graft sewn to each defect, fully covering the raw area.

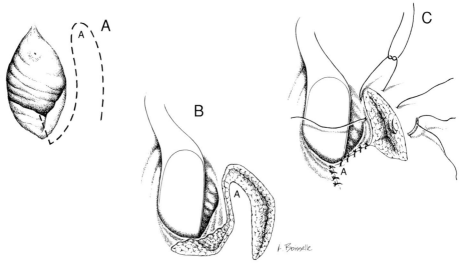

Figure 20.8. Labial cutaneous flap. **A.** The site of a perineotomy and an incision through the full thickness of the labial skin and subcutaneous fat is made (*broken line*). **B.** The base of the flap is wider than the apex. **C.** The flap has been freed from the underlying fascia, swung into the defect created by the perineotomy, and fixed in place by a few interrupted stitches. The labial defect is closed. Note the change in location of the tissue marked with an *a*. Transplanted hair growth is minimal.

together, inverted into the tunnel of the neovagina, and held there by a glass obturator until fixed to the walls of the cavity.

When a major stricture or atresia of the lower half of the vagina is encountered that is more extensive than can be relieved by simple midline perineotomy closed transversely, a modification of the Graves procedure is useful. In this modification two full-thickness flaps of an appropriate size are mobilized from the medial surface of each thigh and swung into the vagina to cover the site of a fresh midline episiotomy (Fig. 20.9). Polyglycolic acid-type suture is used throughout.

Technique of Vulvovaginal Skin Flap Rotation (Modified Graves Operation)

1. The perineum and the medial skin of each thigh are thoroughly infiltrated by subcuticular 0.5% lidocaine in 1:200,000 epinephrine solution. Approximately 100 ml is used.
2. A deep midline episiotomy is made with the skin edges separated widely enough to establish the desired vaginal diameter.
3. Skin flaps are marked off with indelible stain to a size sufficient for each to fill half of the space created by the unrepaired episiotomy.
4. Full-thickness flaps are cut all the way to the underlying fascia, leaving the subcutaneous fat attached to the undersurface of the flap.
5. The residual skin of the thigh is undermined preparatory to its approximation.
6. The flaps are swung medially to meet in the midline, where their medial edges are approximated with interrupted sutures.
7. Incisions in the thigh are closed from side to side, and the apex of the now united flaps is sewn to the apex of the episiotomy. Any excess adipose tissue is trimmed from the underside of the flap.

8. The lateral margins of the flap are fixed to the edges of the episiotomy with a few interrupted sutures.

9. A Penrose drain is inserted beneath the skin of each thigh, a Foley catheter is inserted in the bladder, and a splinting obturator is inserted into the vagina.

10. The obturator and the Foley catheter are removed on the fourth postoperative day, and the flaps and vagina are thoroughly inspected to determine healing. The obturator is replaced, to be removed each time the patient voids. After 2 or 3 weeks, the mold is worn for several months only at night until healing has been completed.

When the vagina is both too short and too narrow and generally inelastic consequent to fibrosis and scarring from previous surgery, the vulvovaginoplasty of Williams (14) may be of use if the labia are thick and well developed; but if atrophic and thin, vaginectomy followed at the same operation by construction of an Abbe-McIndoe-type neovagina is useful (see Chapter 21).

Long-term postoperative estrogen replacement is of value when indicated, and frequent wearing of a suitable obturator is often desirable to maintain both vaginal depth and width.

EVERTED SHORTENED VAGINA

One will occasionally encounter the multioperated patient with total eversion of a shortened vagina—too short, in fact, to reach the bony pelvis for direct colpopexy. In this event there are several additional surgical treatment alternatives from which to choose.

1. Ingram-Frank dilators (5) lubricated with estrogen cream may be used to lengthen the vagina until it will reach the sacrospinous ligament, at which time sacrospinous colpopexy may be performed.

2. Transabdominal sacrocolpopexy may be performed using an intermediate bridge of fascia lata or of a synthetic plastic material.

3. Sacrospinous colpopexy may be performed, creating deliberate suture bridges of nonabsorbable synthetic monofilament suture material, such as Prolene, Surgilene, or NovaFil.

4. If the labia are of sufficient size, a Williams vulvovaginoplasty (14) may be added to provide a supplemental depth of an additional 1-1/2 or 2 inches of vaginal length coincident with the above procedures.

Figure 20.9. A. The modified Graves vulvovaginal skin flap rotation. The small opening into the vagina illustrates the vaginal diameter for the lower half of the vagina. A cross section of the vagina (*right*) shows the extent of the stricture (*arrows*). **B.** The perineum and skin of the medial thighs have been infiltrated with lidocaine-epinephrine solution. A large midline episiotomy will be made (*broken line*) that extends halfway up the posterior vaginal wall to above the stricture. The lower vagina must accommodate three finger breadths in diameter. **C.** The large midline episiotomy has been made. Skin flaps are marked out of such a length and width so that, when united, they will fill the raw area of the episiotomy. **D.** The full-thickness flaps are cut, including the fat and subcutaneous tissue down to the fascia. The residual skin of the thigh is undermined as shown by the *dotted lines*. **E.** The medial margins of the flaps are sewn together in the midline. The apex of the now united flaps is held by a single stitch, which will be sewn to the apex of the episiotomy. Excess subcutaneous fat beneath the flaps is trimmed. **F.** The lateral edges are sewn to the sides of the episiotomy, and the skin of the thigh is approximated as shown. Penrose drains have been placed beneath the skin flaps on the thigh, a Foley catheter placed in the bladder, and a plastic obturator inserted into the vagina. **G.** The end result after removal of the drains and the obturator.

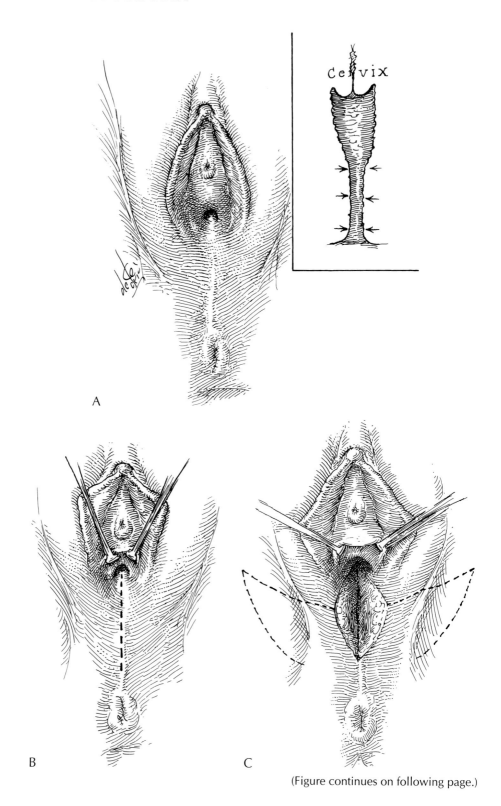

A

Cervix

B

C

(Figure continues on following page.)

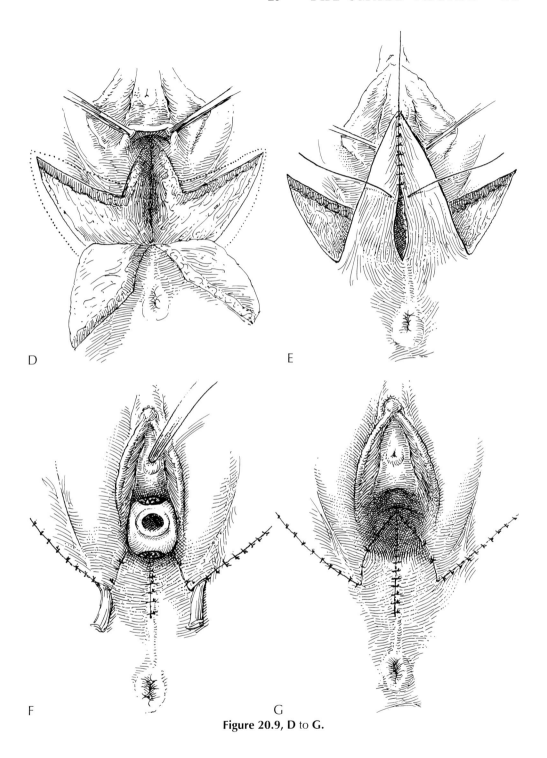

Figure 20.9, D to **G.**

References

1. Amreich J. Äetiologie und Operation des Scheidenstumpf prolapses. Wien Klin Wochenschr 1951;63: 74–77.
2. Becker DW, Massey FM, McGraw JB. Musculocutaneous flaps in reconstructive pelvic surgery. Obstet Gynecol 1979;54:178–183.
3. Frank RT. The formation of an artificial vagina without operation. Am J Obstet Gynecol 1938;35:1053.
4. Graves WP. Operative treatment of atresia of the vagina. Boston Med Surg J 1910;163:753.
5. Ingram JM. The bicycle seat stool in the treatment of vaginal agenesis and stenosis. Am J Obstet Gynecol 1981;140:867–871.
6. Martin LW, Sutorius DS. An improved method for vaginoplasty. Arch Surg 1969;98:716.
7. McGregor IA. Fundamental techniques of plastic surgery. Edinburgh: Churchill-Livingstone, 1972:181.
8. Morley GW. Massive eversion of a shortened vagina. In: Nichols DH, DeLancey JOL. Clinical problems, injuries and complications of gynecologic and obstetric surgery. 3rd ed. Baltimore: Williams & Wilkins, 1995:197–199.
9. Morley GW, DeLancey JOL. Full thickness skin graft vaginoplasty for treatment of the stenotic or fore-shortened vagina. Obstet Gynecol 1991;77:485–489.
10. Morton KE, Davies D, Dewhurst J. The use of the fasciocutaneous flap in vaginal reconstruction. Br J Obstet Gynaecol 1986;93:970–973.
11. Nichols DH. Postoperative vaginal fibrosis and contracture following Abbe-McIndoe procedure. In: Nichols DH, DeLancey JOL. Clinical problems, injuries and complications of gynecologic and obstetric surgery. 3rd ed. Baltimore: Williams & Wilkins, 1995:137–138.
12. Vecchietti G. Le néo-vagin dans le syndrome de Rokitansky-Kuster-Hauser. Rev Med Suisse Romande 1979;99:593–601.
13. West JT, Ketcham AS, Smith RR. Vaginal reconstruction following pelvic exenteration for cancer or postirradiation necrosis. Surg Gynecol Obstet 1965;118:788.
14. Williams EA. Congenital absence of the vagina: a simple operation for its relief. J Obstet Gynaecol Br Commonw 1964;71:511.

CHAPTER 21

Creation of a Neovagina

A neovagina may be developed through a number of techniques, depending on the circumstances, needs, and motivations of the individual patient. Although the most common etiologic factor is vaginal agenesis with the Mayer-Rokitansky-Küster-Hauser syndrome, which occurs in one of about 5000 female births, replacement of the vagina may also be considered after vaginectomy, as from cancer, after extensive scarring from trauma or infection, or in the case of male-to-female transsexual surgery (15). Depending on the circumstances, surgery may range from construction of the entire length of a vagina to the supplement of only a portion of vagina.

TIMING OF TREATMENT

Development of a neovagina need not wait until the time of anticipated marriage or coitus, since several months may be required for the postoperative swelling, edema, pain, and tenderness to subside. When the possible need for construction of a neovagina has been determined, it is time to introduce the patient and her companion or family to the mechanics of surgery and postoperative care for the various solutions, with a thoughtful and detailed discussion of the techniques of aftercare and probable length of time involved. Because the length of postoperative convalescence is unpredictable, an ideal time for this construction is at the beginning of the patient's summer vacation. Because the entire treatment concept is weighted with psychological overtones, the need for emotional maturity on the part of the patient is great. Her understanding of the necessary aftercare and its critical importance in determining the success of the procedure requires coincident strong patient motivation after a realistic description of the entire procedure and process and the alternative methods of treatment have been presented. Some positive assessment of her personal commitment, willingness, and motivation must be appropriately developed for there to be a probable long-term success of her treatment. The patient must be given ample time to consider the treatment alternatives and her personal commitment to the success of the venture and to develop a realistic appraisal of her personal long-term goals concerning the operation. There must be opportunity for her to develop and ask relevant questions and to obtain appropriate answers before a final decision is implemented.

Empathy, understanding, patience, and kindness on the part of the surgeon are part of a friendly and effective doctor-patient relationship. If the patient fails to demonstrate emotional maturity, a surgical plan to implement the goals should be postponed and the patient referred for psychological and social counseling. Treatment usually should not be started until any serious relevant psychological problems have been successfully addressed.

It is now commonly agreed that the timing of reconstructive surgery for congenital absence of the vagina, which was previously assigned to the premarital state, should be offered at the time of endocrine maturity irrespective of the patient's current social status. This presumes that the patient requesting treatment has the maturity to comprehend the social, economic, convalescent, and psychological dimensions consequent to *her* decision concerning treatment. Some male-to-female transsexuals will request neovaginal construction.

CHOICE OF PROCEDURE FOR CONSTRUCTION OF THE NEOVAGINA

There are many effective treatment options from which to choose, and these depend upon the following variable factors:

1. The perceived wishes and plans of the patient
2. The motivation of the patient and her degree of emotional maturity
3. An accurate estimate of the patient's ability to participate effectively in the necessary follow-up program
4. The familiarity and experience of her surgeon with each of the treatment techniques, both surgical and nonsurgical
5. The support of the patient's loved ones

At times, various combinations of treatment may be advised for a particular patient, depending upon her specific needs.

There are at least 11 different procedures currently in use to create a neovagina and to fulfill a variety of clinical indications and circumstances. There are specific indications for each, and the responsible gynecologic surgeon owes it to each patient to be familiar with a number of these techniques so that the surgeon can choose, with her, the one that is most likely to benefit her.

For some persons, a full-length neovagina will be required; for others, a supplemental or additional length is needed. Occasionally, partial or complete vaginectomy followed by creation of a neovagina is indicated, as with total vaginal stenosis or after extirpation for malignant disease (8, 32).

Various options of interest to a particular patient may be described, and a broad range of questions anticipated and solicited to which the surgeon provides practical answers. The patient's views concerning herself, her problem, and her attitude toward a particular treatment strategy should be determined, as best as she can predict. This broad-ranged discussion should be realistic in its appraisal, and assurances should be empathetic and unhurried. It will likely involve more than one discussion.

The patient's understanding of the problem and its solution should lead to objective interpretation of its personal and psychosocial significance to her own social environment or plans for personal sexual intimacy. Her willingness and determination to become involved in a realistic sequence of postoperative planning must be confirmed.

As already mentioned, the surgeon must evaluate the patient's motivation and psychological maturity. This will have a direct bearing on her probable aftercare and follow-through, which might differ with each of the treatment options offered. Whatever method is selected, it is helpful for the gynecologist to maintain a list of previous patients who might be willing to discuss with the new patient their experience concerning neovaginal reconstruction.

Preliminary Work-up

Meanwhile, a necessary work-up, if not already accomplished, is undertaken. This consists of a thorough physical examination, including appraisal of secondary sex characteristics and any possible endocrinopathy, rectal-abdominal examination and deep abdominal palpation, karyotyping, and evaluation of any pelvic masses. Abdominal ultrasound or intravenous pyelography is required to locate conclusively the number, size, and placement of the patient's kidneys, and to determine the possibility of a pelvic kidney or of a hematometra.

Specific Options

A procedure can be chosen from among the following current operations. Under various circumstances, a combination of two or more may be of advantage to a particular patient.

When a strongly motivated patient with a recognized perineal indentation or shortened vagina is anxious to pursue a nonsurgical development of a neovagina, the Frank-Ingram pressure-by-obturator method can be remarkably effective (14, 21).

The simplest of the surgical approaches is the Williams vulvovaginoplasty (44). The surgeon creates a pouchlike vagina by sewing together vulvar skin incisions overlying the labia majora.

Of the transperineal surgical procedures that may be considered, that of Wharton (43) is probably the least complicated. The cavity of a neovagina is created by surgical dissection, bleeding is carefully controlled, and an obturator is inserted. The obturator will be worn most of the time until the cavity has been thoroughly epithelialized, which requires a space of several months. Postoperative use of an obturator for a long time is essential to maintain adequate width. The inconvenience of a chronic bloody discharge during most of this period of time is a disadvantage and inconvenience, and there will be abundant scar tissue formation around the neovagina as time goes on, which will tend to produce vaginal stricture if the lumen is not kept open by frequent wearing of an obturator.

For many years, this has been often replaced by the Abbe-McIndoe operation (1, 25, 37) in which the cavity described above has been lined by a split-thickness skin graft. This requires postoperative attention to the donor site, as well as the wearing of an obturator for many months, taking it out only for a bowel movement or to empty the bladder, and wearing it nightly during sleep for an additional 6 to 12 months, the frequency depending upon the stability of the vaginal size. Tissue expansion techniques can be employed to create vulvar skin flaps for vaginoplasty (23). Cali and Pratt (5) reported that 18 percent of patients with vaginal agenesis treated by an Abbe-McIndoe operation and followed for longer than 10 years demonstrated a complete stenosis of the neovagina.

Much the same effect appears to be achieved by lining the cavity with human amnion (12, 36), usually obtained from a cesarean section delivery. The amnion, mesenchymal side out, is placed around the intravaginal obturator and left in place for 5 postoperative days, at which time the obturator is removed. It is covered with a new layer of amnion, and reinserted. After 5 more days, the obturator is taken out only for voiding and passage of stool, and replaced for most of the time. Granulation tissue is minimal, since there are areas effectively covered by amnion, and epithelialization gradually develops beneath the amniotic membrane. It has been shown that Interceed absorbable fabric (Johnson & Johnson, New Brunswick, New Jersey), made of oxidized regenerated cellulose, can be substituted for the amnion (22) to remove any theoretical risk of unexpected virus transmission to the patient. It rapidly adheres to the raw wall of the newly dissected neovagina and forms a gelatinous, nonadherent layer between the wall and the obturator. This permits epithelialization by skin migration from the perineum. The stent is removed after 5 days and replaced for another 5 days. It is only removed during defecation until the vagina has become fully epithelialized, usually within 3 to 6 months. Nightly insertion of an obturator is necessary until the vaginal size has stabilized and the patient is sexually active. Failure to wear the obturator long enough can result in a rapid contraction of the neovagina during this healing phase.

The Vecchietti (29, 30, 39–41) transabdominal procedure is another technique. The elastic pseudohymenal tissues are stretched using traction from above to create a neovagina.

In years past, the Baldwin procedure, which uses a loop of small intestine to line a newly created neovagina, has been used, but the amount of mucous discharge has been so great as to be uncomfortable and inconvenient for the majority of patients, and the method is no longer used.

In the Schubert operation, the rectum was transplanted to the site of the neovagina, and the large intestine brought down to form a new rectum. Better results have been obtained by the Ober-Meinrenken operation (4, 16, 19, 28, 31), in which a loop of colon is mobilized by a transabdominal approach, and brought down to line a fresh neovaginal cavity that has been made to open into the peritoneal cavity. A major advantage of this procedure is that it does not require postoperative stretching and wearing of an obturator as is necessary with the Abbe-McIndoe operation, although introital stricture at the mucocutaneous junction is a complication that must be avoided by periodic dilation of this site until healing has been completed. The procedure has an obvious disadvantage in that it requires assumption of the operative risks and convalescence coincident with a large bowel resection and anastomosis. It is particularly helpful when the surgeon wishes to replace the upper vagina that had been removed by cancer surgery or after radiation therapy. It provides a usable supplement to the size of an otherwise uncomfortably small vagina. The surgeon must transfix the abdominal end of the colon to lessen the small risk of prolapse.

It is possible to line the vagina with a transplant of skin made by bivalving pedicles from the labia minora and inner surfaces of the thigh-modifications of the Graves operation (20, 24) (see Chapter 20). This does provide some sensory coital perception within the neovagina (34). It is important that these pedicles be held in place by a suitable obturator and that the length of the pedicle be no greater than three times the width, lest the vascular supply of the pedicle be disturbed (26).

In some centers a combined abdominal-perineal approach, the Davyoff operation, is employed, in which the undersurface of a cylinder of peritoneum is dissected from within the pelvis, brought down into a fresh neovagina, and attached to the vulvovaginal skin by a circumferential placement of sutures (7). The abdominal portion of the operation also can be accomplished translaparoscopically (2). The "vaginal vault" of peritoneum is closed by a transabdominally placed pursestring stitch, and over a period of months epithelialization develops beneath the peritoneum.

It is thus clear that in various parts of the world surgical community a number of operative approaches to the construction of the neovagina are currently being performed. There are advantages and disadvantages to each, and the selection of an appropriate procedure must take into account the patient's willingness to participate in the necessary postoperative follow-up program, the depth of her maturity, and her perception of herself. For most of the techniques, the timing of the operation seems best when the patient can afford adequate postoperative convalescence and develop obturator use experience. Therefore, the most popular time for surgery with the mature, school-aged patient is early in the spring or summer vacation.

NONSURGICAL TREATMENT

About one-third of patients who have a dimple at the site of the absent vagina can use the Frank-Ingram dilator method. It takes about 9 months of daily dedicated and concentrated use to achieve a satisfactory vagina. This reestablishment of vaginal depth and width by a program of continued pressure using progressively longer and wider firm obturators has been advocated by Frank (14) and more recently by Ingram (21) for the strongly motivated and cooperative patient. Success requires daily applications of significant pressure of the obturator to the site of vaginal construction, totaling about

2 hours per day using graduated-sized dilators (first, to achieve depth, then to achieve width). The patient should be seen for examination, reassurance, and reinforcement every 2 to 4 weeks, and the size of the obturator exchanged for the next larger size as vaginal deepening develops. If she should decide later that she is unwilling to continue this approach, an alternate surgical plan can be offered at any time. Given an enthusiastic patient and therapist, successful results may be achieved over a period of 6 to 9 months.

Ingram (21) has also developed a unique program in which obturator pressure to the site of the neovagina is maintained for a total of 2 hours each day by the act of sitting on a specially designed bicycle seat (Fig. 21.1), which frees the patient's hands. The obturator length is increased progressively to a maximum of 10 cm, after which successively wider obturators are introduced. It appears that this neovagina does not become constricted.

SURGICAL TREATMENT

It is often economically convenient to initiate surgical creation of a neovagina near the age of 18 years before the parents' medical insurance for their child runs out.

Our primary surgical approach for vaginal agenesis is one of the following alternatives:

1. The Abbe-Wharton-McIndoe operation using a split-thickness skin graft or the use of a graft of human amnion or a lining of Interceed
2. The Vecchietti operation
3. The transplantation of a segment of sigmoid colon
4. The Williams vulvovaginoplasty
5. The Davyoff colpopoiesis

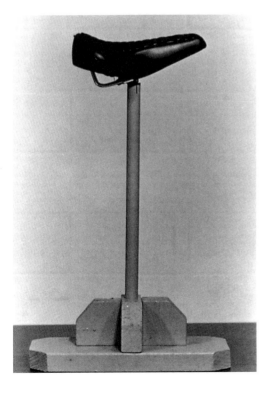

Figure 21.1. The banana-type bicycle seat described by Ingram may be mounted on a stand as shown, permitting the patient the free use of her hands for other purposes while she is sitting upon the seat, obturator in place. (From Ingram JM. The bicycle seat in the treatment of vaginal agenesis and stenosis: a preliminary report. Am J Obstet Gynecol 1981;1:867. Used with permission.)

Which technique is chosen depends on the patient's ability to wear a necessary obturator postoperatively. One need not wait until marriage has been announced before offering a surgical relief.

The treatment of choice for a failed neovagina is to remove the neovagina and replace it with a new one. Grafted skin, Interceed, amnion, or colon may be used.

When one has encountered a vagina that is too short or narrow for marital comfort, one must aim to create a proper depth for a neovagina, sufficient to contain the patient's coital partner. An ideal length is 12 cm with a width of 3.5 cm.

The Abbe-Wharton-McIndoe Operation

The construction of a neovagina by the Abbe-McIndoe technique is particularly useful, but only if the patient is willing to follow instructions concerning the postoperative, long-term wearing of an obturator (1, 6, 10, 25, 37). A tunnel is formed by sharp and blunt dissection between the rectum and the urethra and bladder (Fig. 21.2). The surgeon should expose only a small portion of the peritoneum during the transvaginal operation to lessen the chance of subsequent enterocele. The cavity, thus produced, is lined by a split-thickness skin graft obtained from an area covering the buttocks or lower abdomen normally concealed by the patient's undergarments.

A flap of skin about 19/1,000 of an inch thick should measure about 10 by 13 cm and is easily obtained with the Reese electric dermatome. Our preference (27) is from the suprapubic area of the anterior abdominal wall (9, 35). Before the graft is harvested, the surface of the skin is shaved, and multiple subcutaneous injections of sterile saline, totaling 200 to 300 ml, are made to flatten the skin surface, allowing for a graft of uniform surface dimension and thickness. The skin of the donor site is painted with sterile mineral oil, the graft removed and wrapped in saline-soaked dressings, and a xeroform dressing applied to the donor site. The use of this donor skin has several advantages:

1. Because of the graft's anterior location, the patient is not required to endure the pain and discomfort of sitting or resting upon the donor site during the long healing phase.
2. Because the graft is cut superficial to the hair follicles, there is prompt regrowth of hair of the escutcheon covering much of the donor site, thus making the donor site more cosmetically acceptable to the patient (there is no hair growth within the graft, since the hair follicles are not contained in the split-thickness graft).
3. Pigmentation of the donor site is minimal, and any that is present is mostly covered by pubic hair regrowth.
4. A thicker split-thickness graft is less likely to shrink postoperatively than a thinner graft.

Next, 100 ml of sterile milk, infant formula, or sterile saline deeply colored with indigo carmine is instilled into the bladder through an indwelling, clamped Foley catheter. The bladder will be palpable during subsequent dissection of the neovagina. The bulb of the Foley catheter can be palpated and any unwanted penetration of the bladder recognized by prompt appearance of dye or milk in the operative field.

The surgeon then injects 100 ml of sterile saline beneath the wall of the vaginal vault and upper vagina to compress sites of venous bleeding and to make the dissection of the vagina from the surrounding tissues and scar safer. The operator then proceeds in a somewhat conical direction to the peritoneum of the cul-de-sac of Douglas, which may be exposed for no more than 1 to 1.5 cm (lessening the chance for future enterocele

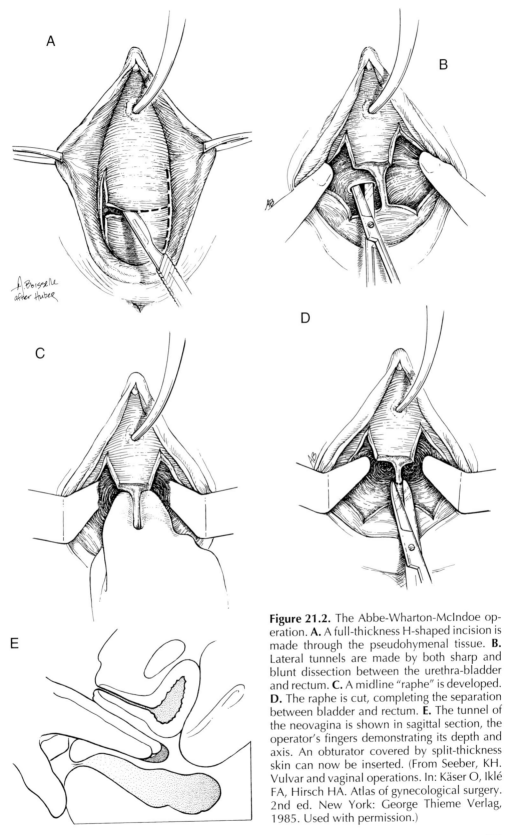

Figure 21.2. The Abbe-Wharton-McIndoe operation. **A.** A full-thickness H-shaped incision is made through the pseudohymenal tissue. **B.** Lateral tunnels are made by both sharp and blunt dissection between the urethra-bladder and rectum. **C.** A midline "raphe" is developed. **D.** The raphe is cut, completing the separation between bladder and rectum. **E.** The tunnel of the neovagina is shown in sagittal section, the operator's fingers demonstrating its depth and axis. An obturator covered by split-thickness skin can now be inserted. (From Seeber, KH. Vulvar and vaginal operations. In: Käser O, Iklé FA, Hirsch HA. Atlas of gynecological surgery. 2nd ed. New York: George Thieme Verlag, 1985. Used with permission.)

481

development, as would be risked were the peritoneal exposure made greater). Lateral relaxing incisions in the vestibule or medial border of the pubococcygei are made to help the patient contain the obturator postoperatively (10). Bleeding points are clamped and coagulated or tied. Venous oozing may be controlled with tight vaginal gauze packing placed for a few minutes.

The edges of the split-thickness graft (raw side out) are draped over the polyethylene foam obturator (no covering condom is necessary). Alternatively, the appropriate sized Heyer-Schulte "inflatable" obturator can be used.

A precut polyethylene foam cylinder (38), 5 by 15 cm and rounded or tapered at the proximal end, is prepared. The graft edges are then approximated over the mold with fine absorbable sutures.

For the partial Abbe-Wharton-McIndoe operation to construct an upper vagina, a full-thickness abdominal skin graft obtained by the technique shown in Chapter 20 may be substituted for the split-thickness graft. Interceed or amnion may be substituted for skin (22).

The graft-covered obturator is inserted into the neovagina and the vaginal orifice closed temporarily by two or three heavy silk sutures in the labia majora, loosely tied, to hold the mold in place for the next 7 to 8 days.

The donor site is covered by xeroform and left in situ until it spontaneously disengages.

The Foley catheter (or suprapubic catheter, if desired) is connected to a drainage system. The patient is placed on a low-residue diet and bedrest and given prophylactic medication to curb intestinal activity. About the seventh postoperative day the vulvovestibular stitches are cut and removed, the mold gently removed under anesthesia if necessary, and the neovagina inspected.

Vulvar squamous epithelium will gradually grow in beneath the adherent amnion or Interceed. The smooth surface of the neovagina 1 month postoperatively is deceptively smooth and shiny. It must be remembered that this covering is essentially a temporary membrane, and is not as yet mature squamous epithelium. Therefore, it retains a great capacity for accelerated shrinkage, and the patient must make adequate use of the obturator, dilator, or stent postoperatively. In most instances, this will require wearing it constantly for 12 months, removing it only to void or for a bowel movement, until the neovagina is well covered by mature squamous epithelium and subepithelial cicatrization has been stabilized.

After 12 months, a new obturator made of firm plastic or balsa wood covered by rubber, measuring 15 cm in length and 12 cm in circumference, is inserted. Alternately, the Heyer-Schulte mold may be used again. The patient is promptly ambulated and instructed in the removal and replacement of the obturator, which may be generously lubricated with estrogen cream. The patient is then discharged.

The mold should be removed only when the patient goes to the toilet, then promptly replaced. Any help that is needed holding the obturator in place may be given by the support of a sanitary napkin worn beneath the patient's underpants.

After a postoperative month, the vagina is reinspected in the surgeon's office, any granulation tissue coagulated with silver nitrate, and permission given the patient for coital activity, if appropriate. The new instructions are to wear the obturator nightly and for 2 hours during the daytime. After 6 postoperative months, if there is no evidence of vaginal stricture, the patient may be asked to wear the obturator nightly three times per week, more frequently if any obstruction to its insertion is observed.

For the strongly motivated patient with congenital absence of the vagina who balks at the thought of a bowel resection or of a skin graft donor site for an Abbe-McIndoe operation, one may use an isograft of posteriorly attached vestibular and perineal skin inserted as a lining into a tunnel dissected between the bladder and the rectum in the

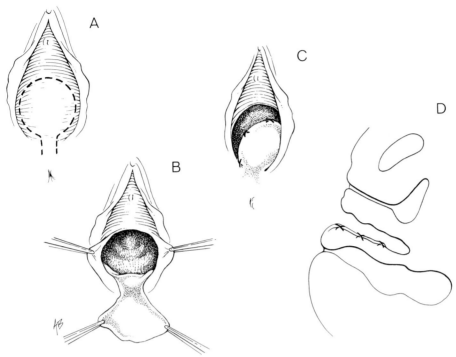

Figure 21.3. The Sheares operation. **A.** A racquet-shaped, full-thickness incision is made inside the labia minora. **B.** The skin flap is dissected from the underlying tissues, preserving its attachment at the base of the "handle." The flap is displaced posteriorly and the tunnels for the neovagina are created by both blunt and sharp lateral dissection. They are united by incising the raphe between them to separate the bladder from the rectum. **C.** The flap isograft is unfolded into the new tunnel so as to cover its lower and posterior surface. The flap is then fixed in place, underside down, by some interrupted sutures. **D.** Sagittal section showing the sutures. An obturator or form is inserted and held in place by suturing together the labia majora.

manner of Sheares (33). This procedure has been reported with enthusiasm by Fleigner (13). This is a useful modification of the Wharton (43) procedure. Epithelialization of the neovagina occurs from the edges of both isograft and vaginal orifice. The technique is illustrated in Figure 21.3. At the conclusion of the operation a vaginal form made of a condom tightly packed with foam rubber is inserted into the neovagina, the labia majora loosely stitched together, a transurethral or suprapubic catheter placed in the bladder, and the patient given a nonresidue diet. The mold is removed on the 14th day and the patient given a solid obturator to be lubricated with estrogen cream and worn most of the time with pressure to the point of discomfort for 3 months, at which time coitus may be initiated. Once fully epithelialized, this neovagina is not as vulnerable to postoperative contraction as is that lined by a split-thickness skin graft, though its size should be tested frequently by the use of the solid obturator, which may be reintroduced from time to time as necessary.

VAGINECTOMY WITH CONSTRUCTION OF A NEOVAGINA

A massively scarred and nonfunctional vagina may be removed by vaginectomy (Fig. 21.4) and replaced by a neovagina. Successful vaginal reconstruction can be

Figure 21.4. Sagittal section showing a massively scarred vagina. A Foley catheter is in the bladder. The entire vagina is excised by sharp dissection along the plane indicated by the *broken line* (1), starting laterally, then posteriorly, and finally anteriorly, beneath the urethra and bladder. An obturator, suitably covered with a split-thickness skin graft, will be placed in the tunnel.

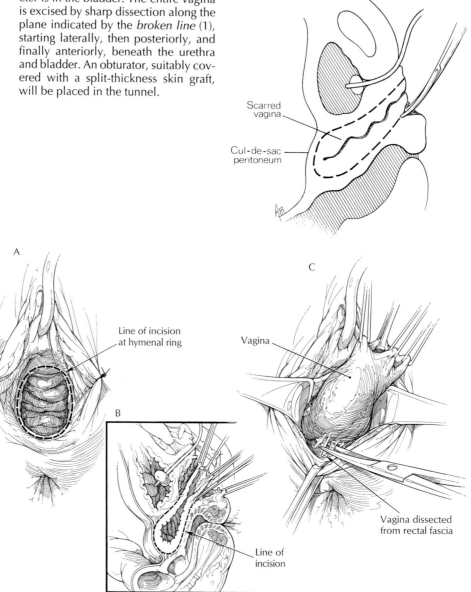

Figure 21.5. Total transvaginal vaginectomy. This may be particularly valuable as the first step in constructing a neovagina for a patient whose vagina has been occluded by scar tissue. **A.** A Foley catheter is inserted into the bladder and 60 ml of indigo carmine solution instilled. An incision is made circumferentially through the full thickness of the vagina and surrounding scar tissue along the path indicated by the *dashed line*. **B.** By sharp dissection this mobilization of the vagina is carried toward the vault, first on one side of the vagina, then on the other, and finally in the midline. The operator separates the bladder by careful sharp dissection, being mindful for any appearance of violet-stained tissue in the course of the dissection, which would indicate proximity of the bladder. **C.** The posterior midline dissection. This can be best accomplished with the operator's finger in the patient's rectum to identify the latter and avoid unwanted penetration. (*Continues on following page.*)

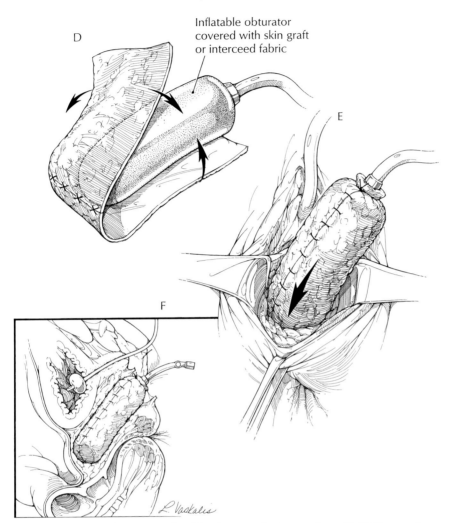

Inflatable obturator
covered with skin graft
or interceed fabric

Figure 21.5 (continued). D. An inflatable obturator is chosen that will fill the newly created vaginal cavity. It is covered by a full thickness of skin obtained from the patient's abdomen or a split-thickness of skin obtained from a donor site. **E.** The edges of the graft are sewn with the rough side out. It is compressed by squeezing to reduce the size of the obturator. The valve at the tip occludes the tubing while the obturator covered with its graft is inserted into the neovaginal cavity. **F.** The obturator is now permitted to expand. If necessary it can be held in place during the initial healing process by several temporary stitches placed through the labia majora. The graft and obturator are left in site for 5 days, after which the retention stitches are cut, the obturator removed, and the vagina carefully inspected.

achieved even years after initial therapy in patients who develop vaginal obliteration from previous radiation or surgery (3, 8, 32, 42). Stenosis may also be seen following radical hysterectomy and vaginectomy, and a neovagina can be used as treatment patients undergoing pelvic exenteration. The reconstruction procedure is as follows:

The scarred vagina is excised by scissor dissection beginning lateral and peripheral to the scar, which provides the least chance for inadvertent damage to the bowel or bladder (Fig. 21.5). When this has proceeded close to the vaginal vault, one of the surgeon's fingers is inserted into the rectum to facilitate posterior dissection, and the freed space is made to communicate with the lateral spaces. A Foley catheter is instilled into the bladder which is emptied of urine, and 60 ml of saline heavily colored with indigo carmine or methylene blue is instilled into the bladder through the Foley. The dissection is carried anteriorly carefully avoiding the violet-stained vesical mucosa. Hemostasis is achieved, and an obturator, covered by amnion, Interceed or harvested skin, is inserted.

The Vecchietti Operation

In this operation, a retroperitoneal loop of suture is introduced from the abdomen to the vulva, where it is threaded through a 2-cm plastic olive (29, 30, 39–41). The abdominal ends of the suture are attached to adjustable tension springs in a metal frame that lies on the patient's abdomen and that applies constant traction to the perineal olive. The upward pressure stretches the elastic vestibular skin, with which it migrates upward over a period of several days, creating a vaginal cavity of the desired depth. The tension of the springs is adjusted daily to produce a 1-cm upward daily migration of the olive. This seems to create a vagina of sexually usable depth in a period of about 7 or 8 hospital-based days. Progressively wider obturators are inserted to develop vaginal width, and persistent frequent sexual activity or wearing of an obturator is required to maintain vaginal depth and patency. We have performed the operation occasionally and enthusiastically in recent years, and also offer it translaparoscopically (11, 18) (using three ports— one to either side of the rectus muscles, and the third subumbilical) to save the patient the discomfort and disfigurement of a laparotomy incision and scar. The procedure is illustrated in Figure 21.6.

Transplantation of a Segment of Colon

There is a place for the Ober-Meinrenken operation (28) (sometimes popularly called the "Schubert-Schmidt" operation), which uses a loop of transplanted colon for the neovagina of the patient whose vagina is shortened after a cancer operation such as exenteration. In these circumstance it may be added as part of the original exenterative procedure. It is also of value in the patient who is neither psychologically nor socially able or likely to use dilators of the neovagina regularly in the postoperative period and who is not sexually active (19, 28, 31). If the distal bowel segment is of too small a diameter to permit coitus, it may be incised for its full thickness at the 3 and 9 o'clock positions, and the lateral raw areas of the distal vagina covered by a flap of filleted labia minora as seen in Figure 21.7. This may also be of use if the bowel segment is too short to be brought all the way to the perineum without tension. It is a technique that may relieve introital stricture, whatever the cause. The diameter of the colonic neovagina will not shrink postoperatively, although contraction at the mucocutaneous junction must be prevented by frequent dilation at this site until healing is complete.

The creation of a colonic neovagina results in a long-term, anatomically satisfactory situation, and with adequate counseling and follow-up, postoperative sexual and social adjustment is good. The patient must understand the risks involved in this surgery because they include the uncommon but possible complications of an elective bowel resection, which therefore include the small risk of leakage at the point of anastomosis, with accompanying postoperative peritonitis. The neovagina retains its gross characteristics of intestinal mucosa. After final healing of the mucocutaneous junction at about the eighth postoperative week, the patient is not required to wear a dilator postopera-

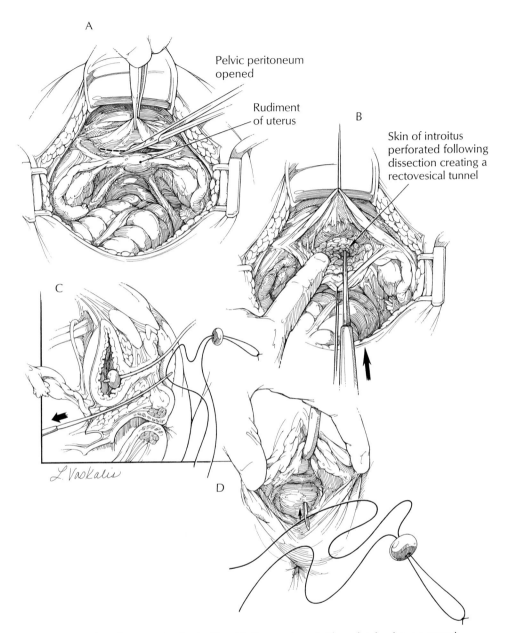

Figure 21.6. Creation of a neovagina by the Vecchietti procedure. **A.** The pelvis has been exposed. A rudiment of uterus is identified, as are normal fallopian tubes and ovaries. The pelvic peritoneum is incised transversely. **B.** Guide sutures are placed through the peritoneum, and a site is developed for construction of a rectovesical tunnel. With a Foley catheter in the bladder and 50 ml of indigo carmine instilled, a long ligature carrier is pushed, as shown, until it perforates the skin of the introitus. **C** and **D.** A suture that has been threaded through a plastic olive is threaded also through the tip of the ligature carrier and withdrawn as shown. The suture is disengaged and the ligature carrier reintroduced parallel to the same tunnel, but perforating the perineal skin about 1.5 cm lateral to the original perforation. The suture has been passed through the plastic olive and the free end threaded to the ligature carrier and withdrawn so that there is a bridge of perineal skin between the two sutures. To aid in later extraction of the olive, a second suture had been threaded through the olive in an opposite direction. (*Continues on following page.*)

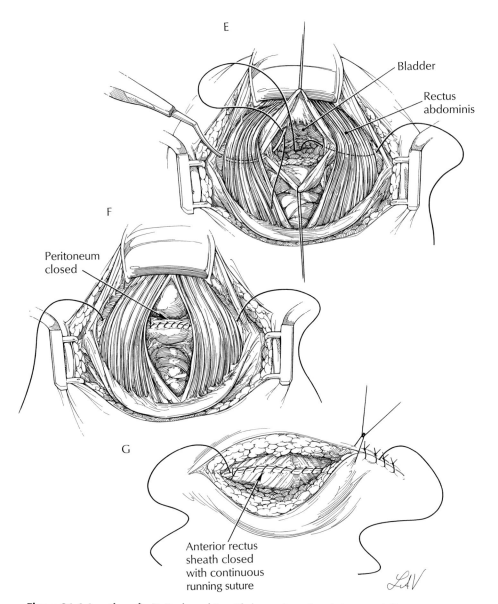

Figure 21.6 (continued). E. Each end is withdrawn into the abdomen. A ligature carrier is introduced lateral to the rectus abdominis on each side, following the path of the round ligament, to appear at the peritoneal opening. When the suture has been threaded to it, the carrier is withdrawn and the retroperitoneal sutures exit the abdomen lateral to the rectus sheath on each side. **F.** The initial transverse incision in the pelvic peritoneum is closed, and the abdomen is closed. **G.** The ends of the suture exit the fascia, and the skin is closed. (*Continues on following page.*)

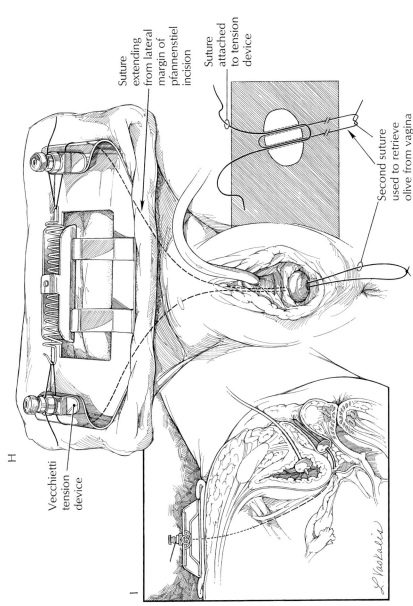

Suture extending from lateral margin of pfannenstiel incision

Suture attached to tension device

Second suture used to retrieve olive from vagina

Vecchietti tension device

H

I

Figure 21.6 (continued). H. A sterile padded dressing is placed over the incision, the Vecchietti tension frame placed on the abdomen, and the thread on each side is looped through the spring and fixed in place by a locknut as shown. **I.** With daily traction to the abdominal end of each thread, the tension is adjusted in such fashion that the olive will advance along the path of the neovagina about 1 cm per day. After 8 to 10 days, the vagina should measure about 10 cm in depth. The abdominal sutures are cut, flush with the skin surface, the Vecchietti device is removed, and the olive and sutures are withdrawn through the vagina using the looped second suture that had been placed as shown in the *inset*. The patient will be given a set of graduated vaginal dilators to apply daily to preserve neovaginal depth. By exchanging them for dilators that are progressively wider, the patient will increase vaginal diameter.

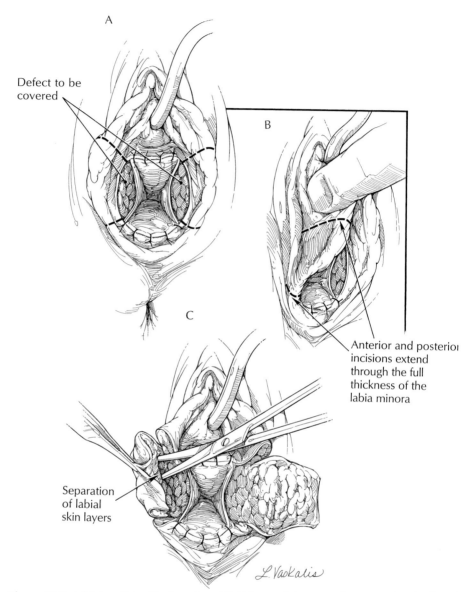

Figure 21.7. Labial pedicle skin flap. **A** and **B.** When a defect must be covered at the 3 and 9 o'clock positions following construction of a neovagina, a stricture-free coverage may be provided by sectioning the full thickness of the labia minora as indicated by the *dashed line.* **C.** The inner surface of each of the labia minora is incised and filleted. (*Continues on following page.*)

tively, and secretions from this area are minimal, particularly if the intestinal graft was placed in the antiperistaltic direction.

The Williams Vulvovaginoplasty

In the patient with thick and well-developed labia majora, the vulvovaginoplasty of Williams (10, 44) is useful. Postoperative stricture and contraction are not common, and

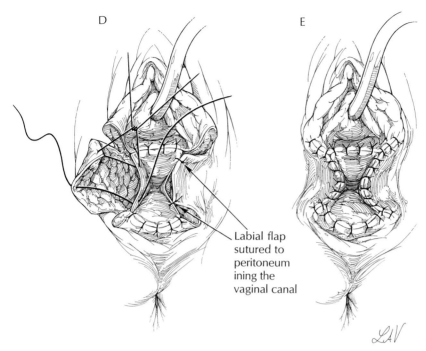

D

E

Labial flap
sutured to
peritoneum
ining the
vaginal canal

Figure 21.7 (continued). D. The margins of the now filleted labium minora are sewn to the free edge of material lining the neovaginal canal. **E.** The raw area of the transected labium is covered by a series of interrupted sutures.

the constant wearing of an obturator is not required. A neovagina several inches deep is constructed as shown in Figure 21.8. When the patient is sexually active, or by the use of an obturator when she is not, the depth of the neovagina should be progressively increased, and a gradual change in the vaginal axis may occur, which with time and sustained sexual use may approximate the normal.

The Davyoff Colpopoiesis

Pelvic peritoneum may be mobilized to cover the raw surface of a neovagina either for the total depth of the vagina (2, 7) or for the upper part, as in the case of a vaginal-lengthening procedure. The technique is illustrated in Figure 21.9. A transperineal translaparoscopic modification (2) of the Davyoff operation (7) for colpopoiesis (championed by Adamyan) using pelvic peritoneum to cover the raw surfaces of the neovagina is shown in Figure 21.10. If the peritoneum from the Davyoff procedure cannot be brought to the perineum without undue tension, filleted labia minora (see Fig. 21.7) may be used to bridge the gap.

COMPLICATIONS OF THE NEOVAGINA

If an introital stricture is found at the conclusion of any surgical construction of a neovagina (particularly with the colon transplant or the Davyoff peritoneal transloca-

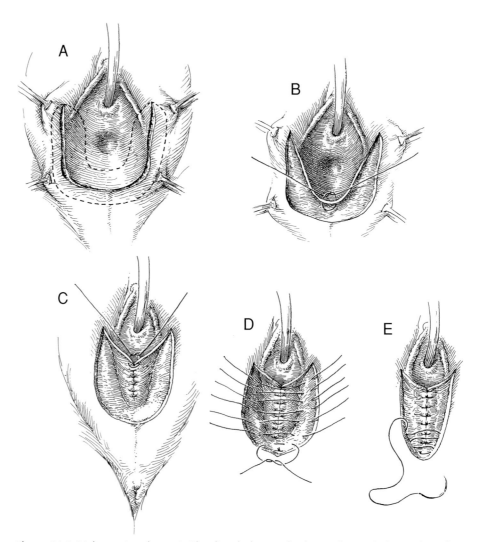

Figure 21.8. Vulvovaginoplasty. **A.** The dimpled area of softening beneath the urethra identifies the site of the missing vagina. Following thorough infiltration with 0.5 percent lidocaine in 1:200,000 epinephrine solution, a U-shaped incision is made along the inner surface of the labia majora about 4 cm lateral to the urethra and undermined as indicated by the *broken line.* **B** to **D.** The medial margins of the incision are united by interrupted sutures (B) and (C) and the subcutaneous tissue by a separate layer (D). **E.** The lateral incisional margins are approximated separately. (*Continues on following page.*)

tion), it can quietly be remedied by the use of bilateral pedicles from the labia minora fashioned as shown in Figure 21.7.

Eversion or prolapse (17) of the vault or stricture of the neovagina is uncommonly seen, but must be addressed promptly if the vagina is to be salvaged. Eversion may be a consequence of the natural absence of strong natural tissues supporting the vault of the neovagina. This weakness is made greater if the underside of too much peritoneal cul-de-sac is exposed during creation of the tunnel.

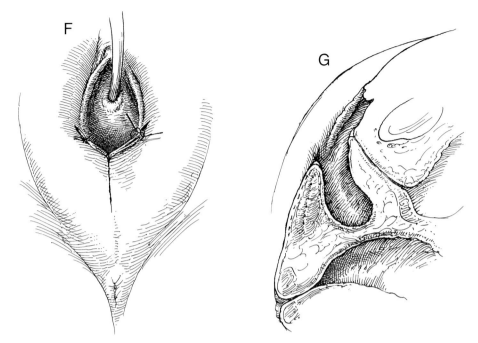

Figure 21.8 (continued). F. Frontal view of vulvovaginoplasty at the completion of the operation. **G.** Sagittal view. (From Capraro VJ, Capraro EJ. Creation of a neovagina. Obstet Gynecol 1972;39:544. Used with permission.)

In making the Abbe-McIndoe neovaginal cavity, the tip of the cavity should come to a point as it nears the abdominal peritoneum to lessen the chance of postoperative —enterocele and eversion of the neovagina. If a wide area of cul-de-sac peritoneum is exposed through the neovagina, the risk of postoperative eversion of the neovagina with enterocele is considerable, which then might require a separate future secondary operation for support. An everted vault must be supported surgically by reoperation.

In the patient with eversion of a neovagina, the surgeon should carefully evaluate the patient for the presence of a pelvic kidney, since this will determine whether or not there is operative room for a transabdominal sacral colpopexy. When room is lacking, a transvaginal surgical remedy can be offered. For a transvaginal surgical colpopexy, the neovagina may be sewn to the sacrospinous ligament or to the "white line" (arcus tendineus) just anterior to the site of the ischial spine.

Stricture or contraction of a neovagina develops after infection and scarring and when the patient has been remiss in wearing the postoperative mold during the required time. It may develop literally overnight. In the instance of a postoperative shrinking neovagina, which is too uncomfortable to permit progressive stretching as by an obturator, the condition may be remedied surgically by lateral incisions in the 3 and 9 o'clock positions that meet at the top of the vagina and extend across the vault. This is followed by the wearing of an obturator (Fig. 21.11) postoperatively until epithelialization and healing have taken place, and until the patient becomes sexually active. During the healing interval, the patient must wear an obturator as instructed.

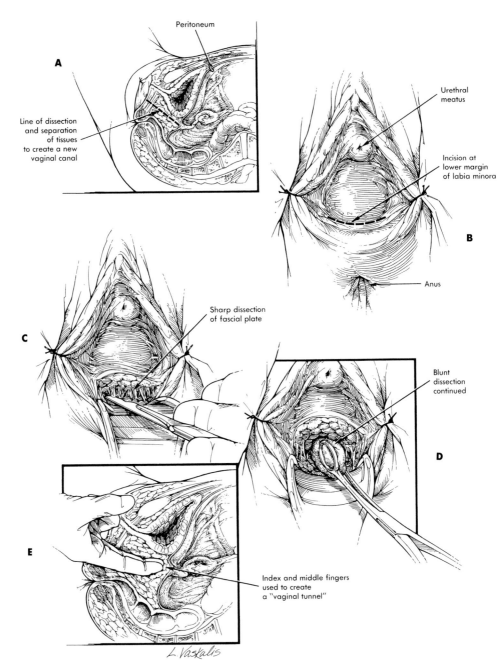

Figure 21.9. One-stage colpopoiesis using peritoneum to line the new vagina. **A.** Sagittal view of a patient with vaginal agenesis. The pathway of dissection to create a new vagina is shown by the *broken line*. **B.** A transverse incision between the lower edges of the labia minora is made at the site indicated by the *broken line*. **C.** Sharp dissection of the sub-epithelial fascial plate begins as shown. **D.** The dissection is continued bluntly in a cranial direction. **E.** The tissues between the bladder and rectum are divided by dissection using two fingers, palm side up. (*Continues on following page.*)

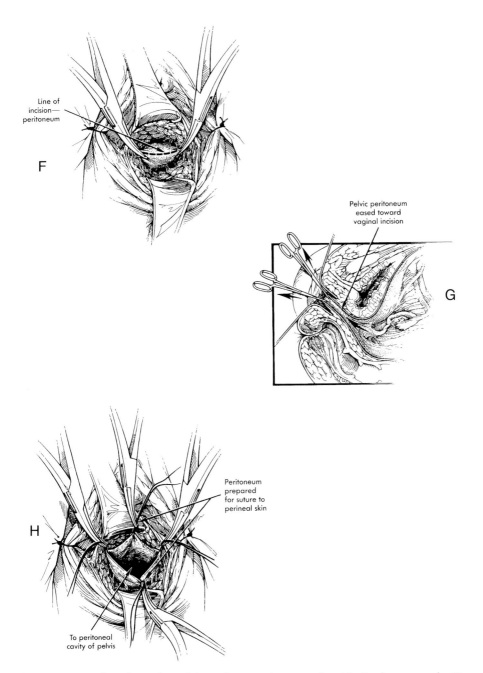

Line of
incision—
peritoneum

F

Pelvic peritoneum
eased toward
vaginal incision

G

Peritoneum
prepared
for suture to
perineal skin

H

To peritoneal
cavity of pelvis

Figure 21.9 (continued). F. The pelvic peritoneum is exposed and incised transversely. **G.** The circumference of peritoneum is gently drawn into the canal of the neovagina. **H.** The edges of peritoneum are sewn to the skin of the vaginal orifice. (*Continues on following page.*)

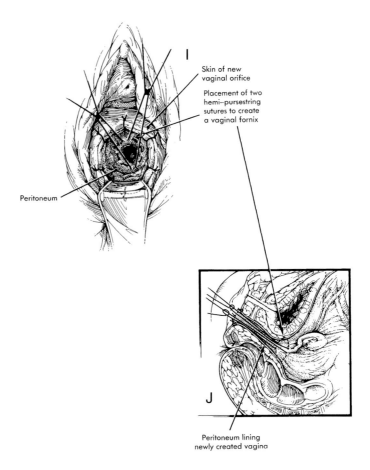

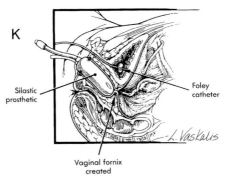

Figure 21.9 (continued). I. The peritoneal cavity is closed by two hemi-pursestring sutures placed high in the neovagina. **J.** Sagittal section showing closing of the peritoneal cavity. **K.** A Foley catheter is inserted into the bladder, and a prosthesis is inserted into the vagina. (From Nichols DH, ed. Gynecologic and obstetric surgery. St. Louis: Mosby-Yearbook, 1993. Used with permission.)

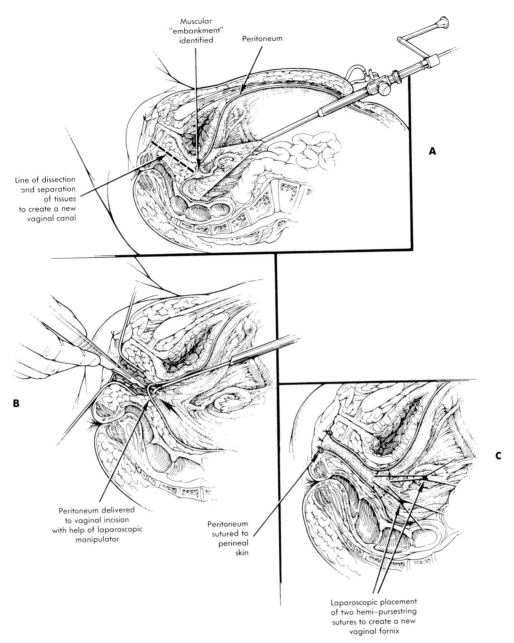

Muscular "embankment" identified

Peritoneum

A

Line of dissection and separation of tissues to create a new vaginal canal

B

Peritoneum delivered to vaginal incision with help of laparoscopic manipulator

Peritoneum sutured to perineal skin

C

Laparoscopic placement of two hemi–pursestring sutures to create a new vaginal fornix

Figure 21.10. Laparoscopically assisted colpopoiesis. **A.** Laparoscopic examination of the pelvis is performed. The site of transvaginal dissection for creation of a neovagina is shown by the *dashed line*. **B.** Using a laparoscopic probe or manipulator may help to deliver the peritoneum to the new tunnel. **C.** The peritoneum is opened transversely. The cut edges of peritoneum are sewn to the skin of the vaginal orifice, and the peritoneal cavity is closed by two hemi-pursestring sutures placed through the laparoscope. (From Nichols DH, ed. Gynecologic and obstetric surgery. St. Louis: Mosby–Year Book, 1993. Used with permission.)

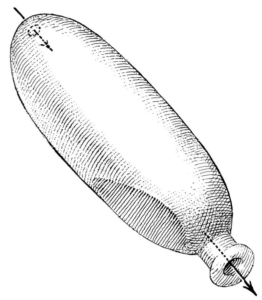

Figure 21.11. The Counseller-type silicone plastic mold. The mold is hollow, and the *arrows* indicate openings that permit drainage through the center of the mold. (Bioteque America, Langhorne, Pennsylvania 19047.)

References

1. Abbe R. New method of creating a vagina in a case of congenital absence. Med Rec 1898;54:836–838.
2. Adamyan LV. Colpopoiesis in vaginal and uterine aplasias. In: Nichols DH, ed. Gynecologic and obstetric surgery. St. Louis: Mosby-Yearbook, 1993:1178–1182.
3. Berek JS, Hacker NF, Lagasse LD, et al. Delayed vaginal reconstruction in the fibrotic pelvis following radiation or previous reconstruction. Obstet Gynecol 1983;61:743–748.
4. Bürger RA, Riedmiller H, Knapstein PG, Friedberg V, Hohenfellner R. Ileocecal vaginal construction. Am J Obstet Gynecol 1989;161:162–167.
5. Cali RW, Pratt JH. Congenital absence of the vagina: long-term results of vaginal reconstruction in 175 cases. Am J Obstet Gynecol 1968;100:752.
6. Counseller VS, Davis CE. Atresia of the vagina. Obstet Gynecol 1968;32:538.
7. Davyoff SN. Peritoneal colpopoiesis. In: Eicher W, ed. Plastic surgery in the sexually handicapped. Berlin-Heidelberg: Springer-Verlag, 1989:74–78.
8. DiSaia PJ, Rettenmaier MA. Vaginectomy. In: Sanz LE, ed. Gynecologic surgery. Oradell, NJ: Med Economics, 1988:151–157.
9. Dudzinski MR, Rader JS. The mons pubis: an excellent graft donor site in gynecologic surgery. Am J Obstet Gynecol 1990;162:722–725.
10. Evans TN, Poland ML, Boving RL. Vaginal malformations. Am J Obstet Gynecol 1981;141:910.
11. Fedele L, Busacca M, Candiani M, Vignali M. Laparoscopic creation of a neovagina in Mayer-Rokitansky-Küster-Hauser syndrome by modification of Vecchietti's operation. Am J Obstet Gynecol 1994;171:258–259.
12. Feroze RM, Dewhurst CJ, Welply G. Vaginoplasty at the Chelsea Hospital for Women: a comparison of two techniques. Br J Obstet Gynaecol 1975;82:536.
13. Fleigner JR. Congenital atresia of the vagina. Surg Gynecol Obstet 1987;165:387–391.
14. Frank RT. The formation of an artificial vagina without operation. Am J Obstet Gynecol 1938;35:1053.
15. Freundt I, Toolenaar TAM, Huikeshoven FJM, et al. Long-term psychosexual performance of patients with a sigmoid neovagina. Am J Obstet Gynecol 1993;169:1210–1214.
16. Freundt I, Toolenaar TAM, Huikeshoven FJM, Drogendijk AC, Jeekel H. A modified technique to create a neovagina with an isolated segment of sigmoid colon. Surg Gynecol Obstet 1992;174:11–16.
17. Freundt I, Toolenaar TAM, Jeekel H, Drogendijk AC, Huikeshoven FJM. Prolapse of the sigmoid neovagina: report of three cases. Obstet Gynecol 1994;83:876–879.
18. Gauwerky JFH, Wallwiener D, Bastert G. An endoscopically assisted technique for construction of a neovagina. Arch Gynecol Obstet 1992;252:59–63.

19. Goligher JC. The use of pedicled transplants of sigmoid or other parts of the intestinal tract for vaginal construction. Ann Roy Coll Surg Engl 1983;65:353–355.
20. Graves WP. Operative treatment of atresia of the vagina. Boston Med Surg J 1910;163:753.
21. Ingram JM. The bicycle seat in the treatment of vaginal agenesis and stenosis: a preliminary report. Am J Obstet Gynecol 1981;1:867.
22. Jackson ND, Rosenblatt PL. Use of Interceed absorbable adhesion barrier for vaginoplasty. Obstet Gynecol 1994;84:1048–1050.
23. Lilford RJ, Sharpe DT, Thomas DFM. Use of tissue expansion techniques to create skin flaps for vaginoplasty. Br J Obstet Gynaecol 1988;95:402–407.
24. Martin LW, Sutorius DS. An improved method for vaginoplasty. Arch Surg 1969;98:716.
25. McIndoe AH, Banister JB. An operation for the cure of congenital absence of the vagina. J Obstet Gynaecol Br Commonw 1938;45:490–494.
26. Morton KE, Davies D, Dewhurst J. The use of the fasciocutaneous flap in vaginal reconstruction. Br J Obstet Gynaecol 1986;93:970.
27. Nichols DH, ed. Gynecologic and obstetric surgery. St. Louis: Mosby–Year Book, 1993:416–417.
28. Ober KG, Meinrenken GH. Allgemeine und spezielle chirurgische operationslehre. In: Kirschner M. Gynakologische Operationen. Berlin: Springer, 1964. Quoted in Käser O, Iklé FA, Hirsch HA. Atlas of gynecological surgery. 2nd ed. New York: Georg Thieme Verlag, 1985.
29. Pelzer V. Anlage einer Neovagina nach Vecchietti in der Düsseldorfer Modifikation. In: Pelzer V, Beck L. Aktuelle Fragen aus der Kinder und Jugendgynäkologie 2. Düsseldorfer Symposium. Stuttgart-New York: Georg Thieme Verlag, 1990.
30. Pelzer V, Graf M. Das gegliederte Steckphantom zur Bildung einer einer Neovagina nach Vecchietti. Geburtshilfe Frauenheilkd 1989;49:977–980.
31. Pratt JH. Use of the colon in gynecologic surgery. In: Sturgis SH, Taymor ML, ed. Meigs and Sturgis, progress in gynecology. New York, Grune & Stratton, 1970;4:435–446.
32. Rettenmaier MA, DiSaia P. Understanding current vaginectomy techniques. Contemp Obstet Gynecol 1987;30:109–117.
33. Sheares BH. Congenital atresia of the vagina—a new technique for tunnelling the space between the bladder and rectum and construction of a new vagina by a modified Wharton technique. J Obstet Gynaecol Br Emp 1960;67:24–31.
34. Song R, Wang X, Zhou G. Reconstruction of the vagina with sensory function. Clin Plast Surg 1982;9:105–108.
35. Stal S, Spira M. Mons pubis as a donor site for split-thickness skin grafts. Plast Reconstr Surg 1985;75:906.
36. Tancer ML, Katz M, Veridiano NP. Vaginal epithelialization with human amnion. Obstet Gynecol 1979; 54:345–349.
37. Thompson JD, Wharton LR, TeLinde RW. Congenital absence of the vagina. Am J Obstet Gynecol 1957; 74:397.
38. Tolhurst DE, van der Helm TWJS. The treatment of vaginal atresia. Surg Gynecol Obstet 1991; 172:407–414.
39. Vecchietti G. Die Neovagina beim Rokitansky-Küster-Hauser-Syndrom. Gynäkologie 1980; 13:112–115.
40. Vecchietti G. Le néo-vagin dans le syndrome de Rokitansky-Küster-Hauser. Rev Med Suisse Romande 1979;99:593–601.
41. Vecchietti G, Ardillo L. La sindrome di Rokitansky-Küster-Hauser Fisiopatologia e Clinica Aplasia vaginale—Corni uterini rudimentale. Rome: Societa Editrice Universo, 1970:1–132.
42. West JT, Ketcham As, Smith RR. Vaginal reconstruction following pelvic exenteration for cancer or postirradiation necrosis. Surg Gynecol Obstet 1965;118:788.
43. Wharton LR. A simplified method of constructing a vagina. Ann Surg 1938;107:842–847.
44. Williams EA. Congenital absence of the vagina: a simple operation for its relief. J Obstet Gynaecol Br Commonw 1964;71:511.

CHAPTER 22

Postoperative Care

Postoperative care begins the minute the patient leaves the operating room. The patient's loved ones should be promptly informed of the details of surgery, told when it is likely that they may see the patient, and what to expect.

GENERAL GUIDELINES

Postoperative monitoring of the patient's vital signs begins immediately following surgery. Measurements of pulse, blood pressure, and respiratory rate should be taken and recorded every 15 minutes during the first hour, then every 30 minutes for 2 hours, every 60 minutes for 8 hours, and every 4 hours thereafter. Any unexpected drop in blood pressure, especially if accompanied by tachycardia, may indicate continued blood loss and call for serial hematocrit and hemoglobin determinations. The urine output is measured hourly until the morning following surgery and every 4 hours thereafter (26). Any marked or persistent discrepancy is reported, evaluated promptly, and treated appropriately. Postoperative fluid and electrolyte administration is carefully calculated to fit the patient's specific needs, taking into account the fluid balance during surgery. Routine hematocrit, hemoglobin, and often creatinine levels are determined the morning of the second postoperative day.

Extended visits with the patient should be discouraged during the first few postoperative days, when the patient needs ample opportunity to rest. Pain relief should be offered as necessary, preferably by the use of small doses of medication repeated at frequent intervals in order to avoid an accumulative effect and a systemic or respiratory depression. Because periods of rest should be carefully interspersed with periods of ambulation and physical activity, it is important to avoid oversedation. Regular periods of deliberately deepened breathing should be encouraged as soon as the patient becomes conscious, and frequent repetition of deep inspiration or incentive spirometry has proved effective in reducing postoperative pulmonary problems.

Little seems to be gained by having a patient dangle her legs over the edge of the bed the evening following surgery; in fact, this may even increase venous stasis. However, the patient should be encouraged to begin flexing her legs, bending her ankles, and gently moving from side to side and changing position in bed soon after awakening from surgery, and to continue these movements throughout the entire postoperative period. Beginning the day after surgery, she should be helped to a bedside chair for a few minutes three or four times daily. This may improve the transit time of intestinal gas. Sitting on a rubber doughnut is not recommended, because stretching of unsupported tissues through the hole in the center may strain new sutures, However, a soft pillow is an acceptable substitute. If the patient is willing, warm sitz baths or showers can be started on the second or third postoperative day. When elastic stockings have been applied preoperatively and the patient is resuming physical activity in a satisfactory manner, the stockings can be removed, usually by the third or fourth postoperative day.

Postoperative intravenous fluids should be continued until one is assured that the patient will take and retain by mouth sufficient fluids, at which point the intravenous route should be discontinued. Liquids by mouth are usually permitted as soon as the patient has recovered from anesthesia, but in sips rather than by glassfuls, and preferably tea or tap water. Carbonated beverages, milk products, and fruit juices should be avoided initially to decrease the production of intestinal gas (21). When frequently repeated, this regime will usually ensure the ingestion of an adequate 2 quarts of liquid per day. Solid foods can be offered as soon as the patient is interested; but, other than an occasional nibble, a significant intake is unlikely until the patient's appetite returns, usually on the second or third postoperative day. There are exceptions, of course, particularly after the repair of rectovaginal fistula or an old fourth-degree laceration, in which instance the patient is best maintained on an initial clear liquid nonresidue diet, followed during the second week after surgery by a low-residue diet.

Sufficient opiate analgesia to afford relief from severe pain is administered and carefully monitored. Patient-controlled analgesia (PCA) is useful during the first 2 postoperative days because it can be adjusted to patient variability and pain severity. By the second or third day it can be replaced by nonopiate analgesics, usually acetaminophen (Tylenol) or aspirin with or without codeine, ibuprofen (Motrin, Advil), or for relief of more severe pain, ketorolac tromethamine (Toradol) is useful.

Collagen is important in wound strength. Early gel-like wound collagen must be broken down and resynthesized into stronger collagen, a process in which collagen lysis and collagen synthesis occur simultaneously. Normally these rates are balanced, but malnutrition and oxygen deficiency may tip the scale in favor of collagen lysis, producing a weak wound, particularly in the absence of ascorbic acid. For this reason, ascorbic acid is prescribed for 3 months (550 mg daily) to inhibit the elaboration of collagenase and hopefully improve wound strength (10).

For the patient taking cortisone, supplemental vitamin A may reverse the inhibitory effect of cortisone on wound healing (9).

Antibiotics or antibacterials to "cover" the bacteria often associated with the use of an indwelling bladder catheter need not be started until the day the catheter is to be removed. This sequence seems to avoid or retard the development of an antibiotic-resistant type of urinary tract infection such as often intrudes when antibacterial "coverage" is instituted immediately postoperatively and continued through the patient's postoperative course. (The exception will be after urinary fistula repair, in which one would wish to "sterilize" the urine during the early healing phase.) A urine culture and sensitivity study should, of course, be obtained the day the catheter is removed; when a positive culture is reported, the most appropriate antibiotic should be used until the culture becomes negative. Gentle percussion of the costovertebral angles should be accomplished postoperatively the evening after surgery and for the next several days. Unexpected or pronounced unilateral tenderness should be promptly investigated by prompt "single-shot" infusion intravenous pyelography to exclude ureteral obstruction.

RESUMPTION OF BOWEL FUNCTION

Bowel movements should be resumed by the third postoperative day. The administration of a gentle laxative with a stool softener (such as casanthranol and dioctyl sodium sulfosuccinate [Peri-Colace]), beginning when the patient starts to eat solid food, is often helpful. If no movement has occurred by the evening of the third postoperative day, 30 ml of milk of magnesia and 4 ml of cascara are given; if this is ineffective, an irritant suppository, such as bisacodyl (Dulcolax), or a saline enema is ordered. If this does not bring about a bowel movement, a gentle rectal examination is necessary to rule out a fecal impaction. Any fecal impaction is gently broken digitally, and an oil retention enema is given, followed by a saline enema. If this is unsuccessful, the impaction can be broken up under general anesthesia either digitally or by using a standard domestic teaspoon (7).

The cessation of smoking in a postoperative patient may inhibit intestinal peristalsis because of the withdrawal of nicotine, so some extra problems with bowel function such as constipation should be anticipated. Stool softeners and laxatives may be particularly appropriate for patients who have undergone a posterior colporrhaphy or perineorrhaphy.

Under no circumstances should the patient recovering from gynecologic surgery be permitted to sit up to strain on a bedpan in an effort to accomplish a bowel movement without an enema. Surgery in the female pelvis is not infrequently followed by thrombosis in relatively large veins that communicate with the internal iliacs and vena cava. The suddenly increased intra-abdominal pressure that occurs as a result of a patient's efforts to accomplish a bowel movement may lead to thromboembolism in the iliacs and vena cava, occasionally with disastrous results. This risk can be reduced by (a) early ambulation of the patient, (b) prohibition of any major postoperative straining efforts to accomplish a bowel movement, and (c) the use of stool softeners and enema to ensure postoperative bowel movement without exertion or strain.

The surgeon should make daily unhurried visits to the patient to assess her response to healing and therapy and to recognize and respond to her psychological concerns, and also to begin the process of discharge planning. The surgeon should give notice of his or her availability for advice and detailed notification of changes after discharge from the hospital, such as unexpected bleeding or fever, that should be brought to the surgeon's attention. The patient should be told how to find her surgeon after discharge from the hospital. The duration of convalescence should be outlined, with questions solicited and a plan made for postoperative examination. Verbal instructions are so often forgotten that written communications or instructions, even if brief, are desirable.

During her postoperative course, it is well to review on several occasions the patient's ingestion of all medications, for conflicting or unnecessary orders may be recognized for which timely correction can be made. Any preexisting medical conditions under treatment (e.g., hypertension) should be frequently reevaluated, the postoperative routine modified, and appropriate therapy reinstituted as necessary.

Appropriate blood studies should be obtained before a patient is discharged from the hospital. A stable postoperative hemoglobin of 9 g/ml or greater and a hematocrit of at least 27 in a patient without cardiovascular disease will respond to oral therapy, and transfusion is unnecessary.

PARTICULAR POSTOPERATIVE CONSIDERATIONS FOR THE OLDER WOMAN

The postoperative hospitalization of the elderly patient is not longer than that of the younger patient (6, 8, 16, 20). Surgical morbidity and mortality do not appear to be related to the length of an operation (15), although the risks of spinal anesthesia suggest that it is best to use this type of anesthesia only when the planned surgery is likely to be 2 hours or less. Epidural anesthesia is a suitable alternative if the surgery is expected to take longer or if there is some concern about the patient's cardiovascular stability. General anesthesia is also a legitimate choice for the elderly patient, since it provides excellent control of patient oxygenation (1). The anesthesiologist's preoperative evaluation and discussion with the patient are of inestimable value in making the final decision.

It is advisable to apply elastic stockings preoperatively onto both the patient's legs from the ankle to the upper thigh. If the legs are not so wrapped, the rapid return of blood to the lower extremities may reduce the patient's blood pressure alarmingly a short time after the legs are lowered postoperatively. During surgery on the elderly and often hypertensive patient at risk, monitoring the pulmonary wedge pressure appears to be a more dependable means of interpreting blood pressure changes than is monitoring central venous pressure. Furthermore, a higher pulmonary capillary wedge pressure may be necessary in the elderly to maintain preload and cardiac output (22).

Postoperative care of the elderly patient should emphasize pulmonary recovery through deep breathing, incentive spirometry, and early ambulation. The lack of pain in an abdominal incision promotes effective patient cooperation, although it may be necessary to remind the patient to perform these activities. Tachycardia and tachypnea are often unreliable indications of hypoxia in the elderly. Any significant change in the arterial blood gas levels or the concentration of circulatory hemoglobin may be an indication for supplemental oxygen therapy, however.

Because it affects the calculations of appropriate dosages of medication, the decrease in the glomerular filtration rate is the most important renal change that occurs with advancing age. The surgeon should prescribe low dosages of those medications that are excreted primarily in the urine (12, 22); in addition, to minimize adverse drug reactions, the surgeon should carefully limit the number of drugs that are used. Any interference with tubular resorption diminishes the ability of the kidneys to concentrate urine. These factors, combined with a decreased renal blood flow, inhibit the prompt restoration of fluid and electrolyte balance. Therefore, fluid intake and urinary output must be carefully measured and balanced. The oral ingestion of 2 liters of fluids per day provides quantity, but because age blunts the sense of thirst, the elderly patient must be under continuous surveillance to ensure that she actually consumes an adequate quantity.

The older patient may require as much as 5 days to recover her full mental function after anesthesia (2). A subtle change in mental status may be the first sign of hypoxemia, acidosis, myocardial infarction, acute infection, or impending septic shock (12, 21). Careful observation of the patient's breath and breathing helps to clarify her status. Pain is less a symptom of acute illness in the older patient than in the younger patient, so monitoring her during daily rounds is necessary for her progressive recovery.

If the patient is postmenopausal and sexually active, oral ingestion of an estrogen can be started as soon as the patient is taking fluids by mouth. This can be supplemented by nightly and later weekly instillations of an intravaginal estrogen (5) to aid wound epithelization, help preserve vaginal blood supply and elasticity, and reduce vaginal atrophy that would otherwise become even more evident with postoperative contraction of the vaginal incision. Caution is necessary in the use of estrogen supplementation in these postmenopausal patients, however. The mechanics of intravaginal insertion of the applicator itself may inhibit the development of postoperative adhesions between the anterior and posterior walls of the vagina.

PROTOCOL FOR REMOVAL OF THE CATHETER

Special attention is needed concerning removal of the catheter in someone recovering from reparative surgery.

A useful protocol concerning patient management after removal of a transurethral catheter is as follows: Between 7:00 and 8:00 a.m., a urine culture is obtained, and the patient is started on an antibacterial, such as nitrofurantoin (50 mg of Macrodantin three times daily), methenamine (24) (1 g three times daily), or trimethoprim sulfa. An alpha-adrenergic blocker (such as 10 mg of phenoxybenzamine) is given by mouth.

One must recall that the bladder neck is well supplied with alpha-adrenergic receptors. When stimulated, these receptors tend to cause smooth muscle contraction in this area, in contrast to beta receptors, which tend to produce relaxation of the bladder neck and trigone in the presence of low amounts of noradrenaline (23). Alpha-adrenergic blocking agents, such as phenoxybenzamine or prazosin, will thus selectively block spasm resulting from alpha-adrenergic receptor stimulation in this area. Success has been reported (14, 18) from the use of the alpha-adrenergic blocking agent phenoxybenzamine (Dibenzyline) in a dose of 10 mg by mouth 4 to 5 hours after surgery and repeated, if necessary, once or twice during the first 24 hours. The drug is given to the catheterized patient coincident with catheter removal. The author's experience with this drug for this circumstance has been favorable. One must remember that any beta blockers, such as propranolol hydrochloride (Inderal), may not only stimulate detrusor tone, inducing a hypertonia, but, by selective blocking, may induce some spasm of the bladder neck.

At the time that a transurethral Foley catheter is removed, the nursing staff should be instructed to catheterize as necessary if the patient is unable to void. An alternate is to catheterize two or three times daily immediately after voiding until a postvoiding residual of no more than 100 ml has been recorded on two consecutive occasions. The amount that the patient voids is usually of prognostic significance, even when the initial urinary residual volume may have been undesirably high. It is of greater significance and much more encouraging if a patient is voiding 100 to 200 ml with a residual of 200 to 250 ml than if the patient is voiding only 10 to 20 ml at a time with a residual volume of 200 to 250 ml. In the first situation, one would expect the amount voided to increase in relative amounts as the quantity of residual urine decreases.

Residual urine volume can also be measured noninvasively by using a portable battery-operated bedside ultrasound unit. The BladderScan (Bard Patient Care Division, Murray Hill, New Jersey) (Fig. 22.1) provides an instantaneous, numerical measurement. It is accurate (3, 4, 19) and saves the patient the discomfort of routine catheterization. It also eliminates the risk of catheter-induced bacterial cystitis (17). This simple bedside scan can be repeated as often as necessary until the residual volume is less than 100 ml on two consecutive determinations. It does not decrease nursing time from that required for catheterization, but it will decrease the number of invasive transuretheral catheterizations, thus reducing the potential for nosocomial infection.

POSTOPERATIVE DIFFICULTIES IN VOIDING

The patient who is unable to void can be taught the technique of self-catheterization, or an indwelling transurethral catheter can be reinserted (see Chapter 10).

The amount that the patient voids is usually of prognostic significance, even when the initial residual volume may have been undesirably high. It is of greater significance and much more encouragine if a patient is voiding 100 to 200 ml with a residual of 200 to 250 ml that if the patient is voiding only 10 to 20 ml at a time with a residual volume of 200 to 250 mi. In the first situation, one would expect the amount voided to increase in relative amounts as the quantity of residual urine decreases. Those factors that inhibit the physiologic obliteration and descent of the posterior vesicourethral angle play a role. For example, very few women can void while a tight vaginal packing is in place (Fig. 22.2), and treatment of this etiologic circumstance is the removal of any mechani-

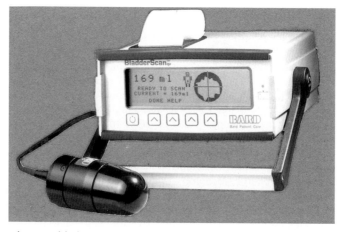

Figure 22.1. The portable battery-operated BladderScan (Bard Patient Care Division, Murray Hill, New Jersey) ultrasound unit to measure residual urine volume. The hand-held probe, seen on the *left side* of the photograph, is applied suprapubically, and the numerical volume of residual urine given, as well as an image of the fluid within the bladder.

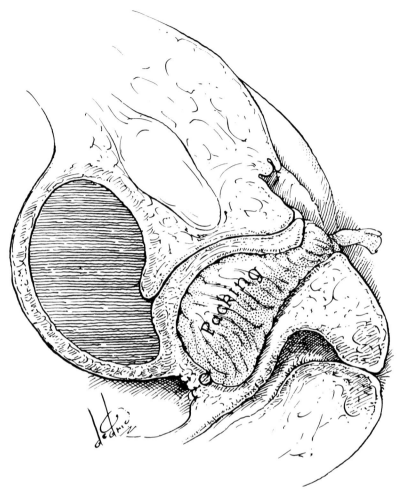

Figure 22.2. Spontaneous voiding after surgery may be inhibited if the vagina is so tightly packed with gauze that physiologic descent of the vesicourethral junction is precluded. (From Nichols DH. Getting the postoperative patient to void. Contemp Obstet Gynecol 1978;12:41–45. Used with permission.)

cal obstruction of the vagina or urethra. It is important that overhydration is avoided at the time an indwelling catheter is to be removed, since overhydradion, although frequently urged by some nursing staff, exaggerates any difficulties that may be present and produces rapid and unnecessary overdistention of the bladder.

Overdistention of the bladder (urine volume >500 ml) is to be avoided at all costs. Not only is overdistention painful, but it appears to interfere temporarily with the blood supply of the bladder and thus to reduce local resistance to infection (13). In addition, overdistention may cause a transient paralysis of the detrusor that can require days to overcome.

Prevention

Prevention of any postoperative voiding difficulty is of prime importance. The circumstances under which the patient is expected to void must be as private and comfortable as possible, and there is no substitute for promptness and calm on the part of the patient's attendants. Von Peham and Amreich (25) wrote years ago of the difficulty some encounter of voiding in the recumbent position. It at all possible, the patient should be permitted to void in a natural sitting position, using a nearby toilet if feasible, a portable commode if not, or sitting on a bedpan if confined to bed. However, some postoperative patients can void more comfortably at first from a semistanding position, probably because it reduces the likelihood of levator spasm. Others may find manual suprapubic compression over the bladder helpful once voiding has begun, and this technique is more effective when the patient leans somewhat forward during the voiding process.

Causes

The bladder has a triple nerve supply—somatic, sympathetic, and parasympathetic—and the perception and balance between these sometimes opposing influences vary from patient to patient and from time to time. Because this harmony is easily disturbed, it is not surprising that postoperative resumption of voiding is a rather common problem, but not often predictable with any degree of certainty. Difficulty in this area may occur after any surgical procedure, but especially after those involving the abdominal and pelvic muscles and overlying skin (e.g., episiotomy, colporrhaphy, hysterectomy, herniorrhaphy, hemorrhoidectomy, and laparotomy).

It is known that a postoperative voiding difficulty can result from several factors (11). There are almost certain to be additional factors that influence the precess of voiding but cannot yet be predictably or accurately understood or measured. Not the least of these is the patient's motivation. There are some whose confidence in the function of their own bladders is sufficient to overcome almost any disturbance. For those who are experiencing difficulty, however, the calm, optimistic, and serene understanding of their attendants is of utmost importance during the brief time that for them constitutes a disquieting and disabling crisis.

ANXIETY

A powerful cause of inability to void is anxiety on the part of the patient or her attendant staff. Sometimes this is preconditioned by fear, conversation with other patients, hearsay, or observation of other patients. Treatment, of course, includes appropriate counseling, gentle calmness, cheerful confidence, and empathy on the part of the attendant staff, and appropriate sedation and pain relief. The administration of tea or beer has been recommended, the former to induce some detrusor hyperactivity and the latter some general body sedation.

MECHANICAL INTERFERENCE

Local physical factors may interfere with the physiology of voiding. Among these are the presence of vaginal packing, local edema, rectal fullness, or any obstruction of urethra or ureters. Any mechanical factors that interfere with the opening of the internal urethral sphincter may play a role, especially those causing failure of physiologic obliteration of the posterior urethrovesical angle during attempts at voiding.

DRUG-INDUCED EFFECTS

One must consider drug-induced hypotonia, since coincident and often long-term consumption of the common tranquilizing agents may be associated with unexpected and sometimes chronic detrusor hypotonia. This effect should be suspected among patients accustomed to daily doses of diazepam (Valium), chlordiazepoxide hydrochloride (Librium), thioridazine hydrochloride (Mellaril), chlorpromazine (Thorazine), prochlorperazine (Compazine), and meprobamate (Miltown). In many instances, these drugs may have been supplied by other physicians, and the patient may have become so accustomed to taking them that she has forgotten to include her consumption of them in her medical history. Discontinuation of the drug, when it is a factor producing detrusor hypotonia, may result in a rather prompt reappearance of normal bladder tone.

If the patient has a history of long-standing bladder decompensation, as may be associated with the aging large or massive cystocele, some intrinsic detrusor hypotonia can be predicted and bladder tone increased by judicious use of bethanechol chloride (Urecholine) before removal of the catheter and for several days thereafter until comfortable voiding has been reestablished. In obviously anxious patients, preliminary sedation with barbiturates and judicious use of analgesics will be rewarding, with a dose tailored to the needs of the individual patient.

EXTRINSIC REFLEX INTERFERENCES

A major etiologic factor can be related to neurologic reflex interference with the normal physiology of voiding. This may be coincident with levator spasm, as is so often seen after parturition, episiotomy, and hemorrhoidectomy, which may give rise to reflex spastic contraction of both the internal and external urethral sphincters. This is, of course, accentuated by nervousness and patient embarrassment. Sitz baths, analgesia, and time are of the greatest help, because when painful but temporary levator spasm has finally been overcome, the bladder and urethral sphincters will once again begin to relax. Similarly, pain in the rectus abdominus muscles, from laparotomy incision, will often reflexly induce levator spasm, interfering with the physiologic descent of the vesical neck during the voiding process. Again, patience and analgesia will help. Temporary use of an alpha-adrenergic blocker, such as phenoxybenzamine, will often relieve urethral spasm, as mentioned above.

As mentioned earlier, overdistention of the bladder can result in a temporary detrusor paralysis and is therefore to be avoided at all costs. It can develop insidiously in the patient who has been oversedated and overhydrated and has failed to perceive or respond to bladder fullness. Once pathologic overdistention has developed, the treatment is primarily expectant: awaiting the return of bladder tone 1 or 2 days after continuous decompression by an indwelling catheter and prevention of additional or future episodes of overdistention.

INTRINSIC NEUROLOGIC ABNORMALITY

Another etiologic circumstance may be that of primary neurologic defect. Neuropathy giving rise to chronic bladder hypotonia may be associated with diabetes, central nervous system lues, or multiple sclerosis. Sometimes this correlation can be suspected from the patient's medical history. Neuropathy coincident with herniated intervertebral disc may be evident; there is coincident constipation and usually a history of sudden onset. Low discs that involve the cauda equina but are too far caudal to be evident on myelography may be present. Skillful neurologic evaluation is required for appropriate diagnosis. Hypotonia can often be suspected preoperatively, and subtle detrusor stimulation by postoperative bethanechol (Urecholine) may be advisable. Dosages may start as low as 10 mg three times a day but rapidly increase to the point of clinical effectiveness, sometimes to as much as 50 to 75 mg three times daily.

Treatment

Generally speaking, the most comfortable and successful treatments at present are those outlined above. Detrusor hyperactivity induced by deliberate production of a chemical cystitis such as by instilling intravesical Mercurochrome or ether is neither popular nor recommended, since the results are not only unpredictable, but the method may unexpectedly give rise to a long-standing, chronic cystitis, sometimes of massive degree. Some postoperative patients will find that they can at first void more comfortably from a semistanding position, probably one that reduces levator spasm, and others may find comfort from aiding voiding once it has begun by manual suprapubic compression over the bladder, more effective when the patient is leaning somewhat forward during the voiding process.

Patients recovering from suprapubic sling procedures who have been accustomed to emptying their bladders by tightening the rectus muscles to increase intra-abdominal pressure must be instructed not to do so in the future, since voluntary rectus muscle contraction may tighten the sling sufficiently to occlude the urethra. Any significant urethral stricture obstructing normal flow can be relieved by gentle urethral dilatation.

The attitude of the nursing staff is of utmost importance in the management of patients unable to void after surgery. Knowledgeable and friendly confidence, smiles, and infinite gentleness in catheterizing these individuals, already apprehensive with understandably tender tissues, is most likely when personnel are experienced in postoperative urinary tract care.

If, after removal of the catheter, the patient is still unable to void in adequate amounts, she may be taught the technique of self-catheterization using the soft plastic Mentor female catheter (a useful handout sheet that can be given to the patient is reproduced in Chapter 10). Alternatively, she may be discharged with a Foley catheter in place and clamped. The clamp is to be opened and the bladder drained periodically as necessary. It should be explained that the temporary inability to void is by no means rare or unusual and will probably not lengthen or change her convalescence. Another handout sheet is provided to the patient for reference concerning the care of the catheter. One the author has found useful is as follows:

Care of the Catheter

The bladder must be given time to rest and heal, and the swelling and irritation from surgery given time to subside. This involves a variable length of recovery time from person to person, lasting anywhere from a few days to several weeks. The more extensive the need for repair, the greater the scope of the repair, and the longer the period of recovery of comfortable bladder function.

During this recovery period, a person's kidney system continues to work, of course, and it is necessary to drain the urine from the bladder until functional recovery of the bladder has been completed. This outlet is provided by an indwelling catheter inserted in the bladder as at the time of surgery.

When the catheter is inserted through the urethra (the usual external canal between vulva and bladder), the urethral catheter can be clamped, to stop its flow, until there is sufficient fluid in the bladder to produce urgency and the sense of wanting to void, at which time the clamp can be removed and the bladder emptied, then the clamp reapplied. After about 2 weeks of bladder rest, the catheter is removed by cutting it across with clean scissors sometime during the midmorning hours, and the patient is requested to call the office that weekday afternoon to inform us how the bladder is working. If adequate amounts of urine are being passed and at intervals greater than 2 hours between voidings, it is good evidence that comfortable bladder function has returned. There will often be a mild sense of burning or irritation during voiding until the swelling in the urethra from the catheter has subsided, usually within 1 or 2 days. Should urinary burning and frequency increase beyond this point, instead of getting progressively better, be sure to call the office.

SUPRAPUBIC CATHETER

The author has used the suprapubic catheter in two particular instances: one, after repair of a fistula at the vesical neck as a means of keeping the catheter away from the site of the fistula repair; another, after the creation of a neovagina in a patient requiring the postoperative use of a vaginal obturator (Chapter 21). Should the surgeon be an advocate of suprapubic catheterization, a handout concerning care of the suprapubic catheter may be of advantage to the patient:

Care of the Suprapubic Catheter

Under many circumstances, the doctor may wish to put the recently repaired tissues around the urethra, bladder, and vagina at complete rest while they recover from surgery, and a catheter will be placed into the bladder through a tiny incision in the skin of the lower abdomen. This is a temporary way of diverting the urine until the patient's own bladder system is able to function again and does save a patient the nuisance, discomfort, and irritation from repeated catheterization during the healing process.

By the time preliminary healing is under way, usually after the fourth postoperative day, this catheter may be fitted with a screw-type clamp that, when tightened, will stop the flow of urine through the catheter and permit the bladder to fill. When the patient feels bladder fullness and the desire to void, she is encouraged to do so, and following voiding, or if unable to pass water through the urethra at that time, the screw clamp is opened and the bladder drained through the suprapubic catheter. This procedure is continued on a regular basis as long as necessary until most of the urine is being passed naturally through the urethra and less than 2 ounces or two is drained from the suprapubic catheter after each voiding. For this reason, it is important to keep a running account of the amount of urine voided each time and the amount obtained from the catheter after each voiding.

When the amount left behind has remained less than 2 ounces in volume, the suprapubic catheter clamp should be left firmly applied for a full 1 or 2 days to see whether regular urinary voiding remains well established. If so, and at the end of the 2 days, the catheter is removed by extraction after simply cutting across its midpoint. The opening left by the catheter will usually close within a day or two, but a small amount of urine will often drip at first from this opening, requiring a small dressing until the opening has closed.

A word of caution regarding estrogen supplementation in certain hypoestrogenic postmenopausal women: If a postmenopausal patient has not been taking estrogen preoperatively, its introduction during the immediate postoperative phase may be associated with some hyperemia and edema of the vesical neck. This swelling may produce some degree of temporary partial obstruction of the urethra.

DISCHARGE FROM THE HOSPITAL

The probable date of discharge from the hospital should be discussed with the patient a day or two ahead of time to give the patient and her family adequate time to make arrangements and preparations. The patient should be given very specific instructions before discharge as to what she may and may not do during her convalescence. Written or printed postoperative instructions as shown in Fig. 22.3 can be extremely useful.

The patient should also be instructed as to the circumstances (fever, excessive bleeding, etc.) for which she should call for help postoperatively. Many patients will appreciate a summary and an interpretation of the laboratory studies recorded while in the hospital, and every patient should be given specific directions as to when to return to the surgeon's office for postoperative examination.

The patient's care after discharge from the hospital may be just as important as her care during hospitalization. Home visits are seldom necessary, however, and assuring the patient before she leaves the hospital that her gynecologist and her surgeon will be available for telephoned questions and consultation while she is convalescing at home reduces the apprehensions that most frequently account for a home visit request. Such assurances maintain the patient's cooperation and confidence until her recovery is complete and her activities are no longer restricted. A routine telephone call at home from the surgeon or the office nurse a few days after discharge is appreciated and invites relevant questions and appropriate discussion of any concerns.

The wise and considerate surgeon does not permit the delicate, and, at times, very personal relationship with the patient to extend inappropriately beyond the time frame of her convalescence. Although a patient's sense of dependence on her surgeon is highly desirable during the perioperative period, the surgeon should consciously discourage the continuation of such a relationship as the patient resumes her private life and personal

---

INSTRUCTIONS ON GOING HOME

1. Go directly home and rest for the remainder of the day.
2. During the first week at home, increase activity gradually. Expect unanticipated tiredness, and let no day's activities become an endurance contest.
3. Beginning the third week, you may go out of doors and, if able, drive at the end of the month. Rest several times daily during the first week.
4. Please call the office within the first week to arrange for a postoperative appointment.
5. Do not hesitate to call for further advice if you have any questions.

ACTIVITIES

Gradually increase activity for the first 2 weeks. Do NOT engage in heavy lifting, scrubbing, douching, or intercourse until you have checked at the office. A program of Kegel perineal resistive exercises (isometric squeezes of the pubococcygeal muscles) is often helpful in restoration of bowel and bladder control. Try to squeeze these muscles 15 times in a row, 3 seconds each squeeze, 6 times a day.

DIET

You may return to your usual diet. For constipation, drink some prune juice or extra water, or take 1 ounce of milk of magnesia, as necessary. Bran with breakfast is often helpful.

BATHS

You may shower, take tub baths, and wash your hair at any time.

Figure 22.3   Discharge instructions.

responsibilities. Ensuring a successful transition and termination requires intelligent and purposeful application of practical psychology and good patient care. The details are likely to be different for almost every patient. Much of the success of a surgeon's practice depends on the development of skills that elevate the surgeon from the role of mere technical craftsperson to the intended and more effective role of the physician.

References

1. Blake R, Lynn J. Emergency abdominal surgery in the aged. Br J Surg 1976;63:956–960.
2. Blundell E. A psychological study of the effects of surgery on 86 elderly patients. Br Soc Clin Psychol 1967;6:297.
3. Cardenas DD, Kelly E, Krieger JN, Chapman WH. Residual urine volumes in patients with spinal cord injury: measurement with a portable ultrasound instrument. Arch Phys Med Rehabil 1988;69:514–516.
4. Coombes GM, Millard RJ. The accuracy of portable ultrasound scanning in the measurement of residual urine volume. J Urol 1994;152:2083–2085.
5. Elia G, Bergman A. Estrogen effects on the urethra: beneficial effects in women with genuine stress incontinence. Obstet Gynecol Surv 1993;48:509–517.
6. Ellenbogen A, Agranat A, Grunstein S. The role of vaginal hysterectomy in the aged woman. J Geriatr Soc 1981;29:426–428.
7. Goligher JC. Surgery of the anus, rectum and colon. 3rd ed. London: Bailliére Tindall, 1975:412–413.

8. Glenn F. Pre- and postoperative management of elderly surgical patients. J Am Geriatr Soc 1973;21:385–393.
9. Hunt TK, Ehrlich HP, Garcia JA, et al. Effect of vitamin A on reversing the inhibitory effect of cortisone on healing of open wounds in animals and man. Ann Surg 1969;170:633–640.
10. Hunt TK, Van Winkle W Jr. Surgery—wound healing: normal repair. South Plainfield, NJ: Chirurgecom, 1976:26–29.
11. Jeffcoate TNA. Principles of gynecology. New York: Appleton-Century-Crofts, 1967.
12. Johnson JC. Surgery in the elderly. In: Goldman DR, Brown FH, Levy WK, Slap GB, Sussman EJ, eds. Medical care of the surgical patient. Philadelphia: JB Lippincott, 1982:578–590.
13. Lapides J. Neurogenic bladder: principles of treatment. Urol Clin North Am 1974;1:81–97.
14. Leventhal A, Pfau A. Pharmacologic management of postoperative overdistention of the bladder. Surg Gynecol Obstet 1978;146:347–348.
15. Marshall WH, Fahey PJ. Operative complications and mortality in patients over 80 years of age. Arch Surg 1964;88:896–904.
16. McKeithen WS Jr. Major gynecologic surgery in the elderly female, 65 years and older. Am J Obstet Gynecol 1975;123:59–65.
17. Meares EM Jr. Current patterns in nosocomial urinary tract infections. Urology 1991;37(Suppl):9–12.
18. Nichols DH. Getting the postoperative patient to void. Contemp Obstet Gynecol 1978;72:41–45.
19. Ouslander JG, Simmons S, Tuico E, Nigam JG, Fingold S, Bates-Jensen B, Schnelle JF. Use of a portable ultrasound device to measure post-void residual volume among incontinent nursing home residents. J Am Geriatr Soc 1994;42:1189–1192.
20. Pierson RL, Figge PK, Buchsbaum HJ. Surgery for gynecologic malignancy in the aged. Obstet Gynecol 1975;46:523–527.
21. Polacek DJ. Monitoring high-risk and critically ill patients. In: Buchsbaum JH, Walton LA, eds. Strategies in gynecologic surgery. New York: Springer-Verlag, 1986:127.
22. Polacek DJ, Buchsbaum HJ. Surgery in the aged. In: Buchsbaum JH, Walton LA, eds. Strategies in gynecologic surgery. New York: Springer-Verlag, 1986:181–194.
23. Stanton SL. Female urinary incontinence. London: Lloyd-Luke (Medical Books), 1977.
24. Tyreman NO, Anderson PO, Kroon L, et al. Urinary tract infection after vaginal surgery: effect of prophylactic treatment with methenamine hippurate. Acta Obstet Gynecol Scand 1986;65:731–733.
25. von Peham H, Amreich J. Operative gynecology. Philadelphia: JB Lippincott, 1934.
26. Webb MJ. J Ostet Gynecol Scand 1986;65:731–733.
25. von Peham H, Amreich J. Operative gynecology. Philadelphia: JB Lippincott, 1934.
26. Webb MJ, Southorn PA, Kelly DG. Postoperative care. In: Webb MJ. Manual of pelvic surgery. New York: Springer-Verlag, 1994:12–20.

CHAPTER 23

Complications of Vaginal Surgery

PREOPERATIVE REVIEW

Every surgeon must recognize the obligation to acknowledge personal weaknesses and to review them from time to time so as to continually improve and develop his or her skills to prevent less than satisfactory results. One should review the patient's hospital record immediately before surgery to refresh one's memory of significant points in the patient's history and preoperative laboratory findings and the recommendations of consultants. This review should include the findings of medical students, house officers, fellows, and referring physicians. When specific changes in the usual preoperative preparation of the patient are indicated, it is important to be sure they have been performed.

The surgeon's thinking should also have been organized in regard to the whole spectrum of postoperative complications. A surgeon with this knowledge will not only be more competent in managing various complications but will also be called upon increasingly for advice or help by other physicians.

Complications can be grouped conveniently into three general categories: intraoperative, early, and late postoperative.

INTRAOPERATIVE COMPLICATIONS

Aside from the immediate problems associated with the administration of anesthesia, complications that occur during surgery are principally related to hemorrhage or accidental injury of adjacent organs or tissues. Ureteral patency may be ensured by cystoscopy performed with the intravenous administration of 1 ampule of indigo carmine (29, 30, 42, 43).

In the evaluation and control of hemorrhage, it is important to differentiate first between venous and arterial bleeding. Venous bleeding can be usually controlled by extrinsic pressure, whereas arterial bleeding requires prompt and accurate ligation or electrocoagulation. It is essential to be familiar with the circulatory anatomy of the region, including the collaterals. When ligation at the point of bleeding is not possible, ligation should be performed at a site proximal to the site of bleeding. The anesthesiologist should be notified regarding the possible need for transfusion when blood loss becomes excessive. Because blood loss tends to be directly proportional to the duration of the operative procedure, time-saving surgical efficiency is obviously important.

The occurrence of postoperative infection is also directly proportional to the length of the operative procedure, tending to increase when the duration of surgery exceeds 2 hours. Accidental trauma also includes undesirable laceration, avulsion, or unwanted incision of nearby pelvic organs, and it is essential that any suspected injury be evaluated and treated promptly. A problem that is neglected intraoperatively eventually may require one or more secondary surgical procedures, which can be as damaging to the surgeon's reputation as they may be to the patient's health. There is no room for procrastination while hoping that suspected damage did not occur, or that by ignoring the possibility the problem will go away.

All sites of possible trauma should be considered preoperatively. It is useful to maintain a file of literature references on the management of obscure and uncommon complications, such as trauma, avulsion, incision, or transection of the ureter (42), bladder, small intestine, large intestine, and rectum, as well as the pelvic musculature.

Laceration or incision into a pelvic viscus should be repaired as soon as it is recognized. The tissues must be adequately mobilized and the repair accomplished under direct vision. The remainder of the operation should proceed as planned. To manage such problems effectively requires candor, scientific objectivity, and confident surgical technique.

For the repair of visceral injury, we favor two or three layers of fine absorbable suture (3-0 polydioxanone, polygluconate, polyglycolic-acid type, or chromic). An important principle when a mucosal stitch is required is to place the knots within the lumen of intestine or rectum where they may fall away readily when the required support has been developed through healing. In the repair of injuries to the bladder or ureter, knots should be extralumenal to lessen the chance of calculus formation at the site of the suture (Fig. 23.1). The major contribution to support must come as a result of accurate approximation of the submucosal muscular layers (3). Although mucosal sutures are hemostatic, they supply minimal support. A layer of watertight running horizontal mattress sutures in the muscular layer inverts the previous stitches, and another layer of interrupted reinforcing mattress stitches may be added, if desired, to lessen the tension on the deeper layer. Care must always be taken to avoid tying mattress sutures so tightly as to strangulate the tissues involved. The manner of suture placement is identified in Figures 23.2 and 23.3. If the ureteral orifices are near or part of the laceration, ureteral catheters should be inserted. Ureteroneocystostomy should be performed if ureteral integrity cannot be ensured. In the case of traumatic penetration of the wall of bladder near its attachment to the cervix, the adjacent peritoneum can be mobilized and sewn over the site of the repair after the defect in the musculature has been repaired (15), to provide support and added blood supply (see Figs. 23.2D and 23.3). If there is a question of penetration of the mucosa or wall of the rectum, the operator's finger should be inserted

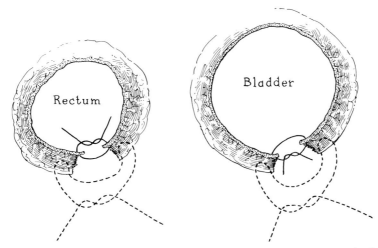

Figure 23.1. Suture placement for a traumatic laceration of a viscus. **A.** The knot of a mucosal stitch is tied within the lumen of the rectum. **B.** This knot is outside the lumen of the bladder. The muscularis is approximated by one or more layers of inverting mattress sutures (*dotted lines*).

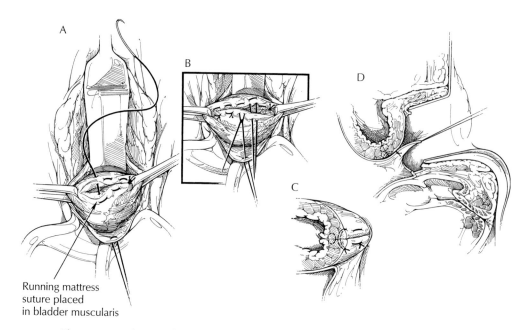

Running mattress
suture placed
in bladder muscularis

Figure 23.2. Closure of accidental cystotomy. **A.** The defect has been identified and widely mobilized. A suture tagging the peritoneum is noted. No mucosal stitch is used. A running mattress suture in the muscularis may be placed as shown, starting and finishing lateral to the defect. **B.** This may be covered by a second layer of interrupted mattress sutures. **C.** A cross section shows that the mattress sutures establish full-thickness reapproximation of the muscularis. **D.** An anterior peritoneal flap is mobilized and tacked in place over the operative repair, providing the security of an additional fresh tissue layer.

immediately in the rectum for confirmation. Any demonstrable defect should then be repaired. A finger in the rectum is often quite helpful as a guide during repair.

When there is a recognizable escape of a urinelike fluid into the vagina during the course of surgery, the possibility of bladder injury should be suspected. It is for this reason that it is desirable to have some urine in the bladder during surgery. We request patients who will undergo vaginal surgery to void shortly before coming to the operating suite and then to be catheterized at the beginning of surgery only if bladder distention is evident on bimanual examination. After repair of a recognized penetration in the wall of the bladder, watertightness may be tested by the instillation of an indigo carmine solution or sterile milk (evaporated milk, sterile condensed canned milk, or sterile infant formula milk from the nursery). Sterile milk has the obvious advantage over dyes in that milk does not stain adjacent tissues if leakage is demonstrated. After additional reinforcing sutures have been placed, the repair should again be tested for leakage. If the ureter is transected, as may occur quite inadvertently when the patient has an undiagnosed duplication of the ureter on one or both sides, the severed ureter can be successfully reimplanted under direct vision (16, 20, 29). Two weeks of postoperative splinting by both ureteral and urethral catheters is desirable.

When grossly bloody urine is found postoperatively and no injury of the bladder wall has been recognized, the bladder should be decompressed by catheter drainage. Generally speaking, in the absence of significant damage to the bladder wall, hematuria should clear grossly within 48 hours, and microscopically within 72 hours. If it is not clear after 72 hours, the bladder should be decompressed by continuous drainage for 10 more days, or the patient can be examined cystoscopically to evaluate and treat the possibility of bladder trauma, such as an unexpected stitch through the bladder wall. The

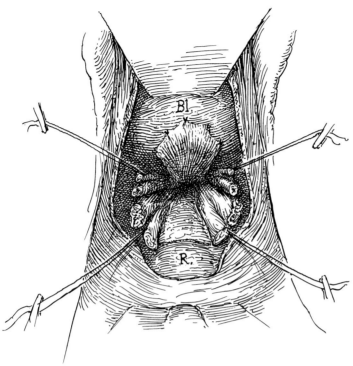

Figure 23.3. Frontal view of the tongue of anterior peritoneum covering the site of cystostomy repair. Vaginal hysterectomy has been completed, and the peritoneal cavity will now be closed in the usual fashion. The positions of the bladder (*Bl*) and rectum (*R*) are noted.

most likely cause is trauma from suture penetration. Even after unrepaired cystotomy, an empty bladder has a remarkable capacity to heal itself. In those instances where adequate surgical exposure is not feasible, 2 weeks of continuous catheter drainage will usually permit a fresh wound to heal spontaneously. But if the traumatized bladder is permitted to distend, a pinpoint opening may fail to close or may even enlarge and, when epithelialized, is likely to give rise to a fistula.

After repair of a laceration of the rectum, 3 days of clear liquid postoperative diet followed by a low-residue diet may be desirable during the first postoperative week, with a rectal tube gently inserted if gas pains or distention develop. A stool softener and gentle laxative should be taken for several weeks postoperatively. In all instances, the patient should be informed of the unexpected trauma and its repair so that she understands the important details of her operation and the need for special postoperative care. This may make her convalescence different from that of others who have had "the same operation." Enema use is inappropriate during the healing phase.

Uncontrolled genital hemorrhage can be treated by tamponade and packing; in rare circumstances, the umbrella pack (7) may be life-saving (Figs. 23.4 and 23.5). The ring and clamp are removed in 12 hours. The surface veil of the pack may be left in place for several days, although gradual removal of its interior packing is usually desirable beginning 24 hours after insertion of the pack. Often the remaining "veil" can best be removed by traction after several days by employing a twisting motion, after gentle irrigation by hydrogen peroxide solution to help separate the veil from any adhesions to it that may be developing.

A gentle bimanual examination is necessary at the completion of every vaginal operation, not only to detect swelling or hematoma but also to determine if the reconstruc-

A

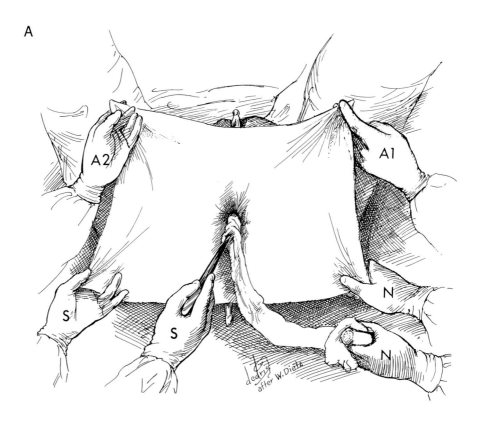

B

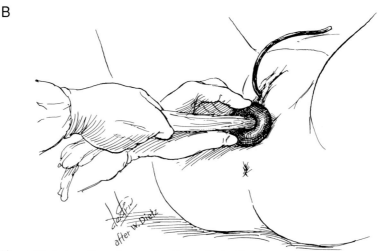

Figure 23.4. Insertion of an umbrella pack. **A.** The four corners of a gauze veil on plastic sheet are supported as shown, with a hand of the assistants indicated by *A1* and *A2*. There is an anterior intraperitoneal retractor in place behind the veil. The nurse (*N*) feeds the gauze packing to the forceps of the surgeon (*S*), who pushes the packing, now covered by the veil, well within the peritoneal cavity, taking the central portion of the veil along with it. **B.** When the pelvis has been thoroughly packed, the four corners of the veil are led through the center of a rubber ring or doughnut pessary, and traction is applied to compress the packing against the source of the bleeding. (After Werner P, Sederl J. Abdominal operations by the vaginal route. Philadelphia: JB Lippincott, 1958. Used with permission.)

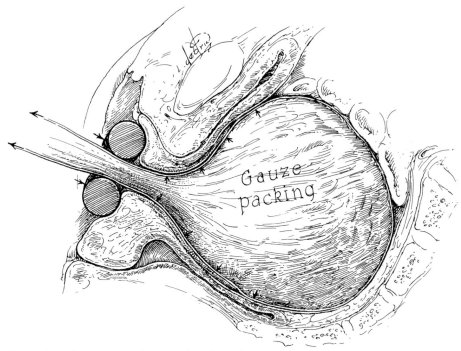

Figure 23.5. Sagittal view showing the effect of compression by the intra-abdominal gauze packing. *Small arrows* denote the areas to which pressure is applied.

tion has been successful. If there is an undesirable ridge in the posterior vaginal wall, it should be corrected immediately, even if it is necessary to reopen the posterior vaginal incision. Such a ridge is likely to be a source of future discomfort or dyspareunia and is likely to become more fibrotic and tender as time goes on. Similarly, any undesirable vaginal stricture or stenosis should be approached aggressively and immediately. These complications result either from the excision of too much vaginal membrane at the time of surgery or excessive plication of slack in the subepithelial fibromuscular connective tissues. Since the anterior and posterior walls of the vagina have received the principal attention during repair, they are also the most vulnerable to future or subsequent trauma.

Individual stenosis should be corrected with relaxing incisions in the lateral walls of the vagina on one or both sides as described in Chapter 20. The vaginal wall may be undermined for a distance of 1 cm along the margins of each incision to enhance the relaxation. The epithelium need not be closed, but it is desirable to place a secure intravaginal pack that should be left in place for 2 days; this should be followed by the regular insertion of a vaginal obturator until healing is satisfactory.

If the defect created in the lateral walls of the vagina by relaxing incisions appears excessive, a full-thickness graft using a portion of the patient's own vaginal wall may be used to fill the defect. At the time of colporrhaphy, the excised pieces or strips of vaginal membrane can be wrapped in sterile sponges soaked with saline and retained temporarily on the nurse's instrument stand for possible grafting later in the procedure.

If excessive blood loss persists at the conclusion of a vaginal operation, adequate inspection should be coincident with accurate hemostasis. If significant venous oozing is noted during the first 24 postoperative hours, a gauze packing of the vagina should be inserted. It will act as a wick in soaking up blood or serum that would otherwise accumulate and will also gently tamponade the operative site and compress the connective tissue spaces. When appreciable bleeding occurs through a pack, however, it usually indicates unsecured hemostasis of some significance, which should be investigated by examination of the patient in the lithotomy position with good lighting and suitable relaxation. When the bleeding point is found, it should be promptly ligated.

When a vaginal pack is in place, the patient will usually experience difficulty in voiding and will need an indwelling Foley catheter. In the absence of bladder trauma or surgical repair, the catheter should be removed at the same time as the intravaginal packing. Bathroom privileges may be permitted then, but daily palpation of the lower abdomen and careful recording of the patient's voiding pattern should be continued during the early postoperative period.

As a last step after conclusion of a vaginal operation, a gentle rectal examination should be performed before the patient is fully awake and before she has left the operating table, so that any unsuspected damage may be identified and repaired. Careful search should be made for any stitches that might have penetrated the rectal mucosa. A penetrating stitch should be exposed with adequate retraction and cut on the lumenal side so that the loose ends will retract into the wall of the rectum. Postoperative difficulty is then unlikely.

Finally, an accurate description of the surgical procedure should be dictated promptly before the details that may later assume considerable importance become less clear or are simply forgotten.

EARLY POSTOPERATIVE COMPLICATIONS

Compartment Syndrome

Prolonged gynecologic surgery—usually over 3 hours duration—upon a patient in the lithotomy position risks compromise of circulation and neurologic function within the legs if external pressure to a fascial compartment is sustained by the position of the supporting stirrups, elevating the pressure within the compartment sufficient to obstruct arteriolar circulation within the contained muscles (11). Ischemia promotes edema, which further compresses the contained nerves, with resultant compromise of function (1, 29). Compression syndrome may be suspected following prolonged surgery if the patient complains of cramping in the lower legs, which are found to be firm and tense although pulsations of the pedal arteries are palpable. Accentuation of the pain is elicited upon passive stretching of the muscles within the fascial compartment. These symptoms may progress, often rapidly, to numbness, burning, and difficulty moving the legs. This may be followed by foot drop and decreased sensation over the feet.

Prompt consultation with a vascular or orthopedic surgeon is desirable. Muscle pressure measurements should be obtained without delay (48), and if the pressure elevated and within the first 12 hours postoperatively, surgical fasciotomy should be performed promptly to decompress the compartment and prevent further damage to its contents. After 12 hours, the risk of infection in tissue now partially necrotic or with circulatory compromise is accentuated and may outweigh the benefits of decompression. To aid circulation within the compartment, the patient's legs should be positioned at the level of her heart.

Prevention of compartment syndrome in surgical cases of long duration in which stirrups are used requires that both legs and thighs be carefully supported by padded stirrups and that special attention be paid to the position of the patient's feet to avoid passive dorsiflexion of the ankle. Passive repositioning of the legs is recommended during the surgical procedure.

The prognosis for recovery is good if permanent nerve and muscular damage has not occurred, although recovery may take several weeks. Significant neuromuscular damage can be suspected in the patient with compression syndrome who develops foot drop.

Neurovascular Complications of the Lithotomy Position

Peroneal nerve injury is characterized by postoperative foot drop, difficulty walking, and inability to abduct or evert the foot (8). There may be numbness of the lateral surface of the leg and dorsal surface of the foot.

Patients with sciatic nerve injury demonstrate weakness of the hamstring muscles coincident with difficulty walking. Treatment is by physiotherapy, including massage and galvanic electrical stimulation of the peroneal nerve. The prognosis is good but recovery is slow, often requiring several weeks or even months.

Neuropathy is prevented by attending to the proper position of the patient's legs in the stirrups, requiring flexion of the knees and hips, and ensuring minimal external rotation of the hips.

Excessive external rotation of the thigh of the patient with legs in "candy-cane" stirrups for operations longer than 1.5 hours invites femoral neuropathy. This is identified postoperatively by the discovery of numbness and paresthesia of the thigh. The knee buckles when the patient stands, and often she cannot walk without assistance (44).

Treatment of femoral neuropathy is primarily by physiotherapy, including massage, active and passive quadriceps exercises, and a great deal of patience. Femoral neuropathy in the patient having vaginal surgery may be prevented by placing lateral supports to the thigh of each leg in stirrups, inhibiting excessive abduction and exaggerated external rotation.

To diagnose arterial thrombosis in a timely fashion, particularly in the patient whose operation was longer than 4 hours, leg pulsations should be checked at the conclusion of surgery and periodically during the first postoperative 24 hours.

These injuries should be recognized and treated promptly to prevent major disability. Prolonged duration of surgery (4 hours or longer) predisposes to these problems, especially when the patient's legs are in stirrups. Direct pressure from stirrups on the calf where the peroneal nerve crosses the fibula can occur even with short operations. The surgeon should be certain that the weight of the leg is on the patient's foot and not on her calf (11, 26).

Postoperative Ileus

Significant intestinal paralysis is less common after vaginal surgery than after abdominal surgery. Patients usually resume an adequate fluid intake and regular diet soon after postoperative nausea subsides following pelvic repairs. Moving about, both in and out of bed, is good prophylaxis; and although the patient is usually not hungry, frequent sips of tap water and occasional small amounts of solid food will usually initiate peristalsis. If postoperative distention and ileus develop, additional days will be required for a return to normal. Intravenous feedings should be continued so long as the abdomen is tympanitic, distended, and relatively silent to auscultation. Peristalsis will eventually return coincident with the expulsion of flatus. If gastric dilation with nausea and vomiting develops, nasogastric decompression should be instituted with an appropriate increase in intravenous fluids.

Intestinal Obstruction

Obstruction of small bowel is usually due to pathologic fixation and kinking of a loop of small intestine, occasionally from a misplaced stitch, but more often the result of attachment to a devitalized tissue surface. It can also be produced by kinking from traction to an unfree adhesion of bowel to adnexa. Obstruction is more common when there are extensive intraperitoneal manipulations or when the patient has sustained adhesions from previous intra-abdominal surgery.

Postoperative obstruction is usually partial at first, and the patient may complain only of anorexia and intermittent colicky pain. Patients who have had previous surgery should be watched with more concern during the first postoperative week, even after resumption of normal peristalsis and bowel function. Tachycardia may occur with only a mild temperature elevation, but peristalsis is usually hyperactive. A flat plate of the abdomen is desirable at this point, and intravenous feeding and intestinal decompression should be considered. Obviously, partial obstruction, when aggravated by postoperative edema, will respond to conservative management, and there will be a gradual return to normal bowel function. When such improvement is to occur, it will usually become evident within 2 or 3 days.

When spontaneous improvement is not apparent, however, the condition of the patient soon changes, with the appearance of projectile vomiting, more frequent and severe crampy abdominal pain, and waves of audible hyperperistalsis coincident with the height of the crampy pain. The patient appears acutely ill, becomes mildly shocky, and develops severe electrolyte disturbances. X-ray studies are now diagnostic, and laparotomy with surgical relief must be undertaken as soon as intravenous feeding and gastric decompression have improved electrolyte imbalance and dehydration. Clinical deterioration can occur in hours. For these reasons, each postoperative patient should be observed by her own physician daily during her hospital stay, and more often when necessary. A 1- or 2-day delay in the diagnosis and treatment of complete intestinal obstruction may result in postoperative mortality.

At laparotomy, the site of the obstruction is usually readily apparent, and blunt dissection by simple finger separation of the bowel from the point to which it has become adherent can be accomplished. The involved loop of bowel should be carefully inspected to ensure its viability and should be observed over a period of several minutes to be certain that both color and peristalsis return. If they do not, resection of the loop may be necessary. If the obstruction cannot be found with ease, a running inspection of the intestines should be performed, beginning with the distal segment of collapsed bowel. If the operative field is obscured by excessive balloonlike intestinal dilatation, this may need to be decompressed by inserting a large-bore hypodermic needle to which suction tubing has been attached. After decompression, the needle is removed, and the point of penetration is closed with a pursestring suture of fine chromic catgut or polyglycolic suture on an atraumatic or intestinal needle (15). When the patient's condition appears critical and will not permit the time necessary for adequate exploration and possible resection, an enterostomy proximal to the point of obstruction may be indicated and should be accomplished without extensive handling of the multiple loops of distended bowel.

FECAL IMPACTION

This may develop insidiously in a postoperative patient who has had no bowel movement within several days of resuming her usual diet. The patient is very uncomfortable, and laxatives and suppositories produce little of substance. The diagnosis is readily made by digital examination of the rectum. Usually the impaction can be broken up digitally, followed by an oil retention enema or even a partial dose of electrolyte bowel cleanser (GoLYTELY or NuLYTELY). When this is ineffective, the patient is by now in severe pain and the rectum should be evacuated under general anesthesia. Goligher (12) states, "This is a tedious and unpleasant operation, the classical instrument for which is the ordinary domestic dinner spoon!" (p. 412). If careful attention is given to bowel habits during postoperative convalescence, this experience should not occur again.

Ogilvie Syndrome

This uncommon syndrome mimics intestinal obstruction but consists of marked dilatation of the distal colon with nausea and vomiting, but without mechanical obstruction. It is an unexpected complication of surgery, especially among older women. It is apparently coincident to a postoperative imbalance between sympathetic and parasympathetic control and the anatomic differences in parasympathetic innervation between the distal and proximal colonic segments. The abdomen is generally very distended but, on examination of a flat radiograph, will demonstrate marked dilatation of the distal colon, at times including the transverse colon and cecum. The condition responds to colonoscopic decompression and a readjustment in the medications the patient is taking postoperatively. If unrecognized and untreated it can be fatal (40).

Postoperative Oliguria

The usual postoperative urinary output is 1 ml per minute; output less than 0.5 ml per minute (30 ml per hour) should be investigated and a determination made as to whether the cause of the oliguria is prerenal (hypovolemia due secondarily to decreased renal perfusion), renal (acute tubular necrosis), or postrenal (ureteral obstruction).

In prerenal oliguria, the urine's specific gravity is high and the urine sodium is very low. With acute tubular necrosis, the ability to concentrate urine is lost and the specific gravity is 10.10 or lower with a rising urine sodium. The treatment of the former is to add parenteral fluids immediately, and if this is not rapidly successful, a dose of 100 ml of 20% mannitol. If this is not effective, 40 mg of furosemide can be given intravenously in an attempt to generate some urinary output. The use of mannitol may decrease intrarenal vascular spasms and prevent the onset of acute tubular necrosis.

With acute tubular necrosis, one must not flood the patient with parenteral fluids lest one risk acute pulmonary edema. The serum potassium gradually rises with progressive oliguria, and any urinary tract infection should be evaluated with cultures and treated appropriately. If the patient fails to respond, indicating renal failure, hemodialysis may be required (40). Postrenal oliguria is generally caused by ureteral obstruction, which should promptly be diagnosed by an immediate infusion intravenous pyelogram and placement of retrograde ureteral catheters with deligation as necessary, or at the least a percutaneous nephrostomy.

Postoperative Infection

Postoperative fever most often originates from problem areas called the "five W's" (their appearance generally in this order according to the number of days postoperatively): Wind (pulmonary), Water (urinary), Wound (abscess), Walk (phlebitis), and Wonder drugs (drug reactions). As has been noted in the review of postoperative complications by Cruse (9), major temperature elevation during the first 48 hours is usually the result of atelectasis, more common if the patient is a heavy smoker. Prompt physiotherapy emphasizing incentive spirometry and prolonged inspiration is the backbone of early treatment. Onset of fever during the 3rd postoperative day is usually from urinary infection. Fever beginning between the 3rd and 5th day is likely to be due to wound infection initiated at the time of surgery. Septic thrombophlebitis may be the explanation of fever originating between the 3rd and 7th postoperative day; between the 10th and 14th day, pulmonary embolism becomes a more likely possibility.

It is especially important that an evening temperature be recorded, because an elevation at this specific time may be the earliest objective evidence than an infection is developing. Costovertebral angles should be percussed the evening of the day of surgery and unilateral discrepancy investigated promptly by infusion pyelography. In the absence of other findings, unexplained ileus should elicit suspicion of unilateral ureteral ligation, and an intravenous pyelogram should be ordered without delay. Acute urinary infection is more likely in the patient with a previous history of urinary tract infections.

Fever persisting beyond the first and second postoperative days will often prove to be from infection within the pelvis, often within the site of an unsuspected pelvic hematoma. Prompt and gentle daily palpation of the abdomen for tenderness or masses and gentle bimanual examination of the pelvis are indicated. Abscess formation should be expected, and the majority of such abscesses will point to and drain into the vaginal vault and be evidenced by a sudden seropurulent discharge followed by almost immediate clinical improvement. Suspected abscess formation may be investigated by rectal examination and gentle digital exploration of the vault of the vagina. Although the natural tendency of this development is to drain spontaneously, this course may be aided easily by gentle digital probing of the suture lines in the vagina over a period of several days. A culture and sensitivity study of any appreciable exudate is desirable.

When the abscess cavity involves or is adjacent to the pelvic peritoneum, signs of pelvic peritonitis usually involve lower abdominal distention, lower abdominal pain, anorexia, and depressed peristalsis. Although adnexal abscess is uncommon after vaginal surgery, this possibility should be suspected when a unilateral pelvic mass is present in a patient in whom ovulation had been occurring regularly. Relatively late development is almost characteristic of this complication, and it may therefore not become evident for days or weeks following discharge from the hospital. Ledger et al. (19) emphasized that the "diagnostic possibility of an adnexal abscess should be considered in any febrile patient readmitted after a recent pelvic operation." Such adnexal abscesses localize relatively high in the pelvis and may not be palpated but may be identified by ultrasound or computerized axial tomography (CAT) scan (18). Spontaneous drainage through the vaginal vault is unlikely, and transabdominal salpingo-oophorectomy or laparoscopic aspiration is usually required. Nondraining retroperitoneal or extraperitoneal abscess as in the retropubic area may be visualized by CAT scan and then drained under ultrasound guidance.

Various studies have demonstrated an increased probability of postoperative infection and morbidity among premenopausal as compared to postmenopausal women undergoing vaginal surgery, probably related to the increased vascularity of their tissues and the increased probability of a hematoma, which becomes a focus of infection. Greater sexual activity increases vaginal bacterial contamination. A larger variety of organisms within the vaginal flora are ready for proliferation under the conditions present after vaginal surgery during the menstrual years, and infection by virulent anaerobic vaginal bacteria may result.

Infection can be minimized by careful anatomic dissection (which minimizes trauma), adequate hemostasis, and provision for drainage when indicated. Also, the short-term use of an appropriate broad-spectrum antibiotic is helpful, given an hour before surgery and repeated if the operation is longer than of 2 hours duration. It is given to those patients in whom it is expected that the peritoneal cavity will be entered during the course of the transvaginal operation, as well as in those less common instances in which the surgery will involve relatively inaccessible although extraperitoneal connective tissue spaces, such as the pararectal, prevesical, or retrorectal spaces, which have no natural path of drainage to the outside.

Anaerobic bacterioid infections are characteristically foul-smelling and result in characteristic systemic reactions. Dangers are greater when a body temperature of 103°F or higher develops along with a white blood count higher than 15,000 or less than 4000/cm. Under such circumstances, any purulent exudate should be cultured for both aerobic and anaerobic organisms, and serious consideration should be given to administration of antibiotics or antibacterials with anaerobic coverage. Antibiotics that will penetrate an abscess include the following:

1. Clindamycin
2. Cefamandole
3. Cefoxitin
4. Metronidazole

SEPTIC SHOCK

Septic shock should be considered when a shocklike state develops postoperatively without evidence of blood loss. Peripheral vascular collapse from endotoxins will often produce subnormal temperature, hypotension, metabolic acidosis, oliguria, and mental confusion. Serial blood cultures should be obtained before antibiotics are started, along with study of the urine and culture and staining of any purulent exudate (45). There will be no response to transfusion. Once the peripheral circulatory collapse has been overcome by intravenous fluids, ideally monitored by central venous pressure or pulmonary wedge pressure measurements, treatment may include norepinephrine and also dopamine and large doses of appropriate combined antibiotics. Search should be made for an abscess cavity. Ultrasound or CAT scan studies may be helpful (18). When found, an abscess should be cultured and excised or drained.

The patient should be transferred to intensive care and vital signs closely monitored.

NECROTIZING FASCITIS

Necrotizing fascitis and synergistic bacterial gangrene are rare, serious, virulent, and toxic infections that can develop subcutaneously at any time (5, 6, 21, 23, 35). The overlying skin is dark, bullae may be present, and thrombosis of nearby blood vessels may precipitate edema of the skin, rendering it anesthetic. Prompt recognition is essential, and the primary treatment is adequate surgical debridement, as extensive as necessary to excise the bacterial inoculum completely (19, 39). Cleansing by immersion in whirlpool tubs may be helpful, as well as placement in a chamber of hyperbaric oxygen (30). Subcutaneous fascial damage is extensive, but muscle may be spared, as would not be the case were crepitant gas gangrene present, as is associated with clostridial infection.

Hemorrhage

Careful observation of the patient's vital signs during the first 2 postoperative days will provide evidence of intraperitoneal bleeding. It is important to monitor the patient's hemoglobin and hematocrit. A coagulation defect should be suspected when the patient shows unexpected ecchymoses or when a sample of venous blood fails to form a firm clot. If external blood loss is insignificant and bleeding seems to be persistent, the patient, who is unusually restless, should be prepared for laparotomy. Bleeding points should be identified and ligated, any hematoma should be evacuated, and a search should be made for the source of bleeding.

If intra-abdominal hemorrhage has stabilized at the end of the first postoperative 24 hours and there is no evidence of further bleeding, operative intervention is seldom necessary unless infection intrudes, at which time a presumed hematoma may become infected and require drainage. Under unusual circumstances in which shock due to blood loss has intervened and massive postoperative hemorrhage is evident within the bases of the cardinal ligaments, aggressive surgery may be required, including bilateral ligation of the hypogastric and ovarian arteries (34). This procedure should not be time-consuming, and the response in arresting an alarming rate of hemorrhage will be dramatic. Every gynecologic surgeon should be experienced with the technique of transperitoneal bilateral hypogastric artery ligation, particularly when the technique can be readily learned by isolation of the hypogastric arteries on fresh autopsy material. Once the arteries have been identified, the relevant surgical anatomy and the position of the ureter and the vein clearly distinguished, and these structures excluded from the operative field, sutures for ligation can be properly placed around the hypogastric artery and below the origin of the superior gluteal artery. The overlying peritoneum is closed with fine absorbable suture, care being taken to avoid the nearby ureter. This practice provides a convenient and easy way to learn or to teach this procedure to oneself or to others, and when the occasion does arise that ligation must be performed as an emergency procedure, the operator can proceed knowledgeably and efficiently with a technique based on some previous personal experience.

Externally evident hemorrhage after vaginal surgery is usually of extraperitoneal origin. When this is mild in quantity and approximates that seen with the menstrual period, firm vaginal packing will usually provide sufficient tamponade to achieve control. If this is insufficient and blood loss appears either accelerated or sustained, surgical intervention may be indicated. When this development is seen during the first postoperative day, the rapidity of blood loss is a reliable indication of the size of the vessel accounting for the bleeding. Suspicion that sustained intraperitoneal bleeding from an unsecured uterine or ovarian artery is accounting for blood loss indicates the need for a prompt surgical approach. Persistent transvaginal bleeding after a vaginal repair will usually arise from a small artery in the edge of a vaginal incision.

Blood loss occurring from the 6th to perhaps the 14th postoperative day is most likely the result of local infection that has hastened suture absorption or has eroded into an adjacent vascular bed. At this stage, tissues are edematous and friable, and additional sutures will not be secure. Dissection will destroy tissue planes and break up established barriers of "inflammatory membrane," thereby resulting in dissemination as well as an increase in the clinical virulence of the infection. Undiagnosed diabetes should be excluded and, if found, appropriate measures employed. Tight vaginal packing may prove effective even in the presence of infection, and broad-spectrum antibiotics should be administered. Local application of the microfibrillar collagen Avitene may be effective. It exerts its hemostatic effect by attracting functioning blood platelets that adhere to the microfibrils, triggering the formation of thrombi in the adjacent tissue. Avitene should not be used near the ureter because it can cause fibrosis with ureteral obstruction. The bladder should be put at rest by an indwelling catheter. If vaginal packing is not effective and a coagulopathy has been excluded, the patient should be returned to the operating room. If transvaginal control of excessive bleeding cannot be achieved, the possibility of bilateral hypogastric artery ligation should be considered. Should this fail, massive hemorrhage may be controlled by percutaneous transcatheter embolization (49).

Transcatheter embolization of the pelvic arteries is an established technique for control of bleeding in patients with massive postoperative hemorrhage, but only if the patient is not in shock and the surgical and radiological team has a window of some 2 hours in which to effect the embolization. It is more difficult in the patient who has had a ligation of the hypogastric artery. In the face of unrelenting postoperative hemorrhage when the patient is in immediate danger, hypogastric ligation may be the procedure of choice. However, if there is a window of 2 or 3 hours, arterial embolization can be recommended, presuming that the hospital and its radiological team are prepared for this treatment and experienced with it (10, 36, 37, 49).

Hematoma formation may be intraperitoneal or extraperitoneal, but occasionally when retroperitoneal it is ominous because it affords an excellent culture medium in proximity to the vaginal or rectal flora and is likely to account for postoperative abscess formation. When a hematoma is palpable and is increasing significantly in size, it should probably be evacuated. Again, it is important to note that a coagulopathy must be excluded.

Small hematomas in the vault of the vagina or beneath a reapproximated tissue plane will generally liquify, and although they may become infected, they usually drain spontaneously through the vaginal suture line. Because these hematomas are more common in the vault of the vagina, the surgeon may wish to leave a small opening in the very center of the vault for drainage at the time of hysterectomy.

Thrombophlebitis

Elastic stockings that have been worn preoperatively and during the operative procedure should be continued for the initial 3 or 4 postoperative days until the patient is comfortably ambulatory. Daily rounds include palpation of the patient's calves and attention to complaint of leg pain, particularly if unilateral. Superficial thrombophlebitis may be treated with elastic stocking compression of the extremity, elevation, and external heat. Phenylbutazone (Butazolidin alka) three times daily for 7 to 10 days will often add to the patient's comfort. Anticoagulation is desirable only when there is evidence of upward expansion of the thrombophlebitis despite the use of the measures already described.

The importance of prophylaxis cannot be overemphasized. All patients should be instructed on the importance of frequently moving their extremities and encouraged to move about in bed freely, starting from the time of recovery from anesthesia. The patient should be encouraged to be up in a chair two or three times daily beginning on the first postoperative day, and should be told clearly that moving her legs will aid her circulation. Oversedation should be avoided.

Of ominous significance is evidence of a thrombophlebitis in pelvic veins, an uncommon development manifested by lower abdominal pain and tenderness to deep palpation without change in hematocrit and without a palpable lower pelvic mass as might be seen with a hematoma. Often accompanied by a high spiking fever and coincident tachycardia, pelvic thrombophlebitis is surprisingly resistant to antibiotic therapy, but it does respond dramatically to anticoagulation with heparin.

When there is a predisposition to thrombophlebitis as indicated by obesity or a history of thrombophlebitis, the increased likelihood of this potentially dangerous development should be anticipated postoperatively. Preliminary preoperative determination of partial thromboplastin time to identify previous unsuspected bleeding disorders will help considerably to prevent the development of thrombophlebitis. If partial heparinization is desired, 5000 units of heparin is given subcutaneously three times daily *beginning the day before the operation* and continued through the first 4 or 5 postoperative days. Because increased operative and postoperative bleeding can be expected, the importance of meticulous surgical hemostasis cannot be overemphasized.

TREATMENT OF SEVERE ACUTE INFLAMMATORY THROMBOPHLEBITIS OF THE LEG

When massive thrombosis occludes practically all of the veins of the leg, the entire leg becomes deeply cyanotic and extremely painful. Total heparinization should be accomplished promptly and thrombectomy should be considered.

TREATMENT OF DEEP VEIN THROMBOSIS

When a deep vein thrombosis of the pelvis or lower extremity has been diagnosed, total heparinization is the treatment of choice; a loading dose of 7500 to 10,000 units of aqueous heparin solution is administered intravenously, and this is followed by a continuous heparin drip providing 5000 units of heparin every 4 to 6 hours via a heparin-well such that the partial thromboplastin time (PTT) is extended from two to two and one-half times normal. A continuous heparin drip has some advantages: PTT can be obtained at any time, and one need not worry about peaks and valleys in anticoagulation. This is usually continued for 6 to 7 days and discontinued after oral anticoagulant therapy has been started. Appropriate medical consultation and follow-up are needed for 3 to 6 months. If embolism occurs despite heparinization, thrombectomy or vena cava ligation should be considered.

Atelectasis and Pneumonia

Atelectasis and pneumonia occur less frequently after vaginal surgery than after pelvic laparotomy, because the absence of an abdominal incision makes it easier for the patient to breathe deeply and to move about comfortably. This tends to reduce diaphragmatic splinting. Routine deep inspiration should be encouraged after any type of pelvic surgery, beginning the day of operation. Incentive spirometry has proven effective in providing good pulmonary aeration, in contrast to intermittent positive pressure breathing devices, which, unless the patient forcefully inhales, often do not provide adequate aeration and may, in fact, increase small airway obstruction. It is important to avoid oversedation, for not only does this tend to depress the respiratory center, but, because it inhibits the sensorium, the patient's voluntary efforts are usually noticeably decreased.

Atelectasis results from occlusion of a part of the bronchial tree as a result of hypoventilation, circulatory stasis, and accumulation of intrabronchial secretions, which are often associated with a preexisting acute or chronic bronchitis. Recent or concurrent upper respiratory infections are distinct contraindications to anesthesia and to elective surgery, because bronchial obstruction is followed by absorption of trapped gases with collapse of the distal segment of lung involved. The patient develops fever, tachycardia, and a noticeable increase in respiratory rate. Cyanosis and air hunger are less common unless there is a massive degree of pulmonary collapse. This complication usually occurs early in the postoperative course. Atelectasis represents one of the more common causes of fever during the first 2 or 3 postoperative days. If unresolved by good pulmonary toilet, bronchial pneumonia and consolidation develop rapidly. The chest x-ray is usually of limited value in making an early diagnosis.

There are two principal types of pneumonia: aspiration and bacterial. The former is initiated during the phase of immediate recovery from anesthesia and the latter from inadequate pulmonary ventilation in the later postoperative period, sometimes after unrecognized or untreated atelectasis. There is gradual development of pleural respiratory pain, and a severe, nonproductive cough is present. Treatment for both must be prompt, and for the former includes clearing of the airway of aspirate, correction of hypoxia, administration of steroids such as Solu-Cortef to diminish pulmonary inflammatory reaction, and administration of prophylactic antibiotics. Bacterial pneumonia is best treated by an aminoglycocide together with clindamycin until the specific pathogen has been identified. Failure to effect adequate treatment of either of these types of pneumonia may result in lung abscess, which may or may not be obvious for several weeks. When lung abscess is diagnosed, prompt and intensive antibiotic therapy is indicated. Failure of resolution requires bronchoscopy, and rarely lobectomy.

Pulmonary Embolism

Pulmonary embolism occurs more frequently in patients with antecedent peripheral venous disease, patients over 50 years of age, those who are obese, and those with known cardiac or pulmonary disease. The latter include a wide spectrum and may be associated with clinically demonstrable pulmonary infarction, so a patient displaying pneumonia, atelectasis, or pleurisy with or without effusion should be watched with particular care. Early diagnosis and aggressive treatment by adequate anticoagulation have been responsible for a noticeable reduction in the mortality rate associated with pulmonary embolism.

Dehydration of the patient with hemoconcentration affects heparin activity. Phenobarbital and chloral hydrate have been shown to antagonize anticoagulants. Oral contraceptives are strongly suspect and should therefore have been discontinued a month or two before elective surgery.

Prophylaxis begins with preoperative recognition of those patients likely to develop difficulty. Every effort should be made to prevent the development of hypotension by maintaining an effective circulating blood volume during surgery. Postoperatively, both active and passive motion of the lower extremities should be ensured on a regular basis, combined with the use of elastic stockings until the patient is ambulatory. All are of proven prophylactic value. In addition, oversedation is to be avoided, and a positive program encouraging voluntary deep breathing exercises should begin on the first postoperative day.

Thrombosis is more likely when swelling of an extremity develops and calf pain and tenderness are localized to the deep venous system than if pain and tenderness are diffuse. When in doubt, x-ray venography, impedance plethysmography, or leg scanning using human fibrinogen labeled with radioactive iodine, may be considered (27).

Intermittent passive venous compression, as by the Kendall boot, can be initiated with surgery upon the patient at unusual risk. Heparin is, of course, contraindicated in patients with a history of stroke, subarachnoid hemorrhage, peptic ulcer, bleeding diathesis, and hypertension.

Prophylactic heparinization should, moreover, be considered only with great caution in the diabetic patient, because the resultant prolonged elevation of plasma-free fatty acid levels in the diabetic may induce hypercoagulability and cardiac arrhythmia, with increased risk of acute myocardial infarction. A massive pulmonary embolism beyond the initial 10th postoperative day (4) may also indicate the use of a thrombolytic enzyme such as streptokinase (250,000 IU as a continuous infusion by syringe pump over 1/2 hour, followed by 100,000 units per hour for the remainder of the 24-hour period) as recommended by Hirsh (13), who mentions cardiac arrest or a second major embolism during treatment as an indicator for pulmonary embolectomy. Streptokinase may be contraindicated during the first 10 postoperative days, since its intense lytic activity may interfere with wound healing and initiate bleeding at the site of the operation. Vena cava ligation should be considered if showers of recurrent or of septic emboli have occurred.

Hirsh also recommends ambulation 5 or 6 days after treatment has been instituted. When the patient is pain-free, she may be gradually switched to oral anticoagulants, which should be continued for some weeks. Should pulmonary embolism be seriously suspected, even though unconfirmed, a single intravenous injection of 10,000 units of aqueous heparin may be given followed by 5000 units subcutaneously every 6 hours for 7 to 10 days or until the patient is ambulatory.

Fatal pulmonary embolism now occurs after major gynecologic surgery about once per 1500 major procedures. Prophylactic low-dose anticoagulation, while possibly reducing the risk of fatal pulmonary embolism, increases the otherwise low incidence of a significant amount of postoperative bleeding. For this reason alone, anticoagulants are usually employed only if the history or the findings suggest a patient at high risk.

Differential Diagnosis between Pelvic Cellulitis and Pelvic Thrombophlebitis

There is little to be found on physical examination that is diagnostic of pelvic thrombophlebitis. Lower quadrant abdominal pain and soreness without cramping are usually present and are aggravated by deep palpation, but when without seemingly related activity in the overlying bowel, are suggestive of the extraperitoneal character of the problem. A sense of fullness may be perceived by the fingers of the examiner, but since some muscle guarding is also present, this is not specific and certainly not pathognomonic. The most characteristic features of the clinical picture are shaking chills accompanying a high spiking fever. A sustained tachycardia does not change even with the abrupt fall in temperature.

In pelvic cellulitis, on the other hand, the pelvic floor is noticeably ligneous and diffusely painful. Chills are usually absent and the temperature elevation is sustained. As the temperature subsides, it does so gradually, and the pulse rate decreases with it.

It is important to make a clinical distinction between infected pelvic thrombophlebitis and pelvic cellulitis because treatment of the two conditions differs in some respects. Although blood cultures are desirable, they are not always positive and conclusive, but fortunately, broad-spectrum antibiotics are indicated in both situations. The role of anticoagulants in pelvic thrombophlebitis is debatable, and many clinicians use anticoagulants only when embolization has developed or when the patient fails to demonstrate favorable response to intensive antibiotic therapy of several days' duration.

The above distinctions apply only to rather classical thrombophlebitis, in which thrombi are infected and the danger of multiple emboli relate to the vascular dissemination of infected loci. Moreover, areas of thrombosis occurring without infection are equally life-threatening and are often totally asymptomatic until uninfected, large, soft thrombi become dislodged to form massive pulmonary emboli.

The indications for vena cava ligation are often debated, but the certainty of the immediate result keeps the desirability of this procedure from being forgotten. Several observers have noted the frequency with which embolization of massive bland phlebothrombosis occurs a week or so after pelvic surgery when an in-bed patient is having a bowel movement on a bedpan. For this reason, we favor both early ambulation and sufficiently frequent stool softeners, laxatives, or enemas to avoid straining at stool during postoperative convalescence.

Other Intra-abdominal Postoperative Complications

The postoperative patient is certainly not immune to an attack of appendicitis, cholecystitis, or diverticulitis, and the characteristic symptoms should never be ignored. Indicated surgery should not be delayed.

LATE POSTOPERATIVE COMPLICATIONS

Evisceration

Dehiscence of the apex of the vagina with extrusion of omentum or intestine, or both, often suggests inadequate reconstruction of the supports of the vault or of the levator plate at the time of surgery, which produces to a faulty vaginal axis. The rarity of posthysterectomy vaginal evisceration must be noted (17). This seems independent of whether the vaginal vault is left opened or closed. Evisceration may occur because the small bowel mesentery is long, and when pathologically long (greater than 15 cm), it permits intra-abdominal contents to exert unusual pressure on the surface of the cul-de-sac in the pelvic floor and vaginal vault. Evisceration may occur with sudden massive increases in intra-abdominal pressure, such as violent coughing or postoperative retching. It may also be seen with extreme overexertion, such as heavy lifting, in which the entire force of increased intra-abdominal pressure is directed to the long axis of the vagina. It may occur with postoperative coitus (38).

Treatment is determined by the viability and integrity of the protruding structure. When loops of intestine protrude, there must be doubt concerning viability (47). At laparotomy, the loops, after cleansing, may be drawn back into the peritoneal cavity, fully inspected, and the pelvic defect repaired, with special attention paid to obliterating the cul-de-sac and any enterocele that might be present. If intestinal viability or the condition of the base of the mesentery is in question, bowel resection is indicated followed by trimming of any necrotic vaginal tissue and transabdominal closure of the vaginal vault defect during the same operative procedure. If the vaginal portion of the bowel is perforated or necrotic, the specimen may be removed by resection per vaginum and after redraping, and the transabdominal anastomosis then accomplished (15, 33).

Forgotten Foreign Bodies

Instruments are not often left behind or lost during and after vaginal surgery. However, it is possible to leave a sponge or pack in the cul-de-sac or in a tissue plane, particularly if there has been noteworthy bleeding during the course of the procedure. A sponge saturated with blood quickly assumes the color of the surrounding tissues when packed into a line of cleavage or beneath a flap or fold of tissue, and it may easily be buried as the tissues are plicated. Periodic sponge counts should be made during the course of a procedure, especially before the peritoneum is closed and again at the conclusion of the operation while the patient is still anesthetized and draped. If a missing sponge is not found in the vagina or in the folds of drapes, an x-ray of the pelvis should be obtained while the patient is still on the operating table. If the patient is obese, it may be necessary to obtain separate films of the lower and upper abdomen. Because only sponges with radiopaque marking should be used in surgery, they will generally be seen on x-ray. Under no circumstances should a sponge be cut in half during the course of an operative procedure, lest a missing but unmarked half be invisible on postoperative x-ray. Because they are so easily lost, small pushers or swabs in the surgical field are never separated from their holding forceps.

Although there are reports of foreign bodies having been found incidentally months or years after they have been left behind, the majority will make themselves known by clinical infection within a few days. Such a patient will usually develop a septic fever unresponsive to any antibiotic combination, and an abscess may form that will point into the vagina. Probing of this abscess may bring forth a few threads of the offending foreign body. The presence or absence of signs of local peritonitis will indicate whether the foreign body is intraperitoneal; if it is and transvaginal removal cannot be accomplished easily, abdominal laparotomy with drainage and culture of the purulent material may be indicated. When there are signs of extraperitoneal infection, gently opening into the tissue planes of the vagina near the site of the suspected abscess will be necessary. In the presence of the local infection, the sutures of a secondary closure, if any, should be spaced so as not to interfere with drainage from the infected area.

A vaginal examination shortly before discharge from a hospital will permit identification of an unsuspected hematoma, intravaginal adhesions to be broken up, or forgotten intravaginal sponges or packing to be removed. When clinically indicated, this examination is too easily forgotten or omitted. An overlooked intravaginal sponge or packing will invariably give rise to a profuse and offensive vaginal discharge and will cause considerable distress for the patient. Fortunately, there is rarely any damage done by a forgotten sponge or packing in the vagina, and the discharge subsides promptly after removal.

Cerebral Changes

Hypertensive patients should be watched postoperatively for any signs of cerebral thrombosis, which, if significant, may include paralysis and coincident discrepancy in pupillary size. More often, however, minor degrees of cerebral insufficiency may be detected only by careful interpretation of the patient's postoperative course. When the effects of postoperative sedation are superimposed, it is easy to miss a slight slurring of speech, fuzziness of thinking, or memory impairment, but those close to the patient are certain to recognize these changes in the later postoperative weeks. Insidious and unhappy acceleration of the cerebral as well as the vascular aging process may occur more often than we anticipate.

Coronary Occlusion

Unexplained postoperative tachycardia, especially when combined with dyspnea and substernal pressure, may be indicative of coronary occlusion, especially in a patient with a history of angina or findings of arteriosclerosis. Any patient with preoperative clinical or cardiographic evidence of coronary insufficiency, with or without additional symptoms, should receive a postoperative electrocardiogram and serial enzyme determinations.

Unexpected Malignancy

The report from the pathology laboratory should be reviewed carefully as soon as available, and preferably before the patient's discharge from the hospital. An unsuspected or more advanced stage of a recognized malignancy occasionally will be demonstrated in the surgical specimen. The patient or a responsible member of her family should be advised promptly of the significance of these findings so that appropriate additional therapy can be instituted when indicated and the advisability and nature of lifetime follow-up studies can be explained. Consultation with an oncologic team is often desirable at this time.

Infection or Exposure of a Vaginal Foreign Body

NEEDLE SUSPENSION OPERATIONS

The removal of the foreign body from an infected Pereyra-type needle suspension procedure is relatively simple, since simply cutting the suture transvaginally and making traction upon the opposite end will usually bring it through. This is not the same with a Stamey type of procedure, in which the bolster must be separately identified and removed, usually transabdominally.

VAGINAL EXPOSURE OF PLASTIC MESH

Rarely, following transabdominal sacrocolpopexy the vagina overlying the position to which it has been fixed to a retroperitoneal plastic mesh may become exposed. If there is no abscess formation, this may be effectively covered by a flap of the vagina mobilized using an inverted U-shaped incision (D. Meyers, personal communication, 1995). If this is not possible, the mesh should be removed, although reinversion of the vagina should be expected and plans made for a future colpopexy.

Prolapse of the Fallopian Tube

Although prolapse of the tube through the apex of the vagina is a rare complication of vaginal hysterectomy (28), it does result in a peritoneal fistula. Fallopian tube prolapse is generally a consequence of a hysterectomy technique in which the vault of the vagina is left open at the conclusion of the procedure and the cut ends of the tube have been sutured along a cut edge of the vaginal vault. Since, in the technique described in Chapter 8, most of the vault is essentially closed in layers, the transected ends of the tubes have been securely buried beneath the wall of the vagina, well away from all vaginal edges. Peritoneal fistulas should be rare, but may be suspected from a watery discharge and by the discovery of a friable soft tissue vaginal vault excrescence that bleeds easily and that, at first, appears to be granulation tissue but fails to heal and disappear after simple cauterization or attempts to curette the suspected granulations away. When local excision fails and discharge persists, salpingectomy may be necessary for cure; otherwise, intermittent hydrorrhea may be reported and a potential route for ascending infection is perpetuated.

A useful transvaginal technique of total salpingectomy for a posthysterectomy fallopian tube prolapse (46) starts with a horizontal incision through the full thickness of the vagina posterior to the prolapsed tube and the vaginal scar (Fig 23.6). The peritoneal cavity is incised horizontally and the peritoneal side of the prolapsed tube is inspected carefully. The tube is mobilized and another horizontal vaginal incision is made anterior to the prolapsed tube, and the entire tube and a collar of vagina between the two incisions are removed; the peritoneum and vagina are closed separately. Alternatively the vaginal portion of the prolapsed tube may be removed as an office procedure by tightly

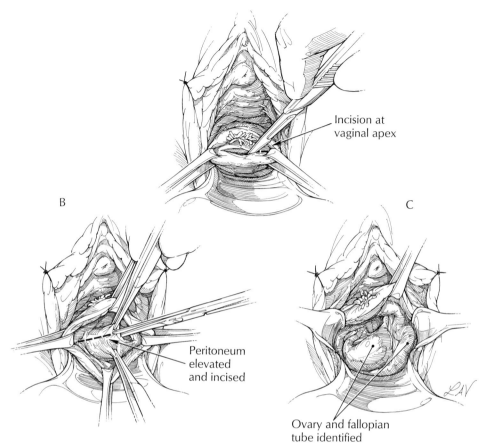

Incision at vaginal apex

B

C

Peritoneum elevated and incised

Ovary and fallopian tube identified

Figure 23.6. Surgical excision of a prolapsed fallopian tube. **A.** Some fimbria of a prolapsed fallopian tube are seen protruding through the site of the scan in the vaginal apex. The apex of the vagina has been grasped between two Allis clamps and an incision made through the full thickness of the vagina posterior to the fimbriated end of the fallopian tube. **B.** The underlying peritoneum is identified, elevated, and incised along the path of the dashed line. **C.** The ovary and full length of the tube through the peritoneal opening are identified. (*Continues on following page.*)

securing an endoloop of 2-0 plain catgut around the base of the mass following application of a benzocaine spray (14).

Depression and Psychiatric Sequelae

A significant degree of depression may develop postoperatively (2). This is attributed to the consequence of a psychological perception of loss or threatened loss of femininity or sexuality, or in the case following hysterectomy, loss of fertility as well. Preoperative discussion and postoperative counseling are valuable. Most psychoses will have been present and demonstrable preoperatively.

Anemia

If the patient has experienced hemorrhage, she should have daily, and, if necessary, more frequent postoperative measurements of hemoglobin and hematocrit. In patients in whom there is no history of operative hemorrhage and no visible postoperative bleeding,

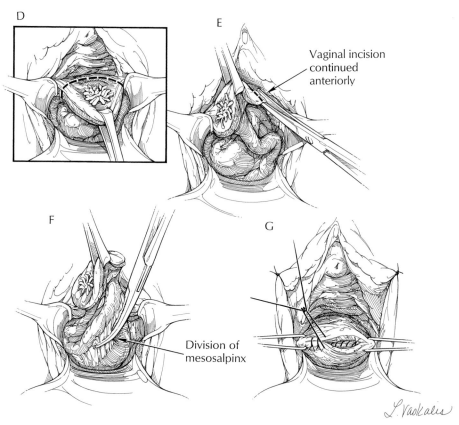

Figure 23.6 (continued). D and **E.** The incision is carried anterior to the site of the tubal pro-lapse along the path of the *dashed line* until the area has been completely circumcised. **F.** The mesosalpinx is clamped and divided, and the tube with adjacent vagina through which it was prolapsed is removed. **G.** Hemostasis is secured, the peritoneum is closed in one layer of run-ning sutures, and the vaginal wall is closed transversely with a layer of interrupted sutures.

hemoglobin and hematocrit determinations should be made on the second postoperative day; and if unexpectedly low when compared with the preoperative values, readings should be repeated during the postoperative period until levels have stabilized or begun to improve. Oral iron supplementation may be indicated both during the course of hos-pitalization and as part of the posthospital postoperative care. If hemoconcentration is present during the first and second postoperative days, a normal or elevated hemoglobin and hematocrit may give a false sense of security. A significantly depressed determina-tion at this time should arouse immediate suspicion and indicate further investigation.

POSTOPERATIVE BLOOD STUDIES IN THE OLDER PATIENT

Older patients tend to lose their sense of thirst with age and may thus live in a state of chronic dehydration and hemoconcentration. At the time of surgery, this is overcome by hydration during anesthesia, and in the immediate postoperative period this may give rise to a hemodilution reflected as a drop in hemoglobin and hematocrit noted on the first or second postoperative day. After a few days and the resumption of the usual reduced voluntary fluid intake, the hemoconcentration tends to return, producing an unexpected rise in the recorded values of hemoglobin and hematocrit of specimens taken beyond the fourth postoperative day.

This phenomenon is different from the condition of concealed retroperitoneal hemorrhage in which the patient's hemoglobin and hematocrit continue to fall. If physical examination is negative, a CAT scan or transvaginal ultrasound examination will establish the diagnosis of retroperitoneal hematoma. The treatment of the latter may be expectant if the size of the lesion and the patient's hemoglobin and hematocrit values have stabilized with no evidence of infection. Packed red blood cell transfusion may be desirable if there is a severe anemia (less than 8 g hemoglobin) to enhance the oxygen-carrying capacity of the circulating blood. If there is a continued fall in hemoglobin and hematocrit, the size of the mass expands, or the hematoma becomes infected, active intervention by drainage of the hematoma is indicated. If the mass is cystic, it may be possible for the drain to be placed under ultrasound guidance. The drain should be left in place until drainage ceases and the mass resolves.

HEMORRHAGE FROM THE ANTERIOR SACRAL FORAMINA DURING SACRAL COLPOPEXY

A stainless steel surgical thumbtack may be placed through the center of a small square of Gelfoam (absorbable gelatine sponge, Upjohn Company, Kalamazoo, MI), which is then tacked over the sacral fenestration.

Arthritis

Acute postoperative monarticular arthritis strongly suggests exacerbation of unexpected gout and should respond to appropriate treatment.

Miscellaneous Problems

Although genital fistulas may become evident at almost any stage of convalescence, a very small one may not become evident until weeks or even months after surgery. Their treatment is discussed in Chapters 12, 18, and 19. Iatrogenic urinary stress incontinence may also be seen, usually as a result of an overcorrection of a cystocele when inadequate attention has been paid to urethral supports or to preservation of a good posterior urethrovesical angle. When this is socially disturbing, it may necessitate additional surgery. Eversion of the vaginal vault is sometimes seen and is considered in Chapter 16. The significance of the postoperatively shortened vagina and the technical means of avoiding this undesirable result are discussed in Chapter 8 on hysterectomy. Vaginal stricture is discussed in Chapter 20.

The atrophic effects of postoperative estrogen withdrawal some years after a satisfactory repair must be anticipated whenever a colporrhaphy is done upon a premenopausal woman. Atrophy of the vaginal membrane can be detected during a lifetime of periodic pelvic examinations, and can be reversed, slowed, or prevented by the long-term regular intravaginal instillation of supplemental estrogen cream once a week, particularly in patients who are sexually active.

SOME CONSIDERATIONS FOR THE OPERATIVE TEAM

Hand Disinfection Four minutes should be adequate for the first scrub of the day, with a 2-minute scrub between cases when using chlorhexidine.

Needle Sticks Double gloving will clearly reduce the incidence of needle perforations. The inner glove should be one half-size larger than that customarily worn by the surgeon, and the outer glove the usual size to which the surgeon is accustomed. No cases of HIV infection have been reported following surgical needle sticks. The small number that have been reported have followed tissue penetration by hollow needles.

References

1. Adler LM, Loughlin JS, Morin CJ, Haning RV: Bilateral compartment syndrome after a long gynecologic operation in the lithotomy position. Am J Obstet Gynecol 1990;162:1271–1272.
2. Bachman GA. Psychosexual aspects of hysterectomy. WHI 1990;1:41.
3. Baum N, Scott FB, Isaza O. Experimental evaluation of bladder closure techniques. Urology 1975;2:194–198.
4. Bell WR. Thrombolytic agents. A better way to treat pulmonary embolism. Consultant 1976;16:39–41.
5. Borkowf HI. Bacterial gangrene associated with pelvic surgery. Clin Obstet Gynecol 1973;16(2):40.
6. Borkowf HI, Mattingly RF. Bacterial gangrenous infection. In: Schaefer G, Graber EA, eds. Complications in obstetric and gynecologic surgery. Hagerstown: Harper & Row, 1981:140–156.
7. Burchell C. The umbrella pack to control pelvic hemorrhage. Conn Med 1968;32:734.
8. Burkhart FL, Daly JW. Sciatic and peroneal nerve injury: a complication of vaginal operations. Obstet Gynecol 1966;28:99–102.
9. Cruse PJE. Complications. In: Beahrs OH, Beart RW, eds. General surgery. Media, PA: Harwal, 1992.
10. Finnegan MG, Tisnado J, Bezirdjian DR, Cho C-R. Transcatheter embolotherapy of massive bleeding after surgery for benign gynecologic disorders. J Can Am Radiol 1988;39:172–177.
11. Fowl RJ, Akers DL, Kempczinski RF. Neurovascular lower extremity complications of the lithotomy position. Ann Vasc Surg 1992;6:357–361.
12. Goligher JC. Surgery of the anus, rectum and colon. 3rd ed. London: Bailliére Tindall, 1975:412.
13. Hirsh J. Venous thromboembolism: diagnosis, treatment, prevention. Hosp Pract 1975;10:53–62.
14. Harris RL, Speights SE, Moore, Jr JL, Hampton HL. Fallopian tube prolapse: a noninvasive technique for correction. J Pelvic Surg 1995;1:47–49.
15. Howkins J, Stallworthy J. Bonney's gynecologic surgery (8th ed.). London, Baillère Tindall, 1974.
16. Janisch H, Palmrich AH, Pecherstorfer M. Selected urologic operations in gynecology. Berlin: Walter de Gruyter, 1979:21–25.
17. Kambouris AA, Drukker BH, Barton J. Vaginal evisceration: a case report and brief review of the literature. Arch Surg 1981;116:949–951.
18. Koehler PR, Moss AA. Diagnosis of intraabdominal and pelvic abscesses by computerized tomography. JAMA 1980;244:49–52.
19. Ledger WJ, Campbell C, Taylor D, et al. Adnexal abscess as a late complication of pelvic operations. Surg Gynecol Obstet 1969;129:963–978.
20. Lee RA. Atlas of gynecologic surgery. Philadelphia: WB Saunders, 1992:304–305.
21. Lee RA. Postoperative necrotizing fasciitis. In: Nichols DH, DeLancey JOL, eds. Clinical problems, injuries and complications of gynecologic and obstetric surgery. 3rd ed. Baltimore: Williams & Wilkins, 1995:52–56.
22. Matsen FA, Krugmire RB. Compartmental syndromes. Surg Gynecol Obstet 1978;147:943–949.
23. Meleney FL. Bacterial synergism in disease processes with a confirmation of the synergistic bacterial etiology for a certain type of gangrene of the abdominal wall. Ann Surg 1931;94:961.
24. Meleney FL. A differential diagnosis between certain types of infectious gangrene of the skin with particular reference to hemolytic streptococcus gangrene and bacterial synergistic gangrene. Surg Gynecol Obstet 1933;56:847.
25. Mitchell GW, Massey FM. Bleeding three hours following vaginal hysterectomy. In: Nichols DH, DeLancey JOL, eds. Clinical problems, injuries and complications of gynecologic and obstetric surgery. 3rd ed. Baltimore: Williams & Wilkins, 1995:242–244.
26. Morrow CP. Discussion of paper by Fowl, Akers, Kempczinski. In: Mishell DR, Kirschbaum TH, Morrow CP, eds. Yearbook of obstetrics and gynecology. St. Louis: Mosby–Year Book, 1994:279–280.
27. Moser KM, Brach BB, Dolan GF. Clinically suspected deep venous thrombosis of the lower extremities. JAMA 1977;237:2195–2201.
28. Muntz HG, Falkenberry S, Fuller AF Jr. Fallopian tube prolapse after hysterectomy. J Reprod Med 1988;33:467.
29. Neuman M, Eidelman A, Langer R, Golan A, Bukovaky I, Caspi E. Iatrogenic injuries to the ureter during gynecologic and obstetric operations. Surg Gynecol Obstet 1991;173:268–272.
30. Nichols DH. Intraoperative and postoperative complications. In: Nichols DH, ed. Gynecologic and obstetric surgery. St. Louis: Mosby-Yearbook, 1993:131–142.
31. Nichols DH. Unanticipated spontaneous vaginal hemorrhage following straining at stool on tenth postoperative day. In: Nichols DH, DeLancey JOL, eds. Clinical problems, injuries and complications of gynecologic and obstetric surgery. 3rd ed. Baltimore: Williams & Wilkins, 1995:245–246.
32. Pettit PD, Petrou SP. The value of cystoscopy in major vaginal surgery. Obstet Gynecol 1994;84:318–320.
33. Powell JL. Vaginal evisceration following vaginal hysterectomy. Am J Obstet Gynecol 1973;115:276–277.
34. Reich WJ, Nechtow MJ. Ligation of the internal iliac arteries. J Int Coll Surg 1971;36:157–168.
35. Roberts DB, Hester LL Jr. Progressive synergistic bacterial gangrene arising from abscesses of the vulva and Bartholin's gland duct. Am J Obstet Gynecol 1972;114:285.

36. Rosenthal DM, Colapinto R. Angiographic arterial embolization in the management of postoperative vaginal hemorrhage. Am J Obstet Gynecol 1985;151:227.
37. Smith DG, Wyatt JR. Embolization of the hypogastric arteries in the control of massive vaginal hemorrhage. Obstet Gynecol 1977;49:317–322.
38. Somkuti SG, Vieta PA, Daugherty SF, et al. Transvaginal evisceration after hysterectomy in premenopausal women: a presentation of three cases. Am J Obstet Gynecol 1994;171:567–568.
39. Stone HH, Martin JD Jr. Synergistic necrotizing cellulitis. Ann Surg 1972;175:702.
40. Surwit EA. Postoperative care of the surgical patient. In: Garcia C-R, Mikuta JJ, Rosenblum NG, eds. Current therapy in surgical gynecology. Philadelphia: BC Decker, 1987:10–13.
41. Thessen CC, Kreder KJ. Ogilvie's syndrome: a potential complication of vaginal surgery. J Urol 1993;149:1541–1543.
42. Thompson JD. Operative injuries to the ureter: prevention, recognition, and management. In: Thompson JD, Rock JA, eds. Te Linde's operative gynecology. 7th ed. Philadelphia: JB Lippincott, 1992:749–783.
43. Thompson JD, Benigno BB. Vaginal repair of ureteral injuries. Am J Obstet Gynecol 1971;3:601–610.
44. Tondara AS, et al. Femoral neuropathy: a complication of lithotomy position under spinal anesthesia. Can Anaesth Soc J 1983;30:84.
45. Webb MJ, Southorn PA. Postoperative complications. In: Webb MJ. Manual of pelvic surgery. New York: Springer-Verlag, 1994:31–49.
46. Wetchler SJ, Hurt WG. A technique for surgical correction of fallopian tube prolapse. Obstet Gynecol 1986;67:747–749.
47. Wheeless CR Jr. Vaginal evisceration following pelvic surgery. In: Nichols DH, DeLancey JOL, eds. Clinical problems, injuries and complications of gynecologic and obstetric surgery. 3rd ed. Baltimore: Williams & Wilkins, 1995:203–213.
48. Whitesides TE, et al. A simple method for tissue pressure determination. Arch Surg 1975;110:1311.
49. Younes N, Bakri N, Linjawa T. Angiographic embolization for control of pelvic genital tract hemorrhage. Acta Obstet Gynecol Scand 1992;71:17–21.

Horizons and Miscellaneous Conditions

Reconstructive vaginal surgery is a dynamic discipline, constantly being refined. The last word has yet to be said concerning the indications and techniques for reconstructive gynecological surgery. It is essential that the gynecologic surgeon appreciate the phenomenon of individual patient-to-patient anatomic variation, particularly in terms of the branches of the blood vessels and the relative strengths of muscular and connective tissue components of the individual's pelvic supporting tissues. For example, Norton et al. (35) have shown that women with joint hypermobility have a significantly higher prevalence of genital prolapse than women with normal mobility. This suggests that an underlying connective tissue abnormality may be one etiologic factor of genital relaxation. Jessee et al. (19) found clinical joint hypermobility to be present in 10 percent of women in a sample of 637 healthy female white American blood donors.

EFFECTS OF ESTROGEN

There are also variations related to a relative deficiency or to the adequacy of estrogenic effects in the pelvic tissues of the woman needing a gynecologic repair. Estrogen and progesterone receptors have been demonstrated in the nuclei of both connective tissue cells and striated muscle cells of the levator ani (42). Although some problems relating to obstetric trauma may come to surgery long before estrogen deficiency is a likely contributing factor, more women develop increased and symptomatic degrees of prolapse during the climacteric and postmenopausal years. It has not been determined to what extent the elastic tissue of the pelvis is dependent upon estrogen and whether its age-related reduction is preventable or reversible by perimenopausal or postmenopausal estrogen supplementation.

The appearance of postmenopausal atrophic changes in the vaginal membrane is not a reliable indication of a woman's chronologic age. Atrophic changes associated with estrogen deficiency are not to be assumed even several years after a physiologic menopause. Evidence of an estrogenic deficiency effect may be noticeable in the vaginal cytology of less than 50 percent of women even 5 years after spontaneous cessation of their menstrual periods. Thus it is evident that a wide range of individual variation must be taken into consideration. Clinically evident tissue change associated with "atrophic vaginitis" becomes symptomatic in no more than 15 to 20 percent of postmenopausal women.

There appear to be racial differences as well, for atrophic vaginitis appears to be distinctly less common in the black woman than in the white. There may be many biochemical and biologic differences that have not been recognized but that exist between the black and the white people of the world. Such considerations require fundamental molecular biochemical studies as well as clinical observations that might have broad clinical significance, possibly suggesting means by which the individual's endocrines might be manipulated to retard the effects of aging. When the vaginal membrane is noticeably atrophic, the gynecologic repair will be technically easier and healing will be accentuated if the tissues have been primed preoperatively with exogenous estrogen until the vascularity improves. Exogenous and vaginal applications of estrogen should be resumed throughout the postoperative period, in a dosage adequate to produce a full-blown estrogenic effect and a desirable degree of vascularity and elasticity, at least until healing is complete and the vaginal caliber has stabilized.

In one's assessment of the tissue of the postmenopausal woman, it is important to recognize that bilateral oophorectomy does not deprive many castrates of all estrogenic effects. Interstitial cells in the nonremoved pedicle portion of the ovary, as well as in the adrenal glands, produce androgens that may be converted into significant amounts of estrogens for not less than 40 percent of castrates. Androstanedione is converted in fat tissue to estrogen in a quantity proportionate to the amount of obesity present, probably due to the ability of fat to aromatize androgens (43). Sex hormone–binding globulin is suppressed in the obese, further increasing free estrogen levels (39). Therefore, symptoms and findings of estrogen deprivation are more likely to be seen in thin women than in the obese. This conversion helps to account for the failure of many women to develop atrophic changes over periods of from 5 to 10 years after oophorectomy. The effectiveness of such continuing estrogenic effects for years after the woman's menopause may be a factor in slowing the individual's aging process, but this effect has yet to be proven.

We do not know the extent to which atrophy and attenuation of elastic tissue might be arrested or reversed by such supplementation or replacement, nor do we know the specific steroid or combination of steroids that are most effective in terms of slowing the more undesirable effects of aging.

There are few data on the suspected long-term effects of the oral progestational agents or "birth control pills" on the ultimate development of the various manifestations of genital prolapse and whether that effect, if any, is related to the intensity of the dose or to the chemical composition of the specific compound. For that matter, we do not know whether the soft tissue components of the pelvis are affected equally or selectively in the attenuating effects of the aging process, just as we cannot accurately predict the individual's tissue response to hormone supplementation or replacement. The degree to which locally applied estrogen equals the efficacy of systemic estrogen replacement certainly must depend upon the effectiveness of the individual's absorption, again emphasizing the importance of the individual's response rather than the magnitude of the dosage given.

Brincat and colleagues (4) have shown that the decline in skin collagen and thickness after the menopause is related to the loss of ovarian estrogens. Comparing skin thickness and collagen content in a group of postmenopausal women treated with sex hormone implants with an untreated group of similar women, they observed

an inverse relation between skin collagen content and years since the menopause, independent of the actual age of the patient. This suggests that the decline in skin collagen is due to the loss of ovarian estrogens. That effect is lost in the treated group of women indicating treatment with sex hormones prevents or reverses the loss of skin collagen after the menopause.*

* From Brincat M, Moniz CJ, Studd JWW, et al. Long-term effects of the menopause and sex hormones on skin thickness. Br J Obstet Gynaecol 1985;92;256–259. Used with permission.

Postmenopausal Estrogen Supplementation after Hysterectomy

Supplemental estrogen appears to lessen the incidence and seriousness of ischemic heart disease if the ovaries have been removed at the time of hysterectomy. This commendable goal may be reduced by the use of supplemental synthetic progestins, although there is some evidence that it is not removed by the use of natural progesterone. For the most part, therefore, in the absence of the uterus, one might recommend the protective cardiovascular and antiosteoporotic benefits of postoperative supplemental estrogen without progesterone, when there is no contraindication to the use of estrogen.

PROLAPSE AND DIABETES

There appears to be an increased incidence of prolapse in patients with diabetes. Some observers have suggested that abnormalities in carbohydrate metabolism, as in the diabetic, have an etiologic role in the development of genital prolapse as a result of a characteristic effect on connective tissues. Cohen (5) has discussed the implication of protein glycosylation in the diabetic patient as a possible mechanism of acquired collagen weakness.

Recent years have witnessed a surge of interest in non-enzymatic glycosylation, which is the attachment of free sugar to certain amino acid residues of proteins . . . Hyperglycemia permits increased non-enzymatic glycosylation not only of circulating proteins such as hemoglobin and albumin . . . but also of tissue proteins, thereby providing insight into pathogenetic mechanisms contributory to chronic complications to diabetes . . . non-enzymatic glycosylation can alter the structure and/or function of involved proteins. Thus, the guilt of glucose can no longer be denied, and has prompted an awareness of the importance of long-term maintenance of euglycemia in diabetic patients in an attempt to prevent the development or arrest the progression of chronic complications. The need for long-term control is further underscored by the recognition that proteins in some of the affected tissues have long biologic half-lives, and hence represent situations in which glycosylation could be relatively permanent since the population of proteins is not quickly replaced . . . Collagen is the main fibrous protein of connective tissues and is a principle constituent of basement membranes. Collagenous proteins are rich in lysine and hydroxylysine, generally have a long biologic half-life, and are continuously exposed to ambient levels of glucose in the vascular compartment and extracellular fluid. Since variables such as the number of free amino groups in and the residence time of a protein determine the extent of glycosylation in vivo, there are a priori reasons to suspect that collagen would be highly subject to excess non-enzymatic glycosylation in vivo. Examination of several collagens has confirmed that this is the case, and a two to three-fold increase has been consistently found when non-enzymatic glycosylation of collagens from tissues of diabetic subjects or animals is compared to that in control samples.

In vitro non-enzymatic glycosylation had been demonstrated with virtually every protein that has been examined to date. It is clear that, at least in vitro, non-enzymatic glycosylation can influence physicochemical properties and packing of collagen fibers. This is further supported by the observation that glucose, in vitro, inhibits the formation of collagen fibrils. This decrease in fibril formation correlates with the loss and the ability of collagen to serve as a substrate for lysyl oxidase [24]. [It is possible that] glucoadducts, once formed, would provide a chemical framework for self perpetuating and damaging processes that can continue even if strict diabetic control is instituted. This hypothesis, if correct, provides one of the strongest arguments in favor of early aggressive therapeutic intervention with intensified regimens to establish and maintain normal normoglycemia.*

Whether because of a relatively high fat content or a specific weakening of elastic tissues, the diabetic frequently seems soft rather than "lean and hard." Certainly, the attenuation of elastic tissue strength in the diabetic is not related to a decreased vascularity related to a declining estrogen effect, for studies have clearly shown that the diabetic, like the person suffering from obesity, stores estrogens more efficiently and metabolizes

---

* From Cohen MP. Diabetes and protein glucysylation. New York: Springer-Verlag, 1986. Used with permission.

them slowly. As a rule, the diabetic, like the obese individual, tends to continue menstrual-like bleeding at ages beyond that of the average climacteric. Such bleeding is usually anovulatory and related more to the individual's slow metabolism of estrogens rather than to an increased or prolonged production by either the ovary or the adrenal.

MISCELLANEOUS PREDISPOSING FACTORS

The still poorly understood role of lymphangiectasia as an etiologic factor in the markedly hypertrophic changes sometimes seen with genital prolapse needs to be clarified, for it must be related to the metabolic effects of venous stasis and chronic congestion.

When fascial layers are attenuated and barely demonstrable, subepithelial homografts, collagen injections, or implantable plastic materials may be useful, but to what extent has not been determined. Evaluation must, of course, be correlated with the predictable connective tissue changes that can be expected as a result of scarring and fibrosis in the later stages of postoperative healing.

Much information concerning individual variations in pelvic architecture can be learned from careful and detailed examination in the morgue. A question that warrants reconsideration from time to time is the extent to which the techniques of surgery can be visualized and developed and improved using postmortem material. In our own experience, certain anatomic questions can best be answered from examination and radical dissection of the fresh postmortem material of many cadavers.

When elongation of the uterus is noted as an apparently dominant feature of genital prolapse, is it the cervix that is actually elongated or is it the lower uterine segment? Is such elongation the result of interference with blood or lymphatic circulation, or both, largely because venous and lymphatic channels are compressed as the prolapsed part descends through the genital hiatus and is squeezed between the lateral pelvic soft tissues? Study of the point at which the major branches of the uterine artery enter the cervix should demonstrate whether this elongation is cervical or really represents elongation of the lower uterine segment. Does the site of attachment of the cul-de-sac peritoneum to the surface of the uterus provide a reliable indicator of where the elongation actually begins? A criterion of considerable help to the gynecologic surgeon in making his or her preoperative appraisal would be a reliable means of determining the actual location of the internal cervical os.

What, if any, are the effects of premature labor, induced labor, or subsequent pregnancy on the integrity of cervical elastic tissue? The clinically incompetent cervix is not always a posttraumatic entity. In instances where conization or cervical amputation has been performed, are the effects on a subsequent pregnancy dependent upon whether the integrity of the internal os was inadvertently damaged?

Although there is documentation of certain positive effects from the voluntary perineal resistive exercises described by Kegel (20), the permanent value of employing galvanic electrical stimulation to the musculature of the pelvic floor and urogenital diaphragm is being clinically established. The stimulation method would seem to provide a more efficient exercise program than the original Kegel-type exercises and may be of greatest value in those patients who seem unable to demonstrate voluntary contraction of the pubococcygeus possibly secondary to a pudendal neuropathy. Huffman and Sokol (17) suggested that a positive effect from a course of galvanic electrical stimulations was the result of stimulation of *both* smooth and striated muscle, in contrast to the voluntary Kegel perineal resisting exercises, which use only striated voluntary muscles.

The beneficial effect of pelvic floor training continues for years. Klarskov et al. (22) pose the question of whether all patients with genuine stress incontinence should be offered physiotherapy as a first therapy. Should all patients undergoing surgery for the correction of urinary incontinence have physiotherapy first to optimize results? Should it be used postoperatively? Indefinitely? Only future study will tell. Injection of biodegradable collagen (GAX) (see Chapter 17) will effectively treat incontinence from intrinsic urethral sphincter dysfunction in many persons, providing there is no urethral hypermobility. How long will it last?

URETHROCOLPOPROCTOGRAPHY

Although much has been written about the significance of defects of the urethrovesical angle and urinary stress incontinence (9, 14, 41), such factors as a relative deficiency in the support of the levator plate, the course of the pelvic diaphragm, the integrity of the perineal body, and its location may each be of importance in the maintenance of urethral position and tone. By simply applying a thin coating of barium paste within the vagina at the time of bead-chain urethrocystography, one can objectively compare preoperative information with similar postoperative studies concerning deficiencies in each or any combination of the following separate systems: the urogenital diaphragm, the bladder base plate, the pelvic diaphragm, the levator plate, and the perineum (6) (Fig. 24.1). A small amount of barium paste may be instilled into the rectum as well if there is reason for studying abnormalities in its configuration. Comparison of preoperative and postoperative films may demonstrate objectively the possible role of a coincident posterior colporrhaphy and a perineorrhaphy in the development of a satisfactory

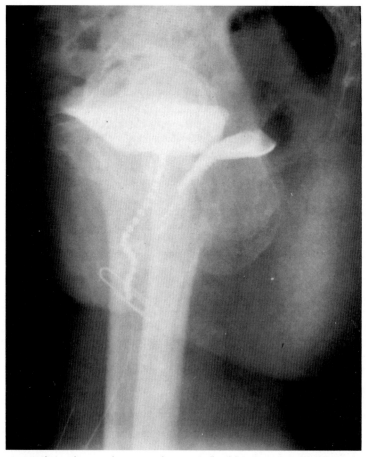

Figure 24.1. Urethrocolpography. **A.** Radiopaque fluid has been instilled into the bladder, a urethral marking chain inserted, and the vagina lightly coated with barium cream. A lateral standing radiograph of the patient at rest is obtained, and the organ relationships to one another and to the bony pelvis are observed.

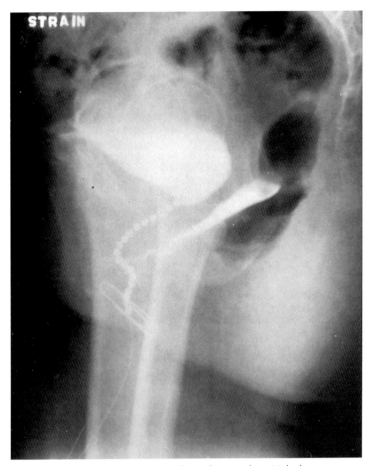

Figure 24.1. B. The patient is asked to strain or bear down as by a Valsalva maneuver and the altered relationships are observed. Note that there is flattening of the posterior urethrovesical angle with some rotational descent of the bladder neck. The vaginal axis is altered, indicating tipping of the levator plate beneath it. (Courtesy of the X-ray Department, St. Francis Hospital, Buffalo, NY, Dr. Paul deMarsovszky, radiologist. Used with permission.)

result. Computerized axial tomography, dynamic ultrasound, or magnetic resonance imaging (MRI) studies may permit dynamic analysis of all the relevant pelvic supporting tissues. Observations can be made without the diagnostic use of ionizing radiation through MRI, which makes visible the soft tissue organs themselves, as seen in Figure 24.2 (16, 26). What effects will these examinations have on anatomic and physiologic studies and clinical diagnosis and relevance?

Although few people seem to question the functional importance of the pubococcygeus portion of the levator ani muscle in the normal voiding process, there remains considerable question as to the role of this muscle and its possible deficiencies in the etiology of urinary stress incontinence.

THE LOW-PRESSURE URETHRA

The optimal clinical management of the low-pressure urethra (maximum urethral closure pressure less than 20 cm of water) remains complex, particularly since it is not always associated with incontinence. It is found at times unexpectedly during uro-

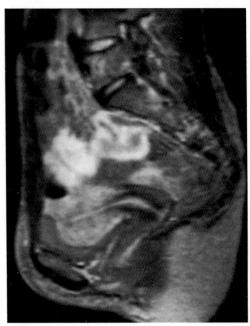

Figure 24.2. MRI of sagittal section through the pelvis, showing uterus and vagina and adjacent organs. Note the relatively thin endometrium. (From McCarthy S, Tauber C, Gore J. Female pelvic anatomy: MR assessment of variations during the menstrual cycle and with use of oral contraceptives. Radiology 1986;160:120.)

dynamic evaluation and not infrequently in postmenopausal prolapse patients. Incontinence is more common among those otherwise continent women whose dislocated vaginal vault has been temporarily replaced within the pelvis, as by a pessary, and is the consequence of straightening of a kinked urethrovesical junction. An element of the latter may be present, but that explanation is simplistic. At the present time, the addition of a urethrovesical sling procedure to a pelvic reconstructive operation (see Chapter 17) has in our hands produced the most successful response. However, it is possible that less formidable surgical procedures will be identified as consistently successful. Among the latter are submucosal collagen or fat injections, urethrocliesis (full-length urethral plication), and a Kelly-type vesicourethral plication stitch coincident with plication of the urogenital diaphragm (see Chapter 10). For the postmenopausal patient, estrogen replacement therapy through the use of long courses of intravaginal estrogen and Kegel pubococcygeal resistive exercises are recommended empirically.

The diagnosis of low urethral closure pressure currently requires sophisticated urodynamic assessment, which is, at times, inconvenient, unavailable, or prohibitively expensive. For these reasons, we have been actively seeking an alternate method that can be employed in the examining room as well as in the operating room. Since 1992, we have used a catheter pull-through test with satisfaction, and with considerable correlation in almost all prolapse patients. The technique is as follows: A no. 8 pediatric Foley catheter whose inflatable bulb normally holds 3 ml of fluid is inserted into the urethra and the bulb is partially inflated with 1 ml of saline. Gentle traction to the catheter is made to see if the catheter bulb can be drawn through the urethra. If so, this suggests a probability of low-pressure urethra. If the bulb cannot be drawn through with 1 ml of saline in the bulb, the bulb is deflated and reinflated using 0.5 ml of saline. The test possibly is positive if gentle traction to the catheter draws the bulb through the full length of the urethra. Whether this "test" is diagnostic of the low urethral closure pressure, or indicative of significant but previously undiagnosed urethral funneling, and/or whether these are basically the same condition, is as yet unclear.

If such a patient had been determined preoperatively to be incontinent when the displaced vault was temporarily replaced within the pelvis, a coincident suburethral sling operation is added to the surgical procedure. If incontinence has not been demonstrated, urethrocliesis (7, 37) or Kelly-type vesical neck plication with coincident plication of the urogenital diaphragm will be performed along with the vaginal vault reconstructive procedure and colporrhaphy. The clinical results to date are most encouraging, but future correlation with the results of conventional urodynamic assessment and with long-term clinical observation is necessary. Such studies are currently under way.

NEUROGENIC DEFECT AND IMBALANCE AS A FACTOR IN GENITAL PROLAPSE

There appears to be considerable variation in the innervation of the voluntary muscles of the pelvis. Although the pudendal is the principal nerve to the levator ani, it is inconstant in its distribution, since there is usually an independently arising and variously located accessory pudendal nerve that assumes a variable share of total pudendal nerve function. When viscera possess a triple innervation (i.e., the somatic, sympathetic, and parasympathetic nerve supply of the bladder), the opportunity for physiologic imbalance is very great. This may be influenced not only by congenital defect, but also by conditioned reflex as well as the trauma of surgery (13). Sensitive direct electromyography may provide objective information of both muscular and neuromuscular efficiency in a particular situation, and thereby provide a more logical basis for the choice of operation and improvement in the prognosis.

Several questions immediately come to mind: Is there a difference between the interpretation of direct and of indirect electromyography? To what extent is genital prolapse caused by secondary damage to the structures or nerves involved (26, 36, 38), and when might it result from a primary or congenital defect in muscle innervation? Can such a possible etiology and pathology of genital prolapse be studied and perhaps effectively measured by electromyography (21)? Is a correlation possible between an abnormal electromyogram and the results of reconstructive surgery? What anatomic or endocrine factors influence pudendal nerve latency transmission rates? Can these rates be correlated with functional disorders? Can the rates be altered by treatment?

To be valid, the long-range effectiveness of transvaginal surgical denervation of the bladder (Fig. 24.3) to relieve socially disabling and medically refractive detrusor instability must be established by *long-term* follow-up of a large number of patients before its place can be determined as a treatment for this condition. To what extent does nerve regeneration reduce the long-term effectiveness of the procedure? The results of such a surgical approach must be compared prospectively to the effectiveness of treatment by drugs and by bladder retraining.

GENITAL FISTULAS

Vesicovaginal Fistula

The selection of surgical treatment technique and its effectiveness may depend partly upon the relationship between the fistula location and the vesicovaginal space. At the very vault of the vagina, there is no vesicovaginal space, since the vagina and bladder capsule are fused to one another at this point. A fistula location more distal in the vagina and through the vesicovaginal space gives the option of separate closure of the wall of the bladder and of the wall of the vagina.

A fistula located near the base of the trigone will likely be in a nonexpansile layer of the bladder, thus influencing the time at which an indwelling catheter may be safely

Figure 24.3. Bladder denervation. An inverted U-shaped incision has been made through the full thickness of the anterior vaginal wall, and by dissection between the bladder pillar and the pelvic diaphragm, the hypogastric plexus has been exposed deep in the wound on the patient's left. The fibers, along with branches of the inferior vesical artery if necessary, are clamped between two forceps, cut, and ligated. A similar procedure can be performed on the patient's right, if necessary, and the vaginal incision closed using interrupted sutures.

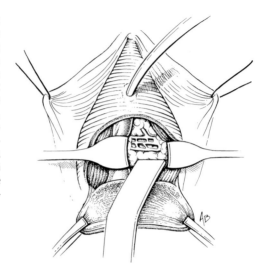

removed postoperatively. If the fistula is in a nonexpansile area, the catheter may theoretically be removed after 48 hours, but if it is in an expansile area, the bladder should be decompressed for 14 to 21 days. If the vesicovaginal fistula transgresses the vesicovaginal space, the postoperative physiology will be closer to normal if the walls of the vagina and of the bladder are closed separately. This is true when the fistula is found distal to the vault of the vagina. A fistula located at the vaginal vault will normally be in an area cranial to the vesicovaginal space. Whether this is closed in one layer or two, it will postoperatively fuse during the course of healing to become a single layer of scar unless an intermediate layer of insulation such as peritoneum, omentum, or a bulbocavernosus muscle fat pad transplant is brought in.

SUTURE PLACEMENT AND KNOT SECURITY

Should the placement of sutures and the security of the knots that are tied in such sutures take into account (*a*) tissue edema preceding repair, (*b*) tissue edema at the time of the repair, and/or (*c*) tissue edema after the repair?

When sutures are placed in edematous tissue, there are two risks to the integrity of the suture line. (*a*) When the edema has subsided, these stitches will no longer be holding the edges in firm apposition.(*b*) If one attempts to overcome this by tying the knots tightly or pulling the sutures too tightly, there is a risk of increasing the edema rather than decreasing it, yielding "necrosis" at the suture line. Therefore, one would not ordinarily operate on tissues that are edematous if a reduction in edema is likely during the time that healing is taking place. What is the place of elastic monofilament permanent sutures that will stretch when edema develops and contract when the swelling is gone? Does this phenomenon give a stronger wound closure?

Because vaginal fistulas represent the development of communication by an epithelialized tract between two organs, might this be effectively treated by simple excision of the epithelialized tract at a site other than at the vaginal vault and watertight but gentle approximation of the freshly trimmed vaginal edges without tension by some simple device such as the Wachenfeldt clip applied by an applicator suitably modified by a 90-degree bend in its tip (Figs. 24.4 and 24.5)? Any tension developed by the approximation of the vaginal edges could be relieved by suitable relaxing incisions in the lateral vaginal walls. After how many days should such clips be removed? Would this not be the essence of the Sims closure?

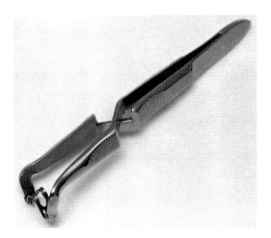

Figure 24.4. The modified Wachenfeldt clip forceps.

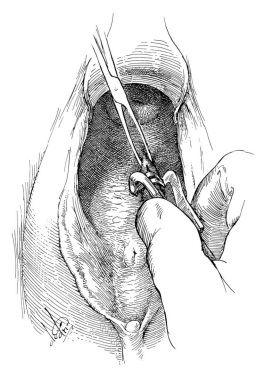

Figure 24.5. Application of the forceps. The patient is in the knee-chest position and a urinary fistula has been excised. The vagina is being closed using the modified Wachenfeldt clip forceps, bringing the freshened edges of the cystotomy in contact with one another.

Cervicovaginal Fistula

This may be seen after traumatic dilatation and curettage or elective pregnancy terminations in which the forces of induced labor have pushed the products of conception into the vagina through the upper and often posterior wall of an otherwise insufficiently dilated cervix. The endocervix protrudes and bulges through the fibromuscular wall of the upper cervical laceration. The fistula should be excised and the cervix closed over a no. 3 Hegar dilator. Because there is considerable tension upon the outermost sutures, they should be of a long-acting synthetic material such as 00 polydioxanone (PDS) or polyglyconate (Maxon). For patients with no desire for further childbearing, Martius

(25) suggests cervical amputation at the level of the fistula, possibly covering the raw wound with a Sturmdorf suture.

The effectiveness, dosage, and patient convenience of newer antibiotics and antibacterials need adequate assessment, particularly for the patient with demonstrated sensitivity to penicillin. Are intravenous doses or rectal suppositories (18) of metronidazole (Flagyl) an effective substitute?

Rectovaginal Fistula

The vast majority of rectovaginal fistulas today are the consequence of the obstetric lacerations that have improperly healed even following primary repair. Most of the residual damages and coincident perineal defects from other mechanical causes can be satisfactorily remedied by the procedures described in Chapter 12, but on occasion, for the patient without residual anal sphincter damage, a simpler solution may be found to be equally effective depending upon the absence of coincident restorative surgery that should be done at the same time (e.g., perineorrhaphy with or without anal sphincter plication). This is described as follows.

A TECHNIQUE FOR ENDORECTAL REPAIR

The direct endorectal approach using the obliterative suture of Block (3) has been useful on occasion for relatively simple closure of a small rectovaginal fistula, providing that the fistulous tract has been transected and the rectum carefully separated from the vagina, restoring the rectovaginal space at this site. The operation can be done in about 15 minutes, and our results to date have been quite satisfactory for the smaller rectovaginal fistula, especially that which is near the vaginal vault and is otherwise of difficult operative exposure. The success depends upon a side-to-side coaptation of the strong intestinal submucosa.

A suitable mechanical bowel preparation is given consisting of 2 days of preoperative liquid diet followed by an electrolyte-type catharsis (NuLYTELY, GoLYTELY, or CoLYTE) and a short-acting general or regional anesthetic.

Through a Fansler rectal retractor, each side of the now mobilized rectal wall containing the rectal side of the fistula is grasped by an Allis clamp, and the full thickness of the wall including the fistulous tract is approximated longitudinally by a running locked, size 00, absorbable polyglycolic acid-type suture such as Dexon or Vicryl (Fig. 24.6). The suture should start caudal to the fistula and end cranial to it. No anal sikin is included. When the top stitch has been placed, the suture is tied, and a second running locked layer of suture is passed through the same tissue from a cranial to distal direction and tied. Great care is taken to ensure that no part of the vaginal wall is included in this suture. The vaginal wall at the site of the fistula is approximated by a separate single interrupted suture. This allows for unobstructed, postoperative drainage, but by narrowing of the vaginal ostium provides a smaller area that must fill in by reepithelialization.

Preoperative and postoperative care is the same as for other repairs, with several days of a liquid diet followed by a month of low-residue diet and daily stool softeners. The hospitalization may be only overnight. In about 10 days, the patient likely will experience passage of a modestly increased, bloody, rectal discharge, coincident with slough of the suture line and the tissue it embraces after reunification of the submucosa and other layers have occurred. When the patient is seen for postoperative examination 4 weeks later, both rectal and vaginal walls should be once again intact.

This is not a repair suitable for the patient requiring coincident perineorrhaphy or plication of the external anal sphincter. This obliterative repair is by nature entirely different from the more formidable vaginal or endorectal flap-sliding operation. We have performed this operation a few times to determine its feasibility and are awaiting analysis of a larger number of cases. In addition to its relative simplicity, it is one that can usu-

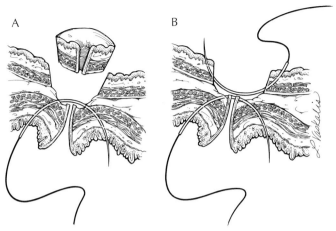

Figure 24.6. Endorectal repair of rectovaginal fistula. **A.** Simple closure of the rectal side of the fistula. A plate of full-thickness vaginal wall surrounding and including the vaginal end of the fistula tract is excised. It is important that the needle includes no part of the vaginal wall and that the rectal vaginal space is carefully identified so that the obliterative suture can be placed through the full thickness of the rectal wall, including the submocosal layer. **B.** After the rectal opening of the fistula has been obliterated in its entirety by two layers of a running locked stitch, the freshened edges of the vaginal incision may be united by one or two interrupted stitches that do not include the rectal wall. This will leave enough room for any transvaginal drainage of this space and yet reduce the size of the vaginal area that must fill in by granulation and reepithelization.

ally be offered to the patient when she is first seen, presuming there is no local necrosis present, and in anticipation of a more formal repair in some weeks in the event that the endorectal repair is unsuccessful.

OBSTETRIC PRACTICE

Inelasticity and Soft Tissue Damage

Current obstetric practices are being subjected to even greater skepticism and modification than is evident in the care of women with gynecologic complaints. Will an increased popularity of home delivery and of spontaneous delivery without episiotomy, particularly among the current older group of parturients in whom tissue elasticity may be compromised as a consequence of aging, result in significant increases in soft tissue damage from delivery and in a greater need for gynecologic repairs in the future?

Chronic Inversion of the Uterus

Under certain circumstances, usually postpartum, the uterus can turn inside out. When the condition is acute, there may be accompanying shock, and the uterus can be reverted by intravaginal manipulation. Rarely, when the patient has survived this event and the diagnosis not previously established, the condition may be discovered months later in the course of a pelvic examination to evaluate a chronic bloody discharge. This is so-called chronic inversion and requires surgical relief (11). When the patient no longer wishes to retain the uterus, hysterectomy is offered, usually by the vaginal route. If she wants to retain her fertility, the integrity of the uterus must be surgically restored, and this can be done transvaginally using either the Spinelli technique or the lesser-known Küstner operation (34). Both will be described. The surgeon should choose whichever technique seems to fit best the needs of a particular patient.

The Spinelli technique requires dissection of the bladder from the inverted uterus; however, it poses a more complex surgical problem than does the Küstner. In the Küstner technique, the incision through the cervix and myometrium is made in the posterior wall of the uterus, sparing any dissection of the bladder but putting the repair on the posterior uterine wall instead of the anterior uterine wall. Whether the scar on the back of the uterus is equally strong and resistant to future rupture has not been proven. Adhesion formation may be increased, and the scar is not accessible for palpation during a subsequent pregnancy. The objections are largely overcome when the newer transvaginal Spinelli operation is performed.

The Küstner operation as described by Halban (10) is performed as follows: The cul-de-sac of Douglas is opened by posterior colpotomy. The index finger of the operator's left hand is inserted into the peritoneal invagination of the uterus. The posterior uterine wall is incised (Fig. 24.7). The surgeon's thumbs make pressure upon the rear wall of the uterus leading to reversion, restoring it to its normal position within the pelvis. The corpus is flipped through the posterior colpotomy and the incision in the posterior uterine wall is repaired, with any myometrium trimmed if necessary to achieve reapproximation of the serosal surface. The uterus is replaced within the pelvis and the colpotomy is closed.

The technique of the Spinelli operation for treatment of chronic inversion of the uterus (Fig. 24.8) was described by Graves (8):

A transverse anterior vaginal incision is first made and the bladder separated from the uterus, as described for anterior colpotomy. A median incision is then made through the cervix, dividing completely the constricting ring. This incision should be carried toward the fundus, through the anterior uterine wall, until a point is reached which will allow the reversion of the inverted uterus. It is, as a rule, necessary to continue the incision as far as the fundus.

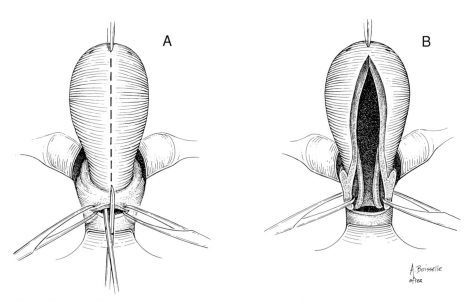

Figure 24.7. The Küstner operation for chronic inversion of the uterus. **A.** The posterior cul-de-sac has been opened, and the cervix and posterior wall of the uterus should be incised along the path of the *broken line*. **B.** When this has been completed, thumb pressure along the sides of the uterus produces reversion, the wounds are closed with interrupted sutures, and the uterus is replaced in the pelvic cavity. The colpotomy is then closed.

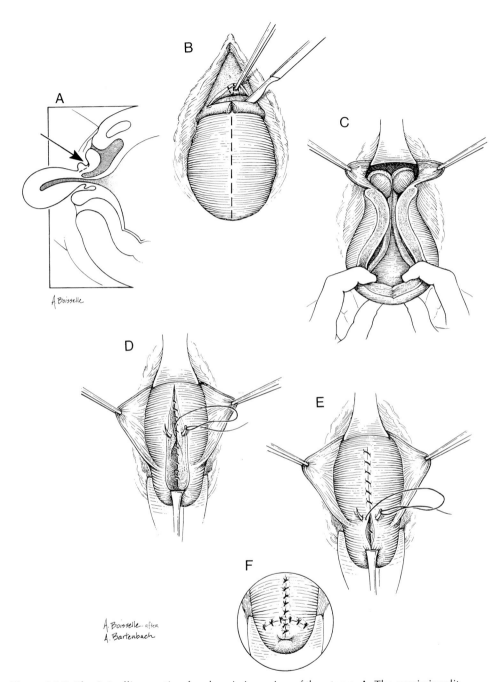

Figure 24.8. The Spinelli operation for chronic inversion of the uterus. **A.** The cervix is split in the midline and carefully separated from the bladder as shown by the *dotted line*. **B.** The anterior wall of the everted uterus is split along the path of the *dotted line*. **C.** By pressure with the operator's index fingers and thumbs, the uterus is turned outside in. **D.** The myometrium is reapproximated by two layers of running PGA suture. **E.** The serosal surface is reapproximated by a single layer. **F.** The vaginal skin is reapproximated with interrupted sutures, as is the full thickness of the cervix.

The uterus is reverted by placing the forefingers at the cervix for counterpressure, and forcing the fundus upward by the thumbs in the manner that one would naturally use in turning a tennis ball inside out through a cut in its side.

When the uterus has been restored to its original form the next step is to close the incision in its wall. It will, however, be found that, owing to the shrinking which the peritoneum has undergone in its inverted position, it cannot be approximated, the tissue of the uterine wall pouting out in the manner of an ectropion. The excess of tissue must be trimmed away in the form of longitudinal wedges, when the peritoneal edges may be coaptated without difficulty. The wound of the uterine wall is closed with two rows of continuous sutures. The first suture includes and firmly unites the muscular wall; the second is superficial and approximates the peritoneal surfaces. The wound of the cervix is closed with interrupted sutures . . . The vaginal wound is sutured.*

Because of the risk of uterine rupture, future obstetric delivery, in most instances, should be by elective cesarean section 2 weeks before term in patients who have experienced such a hysterotomy (34).

MISCELLANEOUS PROCEDURES

Use of Fibrin Glue

This compound is composed of equal parts of cryoprecipitate and bovine thrombin (1000 U/ml) that may be simultaneously sprayed from plastic syringes onto a bleeding site for the control of hemorrhage (30). It also has considerable use in reconstructive surgery because it promotes instant adhesion between surfaces and is biodegradable. It may have application to the retropubic operations for the correction of urethral hypermobility. The fibrin fibers act as a framework for the rapidly ingrowing fibroblasts from which connective tissue is formed (2). It has been used successfully in the repair of recurrent small rectovaginal fistulas (1). Although it is not yet available commercially in the United States, it can be made from the patient's own blood to avoid any possible transmission of unwanted, unrelated virus particles.

TECHNIQUE FOR PREPARATION

Abel et al. (1) have described a technique for making autologous fibrinogen.

Within 8 hours of the blood donation, the plasma is separated and frozen. The freezing process takes about 24 hours. This frozen plasma is then thawed slowly to 1 to 6°C, and through this method of cryoprecipitation the insoluble proteins sink to the bottom of the unit. These heavy proteins are then spun down and are reconstituted with 10 to 15 ml of the patient's plasma. The product is then frozen again until is used. This method of precipitation recovers 20 to 40 percent of the fibrinogen in a unit of plasma and yields 10 to 35 mg/ml of fibrinogen concentrate. Prior to surgery, the concentrate is warmed to 37°C in a water bath, requiring approximately 15 minutes. Overheating is to be avoided since it will denature the proteins. Once the fibrinogen concentrate is opened, it should be used within 4 hours. In a separate syringe, the thrombin (Thrombinar) is reconstituted at 1000 U/ml.

Separate syringes are filled with equal volumes, and the thrombin and fibrinogen are attached to a plastic Y connector. A 14-gauge plastic catheter cut short for easier placement, is attached to the Y connector, completing the administration set. The fibrinogen concentrate and thrombin are dispensed simultaneously and injected into the prepared space. A coagulum is immediately formed. Since the concentration of fibrinogen in the cryoprecipitate is unpredictable, the rate of coagulation should be assessed away from the surgical site prior to the application of the fibrin

* From Graves WP. Gynecology. 4th ed. Philadelphia: WB Saunders, 1928:841–844. Used with permission.

glue. This coagulation rate ideally is similar to the hardening of melted candle wax. To achieve this rate of solidification, the rate of fibrinogen and thrombin administration may have to be varied. The 14-gauge dispensing catheter and, on occasion, the Y connector become occluded and should be replaced if necessary.*

Laparoscopic-Assisted Hysterectomy

The author has elsewhere (32) noted the following:

It has been demonstrated that all variety of gynecologic surgery can be done through the laparoscope, but it must be proven that such laparoscopic surgery is not only better for the patient but is cost effective for society in general, and furthermore, that it can be taught effectively to willing gynecologic surgeons. Measurements of this efficacy must coincide with development and implementation of a credentialing process for such surgery that will safeguard the best interests of the patient. Further new techniques will evolve, and they must be adequately tested before they are made available widely. Since the needs of women are so similar in so many nations and cultures throughout the world, politically free cooperation between physicians and surgeons including the exchange of both teaching and learning personnel and implementation of ideas and significant concepts will speed this process immeasurably.

Laparoscopic-assisted vaginal hysterectomy (LAVH) can be an effective substitute for transabdominal hysterectomy. Because it currently embraces a longer operating time and the use of expensive disposable instruments, its cost effectiveness must be determined by large prospective studies (12). Only time will prove whether a presumably shorter length of stay with LAVH compared to that for abdominal hysterectomy will be matched by a significant reduction in operative complication rates (23, 44). Some have shown that the main hospital charge for LAVH is higher than that of either abdominal or vaginal hysterectomy (31, 45). To what extent will the future choice of hysterectomy route be influenced by aggressive marketing, which may influence the patient's preference (46)?

Early Discharge from Hospital Following Hysterectomy

Reiner (40) has reported a series of 40 patients discharged within 24 hours following transvaginal hysterectomy without complications attributable to the procedure or to "early" hospital discharge. Because of this initial success, will endometrial ablation replace hysterectomy for the treatment of chronic abnormal uterine bleeding, or will endometrial regeneration occur in time sufficient for the symptom to recur?

Sacrospinous Colpopexy

Will bilateral colpopexy versus unilateral colpopexy give even better long-term results? Will a combination of permanent monofilament sutures and simultaneously-placed, absorbable but long-lasting, polyglycolic acid sutures prove to be the best combination? Can better, new, safe, and inexpensive ligature carriers or punches be produced for this operation? The spectrum of challenges to be solved is vast, dynamic, and never ending. The need for appropriate solutions is great and expansive: proportionate to the largely increasing number of older persons who would like to make longevity a source of pleasure and not a liability (33).

Other Miscellaneous

The significance of changes in pelvic organ relationships consequent to increased intra-abdominal pressure from unusually heavy work or physical exertion must be considered as a possible etiologic factor in the development of genital prolapse. Equal rights and equal opportunities are certain to bring the sexes to more equal risks and, more frequently, to similar injuries. More women have become involved in performing the heavy physical types of work previously undertaken only by men. When such strains are superimposed upon (a) preexistent tissue damage as a result of childbirth, (b) congenital deficiency, or (c) the secondary attenuations of aging, more realistic guidelines for worker's compensation must be established so that all concerned can be treated fairly and equally. There is need to provide a reasonable basis for recommendations concerning work restrictions in an effort to lessen the development of genital prolapse or to decrease the likelihood of genital prolapse or the likelihood of recurrence after reparative surgery. When such guidelines are established, agreement should also be developed as to the appropriate duration of convalescence after childbirth and the appropriate time to be allowed for recovery after gynecologic reparative surgery. Hopefully, this will take into consideration not only the nature and the magnitude of the operative procedure but also the particular type of work to which the individual will be returning.

We do not, as yet, know the effects of frequent jogging or impact exercises on the integrity of the urogenital and pelvic diaphragms. There are many women with urinary stress incontinence who are finding the condition aggravated by jogging. We suspect but lack objective evidence that the sport significantly aggravates preexisting damage to the supports of the vagina, urethra, or to the pelvic diaphragm, while it may actually strengthen some of the pelvic supports of the patient *without* preexistent damage.

The long-term surgical and economic effects on complications and end results of same-day admission and early discharge, as promoted by third-party payers, must be studied in detail to determine whether or not this policy is in the public interest. Can society continue to support the activities of the surgeon who has an excessive proportion of postoperative complications and increased length of stay? The surgeons consistently obtaining the best results will become busier at the expense of the less successful. Our individual surgical successes will always improve with continued attention to technical precision and knowledge, learning from the experiences of all, and within an affordable framework of compassion, empathy, and understanding.

Surgery for Invasive Cervical Cancer

What is the place for synchronous combined abdominovaginal hysterocolpectomy for cancer of the cervix (15, 47)? The radical vaginal hysterectomy with extraperitoneal lymphadenectomy (28, 29)?

It is conceivable, for example, that the future operation of choice for invasive squamous cell carcinoma of the cervix might be laparoscopic pelvic lymphadenectomy, followed by the Schauta radical vaginal hysterectomy in appropriate cases in which the greatest diameter of the tumor is less than 4 cm. In selected cases, this may provide for the safe removal of the largest amount of tissue in the shortest operating time (32).

Reconstruction of the External Anal Sphincter

What is the place for the paradoxical incision (27) through the external anal sphincter in the reoperation for failed surgery for sphincter restoration of continence?

The Neovagina

In the construction of a neovagina using the Abbe-McIndoe technique, the patient is often annoyed by the pain and cosmetic disfigurement at the donor site. It has been suggested that an alternative method of obtaining skin sufficient to cover the obturator introduced at surgery might be the development of large sheets of squamous epithelium, even those of but one cell thickness, derived from *preoperative* tissue culture of a skin biopsy taken long before the neovaginal construction. This would require an initial donor site of only a tiny biopsy of skin, relieving the patient of the pain and discomfort and cosmetic scarring of a large donor site.

Possible Alternate Treatment for Massive Eversion of the Vagina

Horner (EN Horner, personal communication, 1988) has suggested a method of preserving sexual function in a patient with massive genital eversion treated by hysterocolpectomy. It consists of saving and refrigerating the vaginal mucosa that was removed, packing the raw cavity for 8 days while postoperative fibrosis with firm support develops, and then reinserting the vaginal wall with a stent when the packing is removed. Alternatively, might such a stent be covered with the fabric "Interceed" (see Chapter 21) instead of mucosa with good results?

Prevention of Pulmonary Embolies

We have long been concerned about the effectiveness of low-dose heparin in reducing the incidence of postoperative pulmonary embolus, fearing the increased incidence of intraoperative bleeding and postoperative wound hemorrhage. Preliminary European reports (A Ferrari, M Dindelli, CM Sellardi, personal communication, 1988) of the new compound Defibrotide (Prociclide, Crinos) in the prevention of deep thrombosis are most encouraging. It is a natural polydeoxyribonucleotide extracted from animal tissues. It apparently has no association with increased bleeding, has no anticoagulant effect, and no adverse effect upon blood platelets. Its molecular structure resembles heparin, but its mechanism of action is not yet known. The effective dose seems to be in the range of 200 mg four times daily or 400 mg twice daily for 7 days starting 24 hours before surgery. Because it is not an anticoagulant, no monitoring is necessary. It is not currently available for use in the United States.

Operative Transfusion

Autotransfusion using blood retrieved through the Cell-Saver is apparently not suitable for the vaginal surgical patient because of its probable contamination by vaginal bacteria, but transfusion of homologous banked blood is useful, sparing the patient the risk of unexpected inoculation with the non-A and non-B hepatitis virus, AIDS, and the risk of transfusion reaction. It probably should not be used in the patient with coronary artery insufficiency or liver or respiratory failure.

References

1. Abel ME, Chiu YSY, Russell TR, Volpe PA. Autologous fibrin glue in the treatment of rectovaginal and complex fistulas. Dis Colon Rectum 1993;36:447–449.
2. Adamyan LV. Additional international perspectives. In: Nichols DH, ed. Gynecologic and obstetric surgery. St. Louis: Mosby-Yearbook, 1993:1167–1169.
3. Block IR. Transrectal repair of rectocele using obliterative suture. Dis Colon Rectum 1986;29:707–711.
4. Brincat M, Moniz CJ, Studd JWW, et al. Long-term effects of the menopause and sex hormones on skin thickness. Br J Obstet Gynaecol 1985;92:256–259.
5. Cohen MP. Diabetes and protein glucosylation. New York: Springer-Verlag, 1986.
6. DeMarsovszky PJ, Nichols DH, Randall CL. Urethrocolpography. Arch Gynäkol 1973;215:351–358.

7. Ghaly AFF, Gbolate BA. Urethrocliesis: treatment for genuine stress incontinence? A retrospective study. J Obstet Gynecol 1993;13:259–261.

8. Graves WP. Gynecology. 4th ed. Philadelphia: WB Saunders, 1928:841–844.

9. Green TH. Development of a plan for the diagnosis and treatment of urinary stress incontinence. Am J Obstet Gynecol 1962;83:632–648.

10. Halban J. Gynäkologische Operationslehre. Wien: Urban & Schwarzenberg, 1932:196–197.

11. Hanton EM, Kempers RD. Puerperal inversion of the uterus. Postgrad Med 1964;36:541–545.

12. Hasson HM, Rotman C, Rana N, Asakura H. Experience with laparoscopic hysterectomy. J Assoc Gynecol Lap 1993;1:1–11.

13. Henry MM, Swash M. Coloproctology and the pelvic floor. 2nd ed. Oxford: Butterworth-Heinemann, 1992:252–255.

14. Hodgkinson CP. Stress urinary incontinence. Am J Obstet Gynecol 1970;108:1141–1168.

15. Howkins J. Synchronous combined abdomino-vaginal hysterocolpectomy for cancer of the cervix: a report of fifty patients. J Obstet Gynaecol Br Emp 1959;66:212–219.

16. Hricak H. MRI of the female pelvis: a review. Am J Radiol 1986;146:1115–1122.

17. Huffman JW, Sokal JK. The management of stress incontinence. Geriatrics 1952;7:225–231.

18. Ioannides L, Somogyi A, Spicer J, et al. Rectal administration of metronidazole provides therapeutic plasma levels in postoperative patients. N Engl J Med 1981;305:1569–1570.

19. Jessee E, Owen D, Sher K. The benign hypermobile joint syndrome. Arth Rheum 1980;23:1053–1056.

20. Kegel AH. Progressive resistance exercises in the functional restoration of the perineal muscles. Am J Obstet Gynecol 1948;56:238–248.

21. Kerremans R, Rosselle N. The parameters of the EMG activity of the external anal sphincters and M pubo-rectalis in normal adult and elderly subjects. Electromyography 1968;8:89–104.

22. Klarskov P, Nielson KK, Kromann-Anderson B, Maegaard E. Long-term results of pelvic floor training and surgery for female genuine stress incontinence. Int Urogynecol J 1991;2:132–135.

23. Levy BS, Hulka JF, Peterson HB, Phillips JM. Operative laparoscopy: American Association of Gynecologic Laparoscopists, 1993 member survey. J Am Assoc Gynecol Laparosc 1994;1:301–305.

24. Lien HY, Stern R, Fu JCC. Inhibition of collagen fibrin formation in-vitro and subsequent crosslinking of glucose. Science 1984;225:1489–1491.

25. Martius G. In: Martius G, Friedman EA, ed. Operative gynecology. New York: Thieme-Stratton, 1982:165.

26. McCarthy S, Tauber C, Gore J. Female pelvic anatomy: MR assessment of variations during the menstrual cycle and with use of oral contraceptives. Radiology 1986;160:119–123.

27. Miller NF, Brown W. The surgical treatment of complete perineal tears in the female. Am J Obstet Gynecol 1937;34:196–209.

28. Mitra S. Mitra operation for cancer of the cervix. Springfield, IL: Charles C Thomas, 1960.

29. Navratil E. Radical vaginal hysterectomy (Schaüta-Amreich operation). Clin Obstet Gynecol 1965;8:676.

30. Nelson BE, Schwartz PE. Hemorrhage and shock. In: Nichols DH, ed. Gynecologic and obstetric surgery. St. Louis: Mosby-Yearbook, 1993:211–212.

31. Nezhat C, Nezhat F, Silfren SL. Laparoscopic hysterectomy and bilateral salpingo-oophorectomy using multifire GIA surgical stapler. J Gynecol Surg 1990;6:287–288.

32. Nichols DH. Epilogue. In: Nichols DH, ed. Gynecologic and obstetric surgery. St. Louis: Mosby-Yearbook, 1993:1183.

33. Nichols DH. The future of vaginal relaxations. In: Baden WF, Walker T, eds. Surgical repair of vaginal defects. Philadelphia: JB Lippincott, 1992:253–255.

34. Nichols DH. Inversion of the uterus. In: Nichols DH, ed. Gynecologic and obstetric surgery. St. Louis: Mosby-Yearbook, 1993:1147–1152.

35. Norton PA, Baker JE, Sharp HC, Warenski JC. Genitourinary prolapse and joint hypermobility in women. Obstet Gynecol 1995;85:225–228.

36. Parks AG. Anorectal incontinence. Proc Roy Soc Med 1975;68:681–690.

37. Payne PR. Urethrocliesis: a simple cure for stress incontinence. Br J Obstet Gynaecol 1983;90:662–664.

38. Percy JP, Neill ME, Swash M, et al. Electrophysiological study of the motor nerve supply of the pelvic floor. Lancet 1981;1:16–17.

39. Plymate SR, Fariss BL, Bassett ML, et al. Obesity and its role in polycystic ovary syndrome. J Clin Endocrinol Metabol 1981;52:1246.

40. Reiner IJ. Early discharge after vaginal hysterectomy. Obstet Gynecol 1988;71:416–418.

41. Roberts H. Cystourethrography in women. Br J Urol 1952;25:253–259.

42. Smith P, Heimer G, Norgren A, Ulmsten U. Localization of steroid hormone receptors in the pelvic muscles. Eur J Obstet Gynecol Reprod Biol 1993;50:83–85.

43. Speroff L, Glass RH, Kase NG. Clinical gynecologic endocrinology and infertility. 3rd ed. Baltimore: Williams & Wilkins, 1983:110–111.

44. Stovall TG. LAVH: a timebomb waiting to explode? OBG Management, Sept 1994:51–53.
45. Summit RL Jr, Stovall TG, Lipscomb GH, Ling FW. Randomized comparison of laparoscopy-assisted vaginal hysterectomy with standard vaginal hysterectomy in an outpatient setting. Obstet Gynecol 1992;80:895–901.
46. Tadir Y, Fisch B. Operative laparoscopy: a challenge for general gynecology? Am J Obstet Gynecol 1993;169:7–12.
47. Vidakovic S. The vagino-abdominal approach to the extended operation. Arch Gynakol 1955;186:420.

"Everything should be made as simple as possible,
but not one bit simpler."
Albert Einstein

INDEX